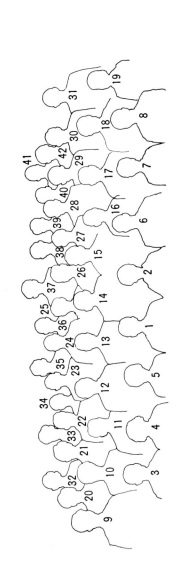

PARTICIPANTS

1. H.I.H. Prince Takamatsu	2. H.I.H. Princess Takamatsu	3. Dr. Tachibana	4. Dr. I. Hellström
5. Dr. G. Henle	6. Dr. Southam	7. Dr. E. Klein	8. Dr. Rauscher	9. Dr. Nishioka
10. Dr. Hayashi	11. Dr. de Thé	12. Dr. Roizman	13. Dr. Ho	14. Dr. Green
15. Dr. K. Hellström	16. Dr. Nakahara	17. Dr. T. Yoshida	18. Dr. Higuchi	19. Mrs. Chen
20. Dr. Suzuki	21. Dr. Takahashi	22. Dr. Moloney	23. Dr. Pope	24. Dr. Nelson
25. Dr. Epstein	26. Dr. Hinuma	27. Dr. Lin	28. Dr. T. O. Yoshida	29. Dr. Fujinaga
30. Dr. Ito	31. Dr. Yang	32. Dr. Yamamoto	33. Dr. Shimojo	34. Dr. Kawamura
35. Dr. W. Henle	36. Dr. Aoki	37. Dr. G. Klein	38. Dr. Tu	39. Dr. Fujii
40. Dr. Takada	41. Dr. Chen	42. Dr. Hirayama		

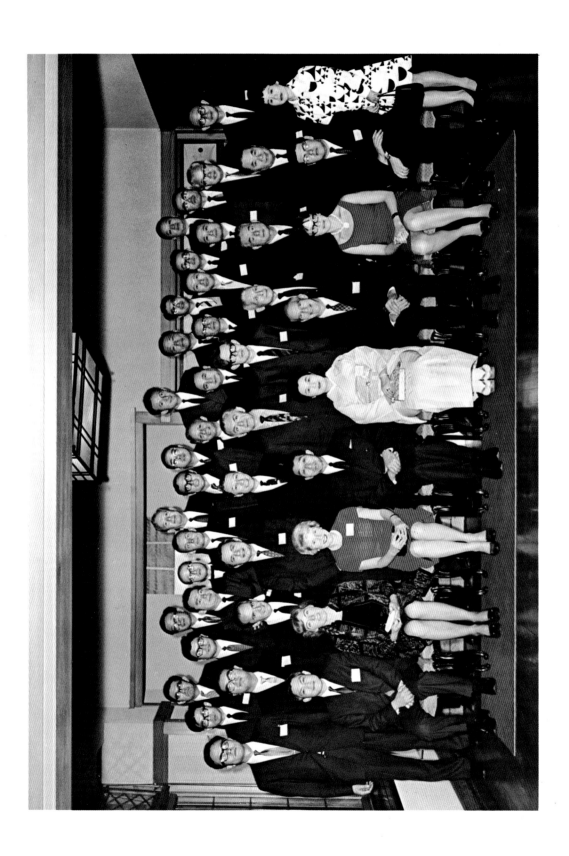

RECENT ADVANCES IN
HUMAN TUMOR
VIROLOGY
AND IMMUNOLOGY

Proceedings of the 1st International Symposium of
The Princess Takamatsu Cancer Research Fund

RECENT ADVANCES IN HUMAN TUMOR VIROLOGY AND IMMUNOLOGY

Edited by

WARO NAKAHARA, KUSUYA NISHIOKA,
TAKESHI HIRAYAMA, and YOHEI ITO

UNIVERSITY PARK PRESS

© UNIVERSITY OF TOKYO PRESS, 1971
UTP No. 3047-67618-5149
Printed in Japan.

Originally published in 1971 by
UNIVERSITY OF TOKYO PRESS

UNIVERSITY PARK PRESS
Baltimore · London · Tokyo
**Library of Congress Cataloging in Publication
Data**
Main entry under title:

Recent advances in human tumor virology and
  immunology.

  Includes bibliographies.
  1.   Oncogenic viruses—Congresses.   2. Immunopathology—Congresses.   I.   Nakahara, Warō,
1894– ed. II. Takamatsu no Miya Hi Gan Kenkyū
Kikin.
RC268.5.R42   616.9′94   70-37741
ISBN 0-8391-0574-6

Princess Takamatsu Cancer Research Fund

Organizing Comittee of the 1st International Symposium

Waro NAKAHARA
    National Cancer Center Research Institute, Tsukiji, Tokyo, Japan
Kusuya NISHIOKA
    National Cancer Center Research Institute, Tsukiji, Tokyo, Japan
Takeshi HIRAYAMA
    National Cancer Center Research Institute, Tsukiji, Tokyo, Japan
Yohei ITO
    Aichi Cancer Center Research Institute, Nagoya, Japan

Participants

Tadao Aoki
National Cancer Institute, National Institute of Health, Bethesda, Maryland 20014, U.S.A.

Hai-Ching Chen
Department of Pathology, National Taiwan University Hospital, No. 1 Chang-Te Street, Taipei, Taiwan, Republic of China

G. Blaudin de Thé
International Agency for Research on Cancer, 16 Avenue Marechal Foch, 69 Lyon (6 eme), France

M. A. Epstein
Department of Pathology, University of Bristol Medical School, University Walk, Bristol B. S. 8, England, Great Britain

Maurice Green
Institute for Molecular Virology, St. Louis University, School of Medicine, 3681 Park Avenue, St. Louis, Missouri 63110, U.S.A.

Genshichiro Fujii
Department of Surgery, Institute of Medical Science, University of Tokyo, Takanawa, Tokyo, Japan

Kei Fujinaga
Laboratory of Viral Oncology, Aichi Cancer Center Research Institute, Nagoya, Japan

Kozaburo Hayashi
Department of Pathology, Institute of Medical Science, University of Tokyo, Takanawa, Tokyo, Japan

Ingegerd Hellström
Department of Microbiology, University of Washington, Seattle, Washington 98105, U.S.A.

KARL ERIK HELLSTRÖM
Department of Pathology, University of Washington, Seattle, Washington 98105, U.S.A.

GERTRUDE HENLE
The Children's Hospital of Philadelphia, Research Department, 1740 Bainbridge Street, Philadelphia, Pennsylvania 19146, U.S.A.

WERNER HENLE
The Children's Hospital of Philadelphia, Research Department, 1740 Bainbridge Street, Philadelphia, Pennsylvania 19146, U.S.A.

YORIO HINUMA
Department of Microbiology, Kumamoto University, Kumamoto, Japan

TAKESHI HIRAYAMA
Epidemiology Division, National Cancer Center Research Institute, Tsukiji, Tokyo, Japan

J. H. C. HO
M. & H. D. Institute of Radiology, Queen Elizabeth Hospital, Kowloom, Hong Kong

YOHEI ITO
Laboratory of Viral Oncology, Aichi Cancer Center Research Institute, Nagoya, Japan

AKIYOSHI KAWAMURA, JR.
Department of Immunology, Institute of Medical Science, University of Tokyo, Takanawa, Tokyo, Japan

EVA KLEIN
Department of Tumor Biology, Karolinska Institutet, S-104 01 Stockholm 60, Sweden

GEORGE KLEIN
Department of Tumor Biology, Karolinska Institutet, S-104 01 Stockholm 60, Sweden

TONG-MIN LIN
Department of Public Health, College of Medicine, National Taiwan University, No. 1 Jenai Road, Section 1, Taipei, Taiwan, Republic of China

CHEN-HUI LIU
Department of Internal Medicine, National Taiwan University Hospital, No. 1 Chang-Te Street, Taipei, Taiwan, Republic of China

J. B. MOLONEY
National Cancer Institute, National Institute of Health, Bethesda, Maryland 20014, U.S.A.

WARO NAKAHARA
National Cancer Center Research Institute, Tsukiji, Tokyo, Japan

DAVID S. NELSON
Department of Bacteriology, University of Sydney, Sydney, Australia

KUSUYA NISHIOKA
Virology Division, National Cancer Center Research Institute, Tsukiji, Tokyo, Japan

J. H. POPE
Queensland Institute of Medical Research, Herston Road, Herston Brisbane, Queensland, Australia

FRANK J. RAUSCHER, JR.
National Cancer Institute, National Institute of Health, Bethesda, Maryland 20014, U.S.A.

BERNARD ROIZMAN
Department of Microbiology, The University of Chicago, 939 East 57th Street, Chicago, Illinois 60637, U.S.A.

HIROTO SHIMOJO
Department of Tumor Virus Research, Institute of Medical Science, University of Tokyo, Takanawa, Tokyo, Japan

CHESTER M. SOUTHAM
Division of Medical Oncology, Department of Medicine, Jefferson Medical College, Thomas Jefferson University, 1025 Walnut Street, Philadelphia, Pennsylvania 19107, U.S.A.

HARUO SUGANO
Department of Pathology, Cancer Institute, Toshima-ku, Tokyo, Japan

IKUO SUZUKI
Department of Ultrastructure Research, Aichi Cancer Center Research Institute, Nagoya, Japan

TAKEHIKO TACHIBANA
Virology Division, National Cancer Center Research Institute, Tsukiji, Tokyo, Japan

MITSURU TAKADA
Department of Virology, Kitasato Institute, Minato-ku, Tokyo, Japan

MORINOBU TAKAHASHI
Department of Molecular Immunology, Kanazawa University Cancer Institute, Kanazawa, Japan

SHIE-MIEN TU
Department of Otorhinopharyngology, National Taiwan University Hospital, No. 1 Change-Te Street, Taipei, Taiwan, Republic of China

TADASHI YAMAMOTO
Department of Oncology, Institute of Medical Science, University of Tokyo, Takanawa, Tokyo, Japan

CZAU-SIUNG YANG
Department of Bacteriology, College of Medicine, National Taiwan University, No. 1 Jenai Road, Section 1, Taipei, Taiwan, Republic of China

TAKATO O. YOSHIDA
Laboratories of Viral Oncology, Aichi Cancer Center Research Institute, Nagoya, Japan

Observers

H. I. H. Prince Masahito Hitachi, Cancer Institute

Miki Aizawa, Hokkaido University

Kaneyoshi Akazaki, Aichi Cancer Center Research Institute

Yuzo Aoyama, Institute of Medical Science, University of Tokyo

Shaoyuan Chang, National Cancer Center Research Institute

Hideya Endo, Kyushu University

Fumiko Fukuoka, National Cancer Center Research Institute

Atushi Gotoh, Institute of Medical Science, University of Tokyo

Kenji Hamajima, Institute of Medical Science, University of Tokyo

Yoshiyuki Hashimoto, Tokyo Biochemical Institute

Hidematsu Hirai, Hokkaido University

Masaharu Hitosugi, National Cancer Center Research Institute

Shen-Wu Ho, National Taiwan University

Akira Hoshino, Aichi Cancer Center Research Institute

Ming-Nan Huang, Institute of Medical Science, University of Tokyo

Heizaburo Ichikawa, National Cancer Center Hospital

Noriaki Ida, Toyo Kogyo Hospital

Tsuyoshi Iida, Sankyo Co.

Yoji Ikawa, Cancer Institute

Husahiro Ikuta, Niigata University

Kuniyuki Imai, Aichi Cancer Center Hospital

Masaharu Inoue, National Cancer Center Research Institute

Masahide Ishibashi, Osaka University

Yukio Ishibashi, Institute of Medical Science, University of Tokyo

Nakao Ishida, Tohoku University

Motoi Ishidate, Cancer Institute

Akinori Ishimoto, Aichi Cancer Center Research Institutute

Reiko Irie, National Cancer Center Research Institute

Shiro Kasahara, Kitasato Institute

Ken Katagiri, Shionogi and Co. Ltd.

Shiro Katoh, Osaka University

Yoshitaka Kawabe, Aichi Cancer Center Research Institute

Ikuo Kimura, Aichi Cancer Center Research Institute

Ren Kimura, Kyoto University

Masayasu Kitagawa, Osaka University

Opening Address

H.I.H. Princess Kikuko Takamatsu

It gives me much pleasure to be present at the opening meeting of the International Symposium on Virology and Immunology of Human Tumors, to greet all the participants, and especially to extend my cordial welcome to those who have come from abroad to complete the international list of active workers on the subject.

Ever since I lost my mother through cancer many years ago, it has been my earnest desire to do something toward the conquest of this dread disease. This desire led me to the idea of forming a Fund which may be useful for the promotion of cancer research. Through the co-operation and assistance of my many friends, this objective has been realized recently in the form of the Fund for Cancer Research which bears my name.

It is my strong conviction that, at the present time, our fight against cancer can hope for the best ultimate result by promoting scientific research, and the Board of Directors of the Fund has decided the current activities of the Fund on three major lines, that is, to give grants-in-aid of research, to award prizes in recognition of meritorious research accomplishments, and to hold international symposia for discussing problems of importance in cancer research.

The present Symposium on Virology and Immunology of Human Tumors was planned as the first venture of the Fund in this direction. I am told that this is the first meeting of the World's most active experts on Burkitt's lymphoma and certain nasopharyngeal carcinoma, both of which seem to be associated with specific viruses. These two virus-associated tumors are being most intensively investigated at the present time, and, pending the final conclusion, it seems very profitable for investigaters to get together and compare their data and exchange their opinions. My scientific advisers suggested the subject as most appropriate and timely for the First International Symposium of our Fund, and I have the pleasure of acting upon their suggestion.   In this connection, I have to thank members of the Organizing Committee for making all the necessary arrangements for the Symposium.

Here are my best wishes for the success of the Symposium.   May your discussions be fruitful and be productive of better understanding of the complex problems in tumor virology and immunology.

Dr. Waro Nakahara

In appreciation of the gracious words of Your Imperial Highness, I wish to say that all the participants in the Symposium will make the best use of this opportunity for the elucidation of the problems in virology and immunology of human tumors. Burkitt's lymphoma and nasopharyngeal carcinoma, and EB virus associated with these diseases will form fit subjects to serve as entering wedges.   If I may be allowed to use the terminology of baseball game, I feel certain that there will be a few hits at least, even if we do not make a homerun.

Dr. Klein, may I asky you to represent the participants from abroad and say a few words in answer to Her Imperial Highness?

Dr. George Klein

Our Imperial Highness, Prof. Nakahara, Members of the committee, in the name of all participats, I should like to express our deep thanks to you for having organized this Symposium and for having invited us.   This is the first international symposium on human tumor immunology and virology.   It will show the results of international collaborations and will no doubt initiate new international collaborations.

The other evening, in my hotel room, I read a small book, called : " The teachings of Buddha ".   I found that there were 3 precepts to remember if one wished to follow the road from Delusion to Enlightenment : the use of right practices, the concentration of mind and the attainment of wisdom.

The use of right practices must mean, in our terminology, the use of right materials and methods.   Important materials in human cancer are distributed in very different ways in different parts of the world.   One function of international collaboration is to allow scientists in different countries to cooperate in securing the tumor and serum materials important for their study.   The Japan-Taiwan collaborative study is an important example that will be discussed at this symposium ; together with others.

Another fact is that methodology applied in different laboratories is very different.   By collaborating across national boundaries, scientists can work together in a way where each laboratory does what it is best qualified to do.   This is much better than competing, as otherwise often is the case.

Concentration of mind is also much easier, very often, in international collaboration.   We are all entangled with our academic organizations and institutions and sometimes, on the national level, we tend to think more of the organizational problems than about the scientific problem.   In international collaboration this tends to disappear, our mind becomes disentangled from the trivial and concentrates on the important. Many examples of this will appear at this symposium.

The third precept—the attainment of wisdom-will certainly not happen this week, but some steps will be made, some issues will be clarified, new international collaborations will be started, and all this will help to conquer human cancer. It will also promote international friendship and understanding, so important for human development and peace.

Japanese cancer research has great traditions, ever since Yamagiwa and Ichikawa discovered the first experimentally induced cancer. Since then, Japan has been one of the great powers of cancer research. This symposium is entirely in line with that great traditions, for which we would like to express our profound admiration to you.

Dr. Waro Nakahara

Thank you Dr. Klein. With the kind permission of Your Imperial Highness, Ladies and Gentlemen, I now declare open the First International Symposium of the Princess Takamatsu Cancer Research Fund. Let the scientific sessions start, first under the co-chairmanship of Dr. Rausher and Dr. Ito.

Contents

Princess Takamatsu Cancer Research Fund.............................. v

Organizing Committee of the 1st International Symposium vi

Participants vii

Observers xi

Opening Address...................... H. I. H. PRINCESS KIKUKO TAKAMATSU xiii

Human Tumor Virology: A Review

Major Opportunities for Determination of Etiologies and Prevention of Cancers in Man

....F. J. RAUSCHER, JR.   3

Search for Possible Etiological Agent of A Viral Nature in Human Neoplasia

.... Y. ITO   25

Human Tumor Virology: The Problems of RNA Virus

Recent Topics on Type C RNA Virus Oncogenesis

.... L. R. SIBAL, AND J. B. MOLONEY   35

An SR-RSV-induced Mouse Tumor Cell Line Converted into A Murine C-Type RNA Virus Producer

.... T. YAMAMOTO, S. HINO, N. YAMAGUCHI, AND M. TAKEUCHI   43

Discussion   55

Advances in Molecular Virology

Molecular and Submolecular Programming of Viral Oncogenesis
.... M. GREEN, M. ROKUTANDA, K. FUJINAGA, H. ROKUTANDA,
C. GURGO, R. K. RAY, AND J. T. PARSONS   65

Viral and Cellular Gene Expression in Cells Transformed by Human Adenoviruses
.... K. FUJINAGA, M. GREEN, K. SHIMADA, D. TSUEI,
K. SEKIKAWA, AND Y. ITO   87

Changes in Permissiveness for Virus Infection in Cells Transformed by The SV40 Genome
.... H. SHIMOJO   97

Discussion   105

Mechanism of Herpesvirus Infection

Biochemical Features of Herpesvirus-infected Cells
.... B. ROIZMAN   109

Mambrane Changes of Cells Infected with Herpes Simplex Virus
.... K. HAYASHI   139

Discussion   159

Problems in Tissue Culture Study

A New Virus in Cultures of Human Nasopharyngeal Carcinoma
.... M. A. EPSTEIN, B. G. ACHONG, AND P. W. A. MANSELL   163

Discussion   173

EB Virus as A Biologically Active Agent
.... J. H. POPE, W. SCOTT, B. M. REEDMAN, AND M. K. WALTERS   177

Biological Activities of Herpes Type Virus Derived from Nasopharyngeal Carcinoma and Burkitt's Lymphoma
.... M. TAKADA, A. KAWAMURA, JR., AND H. SUGANO   189

Discussion   203

Research on Nasoharyngeal Cancer :   A Review

Present Status of Studies on Nasopharyngeal Carcinoma
.... A. KAWAMURA, JR.   209

Discussion   217

Research on Nasopharyngeal Cancer : Clinical and Pathological Aspects

Clinical Characteristics of Nasopharyngeal Carcinoma in Taiwan
.... S.-M, TU 221

Carcinoma of The Nasopharynx in Japan
...........H. SUGANO, S. SAWAKI, G. SAKAMOTO, AND T. HIRAYAMA 229

Anaplastic Carcinoma of The Nasopharynx
.... H.-C. CHEN, S. YEH, S.-M. TU, M.-M. HSU, T.-C. LYNN,
AND H. SUGANO 237

Discussion 269

Research on Nasopharyngeal Cancer : Its Relation to EBV

Genetic and Environmental Factors in Nasopharyngeal Carcinoma
.... J. H. C. HO 275

Association between A Herpes-type Virus and Nasopharyngeal Carcinoma :
Present Status of The Studies
.................G. DE THÉ, J. H. C. HO, T. GREENLAND, A. GESER,
AND N. MUNOZ 297

Antibodies to Herpes Type Virus in Nasopharyngeal Carcinoma and Con-
trol Group in Taiwan
.... T.-M. LIN, C.-S. YANG, S.-W. HO, J.-F. CHIOU, C.-H. WANG,
S.-M. TU, K.-P. CHEN, Y. ITO, A. KAWAMURA, JR., AND T. HIRAYAMA 309

The Natural History of HTV Infection and Its Clinical, Immunological, and
Oncological Manifestations
.... T. HIRAYAMA, K. NISHIOKA, A. KAWAMURA, AND T.-M. LIN 317

Discussion 337

EBV Intracellular Antigens

Antibodies to EBV-induced Early Antigens in Infectious Mononucleosis,
Burkitt's Lymphoma and Nasopharyngeal Carcinoma
.... G. HENLE 343

A New Antigen Induced by The Epstein-Barr Virus and Its Reactivity with
Sera from Patients with Malignant Tumors
.... Y. HINUMA, T. SAIRENJI, T. SEKIZAWA, AND S. IDA 351

Evidence for A Relation of The Epstein-Barr Virus to Burkitt's Lymphoma
and Nasopharyngeal Carcinoma
.... W. HENLE 361

Discussion 369

EBV-induced Membrane Antigens

Membrane Antigen Changes in Burkitt Lymphoma Cells
. . . . G. KLEIN 379

Immunological Studies on The Cell Membrane Receptors of Cultured Cells Derived from Nasopharyngeal Cancer, Burkitt's Lymphoma, and Infectious Mononucleosis
. . . . K. NISHIOKA, T. TACHIBANA, T. HIRAYAMA, G. DE THÉ, G. KLEIN, M. TAKADA, AND A. KAWAMURA, JR. 401

Discussion 421

Suppression of Antigen in Burkitt's Lymphoma and Human Melanoma Cells Grown in Selected Human Sera
. . . . T. AOKI, G. GEERING, E. BETH, AND L. J. OLD 425

Immunological Interaction of Host and EBV Carrying Cell

Immunological Analysis on Hemadsorption of Cultured Cells Derived from Burkitt's Lymphoma
. . . . T. TACHIBANA, K. NISHIOKA, T. HIRAYAMA, AND A. KAWAMURA, JR. 433

High Incidence of Antinuclear Antibodies in The Sera of Nasopharyngeal Cancer Patients
. . . . T. O. YOSHIDA 443

Discussion 461

Immunoglobulin Production of EBV Carrying Cells

Immunoglobulin Production in Cultured Human Lymphoid Cells Derived from Burkitt's Lymphoma and Other Malignancies
. . . . M. TAKAHASHI 467

Immunoglobulin Production of Lymphoid Cells
. . . . E. KLEIN 479

Discussion 485

Immuno-electron Microscopy Study

Characterization of Antibodies Emerging in Epstein-Barr Virus-associated Disease by Immuno-electron Microscopy
. . . . I. SUZUKI, AND M. HOSHINO 489

Discussion 511

Problems of Cell-mediated and Humoral Immunity in Cancer

Cross-reacting Antibody in Cellular Immunity
. . . . G. FUJII, S. GOTO, T. NISHIHIRA, AND Y. ISHIBASHI 515

Humoral Factors in Cell-mediated Immunity
. . . . D. S. NELSON 529

In Vitro Studies on Immunological Enhancement of Autochthonous and Syngeneic Tumors
. . . . K. E. HELLSTRÖM, AND I. HELLSTRÖM 557

Evidence for Cell-mediated Immunity to Human Tumor Antigens
. . . . I. HELLSTRÖM, AND K. E. HELLSTRÖM 563

Discussion 567

Summary and Prospects

Immunological Research in Human Neoplasia, Present Status and Prospects
. . . . C. M. SOUTHAM 575

Closing Remarks
. . . . W. NAKAHARA 589

HUMAN TUMOR VIROLOGY:
A REVIEW

Chairmen:

Frank J. Rauscher, Jr., Yohei Ito

Major Opportunities for Determination of Etiologies and Prevention of Cancers in Man

Frank J. Rauscher, Jr.

Etiology Area, National Cancer Institute, National Institutes of Health, Bethesda, Maryland, U.S.A.

Dr. Ito, one of our distinguished hosts and colleagues, thought it appropriate and important that within an international symposium entitled " Tumor Virology and Immunology " at least one paper should attempt to present a broad perspective of the impact of cancer, regarding current and projected kinds, rates, incidences, *etc.* for people. And secondly, that it would be worthwhile to discuss the problems and opportunities of other major areas of cancer research as they appear to inter-relate with viral oncology. He is of course correct. Cancer is a group of over 100 different diseases as viewed by the pathologist and over 1,000 different lesions as viewed by the histologist. These diseases most likely have many different etiologies or at least there are many complex cofactors, which together contribute to the induction of the lesions we call cancer.

Our major opportunity and mission is, of course, prevention of cancer in people. Prevention is not new—our colleagues have done this (or have known how to) for many years. Sir Percival Pott's pioneering studies showed that if men stay out of contaminated chimneys their incidence of scrotal cancer decreases; diminution or cessation of tobacco smoking results in a decreased risk of lung cancer; negation or modification of certain industrial products, actinic rays, or X-irradiation result in decreased risk and incidence of some cancers—in effect, prevention.

Many of us feel that viruses are etiologically associated with many of man's cancers. What emphasis and priority, therefore, are we devoting to proof of on-cogenicity and to prevention of viral-induced cancers in people—perhaps even at the " risk " of deemphasizing the mouse, rat, hamster, *etc.*

The purposes of this paper are to try to identify progress highlights towards these goals (etiology and prevention) and to discuss major deterrents to further expedient progress. I will try to accomplish this through discussions of broad aspects of three major areas of cancer research—chemical carcinogenesis, demography, and viral oncology—and, in particular, will attempt to identify leads from chemical carcinogenesis and demography available for virologic exploitation.

Impact of Cancer (U.S. 1970–2000)

Cancer occurs in all parts of the world, but variation in the incidence of specific forms of cancer is the rule rather than the exception.   A range of ten- or twenty-fold is common and for some types of cancer it is far wider.

In general, the rate of cancer mortality in the United States occupies an inter-mediate rank in the worldwide range, but the rank of mortality from specific types of cancer varies markedly.   The white population in the United States has the lowest mortality from cancer of the stomach and close to the highest from cancers of the colon and female breast.   As shown in Table 1, the incidence rates of various cancers in the U.S. are expected to increase from a low of 25% each for leukemias and breast cancer to a possible high of 80% for cancer of the pancreas (1).

Available evidence suggests that environmental agents and social practices, rather than genetic factors, are largely responsible for the variations in the occur-rence of cancer in different populations.   It should therefore be possible to reduce the occurrence of the major types of cancer in the United States to the level of the lowest ranking country for that type.   Such a reduction would cut mortality from cancer by one-third.   This is the minimum goal we should aim for.

A reduction of cancer mortality in the United States by one-third in 1976 would save 115,000 lives (see Table 2).   The total life expectancy of each salvaged life

TABLE 1.   Cancer Incidence : Expected Numbers, 1970–2000 ; Change in Rates, 1970–2000 ; Deaths, 1970

Site	New cases (incidence)		Deaths 1970	Incidence year 2000 % change[a] in rate	Major causation	Means of prevention
	1970	2000				
Lung	68,000	144,000	62,000	52	tobacco smoke air pollution (includ-ing on-the-job)	stop smoking ; reduce pollution less hazardous cigarette
Large and small bowel	75,000	143,000	44,000	40	intestinal flora? heredity diet?	viruses? other insults? identify susceptibles and eliminate their exposure
Breast	69,000	121,000	30,000	25	virus? diet? (hormones) genetic?	vaccines identify susceptibles
Pancreas	19,000	101,000	18,000	80	diet? virus? other insults?	identify etiology identify susceptibles
Prostate	35,000	61,000	17,000	27	hormones? diet?	identify etiology identify susceptibles
Stomach	17,000	5,000	16,000	(80) decrease	diet poor socio-economic conditions	diet modifications sociologic modifications?
Leukemias	19,000	33,000	15,000	25	viruses, radiation, genetic	vaccines, identify susceptibles and limit radiation
Skin	112,000	186,000	5,000	20	actinic rays, genetic	limit radiation exposure identify susceptibles
Miscellaneous	120,000	217,000	75,000	30	multiple	identify extrinsic and intrinsic factors and modify them

[a] Expected change in age adjusted incidence rates.   Year 2000 compared to 1970.

TABLE 2. Summary—Prevention Projections

Year	Projected rate reduction	New cases	Deaths	Lives saved	Economic impact	
					One year	Total earnings
1970	—	652,000	320,000	—	—	—
1976	trend (1970)	747,000	346,000	—	—	—
	reduce 1/3	523,000	241,000	115,000	$575 million	$3.45 billion
2000	trend (1970)	1,085,000	471,000	—	—	—
	reduce 2/3	360,000	157,000	314,000	$1.7 billion	$10.2 billion

All figures are annual and based on observed 1970 trends. Dollars (on the 1970 dollar value) returned to the economy per year as the incidence trends for 1970 are reduced 1/3 by 1976: and 2/3 by 2000. Dollar figures were computed by projecting for each life saved an average of (a) 15 years life expectancy; (b) 6 years productive earning power; and (c) $5,000 annual earnings. The latter figure is deliberately low to compensate for the male-female ratio within the "saved" cohort. Dollar figures do not account for (a) earning losses during illness; (b) diagnostic and medical care costs saved ($1.7 billion in 1970); and "emotional" return to the economy (society).

would be increased by more than 15 years, of which at least 6 years would be during the economically productive years, i.e., ages 20–64. If we figure average annual earnings to be as little as $5,000, the input to the economy by these 115,000 people would be $575 million a year and $3.45 billion during their 6 years of economically productive life. A similar salvage rate in each year after 1976 would have the cumulative effect of adding more than $4 billion to the economy each year.

The foregoing figures make no allowance for the saving of lives that can be achieved through earlier case finding and more effective treatment. By the year 2000, we should be able to reduce the rate of cancer mortality by at least *two-thirds* through the combined effect of preventive programs, earlier case finding, and more effective treatment. This means that in the year 2000 the number of cancer deaths should be no more than 157,000 in contrast to the 471,000 expected if recent trends persist. The input to the economy by the salvaged lives should be in excess of $10 billion dollars a year (1970 dollar).

The foregoing figures do not account for the direct costs for diagnosis, treatment, and care of cancer patients, which currently are in excess of $1.5 billion a year, nor for earnings lost during illness. Neither do they include the substantial economic and sociologic benefit to society through the freeing of health delivery manpower for the control of other chronic diseases of man.

Major Problems and Opportunities

Demography

Cancer can be prevented by identifying its causes and: (a) removing them, and/or (b) increasing the body's defenses against them. Thus, it is important to know not only *what* causes cancer, but also *who* is unduly susceptible or resistant. Susceptibility may be immense. For example, if an identical twin develops leukemia during the first year of life, his co-twin is virtually certain to develop leukemia within weeks or months. This increased risk fades quickly with age, and entirely disappears by 6 years of age (*22, 36*).

Recently there has been a substantial increase in our list of characteristics of persons who are unusually susceptible to leukemia, lymphoma, and other cancers (23, 24). Once such a list has been created, it can be examined for a common denominator. Many items can be explained by a known or possible genetic defect, sometimes extensive enough to cause various abnormalities in the appearance of chromosomes. It should be noted that the only environmental agent known to be leukemogenic in man, ionizing radiation, and the strongest suspect among the chemicals, benzene, produce long-lasting chromosomal abnormalities in somatic cells.

By contrast, persons at high risk of lymphoma (solid tumors of lymph tissue) have inborn immunological deficiencies (ataxia-telangiectasia, Wiskott-Aldrich syndrome, or congenital X-linked agammaglobulinemia) (24). Consistent with these observations is the increase reported in the occurrence of lymphomas among persons given immuno-suppressive drugs following renal transplanation. A sudden upturn in one form of lymphoma, Hodgkin's disease, at about 8 years of age, also suggests a relationship to immunological development. Normally, at this age, there is a marked spontaneous involution of lymphoid tissues throughout the child's body. Lymphoid tissues are centers of immunologic activity. It is tempting to think that some failure in this normal regression accounts for the upturn in the occurrence of the neoplasm.

There are many other inborn defects that carry high risk of cancer of various type. In the aggregate, they do not account for a large proportion of cancer, but they probably do constitute a large percentage of cancers among young people. In this group, prevention or early detection and treatment can provide decades of healthy life. Peaks soon after birth in the frequency of diagnosis of leukemia, neuroblastoma, Wilms' tumor, and certain forms of brain cancer indicate that many of these neoplasms are likely to have been initiated during intra-uterine life.

Knowledge of these relationships permits physicians to examine children with certain defects more closely than usual, since early detection and prompt removal of the these tumors can be life-saving. Scientists, on the other hand, can explore the origins of the tumors in the light of what is known of the associated birth defects. Thus, instead of studying a tumor in terms only of itself, new avenues of approach have been opened. What is learned through these rare mistakes of nature may well apply to prevention of large categories of cancer. In particular, the epidemiologic identification of individuals and populations at increased risk of different cancer patterns should aid the investigator in virology and chemical carcinogenesis in searching for specific etiologies or combinations thereof. As an example, epidemiologically, leukemia in man and in mice is similiar in many respects. Acute lymphocytic leukemia in Caucasian children shows a sharp increase peaking at approximately 3–4 years of age, followed by a precipitous decline to a lower persistent incidence. There is no such peaking in Negro children. Mice of strains AKR and BALB/c also show a peak incidence of leukemia early in life either of "spontaneously" developing leukemia or following deliberate inoculation with a leukemogenic virus. Mice of other strains are highly resistant to the development of "spontaneous" or virus-induced leukemia and show little or no peaking. Newborn mice and rats of all strains tested are more susceptible to virus-induced leukemia than mature animals. In man, the peaking phenomenon at a young age of Caucasian children is consistent with an increased sensitivity to leukemogenic stimuli and a decreased susceptibility of older persons. In mice and in man, lymphoid leukemia occurs earlier and at a higher incidence than myeloid leukemia. There is proportionately more of the acute disease in young than in old individuals. A further similarity to human adult leukemia is apparent from the response of mice inoculated with leukemogenic viruses (*e.g.*, Gross, Moloney) as adults or immediately following thymectomy as newborns. Under either of these experimental conditions, and following a long latent period, mice develop a low incidence of chronic leukemia predominately of the myeloid type. In this regard it is also of interest that intensive abnormal erythrocytopoiesis begins and continues in the liver following splenectomy of humans with erythroleukemia and of similarly diseased mice previously inoculated with murine leukemia viruses (*e.g.*, Friend virus).

Many of the gross hematologic and histologic aspects of the disease in man and laboratory animals are similar. Virtually all types of the disease recognized in man are seen in mice (*e.g.*, lymphoid, myeloid, erythroid, stem cell, reticulum cell, *etc.*), wherein the organs and cell types involved in the neoplastic process are essentially the same. It is also of interest that the six most effective antileukemic drugs used for chemotherapeutic treatment of human leukemia are also effective in murine leukemia.

These similarities together with the very recent finding of a unique viral polymerase in murine, feline, avian, and human leukemias (3, *30–33*, Speigelman *et al.* and Gallo, unpublished) strengthen the probabilities that some human cancers are virus-induced. They also present a rational approach to test the hypothesis of Huebner *et al.* (*14, 15*) (see section on Viral Oncology) which states that the capacity to develop cancer is inherited virtually by all vertebrates as a natural event through vertical transmission of a virus-mediated oncogene.

Chemical carcinogenesis

The observed relation between exposure to certain chemicals and the development of cancer in man has been historically the first step towards knowledge of the etiology of cancer. A listing of agents presently known to produce cancers in man includes some 10 specific chemicals, 12 mixtures and crude products and, in addition, radioactive materials and radiation (including X-rays and ultraviolet light). The number of items is relatively small because studies capable of identifying an agent as directly causative of cancer in man require large-scale and time-consuming epidemiologic studies and have been conducted for a very small proportion of the potential exposures of man. In fact, essentially all materials that have been demonstrated to be carcinogenic for man have also been found to be carcinogenic in animals.

Most chemical carcinogens known from animal studies appear active in a variety of animal species. It is estimated that more than 1,000 chemicals have so far been found carcinogenic in animal bioassays out of about 6,000 that have been tested.

The major types of cancer in man that can be directly related to known carcinogenic exposures are as follows: (a) cancer of the lung related to cigarette smoke and certain other inhalation hazards (particularly asbestos, chromates, and radio-active materials); (b) cancer of the skin related to exposure to a variety of crude tar products and combustion products as well as to ultraviolet light and other forms of radiation; (c) cancer of the bladder related to exposure to aromatic amines and their derivatives ; (d) leukemias related to exposure to radioactive materials; and (e) mesotheliomas related to asbestos exposure. A number of other human cancers have been considered to be related to exposure to environmental carcinogens but the evidence is less clear.

Because of the widespread use of some of these materials, the proportion of the total population exposed and affected is extremely difficult to estimate, with the exception of such materials as cyclamates, DDT, and tobacco smoke. Since it has been estimated that the majority of the present cases of lung cancer in the United States are attributable to cigarette smoking, that factor alone appears to be res-ponsible for a death toll in the neighborhood of 40,000 deaths a year. Current projects to produce a less hazardous cigarette must therefore be expanded.

The development of our knowledge of the causative factors of cancer in man can be projected along the following lines: (a) epidemiologic studies to correlate specific exposures to certain types of cancer in man with particular emphasis on occupational exposures; (b) additional bioassays in animal models which will identify chemicals as carcinogenic in animals and therefore potentially carcinogenic in man; (c) studies of animal-human correlations by comparisons of bioassay results with the results of epidemiologic studies or by bioassays on isolated human tissues by *in vitro* techniques; and (d) by studies of pharmacologic metabolic correlations among species.

The major areas of opportunity and need for progress in cancer prevention through studies in chemical carcinogenesis are: (a) to develop better means for the removal of hazardous chemicals from the environment; (b) to develop means to enhance the ability of the host to detoxify environmental agents; (c) to determine the extent to which chemicals act in synerigistic concert with viruses or with physical carcinogens such as irradiation; and (d) to develope more rapid and more sensitive means to detect and bioassay the cancer-inducing effects of chemicals for man. The latter area of activity is particularly important. For example, it is estimated that approximately 200,000 new chemicals enter our environment each year. If only 500 to 2,000 of these chemicals enter at reasonably high levels, and if only 10% of these are hazardous, then at least 50 to 200 new bioassays must be con-ducted per year. With present assays it takes approximately two years with 200 mice at approximately $200 per animal to test one chemical. It is hoped that newer studies in animal and human tissue cultures such as those being conducted by Drs. DiPaolo, Heidelberger, Sachs, and others will diminish the two years and $40,000 now required to test a single compound.

Viral oncology

The probability is very high that viruses responsible for at least some human and domestic animal cancers have been found and that it will be possible to develop measures (including test vaccines) for the prevention or control of these diseases.

TABLE 3.   Viruses That Induce Neoplasia in Animals

Common name of virus	No. of major isolates	Host origin	Produces neoplasia in :	Tumor type in animals
Mouse leukemia	16	mouse	mice, rats, hamsters	leukemia, lymphoma
Mouse sarcoma	6	mouse	mice, rats, hamsters, cats, TC[a]	sarcomas
Polyoma	2	mouse	mice, hamsters, TC	all types except leukemia
Mammary tumor	2	mouse	mice	carcinoma
Chicken leukemia	4	chicken	chicken, TC	leukemia
Twiehaus	1	chicken	chicken, quail, hamster	reticuloendotheliosis
Chicken sarcoma	9	chicken	chicken, quail, turkey, duck hamster, monkey, snake, TC, etc.	sarcoma
Marek's	1	chicken	chicken	lymphoma
CELO	1	chicken	hamster	sarcoma
Cat leukemia	4	cat	cat	leukemia, lymphoma
Cat sarcoma	3	cat	cat, rat, dog, monkey, TC	sarcoma
G. pig leukemia	1	G. pig	G. pig	leukemia
G. pig herpes	1	G. pig	G. pig	sarcoma
Deer fibroma	1	deer	deer	fibroma
Squirrel fibroma	1	squirrel	squirrel	fibroma
Shope fibroma	1	rabbit	rabbit	fibroma
Shope papilloma	1	rabbit	rabbit	papilloma
Dog sarcoma	1	dog	dog, TC	sarcoma
Dog mast cell	1	dog	dog	carcinoma
Lucké	1	frog	frog	carcinoma
Human adeno	31[b]	man	hamster, mice, TC	sarcoma-lymphoma
Wart	1	man	man	papilloma
Hybrids[c]	7	monkey, man, cat mouse	hamster, cat, TC	sarcoma, lymphoma
Yaba	1	monkey	monkey, man	histiocytoma
H. saimiri	1	monkey	monkey	lymphoma
Simian adeno	6	monkey	hamster, TC	sarcoma-lymphoma
SV 40	1	monkey	hamster, mice, TC	lymphosarcoma
Graffi hamster	2	hamster	hamster	lymphoma, papilloma
Bovine papilloma	1	cow	cow, horse, mouse, hamster	papilloma, fibroma, sarcoma
Bullhead pap.	1	fish	fish (bullhead cat fish)	papilloma
Total	110[b]			

[a] TC, Tissue Culture.

[b] As of May 1970 approximately 12 of 31 human adeno viruses induce malignancies in hamsters. These 12 and the remaining 19 induce discrete foci of transformed (apparently cancerous) cells in tissue cultures.

[c] Hybrid, Genotypic recombinates of 2 different viruses ; e.g., SV 40+Adeno ; cat leukemia+mouse sarcoma.

There are now over 100 viruses (Table 3) which are known to cause virtually all kinds of cancer in every major group of animals including subhuman primates. Many of these viruses will not only replicate, but will induce " cancerous " transformations in human cells grown in tissue cultures (Table 4).   The direct application of this laboratory know-how to human disease has revealed that virus particles of three types can be detected and in some cases isolated from patients afflicted with different types of cancer—Type C, Type B and herpes type (HTV).   Particles

TABLE 4.   "Tumor" Viruses That Replicate and/or Transform Human Cells

	Common name of virus	No. of major isolates	Type	Host of origin	Replication [a] transformation
A.	Known tumor viruses				
	Chicken sarcoma	3	RNA	chicken	T
	CELO	1	DNA	chicken	T
	Mouse sarcoma	2	RNA	mouse	R, T
	Mouse leukemia	1	RNA	mouse	R
	H. saimiri	1	DNA	monkey	R
	Yaba	1	DNA	monkey	T
	SV 40	1	DNA	monkey	R, T
	Hybrids[b]	7	DNA	monkey-man	T
	Cat sarcoma	2	RNA	cat	R, T
	Cat leukemia	1	RNA	cat	R
	Human adeno	1	RNA (12)	man	R, T
	EBV	2	DNA	man	R, T
B.	Suspect tumor viruses[c]				
	Influenza	2	RNA	man	R
	Sarcoma particle	2	("C")	man	R
	Herpes-2	1	DNA	man	R
	Herpes-1	1	DNA	man	R
	Human breast particle	3	"RNA"	man	R
C.	Other				
	Shope papilloma[d]	1	DNA	rabbit	R
	Monkey breast particle	1	"RNA"	monkey	R

[a] R, Replication of intact detectable virion; T, transformation as represented by nonlytic morphologic alteration and prolonged life.

[b] Genotypic recombinates of 2 different viruses; e.g., SV 40 plus Adeno 12; cat leukemia+mouse sarcoma viruses.

[c] Viruses or virus-like particles reported in "consistent" association with cancers or which enhance (or are enhanced) by physical or chemical agents.   See text.

[d] This virus may replicate in man as judged by significant antibody levels and low serum arginase levels in some exposed laboratory personnel.

of one kind (Type C) are identical with those known to induce leukemias and sarcomas in laboratory animals.   Current studies by Huebner and others have culminated in one of the most exciting, unifying hypotheses of cancer etiology yet postulated.   Huebner et al. (14, 15) have painstakingly accumulated data which suggest that the young of all species, including man, may be born with an incomplete virus or an oncogene related to a virus which can predispose or trigger cancer later in life in response to various inborn and environmental stimuli.

A unifying hypothesis of cancer etiology

The highly predictable natural incidence and behavior of most cancer in animals as well as in man, plus a number of new discoveries and the resulting development of new concepts and insights, led some investigators to concentrate on the unique C-type RNA tumor virus genome as the most likely important viral cause of the generality of cancer.   These new concepts and approaches, and the results of studies carried out in 1970 were epochal, since they led to a testable (heuristic) new hypothesis concerning the basic inherited nature of the RNA viral genome as a general cause of cancer and to a unitary theory capable of explaining spontaneous cancer as well as cancer evoked by exogenous environmental pollutants, endogenous physiological aberrations, genetic defects and mutations, as well as cancer clearly induced by viruses in experimental animals.

The hypothesis of Huebner *et al.* (*14*, *15*) proposes that the cells of probably all vertebrates have RNA tumor virus genomes of the C-type, the prototypes of which are the avian sarcoma virus described by Rous and the murine leukemia virus described by Gross. These genomes we postulated must be transmitted from parent to offspring, and from cell to daughter cell, as part of normal inheritance. Host regulator genes and the repressors and various environmental carcinogens were regarded as factors controlling the expressions of the oncogene(s) and virogene(s) of the generally switched off viral genome. This hypothesis therefore views cancer as a natural biological event determined by a spontaneous and/or induced " switch on " or derepression of universally prevalent specific viral oncogenes, thus providing a possible basis for a unifying theory of cancer which is consistent with naturally occurring cancers, as well as with those induced by radiation, chemicals, and viral agents. Genetic defects, mutant genes, inducing agents, and finally the aging process itself, all appear to act to decrease the repression of the endogenous virogene(s) and oncogene(s). Other endogenous host factors, such as the immunological and hormonal systems, are viewed as probably not involved in the oncogenic process at the cell level but they are potent additional determinants of cancer as a clinical entity in the whole animal.

These new observations when viewed in the light of this unitary theory and the assumption of the universality of the genetic code, inevitably may have a radical influence on our thinking and over-all approaches to the prevention and treatment of cancer. Thus, the concept of built in virogenes and oncogenes, the expressions of which are recognized by both the whole organism and the individual cells as " self " very likely explain the failure of current approaches to control the majority of cancers. Contemporary therapeutic efforts based on destruction of transplanted tumors in experimental animals, surgical and radiation treatments, and experimental immunological vaccines might now be viewed as largely palliative and, more frequently than not, temporary in their effects on cancer. Although these therapeutic measures represent enormous advances and are life-giving in a good many instances, the only satisfactory *final* solution will have to start with a recognizable handle on the basic inherited genomic cause of cancer which then leads to the development of methods (a) to repress the built-in oncogene(s) from " doing its thing " in the normal cell, and (b) to devise ways for fortifying and supplementing the body's natural protective immunological mechanisms. Huebner *et al.* (*14*, *15*) believe, therefore, that eventual control of cancer will have to come about at the cellular level through " repressor " control of oncogene expression, and at the organism level through maintenance and/or substitution of specific immunological " bullets " aimed at specific tumor cell proteins which inevitably must be produced as the result of abnormal gene expressions which lead to the neoplastic state.

The significance of the direct evidence for RNA tumor virus group specific antigen expression in virtually all mouse embryos and indirect evidence for similar general expression during prenatal life in cats, hamsters, and chickens must still be determined. While it is impossible at this stage to rule out a " nonsense gene " role for the C-type virus, its involvement in four species and two classes of vertebrates suggests that embryonic expression of the genome is a general biological phenomenon and because of this it is logical to suspect that it must have a functional role in embryonic development. Just what this role might be is wholly undetermined but the stimulating effects of C-type RNA virus infection on cell growth in tissue culture, the cell transforming effects of certain highly oncogenic strains and their frequent tumorigenic activities *in vivo* suggest many possible influences on both normal and abnormal development in the embryo.

Increasing knowledge of the host cell gene controls of the various C-type RNA genome expressions promises to provide some of the keys needed to explain the role(s) of the fascinating genome found with increasing frequency in embryonic and postnatal cells and in abnormal tumor cells later in life.

Intrinsic enzymes of RNA " tumor viruses "

A new series of findings which, among many other things, may contribute to the identification of a " switch " for the Huebner hypothesis are the detection and characterization of preformed enzymes in RNA tumor viruses.

Genetic expression in bacterial cells is known to be mediated by transcription of the genetic information, coded in the form of base sequences in DNA, into RNA molecules followed by translation of the RNA into specific proteins. Until recently the operation of a similar mechanism in mammalian cells was unquestioned. Recently Temin (*33*) and, afterwards, Baltimore (*3*) independently reported that RNA-containing oncogenic viruses contain a polymerase enzyme, which transcribes the genetic information contained in the RNA of these viruses directly into DNA. This finding, and others, have been fully confirmed and extended by Spiegelman *et al.* (*31*, *32*) and Green *et al.* (unpublished) who have shown that the DNA formed is complementary to the viral RNA. More recent studies have revealed the presence of this enzyme in vishna virus and in several simian foamy viruses, (Todaro, unpublished) but not in approximately ten other non-oncogenic RNA viruses of animal and tumor origin (Spiegelman, unpublished). Of further interest and apparent importance are preliminary reports by Spiegelman *et al.* and Gallo (National Cancer Institute; personal communications) that this polymerase was present in peripheral leukocytes from five leukemic patients but not in cells from ten normal persons.

These findings are important because this unique mode of replication of oncogenic viruses, through a RNA-DNA hybrid molecule, provides the possibility of selectively interfering with this step by chemotherapy, utilizing components which may interfere with DNA-RNA hybrid formation. Thus, new avenues for the chemotherapeutic control of virally produced cancer are opened. The polymerase enzyme can be utilized in the laboratory to prepare the DNA complement of the RNA-containing oncogenic viruses. This complementary DNA has been shown by Spiegelman to bind with high selectivity and form a DNA-RNA hybrid with the

RNA of the oncogenic virus. Thus, the DNA made in the laboratory can be used to test for hybrid formation with homogenates of human or other tumor cells and thus probe for the presence of the RNA of a tumor virus in such cells. Early experiments suggest that the method may provide a new sensitivity in the detection of viral genetic material in cancer cells and thus determine the role of viruses in the induction of human tumors.

A *second* category of viruses is of the DNA herpes type. Epstein *et al.* (*9*) in 1964 reported the successful tissue culture propagation of cells from several Burkitt's lymphoma biopsies. This was followed nearly concurrently by Iwakata and Grace (*16*) who were able to culture cells derived from the peripheral blood of a patient with chronic myeloid leukemia. Both patient sources yielded cell lines in which were detected particles having morphologic and other characteristics of herpes type viruses (EBV). Over 200 cell lines from cancer and noncancer patients have been established by investigators in laboratories in England, Australia, New Guinea, Japan, Sweden, Africa, and the United States (*28*). Viruses other than EBV have not been reported in these lines. The cells of nearly all of these cultures are large, mononucleated, and resemble lymphoblasts. They usually do not attach to the surface of the tissue culture vessel and appear to grow best in static suspension cultures.

Comparative immunofluorescent and electron microscopy studies have shown that only 1–5% of the cells of most of these lines are positive at any one time for the virion antigen, (see *28*). This apparently low incidence of infected cells has made it extremely difficult to extract and purify adequate quantities of virus for further characterization work. More recently, however, zur Hausen *et al.* (*37*) have presented convincing evidence that virtually all cells of such cultures contain and maintain the EBV genome. Thus, a covert or silent infection exists with this virus similar to other herpes viruses and, indeed, with oncogenic viruses of the RNA type.

EBV is antigenically different from known agents of the herpes virus group, and antibody evidence of infection by it is widespread in human populations throughout the world as well as in other higher primates. Such evidence is present in 100% of the children thus far studied, with a peculiar type of lymphoma (Burkitt's) highly prevalent in certain regions of Africa; whereas, the specific antibodies are found, in much smaller amounts, in less than 50% of nondiseased children of similar age in the same regions. A very high incidence of antibodies to this virus is also found in patients with postnasal carcinoma, and in 100% of individuals who have had infectious mononucleosis. Other evidence strongly indicates that this virus is a major cause of infectious mononucleosis, a non malignant human disease in which cells of the same type that are involved in leukemia proliferate rapidly and behave for a short while as if cancerous. This raises the question of whether the same virus might not also cause the cancers with which it is highly associated, under certain host circumstances or in joint interactions with other viruses or chemical agents of the environment.

To recap, the following highlight findings regarding EBV strengthen its candidacy as an oncogen for man:

(a) The virus or high levels of antibody to the virus are present in nearly 100% of Burkitt's and postnasal carcinoma patients from six continents. In Africa fewer than 48% of non-Burkitt's (matched for age and geography) controls had antibody to the virus; when antibody was present it was usually of low titer.

(b)   Strong evidence was presented (10) indicating that EBV is the major, if not the sole, cause of infectious mononucleosis in young adults. At the very least this shows that the virus is capable of inducing rapid and for a time uncontrolled proliferation of the same series of cells that are also involved in leukemia and lymphoma.

(c)   It is very difficult to grow cells from the peripheral bloods of individuals whose sera are negative for antibody to EBV. Presumably this indicates no infection with EBV. However, when virus or virus containing non replicating cells is added to leukocytes from antibody free controls, the cells then grow in a rapid and prolonged manner (11).

(d)   Dr. George Klein has reported virus induction of a non virion but virus mediated neoantigen on the surface of Burkitt's lymphoma cells. This is important because if an oncogenic role for this virus is proposed, one must also assume that the virus is capable of integrating and permanently modifying the cellular genome. The induction of a new cellular antigen is good evidence that the virus has in fact modified the cells' genetic apparatus.

(e)   Large quantities of EBV were isolated from tissues of a congenital leukemic and from the mother before an after culture *in vitro* (Jensen *et al.*, Pfizer Co., unpublished data). This is important because it helps to negate the criticism that the virus is present in such cultures only after it is picked up as a serum transmitted or airborne contaminant.

(f)   EBV or a closely related virus was isolated from the tissues of two rhesus monkeys with myeloid leukemia. The virus has not been found in tissues from normal rhesus monkeys (Manaker, unpublished data).

(g)   Unpublished and apparently unconfirmed reports suggest that remissions were induced in several lymphoma patients treated with convalescent infectious mono serum. It is also interesting to note that in six cases of acute lymphocytic leukemia where the patient developed infectious mononucleosis during remission of his leukemia, the remission was twice the duration ordinarily observed in patients on the same chemotherapy. It is possible that EBV may prove valuable in treating patients with leukemia. Reports from the Roswell Park Memorial Institute indicate that two soluble antigens separated and purified to a high degree from cultures of the EBV infected cells were physically characterized. The immunizing potential of these antigens will be determined. This could lead to the development of a vaccine free of cells and virus nucleic acid.

(h)   Patients with postnasal carcinoma have titers to EBV as high as do patients with Burkitt's lymphoma. No other group of malignant diseases has been found that has this serologic reactivity. Unusual antibody patterns to other tested viruses have not been found with sera from these cancer patients.

Many of the points listed above could be explained if one simply assumes that this particular virus (EBV) happens to grow well in cretain lymphoid cells. This could mean that the more cells of this type the more virus, therefore, the more antigen which in turn will provide the high stimulus for the production of high levels of antibody. If this were true the virus would probably represent a passenger rather than an inducer of a specific disease. The determination of which of these and perhaps of other options is real, should be a major emphasis at the present time. Data to date are ambiguous. For instance, sera from patients with non malignant diseases associated with a significant leukoproliferative response (lupus erythematosus, measles, *etc.*) show no higher levels of antibody than the normal background population. Similarly, Burkitt's lymphoma patients with very high antibodies to EBV show no diminution of these levels following remission of their tumors through chemotherapy. These observations suggest that high levels of virion antibody are not dependent on high levels of virus antigen associated with virus replication in these lymphoid cells. Conversely, patients with sarcoidosis in which there is also a high leukoproliferative response show unusually high levels of this antibody to EBV (*13*). This observation, however, appears not to have been confirmed in another study (Henle *et al.*, personal communication).

The question of whether a virus can ever be proven to be oncogenic for man is, of course, very difficult and probably not answerable within our society. The only direct means of proof is not available to us as the inoculation of the newborn of our species will not be done. Consequently, studies on the proof of oncogenicity seem to be diverting to the attainment of enough predictive information to prepare and conduct a field trial with preventive means, such as that containing the candidate virus within a safe and effective vaccine. As with rabies and other viruses of man, proof of etiology is surmised through effective prevention with appropriate inocula containing the specific organism. In regard to infectious mononucleosis, Burkitt's lymphoma, nasopharyngeal carcinoma, and perhaps to some forms of Hodgkin's disease and chronic leukemia, this approach may be feasible in that EBV seems clearly to be a horizontally transmitted agent, and therefore amenable to classic vaccine approaches with the particulate pathogen.

So then, with these formidable deterrents and considerations, is it possible to devise criteria upon which one can reliably assign a role of oncogenicity for any candidate virus? If it is agreed that this can never be done directly, then indirect pieces of information must serve this purpose. With EBV, I believe the data are at hand to firmly assign a role of oncogenicity for man. Viruses which induce tumors do two things that other nononcogenic viruses do not do:

(a) They transform cells. This phenomenon, which can be measured *in vitro* or *in vivo*, is defined as morphologic alteration with prolonged life.

(b) Since cancer is an inheritable disease (from cell to daughter cell), one must therefore assume that any oncogen has the capacity to reprogram a cellular genome, in the sense that, following exposure, the cell produced something or does something that it would not have done prior to exposure. The induction of neoantigens on plasma membranes through exposure to EBV indicates that this virus does indeed have the capacity to command the cell to make a new protein in an inheritable way that it would not have done without exposure to the virus. So far as is known, viruses not known to have an oncogenic capability do not have this capacity. In a genetic sense the probability of EBV as an oncogen is further strengthened by its apparent major etiologic role in infectious mononucleosis and, philosophically, by the induction of neoplastic disease in rabbits (*12*), chickens (*5*), monkeys (*21*), and frogs (*25, 35*) by other herpes viruses.

A similar case seems to exist for the possible involvement in human cancer of one of the previously known members of the herpes virus group (herpes simplex type 2), which has been found to be highly associated with cervical and perhaps penile cancers. The peculiar epidemiology of this cancer suggests that it may be caused by a venerally transmitted agent of which herpes type 2, through studies of Rawls *et al.* (*29*), and Josey *et al.* (*18*), is one requiring further research. In this regard, and most recently, Aurelian (personal communication), Johns Hopkins University, has presented convincing evidence that the cells of the earliest lesions, including dysplasia and carcinoma *in situ*, contain immunofluorescent virion antigen, whereas apparently normal adjacent cells do not.

The paper by Dr. Moloney, as well as others by subsequent speakers of this symposium, will present more detailed aspects of these phenomena.

An exciting and important area of viral oncology which, because of its newness, appears not to be fully covered at this meeting, is that regarding the detection, isolation, and cultivation of new viruses (Type B) from breast cancers of monkeys and humans. These data, largely unpublished, are presented through the courtesy of the investigators named and, in particular, through Dr. W. R. Bryan, coordinator of these activities for the National Cancer Institute.

Breast Cancer Studies

Until recently, research activities in breast cancer have been limited to exploratory studies in search of evidence that viruses might be associated with human breast cancer. The consistent finding by electron microscopy of particles resembling the known RNA tumor viruses in human materials, and the successful isolation and laboratory propagation of three candidate viruses—one from a subhuman primate (Rhesus monkey) and two of human origin—have already led to the supposition that viruses of this type should be considered as major oncogens for animals " higher " than the mouse.

Isolation of a virus from a monkey breast cancer

The most advanced and one of the most significant of the developments in breast cancer is represented by the discovery, isolation, and successful propagation of a C-type virus associated with an adenocarcinoma of the breast of a Rhesus monkey. This development was achieved in collaborative studies between scientists of the Mason Research Institute and of the John L. Smith Laboratory of the Pfizer Company in research activities sponsored jointly by the Breast Cancer Task Force (BCTF) and the Special Virus Cancer Program (SVCP) of the National Cancer Institute (*6, 8, 17, 20*).

This is the first C-type virus of any primate thus far propagated continuously in sufficient quantities to support systematic investigations on its virological, biological, immunological, chemical, and physical characterization. It has been designated as the Mason-Pfizer Monkey Virus (M-PMV).   The M-PM virus grows readily in primary Rhesus monkey embryo and fetal lung cultures, and to a lesser extent in cell lines of chimpanzee lung, human embryo and human lymphoblasts (NC-37).   It could not be propagated in kidney cells from any of the four species tested (including the Rhesus monkey), nor in feline lung, mouse bone marrow, or baboon leukocytes.

The M-PM virus was shown by Chopra *et al.* (*8*) to form from precursor intracytoplasmic A-type particles which bud through the cell membrane, as in the formation from B-type particles of the mouse mammary tumor virus, but not to have the spikes characteristic of the latter.   The mature particle is indistinguishable from C-type particles in ultrastructural morphology, although the nucleoid does not form during budding, at cell membranes, as do all of the other known C-type viruses.   The M-PM virus therefore possesses certain characteristics of both B and C-type viruses.

The nucleic acid is of the RNA type and the virus particles contain RNA-dependent DNA polymerase as do all known oncogenic RNA viruses thus far studied (Spiegelman, unpublished).

Virological studies (unpublished) by Heberling of the Southwest Foundation have failed to identify the M-PMV as one of the previously known simian viruses.

Limited efforts to further characterize the M-PM virus, to determine its host range, and to test its cross-reactivity with other known oncogenic viruses have recently been initiated.

The limited nature of these efforts is due to the fact that the efficiency of the best tissue culture method now available for producing this virus is only about 1/50th that for producing the murine oncogenic viruses, and the quantities available for research are therefore limited.

Stored serum samples from monkeys collected by Bionetics Research Laboratory, Kensington, Maryland, are now undergoing tests for antibodies against the M-PM virus.   Most of the specimens are from Rhesus monkeys but many samples from various other primate species are also included.

In gel diffusion tests on 450 specimens studied to date, 50 showed weak single lines of precipitation.   However, they did not identify with the control line for specific antibody against the M-PMV.   Further studies are necessary to determine the significance of this finding.

Human serum specimens are also being tested for evidence of antibody cross-reactive with the M-PM virus.   In over 200 specimens tested thus far by gel diffusion, none have shown lines of identity with the specific antibody against M-PMV.   However, 32 of the specimens, most of which came from women with some type of breast disease including cancer, showed weak single lines of precipitation with some antigen in the M-PMV reagent used in the tests.   The same reacting sera also reacted with some antigen in normal human cell lines in tissue culture (NC-37 or F-265).   The significance of these results has not yet been determined.

No human candidate breast cancer virus is yet available in sufficient quantities to support seroepidemiological studies, but attempts to scale up production of one of them are underway.   The same bank of specimens used in the M-PM virus tests are on hand to be tested similarly with the human agents as they become available.

Demonstration of an RNA virus in cell lines derived from human breast cancer

Two groups of scientists and Lesfargus and Moore (unpublished) have demonstrated morphologically similar RNA viruses in tissue culture lines derived from two different cases of human breast cancer. The former investigators also reported isolating the same type of virus from two cases of cancer of other types, among a total of 56 specimens from human cancer patients studied.

The virus produces no CPE or other morphological evidence of its presence, but it can be detected both by ^{3}H-uridine incorporation and electron microscopy. The virus is found in appreciable amounts in tissue culture fluids, and can infect other human cell lines (*34*). It resembles the mouse mammary tumor virus (MTV) in that it has peripheral spikes of identical size, spacing, and morphology, but it is only 2/3 the size of the MTV, *i.e.*, 50–75 mμ as compared with 100–140 mμ. Except for its slightly smaller size, therefore, it resembles the only presently known breast cancer virus (MTV).

Moore and associates have reported finding particles resembling the B-type virus of mouse mammary cancer in 5 out of 75 (6.7%) milk specimens from normal women in the Philadelphia area (*26*). In further studies as yet unpublished, much higher frequencies of similar particles have been found in milk from women of the following special population groups:

(a) 6 out of 10 (60%) normal women belonging to high-breast-cancer families (in collaboration with Dr. Michael Brennan, Detroit, Michigan).

(b) 12 out of 30 (40%) normal women of the relatively highly inbred Parsi sect of Bombay, India (in collaboration with Dr. J. C. Paymaster).

Twenty-five additional milk specimens from normal women of the general population have also been studied. Only one of them was found to be positive, bringing the total for the normal population to 6 out of 100 (6.0%).

The characterization of the particles as B-type was based primarily on negative staining electron microscopy, and the identification of peripheral spikes identical with those of the mouse MTV. The human particles were of the same size as the MTV, and many of them had eccentric nucleoids, typical of the majority of MTV particles.

In collaborative studies involving two Special Virus-Cancer Program contractors, Chopra and Feller (*7*) have reported finding particles of the same size and ultrastructural morphology as oncogenic RNA viruses in 1 out of 43 (2.3%) milk specimens from normal women, and in 3 out of 12 (25%) from women who have had breast cancer (1 breast removed). In more recent studies involving 4 additional such cases and an improved virus isolation technique, 3 of the 4 were positive, bringing the total to 6 out of 16 (37.5%). These studies were made by thin section electron microscopy, and since both centric and eccentric nucleoids were observed, these workers did not commit themselves to specific B- or C-type particles, but used the general descriptive terminology—" resembling oncogenic RNA viruses."

Detection of C-type virus-like particles in a continuous cell line derived from human breast cancer

An established cell line derived by Dr. Lloyd Old from the pleural effusion of a metastatic breast cancer case (the Levine 3 line) has been studied in the collaborative project of Feller and Chopra for a period of over one year.   During this period small amounts of virus-like particles resembling C-type oncogenic RNA viruses have been consistently observed in about 25% of the tissue culture preparations examined, indicating that the production of these particles is still continuing.   Benyesh-Melnick and Biswal studied RNA contained in or released by these cells and found that the cells contained a unique double-stranded 18S nuclear RNA with a base composition different from other cell RNA, but similar to that of the oncogenic RNA viruses (4).

The highest priority for the entire breast cancer problem is the development of knowledge and technology for the production and assay of breast cancer viruses in tissue culture.   The mouse mammary tumor virus (MTV) cannot yet be produced or assayed *in vitro* and a major effort on this virus is planned to lead the way in parallel studies involving the similar B-type particles found in human milk, and the C-type found in the Levine 3 line of human orgin.

The facts that breast carcinoma is the cancer of highest incidence among women in the U.S., and that a 25% rate increase is expected by the year 2000, attest to the importance of these studies.   At the very least, the development of virologic reagents and serologic tests may allow identification of women at highest risk so that early diagnosis, prophylactic mastectomy and other means may be employed for prevention or control.

Attempts to induce increased particle production in human cell lines carrying C-type particles, using human hormones

Project by investigators of the Marquette School of Medicine has recently been started for the study of the effects of protein and steroid hormone on the production of virus-like C-type particles observed in the human breast cancer tissue culture line, Levine 3.

These investigators have developed a tropoblastic cell line (Be Wo) (27) which has the capacity of producing various human pregnancy hormones (chorionic gonadotropin (HCG), placental lactogen (HPL), progesterone, and estradiol) in sequences and amounts that can be controlled by the inclusion of specific precursors in the media.   The human hormones HCG and HPL are not otherwise available in sufficient purity for such research, and co-cultivation of the Levine 3 and Be Wo lines will be carried out in attempts to derepress viral oncogenes through various hormonal concentrations and sequences (*e.g.*, specific sequences are essential for the normal control of hormone-dependent functions, and may be important, also, in oncogene derepression).   Attempts will also be made to propagate virus-like particles from human milk in Be Wo cells, under various hormonal conditions and sequences.

DISCUSSION

Between 30 and 90% of cancer deaths in man are preventable.   Mortality statistics from around the world show that if cancer mortality in the United States, site for site, was comparable with that of the lowest country reporting for each site, approximately 100,000 lives would be saved each year.   The major sites in which gains should be made are cancer of the colon and rectum, cancer of the lung, breast cancer, cancer of the cervix and uterus (particularly among non-whites), cancer of the ovary, cancer of the prostate, and probably leukemia.

Information is already in hand to reach these goals for lung cancer and for cancer of the cervix and uterus. These two sites alone would account for 60,000 or more savable lives. A concerted research effort is called for in cancer of the colon, breast cancer, and cancer of the prostate. There is promise of substantial returns for these sites. For example, migrant studies have provided extremely strong evidence that cancer of the colon is a disease with a very strong environmental base. Japanese migrants to Hawaii show a three to fivefold increase in contrast to Japanese on the home islands. When we find those things in the new environment that lead to so large an increase, application of this knowledge to the present United States population could reduce the U.S. incidence by another 25,000–30,000 lives a year.

Thirty % (or 100,000 lives) is a minimum estimate. If we add to the preventable cases (in terms of current knowledge, or knowledge that should be available in the next few years), earlier diagnosis and improved treatment—where prevention has broken down—this number should be easily doubled. For example, if the most recent results of the HIP-NCI (Health Insurance Plan-National Cancer Institute, unpublished) studies on early diagnosis of breast cancer were applied across the country, we might anticipate 12,000 fewer deaths each year from breast cancer alone. If the finding that early pregnancy (before age 20) cuts in half the probability of developing breast cancer, could be translated into a prophylactic treatment for young women (*i.e.*, create the hormonal milieu of pregnancy without actual pregnancy) another substantial reduction in breast cancer deaths would follow.

Current work on identifying the cancer " susceptibles," as it is successful, will lead to the cutting down of cancer deaths in two ways. First, by identifying susceptibles, we will know what people to watch closely and regularly, so that we may diagnose their disease early, and thus treat it successfully. Second, by identifying the cancer susceptibles, it should be possible to protect them from those environmental assaults which could be carcinogenic to them—while essentially innocuous to others.

Ninety % reduction in cancer deaths could be reached within the present century, if, in addition to the current knowledge of prevention, and the universal application of the best diagnosis and treatment techniques, our research uncovered (a) the environmental elements that cause migrants' cancer rates to change toward those of their new countries; (b) those environmental elements which lead to different rates in the different countries of the world; and (c) the susceptibles whom we must and can protect.

While there are major problems in the prevention of virus-induced cancers, not heretofore experienced in other areas of infectious disease, we should anticipate substantial inevitable success in the control (including prevention) of these diseases in man. Table 5 presents summary of progress towards the control of virus-induced cancers in laboratory and domestic animals and in man. These problems include the probable difficulties in using conventional vaccines for prevention if a major means of virus exposure is vertical rather than horizontal. Secondly, the " peaking " phenomenon of acute lymphocytic leukemia in Caucasian children at about four

TABLE 5. Viruses and Cancer—Progress towards Control (September, 1970)

Sequential activities	Major systems of study							
	Chicken	Frog	Mouse	Cat	Dog	Cow	Monkey	Man
Acquisition of materials	1903 1910 1967	1934	1937 1951 1957 1967 1962	1968	1965	1968	1968 1969	1957 1963 1968 1969 1968
Detection					C*			
Isolation								
Replication(Lab.)								C+
Identification							C*	
Replication(pilot)							B	B
Characterization						C*+		H
proof of etiology		H		C* C+			H	
Replication(industrial)	C+ C*							H
Control	H		B C*	P C+				

	Chicken	Frog	Mouse	Cat	Dog	Cow	Monkey	Man
Animal:	Chicken	Frog	Mouse	Cat	Dog	Cow	Monkey	Man
Years:	67 60 3	36	33 19 13 3	8 2	5	2	2 1	13 7 2 1 2
No. viruses:	3 5 1	1	2 3 2 6	3 3	?	2	1 1	3 2 1 1 2
Control by:	isolation genetic vaccine	temperature	vaccine genetic therapy nursing	none	none	sacrifice	none	therapy surgery

H, DNA, herpes type viruses; C, RNA, murine leukemia and sarcoma-type viruses or virus-like particles. B, RNA particles of the mouse mammary tumor type; P, DNA polyoma viruses. *, C-type particles of leukemias; +, C-type particles of sarcomas.

years of age and other similar phenomena suggest that it would take 5–10 years before the results of a preventative field trial were known. Even with a " clustering " disease of relative high incidence, such as Burkitt's lymphoma in equatorial Africa, nearly 1,000,000 children would have to be included in the " treated " cohort observed for 5–8 years to determine whether the expected 40–50 lymphomas would be eliminated or decreased.

These difficulties notwithstanding, opportunities for cancer prevention and control are very bright through the application of existing knowledge and through a priority commitment to seek new information with innovative application for man.

Finally, I believe that one of the major broad elements of progress has been the negation of the so-called " hit and run " phenomenon of viral oncology. As you will recall, this dictum which peaked in about 1963–65 implied that viruses predominantly of the DNA type had the capacity to begin (induce) the neoplastic process, after which they disappeared or were no longer essential for continuation of this process. This led many of us to believe that even if viruses were involved in human cancer, we would never be able to prove it because a " hit and run phenomenon " many years ago may have negated our ability to pick up an incriminatory fingerprint when the cancer developed. We now know that not a single cancer-inducing virus, be it of the RNA or DNA variety, fails to leave its fingerprint or some detectable phenomenon whereby the induced cancer can be related to a specific inducing virus. Most recently, Balduzzi and Morgan (2) and Martin (19) have shown that chicken cells transformed by Rous sarcoma virus can return to a normal state following the implementation of procedures designed to negate the virus or the virus message. This information may help answer one of the most important questions in cancer biology. Does the virus-induced tumor cell exist as a tumor cell because of the continuing presence and activity of an oncogenic virus? If, as these data suggest, such tumors are dependent on the continuing activity of the virus, then it should be possible to interrupt this continuing sequence through the polymerase findings of Temin, Baltimore, Spiegelman, Green *et al*. This, of course, is a tremendous challenge to all of us as viral oncologists. Although we have known about tumor viruses since about 1900 our expenditure of funds and utilization of other resources have, to date, not provided the clinician with sufficient technique and information to modify these diseases in a single patient with a single type of cancer.

SUMMARY

The probabilities are very high that viruses and other oncogens have been and will be identified for man, and that many of their induced diseases can be prevented or controlled. Cancer prevention is not new—we have been able to do this or have known how to do it for many years. The cessation of tobacco usage or the development of a less hazardous tobacco product, the negation or control of industrial materials such as asbestos and the more intelligent use of X-irradiation are but several examples of information through which some of man's cancers can be prevented.

This paper presents progress and highlights of the identification of other carcinogens and of potential preventive means through current studies in three major areas of cancer research: chemical carcinogenesis, demography, and viral oncology. With adequate resources and motivation, further substantial progress in cancer prevention is not only feasible, but because of the steadily increasing rates of certain types of cancer it is mandatory. For example, in the United States approximately 652,000 new cases with 320,000 deaths are expected in 1970. If present trends continue, over 1,085,000 new cases and 471,000 deaths will occur by the year 2000. Through effective application of existing knowledge and the development of new information, it is projected that this incidence can be reduced one-third by 1976 and two-thirds by the year 2000. The rationale and justification for these projections are discussed with particular emphasis on current and anticipated progress in viral oncology.

I wish to express my sincere thanks for the unselfish and timely provision of information and analyses by investigators throughout the world working with the National Cancer Institute, and in particular to the expertise of Drs. W. R. Bryan (etiology), J. B. Moloney (viral oncology), U. Saffiotti (chemical carcinogenesis), M. A. Schneiderman (demography), and G. B. Gori (etiology) and to their associates. Errors of interpretation and reproduction are mine.

REFERENCES

1. Bailar, J. C. III, Axtell, L., and Bois, G. Cancer Deaths and Estimated New Cancer Cases in the United States, 1930–1965, with Projections for 1970–2000 (Unpublished document of the Biometry Branch, National Cancer Institute).

2. Balduzzi, P., and Morgan, H. R. Mechanism of Oncogenic Transformation by Rous Sarcoma Virus. I. Intracellular Inactivation of Cell Transforming Ability of Rous Sarcoma Virus by 5-Bromodeoxyuridine and Light. J. Virol., 5: 470–477, 1970.

3. Baltimore, D. Viral RNA—Dependent DNA Polymerase. Nature, 226: 1209–1211, 1970.

4. Benyesh-Melnick, M., and Biswal, N. Double-Stranded Nuclear RNA in a Cell Line Derived from a Patient with Metastatic Mammary Cancer. Nature, in press.

5. Calnek, B. W., and Hitchner, S. B. Localization of Viral Antigen in Chickens Infected with Marek's Disease Herpes Virus. J. Nat. Cancer Inst., 43: 935–950, 1969.

6. Chopra, H. C. Electron Microscopic Detection of an Oncogenic-Type Virus in a Monkey Breast Tumor. Proc. Amer. Assoc. Cancer Res., 11: 16, 1970.

7. Chopra, H. C., and Feller, W. F. Virus-like Particles in Human Breast Cancer. Texas Rep. Biol. Med., 27: 945–953, 1969.

8. Chopra, H. C., Jensen, E. M., Zelljadt, I., Mason, M. M., and Woodside, N. J. Studies of a Virus from Spontaneous Mammary Carcinoma of the Rhesus Monkey. II. Electron Microscopic Study of Infected Cell Cultures. Cancer Res., in press.

9. Epstein, M. A., Achong, B. G., and Barr, Y. M. Virus Particles in Cultured Lymphoblasts from Burkitt's Lymphoma. Lancet, 1: 702–703, 1964.

10. Henle, G., Henle, W., and Diehl, V. Relation of Burkitt's Tumor-Associated Herpes-Type Virus to Infectious Mononucleosis. Proc. Nat. Acad. Sci., 59: 94–99, 1968.

11. Henle, W., Diehl, V., Kohn, G., zur Hausen, H., and Henle, G. Herpes-Type Virus and Chromosome Marker in Normal Leukocytes after Growth with Irradiated Burkitt Cells. Science, 157: 1064–1065, 1967.

12. Hinze, H. C. Rabbit Lymphoma Induced by a New Herpes Virus. Bact. Proc., 157, 1969.

13. Hirshaut, Y., Glade, P., Vieira, L.O.B.D., Ainbender, E., Dvorak, B., and Siltzbach, L. E. Sarcoidosis, Another Disease Associated with Serologic Evidence for Herpes-Like Virus Infection. New Eng. J. Med., 283: 502–506, 1970.

14. Huebner, R. J., Kelloff, G. J., Sarma, P. S., Lane, W. T., Turner, H. C., Gilden, R. V., Oroszlan, S., Meier, H., Myers, D., and Peters, R. L. Group-Specific (gs) Antigen Expression Genome During Embryogenesis of the Genome of the C-Type RNA Tumor Viruses. Implications for Ontogenesis and Oncogenesis. Proc. Nat. Acad. Sci., 67: 366–367, Sept. 1970.

15. Huebner, R. J., and Todaro, G. J. Oncogenes of RNA Tumor Viruses as Determinants of Cancer. Proc. Nat. Acad. Sci., 64: 1087–1094, 1969.

16. Iwakata, S., and Grace, J. T. Cultivation In Vitro of Myeloblasts from Human Leukemia. N.Y.H. Med., 64: 2279–2282, 1964.

17. Jensen, E. M., Zelljadt, I., Chopra, H. C., and Mason, M. M. Isolation and Propagation of a New Virus from a Spontaneous Mammary Carcinoma of a Rhesus Monkey. Cancer Res., 30: 2388–2393, Sept. 1970.

18. Josey, W. E., Nahmias, A. J., and Naib, Z. M. Genital Infection with Type 2 Herpes Virus Homines: Present Knowledge and Possible Relationship to Cervical Cancer. Amer. J. Obstet. Gynec., 101: 718, 1968.

19. Martin, G. S. Rous Sarcoma Virus: A Function Required for the Maintenance of the Transformed State. Nature, *227*: 1021–1023, 1970.

20. Mason, M. M., Baker, J. R., and Ilievski, V. R. Histopathology of a Spontaneous Tumor in a Macaca Mulatta in Which RNA Virus Particles were Found. Proc. Amer. Assoc. Cancer Res., *11*: 53, 1970.

21. Melendéz, L. V., Hunt, R. D., Daniel, M. D., Garcia, F. G., and Fraser, C.E.O. Herpes Virus Saimiri. II. Experimentally Induced Malignant Lymphoma. Lab. Anim. Care, *19*: 378–386, 1969.

22. Miller, R. W. Deaths from Childhood Leukemia and Solid Tumors among Twins and Other Sibs in the United States, 1960–1967. J. Nat. Cancer Inst., *46*: 203–209, 1971.

23. Miller, R. W. Persons with Exceptionally High Risk of Leukemia. Cancer Res., *27*: Part I, 2420–2423, 1967.

24. Miller, R. W. Relation between Cancer and Congenital Defects; an Epidemiologic Evaluation. J. Nat. Cancer Inst., *40*: 1079–1085, 1968.

25. Mizell, M., Toplin, I., and Isaccs, J. J. Tumor Induction in Developing Frog Kidneys by a Zonal Centrifuge Purified Fraction of the Frog Herpes-type Virus. Science, *165*: 1134–1137, 1969.

26. Moore, D. H., Sarkar, N. H., Kelly, C. E., Pillsbury, N., and Charney, J. Type B Particles in Human Milk. Texas Rep. Biol. Med., *27*: 1027–1039, 1969.

27. Pattillo, R. A., Gey, G. O., Delfs, E., Huang, W. Y., House, L., Garancis, J., Knoth, M., Amatruda, J., Bertino, J., Friesen, H. G., and Mattingly, R. F. The Hormone Synthesizing Tropoblastic Cell *In Vitro*: A Model for Cancer Research and Placental Hormone Synthesi. In the Annals of N.Y. Acad. of Sci., Vol. 172. Art 10, 288–298, Jan. 28, 1971.

28. Rauscher, F. J. Virologic Studies in Human Leukemia and Lymphoma: The Herpes-Type Virus. Cancer Res., *28*: 1311–1318, 1968.

29. Rawls, W. E., Gardner, H. L., and Kaufman, R. L. Antibodies to Genital Herpes virus in Patients with Carcinoma of the Cervix. Amer. J. Obstet. Gynec., *107*: 710–716, 1970.

30. Rokutanda, M., Rokutanda, H., Green, M., Fujinaga, K., Ray, R. K., and Gurgo, C. Formation of Viral RNA-DNA Hybrid Molecules by the DNA Polymerase of Sarcoma-Leukemia Viruses. Nature, *227*: 1926–1028, 1970.

31. Spiegelman, S., Burny, A., Das, M. R., Keydar, J., Schlom, J., Travnicek, M., and Watson, K. Characterization of the Products of RNA-Directed DNA Polymerases in Oncogenic RNA Viruses. Nature, *227*: 563–567, 1970.

32. Spiegelman, S., Burney, A., Das, M. R., Keydar, J., Schlom, J., Travnicek, M., and Watson, K. DNA-Directed DNA Polymerase Activity in Oncogenic RNA Viruses. Nature, *227*: 1029–1031, 1970.

33. Temin, H. M., and Mizutani, S. RNA-Dependent DNA Polymerase in Virions of Rous Sarcoma Virus. Nature, *226*: 1211–1213, 1970.

34. Todaro, G. J., Zeve, V., and Aaronson, S. A. Virus in Cell Culture Derived from Human Tumor Patients. Nature, *226*: 1047–1049, 1970.

35. Tweedell, K. S. Renal Tumor Transmission in Frog Embryos by Subcellular Fractions. Amer. Zool., *5*: 171–172, 1965.

36. Zuelzer, W. W., and Cox, D. E. Genetic Aspects of Leukemia. Sem. Hemat., *6*: 228–249, 1969.

37. zur Hausen, H., and Schulte-Holthausen, H. Presence of Nucleic Acid Homology in a " Virus-Free " Line of Burkitt Tumour Cells. Nature, *227*: 245–248, 1970.

Search for Possible Etiological Agent of a Viral Nature n Human Neoplasia

Yohei Ito

Laboratory of Viral Oncology, Aichi Cancer Center Research Institute, Nagoya, Japan

Recent advances in the concepts and technology of modern virology and immunology have been remarkable enough to tempt viral oncologists to launch a project to search for possible etiological agent(s) of a viral or subviral nature in human neoplasia. Although the ideas were very naive, retrospectively, and came mostly from a simple analogy to the knowledge already available on experimental animal systems, in the early 60's the road ahead looked quite rosy, at least to our hopeful eyes. It was around this time that studies on human material were also initiated in Japan. The purpose of the present paper is to provide a brief summary of the work pertaining to the virological and immunological studies on human cancer material that has been carried out during the past decade.

Early Studies of Gastric Carcinoma

In the first phase, shooting-in-the-dark type experiments were carried out. Examples of studies of this category can be seen in attempts to induce tumorous growth in experimental animals with nucleic acid extracts from human cancer tissues (3, 5). The model was taken from the Shope papilloma-carcinoma complex (15) in which the viral genome derived from the etiological Shope papilloma virus (SPV) could be shown to persist in the transformed malignant cells of the system, i.e., V×7 and V×2 cells (12, 13), for some 20 years and over 150 transplantation generations. This could be understood from the fact that SPV virion antigen is demonstrable by immunofluorescent technique with both V×7 and V×2 carcinoma cells cultured in vitro (9), and also by the findings that the tumorigenic nucleic acid preparations could be extracted from the V×7 carcinoma tissues (4).

Bearing these data in mind, the nucleic acid preparations were prepared from human gastric carcinoma tissues by a phenolic extraction procedure and were inoculated into experimental animals, i.e., rabbits. Rabbits were chosen because of

TABLE 1. Induction of Cutaneous Nodules in Domestic Rabbits with Crude Nucleic Acid Extracts from Tissues of Human Gastric Carcinomas

Experiment No.	Inoculum	No. of rabbits used	Treatment	Cutaneous nodules	
				No. positive sites per No. inoculated	Appeared[a] on day
1	NA (PBS)[b]	3	M C (8)[c]	0/12	—
	Control (PBC)	3	M C (8)	0/12	—
2	NA (PBS)	2	N Q (8)	0/8	—
	Control (PBS)	2	N Q (8)	0/8	—
3	NA (1M NaCl)	1	None	1/8	29
	Control (1M NaCl)	1	None	0/8	—
4	NA (1M NaCl)	7	M C (8)	7/34	17–20
	Control (1M NaCl)	7	M C (8)	0/34	—
5	NA (1M NaCl)	20	N Q (6–8)	6/38	13–22
	Control (1M NaCl)	20	N Q (6–8)	0/38	—
6	NA (1M NaCl)	13	C O (2–7)	8/42	13–15
	Control (1M NaCl)	13	C O (2–7)	0/42	—
7	DNA (1M NaCl)	7	M C (8)	0/42	—
	RNA (PBS)	2	M C (8)	0/42	—
	DNA+RNA (0.5 M NaCl)	2	M C (8)	0/12	—

NA, nucleic acid, crude extract from human gastric carcinoma; PBS, phosphate-buffered saline (pH 7.4); MC, methylcholanthrene; NQ, 4-nitroquinoline-1-oxide; CO, croton oil; DNA, deoxyribonucleic acid, highly polymerized, commercial preparation; RNA, ribonucleic acid, from yeast, commercial preparation.
[a] Days after inoculation.
[b] In parentheses, solution used to resolve nucleic acid preparations or as controls.
[c] In parentheses, initiation of treatment, days after inoculation.

the fact that little spontaneous neoplasia are known to occur in this species of animal. To test the tumorigenic activity of the nucleic acid extracts, inoculations were made in the skin of the ear of the animal. The results obtained from this experiment were puzzling (Table 1). With the additional painting of a submanifestation dose of chemical carcinogens such as methylcholanthrene and 4-nitroquinoline-1-oxide, hyperplastic growth designated as cutaneous nodules appeared at some inoculation sites. The "co-carcinogen," croton oil also showed such an effect. These nodules persisted for a considerable period of time even after the application of the carcinogens was stopped. However, none of them showed signs of progression to genuine neoplastic growth.

Another series of experiments was carried out by inoculating the nucleic acid extracts from the tissues of 16 human stomach-cancer cases into the gastric mucosa of rabbits. In some experiments, cortisone and 4-nitroquinoline-1-oxide were given subcutaneously to the animal to anticipate systemic or remote effect, if any, in accelerating the induction of expectant neoplastic growths. In most cases, however, no additional treatment was performed. The results thus obtained were more difficult to interpret than those of the tests carried out on the skin. By gross observations, lesions reminiscent of gastric ulcer in man (Fig. 1) were seen in ap-

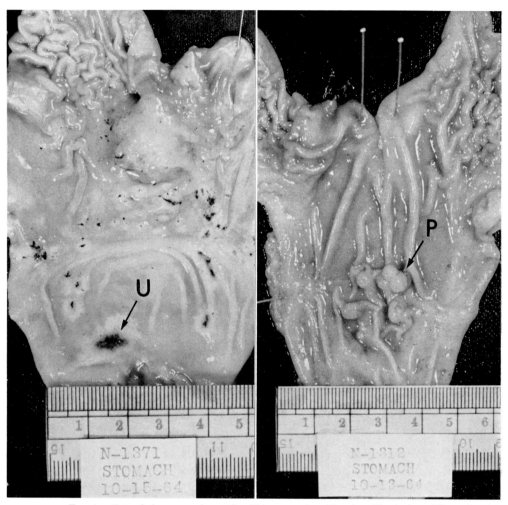

FIG. 1.   Extended preparations of rabbit stomach with ulcer-like lesion (U) and with multiple polyps (P).   The pyloric ring is located beneath the middle portion of the ruler.

proximately one-third of the animals in both the experimental and control groups. The histological and microscopic observations of the lesions also showed no sign of neoplastic growth.   However, a lesion appeared in one animal among 58 in the experimental group which possessed the features of a multiple gastric polyp both by gross and histological observation (Fig. 1).   The growth was detected at the approximate area where the nucleic acid extract had been inoculated and was seen when the rabbit was sacrificed 210 days after the inoculation.

Despite all the effort being put into experiments of this sort, the significance of the data obtained were unfortunately obscured by the fact that adequate controls were not available at the time.   More precisely, the nucleic acid extracts from normal human stomachs had to be tested in a similar fashion.   This was practically very difficult, if not impossible, because 150 to 200 grams of fresh gastric tissue was required as the starting material for the extraction.

Virological Studies on Human Leukemia and Allied Diseases

The second phase of the study on human virus-cancer problems could be represented by a series of experiments carried out on human leukemia and Hodgkin's disease. These were the *in vitro*-transformation-type experiments (*10, 11*). The outline of the procedure employed is shown in Fig. 2.

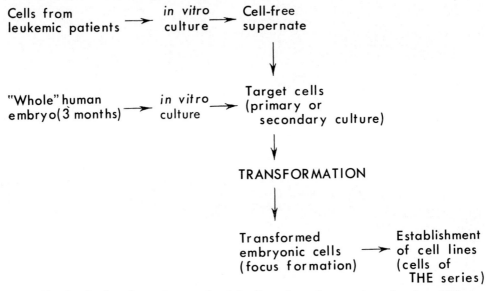

FIG. 2. Outline of procedure employed for " transformation experiment " and establishment of the cell lines.

The human leukemic cells were obtained from the buffy coat of the blood withdrawn from the patients and were cultured *in vitro* for a relatively short period of time such as one to four weeks. The " target cells " were prepared from human embryos approximately three months old. The cell-free supernatant and the target cells were kept in contact for 24 hr at 37°C. After that the cells which settled down on the glass surface of the culture vessel were allowed to grow. The medium was changed periodically and the cells gradually grew to form a monolayer. Approximately four to ten weeks later, the piling-up " foci " of morphologically altered cells were occasionally observed among the fibroblastic cells composing the over-all background of the embryonic culture. These " transformed foci " appeared only in the cultures treated with the leukemic culture fluid and never in the control

TABLE 2. Focus Formation in Human Embryonic Cell Cultures Inoculated with Leukemic Cell Culture Fluid

No. patients examined	Type of leukemia		No. positive cases/total cases	No. positive cultures/ total cultures	Appearance of foci after inoculation (days)
	acute	chronic			
14	10	4	6/14	28/115	23–76

TABLE 3. Some Characteristics of Cells of THE Series

Cell line	Origin	Morphology	Growth	EB virus particle	Chromosome anomaly (C10 marker)
THE–1	epithelioid focus	round	floating clumps	nt	nt
THE–2	round cell focus	round	floating clumps	+	+
THE–3	round cell focus	round	floating clumps	+	+

nt, not tested.

cultures. Some results from this experiment are listed in Table 2 (*10*).

Further attempts were made to isolate and to establish continuously growing cell lines from the foci of the transformed human embryonic cells. Subsequently, three cell lines designated as THE-1, -2 and -3 were established. Some characteristics of these THE cells are shown in Table 3. (*11*).

The results of these experiments became available about the time the herpes-type virus (HTV) came more and more into the picture of the study. Thus, intensive efforts were made in electron microscopic examination of the THE cells, by which the presence of the HTV virions were demonstrated (*7*) for the first time in human material in Japan. Further investigation also revealed the occurrence of the chromosome anomaly known as the C10 marker in these THE cells together with the trisomy of the same chromosome (*8*).

Analogous experiments were carried out with the lymphatic tissues from patients with Hodgkin's disease. A cell line designated as AICHI-4 was eventually established (*6*) and the transformation experiments also turned out to be successful (*14*). However, the establishment of cell lines from the transformed cells in the culture was not achieved.

Immunological Studies as Related to Known Tumor Viruses

Taking advantage of availability of well-refined antigen and antibodies to certain kinds of known tumor viruses, Ishii *et al.* (*2*) looked for the presence of antibodies to such viral antigens in sera of Japanese cancer patients and also of the non-cancer controls. The assays were carried out by the complement fixation (CF) test. The CF antibodies checked were those for V- and T-antigens of adenovirus and SV40, and gs-antigens of the Rous sarcoma virus.

The results showed that the CF antibody titer against both adenovirus V- and T-antigen was significantly higher in the sera of cancer patients than in that of the non-cancer patients and of the normal controls. However, reservation was made in relating this finding to the possible role of the virus in these neoplastic diseases.

Studies as Related to HTV and Human Cancer

The third phase of the study took place around 1968. This could be considered as part of the worldwide research activity which was made possible through the lead created by the Henle's findings on the HTV antibody in human sera (1). Despite the fact that HTV is now considered to be a wide-spread viral agent in man throughout the world, at least three disease entities exhibit extraordinally high HTV antibody titer in their sera.   These are Burkitt's lymphoma (BL), infectious mononucleosis and nasopharyngeal carcinoma (NPC).

Since the endemic area of BL was rather difficult to approach geographically, attempts were made to assess the problems of NPC.   With the cooperative efforts of our colleagues at the National Taiwan University College of Medicine, intensive virological and immunological studies were launched.   These results will be presented in detail.

The present study was supported in part by a contract (NIH-69–96) from the National Cancer Institute under the Special Virus-Cancer Program.   The author is also indebted to Drs. F. Rauscher, J. Moloney, R. Bryan, R. Manaker, and other colleagues at NCI for their continuous encouragement and help for the development of the studies described in this brief review.

REFERENCES

1.   Henle, G., and Henle, W.   Immunofluorescence in Cells Derived from Burkitt's Lymphoma.   J. Bacteriol., *91*: 1248, 1966.
2.   Ishii, K., Koyama, K., Shimojo, H., Kawamura, A. Jr., Aoyama, Y., and Nishioka, K.   Antibody to Oncogenic Viruses in Sera of Cancer Patients.   GANN Monograph, *7*: 157, 1969.
3.   Ito, Y.   Induction of Cutaneous Nodules in Rabbits with Crude Nucleic Acid Preparations from Tissues of Human Gastric Carcinomas.   Oncology, *21*: 129, 1967.
4.   Ito, Y.   Induction of Papillomas in Rabbits with Nucleic Acid Extracts from V×7 Carcinomas.   Brit. J. Cancer, *24*: 535, 1970.
5.   Ito, Y., and Asakuma, R.   Gastric Polyps in a Rabbit: A Preliminary Experiment with Nucleic Acid Extracts of Human Carcinomas.   Oncology, *20*: 267, 1966.
6.   Ito, Y., Shiratori, O., Kurita, S., Takahashi, T., Kurita, Y., and Ota, K.   Some Characteristics of a Human Cell Line (AICHI-4) Established from Tumorous Lympatic Tissue of Hodgkin's Disease.   J. Natl. Cancer Inst., *41*: 1367, 1968.
7.   Kimura, I., Osato, T., Nagano, T., and Ito, Y.   Transformation *in vitro* of Human Embryo Cells by Human Leukemic Culture Fluid.   II. Demonstration of Herpeslike Virus Particles in Transformed Cells.   Proc. Japan Acad., *44*: 95, 1968.
8.   Kurita, Y., Osato, T., and Ito, Y.   Studies on Chromosomes of Three Human Cell Lines Harboring the EB Virus Particles.   J. Natl. Cancer Inst., *41*: 1355, 1968.
9.   Osato, T., and Ito, Y.   *In vitro* Cultivation and Immunofluorescent Studies of Transplantable Carcinoma V×2 and V×7.   J. Exptl. Med., *126*: 881, 1967.
10.   Osato, T., and Ito, Y.   Morphological Alteration of Human Embryo Cells *in vitro* by Treatment with Human Leukemic Culture Fluid.   Proc. Natl. Acad. Sci. U.S., *57*: 1076, 1967.
11.   Osato, T., and Ito, Y.   Transformation *in vitro* of Human Embryo Cells by Human

Leukemic Culture Fluid.   I. Isolation and Establishment of Transformed Cells. Proc. Japan Acad,. *44*: 89, 1968.

12. Rogers, S., Kidd, J. G., and Rous, P.   Relationship of the Shope Papilloma Virus to the Cancer It Determines in Domestic Rabbits.   Acta Union Intern.   Contre Cancer, *16*: 129, 1960.

13. Rous, P., Kidd, J. G., and Smith, W. E.   Experiments on the Cause of the Rabbit Carcinomas Derived from Virus-induced Papillomas.   J. Exptl. Med., *96*: 159, 1952.

14. Shiratori, O., Ito, Y., Takahashi, T., and Imaeda, Y.   Further Studies on the Established Cell Line (AICHI-4) Derived from a Patient with Hodgkin's Disease. GANN Monograph, *7*: 183, 1969.

15. Shope, R. E.   Are Animal Tumor Viruses Always Virus-like?   (Review) J. Gen. Physiol., *45*: Supplement 143, 1962.

HUMAN TUMOR VIROLOGY: THE PROBLEMS OF RNA VIRUS

Chairmen:

Yohei Ito, Frank J. Rauscher, Jr.

Recent Topics on Type C RNA Virus Oncogenesis

Louis R. Sibal, and J. B. Moloney

Etiology Area, National Cancer Institute, National Institutes of Health, Bethesda, Maryland, U.S.A.

Studies on Type C RNA oncogenic viruses have expanded rapidly under the stimulus of applying the information gained from animal tumor virus research to the problems of the viral causation of human malignancies. At present, Type C viruses have been isolated from four animal species and two classes of vertebrates and are established as the causative agents of leukemias, lymphomas, and sarcomas of chickens, mice, cats, and hamsters (*17*). Many of the known animal Type C viruses infect and produce malignancies in closely related animal species (*e.g.* feline sarcoma virus produces tumors in marmoset monkeys) (*3*). The agents replicate in and, in some cases, transform animal and human cells in tissue culture (*e.g.* feline leukemia and sarcoma viruses can be propagated in and transform human embryonic fibroblasts) (*24*) (see Table 1).

Virus particles of similar morphology have been found in association with malignancies of a spectrum of animal species including non human primates, guinea pigs, swine, rats, cattle, woolly monkeys, gibbons, and man (*17*). In certain instances, viruses have been isolated and propagated for limited periods in tissue culture, but at a level too low to determine biological activity (oncogenicity).

Electron microscopic examination of selected malignant tissues has revealed

TABLE 1. Occurrence of Type C Viruses in Various Animal Species

Proven oncogenicity	Unproven oncogenicity	
	Seen on electron microscope examination and isolated in tissue culture	Seen on electron microscope examination only
Chickens (ALV, RSV, strains)	cattle	guinea pigs
Mice (MuLV, MSV, strains)	non human primates (woolly monkeys, gibbons)	snakes
Hamsters (HaLV)	humans	humans
	rats	

the presence of virus particles but to date recovery of active material has not been effected.   Indeed, even with recent modifications in tissue culture technology directed toward virus amplification in cells from naturally occurring lesions, isolation and propagation may not be readily achieved in some animal species (2).

Many of the recent advances which indicate that the Type C RNA oncogenic viruses represent a unique class of viruses have come from extensive immunologic and biochemical investigations at the subviral or molecular level.   Although electron microscopy is an important method in the search for Type C particles, it is less sensitive and consequently less likely to detect small numbers of virions than certain newer immunological and biochemical methods.   This is especially true in primary tumor specimens which may only rarely contain Type C particles or in which the presence of virus infection may be expressed in a way other than the production of mature virions (e.g. defective viral genomes) (2).

This paper presents recent findings on the detection and definition of the role of Type C viruses in oncogenesis.   The immunological and biochemical methods employed could have considerable implications for establishing the etiologic nature of this class of viruses in human neoplasia and for contributing to the understanding of the mechanisms of viral infection and cell transformation.

Immunological Studies

Immunological methods have been of great value in the detection of Type C viruses or virus antigens.   To prepare specific diagnostic reagents, however, it is usually necessary to have sufficient amounts of virus, preferably highly purified virus.   Fortunately, the high concentrations of virus in the blood and tissue of certain experimentally infected, highly susceptible animal strains and in the supernatant fluids of infected cell cultures have provided the necessary starting material to prepare these reagents.   These resources have resulted in the development of several useful serological tests both for the detection of envelope (V) or type specific antigens associated with infectious viruses and for the detection of subviral antigenic components of group specific antigens; specifically: virus neutralization (23), viral hemagglutination (26), complement fixation (14, 24, 25), immunodiffusion (6), immunofluorescence (7), passive hemagglutination (30, 31), and cytotoxicity (22) tests.   In this respect, it is well documented that virus isolates from a single animal species have at least one group antigen in common.

Purified, intact Type C virions derived from murine animals, yield a nucleoprotein core or nucleoid (21), when disrupted by ether, by detergents, or ether-detergent treatment.   This internal structure, which has been shown to contain a *species-specific* group antigen, designated gs-1, is common to all murine leukemia viruses (MLV) (8).   Further purification has shown that this material, with a molecular weight of approximately 26,000, is not antigenic in the host of origin, but antibodies are readily produced when it is injected into other animal species (8, 12, 27).   Studies on avian and feline Type C viruses have yielded similar information.

The detection of this group-specific antigen in cells has been a useful marker for evidence of infection.   Thus, the finding of an MLV group-specific antigen by complement fixation in highly concentrated suspensions of animal tissues or extracts of normal, infected, or tumor cells grown *in vitro* provided a means for Huebner and his colleagues to conduct exhaustive field studies on the natural occurrence of Type C RNA viruses or their expression in chickens, mice, and, more recently, in cats (*17*).   The results suggest that the cells of most vertebrate species have Type C RNA virus genomes which are vertically transmitted from parent to offspring.   Concentration of antigen in the rapidly differentiating tissues of unborn mice suggests further that this material (genome) is implicated in the natural control of cell division.   The role of the host and the effect of certain environmental factors on virus production and/or tumor formation which may develop at some time in the life of the animal must be defined.   Ultimately, control of cancer would then depend on understanding virus expression and the nature of the factors repressing it (*16, 17*).

Very recently, a second group antigen associated with Type C viruses has been demonstrated (*13*).   Preliminary evidence would indicate that it may be an *interspecies-specific* group antigen; it has been referred to as " gs-3 " or " interspec " antigen.   This antigen has already been shown to be present and common among the Type C oncogenic viruses of 3 mammalian species: the mouse, cat, and hamster, but not the chicken (*28*).   Further, this antigen has been detected in highly concentrated extracts of cells from two different human tumors, one of which has at times produced small amounts of a virus resembling animal Type C particles (*28*). At the present time, it is not known if " gs-3 " is antigenic in the host of origin.   It is apparently only weakly antigenic in other animal species, but whether this is due to small amounts of antigen within the virion itself or other intrinsic factors associated with the antigen molecule has not been investigated.   Additional basic immunologic information on this antigen is clearly needed.   If the findings are confirmed, a formidable probe for the presence of virus or viral genome in human cells has been developed.

A somewhat different approach, based on the premise that tumor cells containing a common antigen may indicate a similar viral etiology has been used by other workers.   In particular, the work of Morton and his colleagues exemplifies this type of study (*4, 5, 19, 20, 36*).   In examining the tissues from various human sarcomas, these investigators found particles resembling known animal Type C viruses in at least one liposarcoma.   With continued culture of the tumor, particle production ceased, but indirect immunofluorescence tests using the serums of sarcoma patients revealed that the cells still contained an antigen which is sarcoma-specific.   Cell-free extracts of several sarcoma lines have induced the formation of the sarcoma antigen (SA) in normal cells carried in culture.

The results of epidemiologic surveys by Morton *et al.* (*4, 5, 19, 20, 36*) on the incidence of antibodies to SA in human serums are summarized in Table 2.   A high incidence of serum antibody to SA, as determined by three different serologic tests, was found in patients with various types of skeletal and soft tissue sarcomas and their close associates; a significantly lower incidence was found in normal blood-bank serums.   The antigenic activity is not due to histocompatibility, blood group, or other known human virus antigens and, thus far, appears to be specific for sar-

TABLE 2.   Incidence of Antibody in Human Serums to a Sarcoma Antigen (SA)[a]

Serums from	Percent positive		
	Indirect immunofluorescence	Complement fixation	Complement dependent cytotoxicity
Sarcoma patients	100	95	70
Family members	85	67	58
Normal blood donors	29	25	8

[a] From the data of Morton *et al.* (see references *4, 5, 19, 20,* and *36*).

coma cell lines.   The data suggest that a viral agent may be the etiologic factor in this disease.   Indeed, results of ongoing virologic and immunologic studies will establish a more definite relationship of the antigen to this disease and will certainly contribute to the development of possible control measures for human neoplasia.

Biochemical Studies

In 1964, Temin (*34*) proposed that certain RNA tumor viruses must contain an enzyme which permits the translation of the viral genetic information and subsequent incorporation of this information into the cell genome.   Indeed, more recently Temin and Baltimore (*1, 35*) simultaneously demonstrated that Type C RNA oncogenic viruses contain an RNA-dependent DNA polymerase.   Spiegelman, Green, Todaro, and others (*10, 11, 15, 18, 32*) extended these findings and have reported the enzymatic activity in every RNA tumor virus tested.   Viruses that cause leukemias or sarcomas in chickens, mice, cats, and hamsters as well as mammary tumors in mice, rats, and monkeys have been found to contain the polymerase. By contrast, well-characterized, non oncogenic viruses that contain RNA and develop by cell membrane budding, do not show this activity.   Two exceptions are Visna, a " slow " virus that induces a neurological disease in sheep, and a primate syncytium-forming virus (*29*).   RNA-dependent polymerase activity has been separated from intact virions and is found associated with the nucleoid, its activity can be blocked by antibody in the serum of animals bearing virus-induced tumors (*10*).

Using a synthetic template (dCrG) a second enzyme activity has been demonstrated by Spiegelman and his associates (*33*).   This enzyme, a DNA-dependent DNA polymerase, acts upon the product of RNA-dependent DNA polymerase synthesis.   Because the DNA synthesized in this reaction shows complementarity to Type C viral RNA derived from various animal species and serves as a tool for determining the degree of relatedness among oncogenic viruses, it also is an extremely sensitive device, surpassing electron microscopy by 100-fold as a method for detecting viruses and should thus be useful in searching for covert viral states.

Although Type C RNA viruses have not been clearly associated with human malignancies, the movement to study leukemic cells for the presence of RNA dependent DNA polymerase has been immediate.   If RNA virus particles are present in human leukemic cells, but not detectable by ordinary means, the finding of a unique enzyme system might offer a more sensitive indication of virus infection or expression of the viral genome. Gallo *et al.* (*9*) have already shown that cells of patients with acute lymphoblastic leukemia possess an enzyme activity analogous to the enzymes of the RNA oncogenic viruses which synthesize RNA-dependent DNA. This activity was not found in phytohemagglutinin-stimulated lymphoblasts obtained from the blood of normal donors. The enzyme, which has been obtained in a purified state, uses an RNA template from rat liver and is inhibited by analogues of rifampicin, which also inhibits the enzyme activity found in Type C oncogenic viruses. Using synthetic DNA-RNA hybrids as templates for DNA polymerase enzymes, Spiegelman has found specific activities in the cells of many leukemic patients, but not in normal controls (*33*).

Because the RNA-dependent polymerase is apparently always present in the RNA tumor viruses of animals, its discovery in cells of human leukemics offers good supportive evidence that viruses are associated with cancers in man. Certainly, the presence of this enzyme and the DNA-dependent DNA polymerase will be extremely important for studying the relationship of virus replication to the oncogenic state in both animal and human systems. At this point, however, it is difficult to predict how many key questions these investigations will be able to answer.

REFERENCES

1. Baltimore, D. Viral RNA-dependent DNA Polymerase. Nature, *226*: 1209, 1970.
2. Bryan, W. R., Dalton, A. J., and Rauscher, F. J. The Viral Approach to Human Leukemia and Lymphoma: Its Current Status. Progress in Hematology, *5*: 137, 1967.
3. Deinhardt, F., Wolfe, L. G., Thielen, G. H., and Snyder, S. P. ST-Feline Fibrosarcoma Virus: Induction of Tumors in Marmoset Monkeys. Science, *167*: 881, 1970.
4. Eilber, F. R., and Morton, D. L. Immunologic Studies of Human Sarcomas: Additional Evidence Suggesting an Associated Sarcoma Virus. Cancer, *26*: 588, 1970.
5. Eilber, F. R., and Morton, D. L. Sarcoma-Specific Antigens: Detection by Complement Fixation with Serum from Sarcoma Patients. J. Nat. Cancer Inst., *44*: 651, 1970.
6. Fink, M. A., and Cowles, C. A. Immunodiffusion: Detection of a Murine Leukemia Virus (Rauscher). Science, *150*: 1723, 1965.
7. Fink, M. A., and Malmgren, R. A. Fluorescent Antibody Studies of the Viral Antigen in a Murine Leukemia (Rauscher). J. Nat. Cancer Inst., *31*: 111, 1963.
8. Fink, M. A., Sibal, L. R., Wivel, N. A., Cowles, C. A. and O'Conner, T. E. Some Characteristics of an Isolated Group Antigen Common to Most Strains of Murine Leukemia Virus. Virology, *37*: 605, 1969.
9. Gallo, R. C., and Yang, S. S. RNA-dependent DNA Polymerase of Human Acute Leukemic Cells. Nature, *228*: 927, 1970.
10. Gerwin, B. I., Todaro, G. J., Zeve, V., Scolnick, E. M., and Aaronson, S. A. Separation of RNA-dependent DNA Polymerase Activity from the Murine Leukemia Virion. Nature, *228*: 435, 1970.
11. Green, M., Rokutanda, M., Fujinaga, K., Ray, R. K., Rokutanda, H., and Gurgo, C. Mechanism of Carcinogenesis by RNA Tumor Viruses. (1) An RNA-dependent

DNA Polymerase in Murine Sarcoma Viruses. Proc. Nat. Acad. Sci. U.S., *67*: 385, 1970.

12.   Gregoriades, A., and Old, L. J.   Isolation and Some Characteristics of a Group-specific Antigen of the Murine Leukemia Viruses.   Virology, *37*: 189, 1969.

13.   Hardy, W. D., Geering, G., Old, L. J., de Harven, E., Brodey, R. S., and McDonough, S.   Feline Leukemia Virus: Occurrence of Viral Antigen in the Tissues of Cats with Lymphosarcoma and Other Diseases.   Science, *166*: 1019, 1969.

14.   Hartley, J. W., Rowe, W. P., Capps, W. I., and Huebner, R. J.   Complement Fixation and Tissue Culture Assays for Mouse Leukemia Viruses.   Proc. Nat. Acad. Sci., U.S., *53*: 931, 1965.

15.   Hatanaka, M., Huebner, R. J., and Gilden, R. V.   DNA-polymerase Activity Associated with RNA Tumor Viruses.   Proc. Nat. Acad. Sci., U.S., *67*: 143, 1970.

16.   Huebner, R. J., and Todaro, G. J.   Oncogenes of RNA Tumor Viruses as Determinants of Cancer.   Proc. Nat. Acad. Sci. U.S., *64*: 1087, 1969.

17.   Huebner, R. J., Todaro, G. J., Sarma, P. S., Hartley, J. W., Freeman, A. E., Peters, R. L., Whitmire, C. E., Meier, H., and Gilden, R. V.   " Switched off " Vertically Transmitted Type C RNA Tumor Viruses as Determinants of Spontaneous and Induced Cancer: A New Hypothesis of Viral Carcinogenesis.   Proc. 2nd Int. Symp. on Tumor Viruses, Paris, 1969.

18.   McDonnell, J. P., Garapin, A., Levinson, W. E., Quintrell, N., Fanshier, L., and Bishop, J. M.   DNA Polymerase of Rous Sarcoma Viruses. Delineation of Two Reactions with Actinomycin.   Nature, *228*: 433, 1970.

19.   Morton, D. L., and Malmgren, R. A.   Human Osteosarcomas: Immunologic Evidence Suggesting an Associated Infectious Agent.   Science, *162*: 1279, 1968.

20.   Morton, D. L., Malmgren, R. A., Hall, W. T., and Schidlovsky, G.   Immunologic and Virus Studies with Human Sarcomas.   Surgery, *66*: 152, 1969.

21.   O'Connor, T. E., deThe', G. B., Rauscher, F. J., and Fink, M. A.   Comparison of Rupture of Murine Leukemia Viruses and Myxoviruses on Treatment with Ether and Detergents.   *In* Viruses Inducing Cancer, ed. Burdette, W. J., p. 13, Salt Lake City, 1966.

22.   Old, L. J., Boyse, E. A., Geering, G., and Oettgen, H. F.   Serologic Approaches to the Study of Cancer in Animals and in Man.   Cancer Res., *28*: 1288, 1968.

23.   Rubin, H.   Response of Cell Organism to Infection with Avian Tumor Viruses.   Bact. Rev., *26*: 1, 1962.

24.   Sarma, P. S., Huebner, R. J., Basker, J. F., Vernon, L., and Gilden, R. V.   Feline Leukemia and Sarcoma Viruses: Susceptibility of Human Cells to Infection.   Science, *168*: 1098, 1970.

25.   Sarma, P. S., Turner, H. C., and Huebner, R. J.   An Avian Leucosis Group-specific Complement Fixation Reaction.   Application for the Detection and Assay of Non-cytopathogenic Leucosis Viruses.   Virology, *23*: 313, 1964.

26.   Schäfer, W., and Szanto, J.   Studies on Mouse Leukemia Viruses.   II. Nachweis Eines Virusspezifischen Hämagglutinins.   Z. Naturforsch., *24*: 1323, 1969.

27.   Schäfer, W., Anderer, F. A., Bauer, H., and Pister, L.   Studies on Mouse Leukemia Viruses.   I. Isolation and Characterization of a Group-specific Antigen.   Virology, *38*: 387, 1969.

28.   Schäfer, W., Lange, J., Pister, L., Seifert, E., Noronha, F., and Schmidt, F. W.   Vergleichende Serologische Untersuchungen über Leukämieviren.   Eine Komplementbindungsreaktion zum Nachweis der bei Leukämieviren Verschiedener Säuger

Vorkommenden Gemeinsamen Antigenen Komponente. Z. Naturforsch., *25*: 1029, 1970.

29. Scolnick, E., Rands, E., Aaronson, S. A., and Todaro, G. J. The Divalent Cation Requirements for RNA-dependent DNA Polymerase Activity in Five RNA Viruses. Proc. Nat. Acad. Sci., U.S., *67*: 1789, 1970.

30. Sibal, L. R., Fink, M. A., Plata, E. J., Kohler, B. E., Noronha, F., and Lee, K. M. Methods for the Detection of Viral Antigen and Antibody to a Feline Leukemia Virus (a preliminary report). J. Nat. Cancer Inst., *45*: 607, 1970.

31. Sibal, L. R., Fink, M. A., Vice, J. L., Brandt, B. L., and O'Connor, T. E. Hemagglutination Studies of the Viral Antigen in a Murine Leukemia (Rauscher). Proc. Soc. Exper. Biol. and Med., *122*: 591, 1966.

32. Spiegelman, S., Burny, A., Das, M. R., Keydar, J., Schlom, J., Travnicek, M., and Watson, K. Synthetic DNA-RNA Hybrids and RNA-RNA Duplexes as Templates for the Polymerase of the Oncogenic Viruses. Nature, *228*: 430, 1970.

33. Spiegelman, S. Personal communication.

34. Temin, H. M. Nature of the Provirus of Rous Sarcoma. Nat. Cancer Inst. Monograph, *17*: 557, 1964.

35. Temin, H. M., and Mizutani, S. RNA-dependent DNA Polymerase in Virions of Rous Sarcoma Virus. Nature, *226*: 1211, 1970.

36. Wood, W. C., and Morton, D. L. Microcytotoxicity Test: Detection in Sarcoma Patients of Antibody Cytotoxic to Human Sarcoma Cells. Science, *170*: 1318, 1970.

An SR-RSV-Induced Mouse Tumor Cell Line Converted into a Murine C-Type RNA Virus Producer

Tadashi Yamamoto, Shigeo Hino, Nobuo Yamaguchi, and Mieko Takeuchi

Department of Oncology, Institute of Medical Science, University of Tokyo, Tokyo, Japan

Mammalian tumor cells induced *in vivo* or cells transformed *in vitro* by the sub-group D Schmidt-Ruppin strain of the Rous sarcoma virus (SR-RSV) usually contain the viral genome in a form transmissible to chicken cells, but do not produce any demonstrable infectious virus (*33*). Such cells could be one of the most adequate models for meeting the classic criterion of autonomous growth without additive growth induced by the RNA tumor virus (*37*). To elucidate the role of the viral genome in such tumor cells we have established several strains of SR-RSV-induced ascites sarcomas (*26, 27, 38*) and brain tumors (*12*) in mice. Cell culture lines from these tumors were also prepared (*35, 36*). However, a clonal cell culture line, SR-C3H-2127, originating from an ascites sarcoma of a C3H/He mouse and maintaining the viral genome continuously, was recently found to produce C-type RNA viruses. The present paper will briefly approach the area of RNA tumor virus oncogenesis on the basis of our recent observations on this particular cell line.

The SR-C3H/He Ascites Sarcoma and the SR-C3H-2127 Cell Culture Line

The SR-C3H-2127 cell culture line originated from an ascites sarcoma of a C3H/He mouse, SR-C3H/He ascites sarcoma, at its 17th transplant generation and has been cloned three times by the single cell clone technique (*35, 36*) described by Puck *et al.* (*20*). The original ascites sarcoma was prepared after the neonatal inoculation of SR-RSV-infected chicken tumor cells into a C3H/He mouse and subsequent conversion into the ascitic form (*38*). It was also cloned three times *in vivo* employing thymectomized suckling mice (*26*). During these *in vivo* clonings, the Th11C line was found, after the second cloning, to possess virus particles in cytoplasmic vacuoles and, at the same time, the tumor-bearing mice showed contamination of plasma lactate dehydrogenase elevating virus or Reiley virus. Fortunately, at that time, the virus particle and Reiley virus activity were altogether eliminated

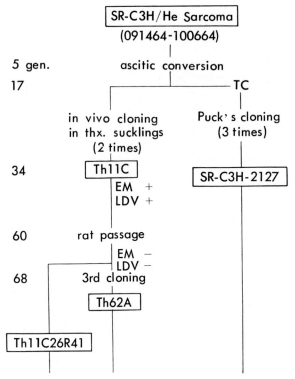

FIG. 1.   Diagrammatic outline of the SR-C3H/He ascites sarcoma and its allied clonal cell lines. thx, thymectomized; EM, electron-microscopically detectable particles; LDV, lactate dehydrogenase-elevating virus.

after a rat passage of the ascites sarcoma cells.   At the 10th and 20th transplant generations after the rat passage, the Reiley virus activity remained negative.   The Th62A line, which we will later compare with the SR-C3H-2127 cell culture line, was prepared after one more cloning in thymectomized mice (Fig. 1).

Last year, when Prof. Takuzo Oda of Okayama University School of Medicine again showed the existence of virus particles in cell culture preparations derived from the Th11C26R41 ascites sarcoma at the 41st transplant generation after rat passage, we at first thought the particles might be a contaminant during the course of mouse passages like our experience with Reiley virus.   However, the SR-C3H-2127 cell line, which had been transferred *in vitro* from a much earlier transplant generation, was also revealed to produce a considerable quantity of virus particles. As shown in Fig. 2, C-type virus particles, including budding forms from the plasma membrane and containing a significantly larger nucleoid than that of the SR-RSV, were clearly demonstrated.

The SR-C3H-2127 cell line showed some particular properties from the beginning of its establishment.

Typical chicken sarcomas usually develop after the back transplantation of SR-RSV-induced mammalian tumor cells, when the cells contain the viral genome in masked form.   However, the development of chicken tumor was much less ef-

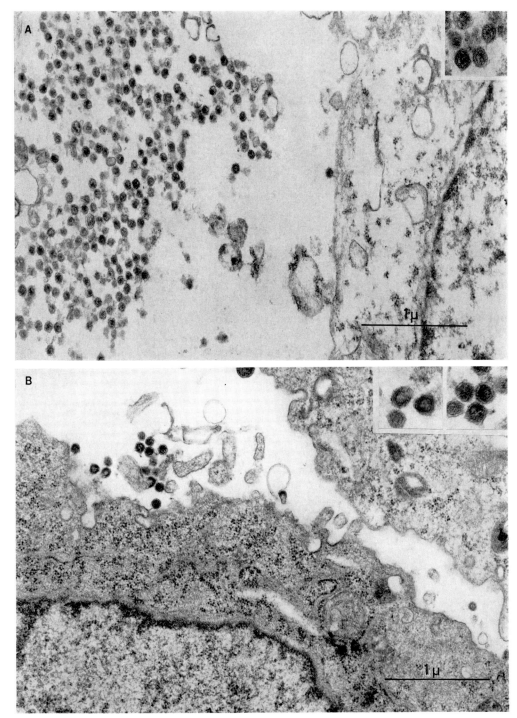

FIG. 2. Budding (A) and mature virus (B) particles from SR-C3H–2127 cells. Double fixation with glutaraldehyde and osmium. Double stain with alcoholic uranyl acetate and lead citrate. Prepared through the courtesy of Prof. Takuzo Oda.

ficient when inoculated back into chicken wing webs with cells from this particular cell line.   Tumors were induced in only 10 to 15% of the chickens inoculated with 10^7 cells and no tumor resulted from inoculations with 10^6 cells, while the Th62A ascites sarcoma cells induced chicken tumors in all the chicknes with 2×10^6 cells and in 40% with as few as 2×10^5 cells (*36*).

Contact culture of SR-RSV-induced mammalian tumor cells with permissive chick embryo cells usually produces infectious SR-RSV, as can be seen in the case of Th62A ascites sarcoma cells, but the 2127 cells did not produce any SR-RSV during 48 days' observation with several transfers of culture (*35*).   Nevertheless, when combined with the cell fusion reaction (*17*) of the 2127 cells and chick embryo cells by the aid of UV-irradiated HVJ (Hemagglutinating virus of Japan), the contact culture always yields infectious SR-RSV.   Moreover, the rate of the rescue of this viral genome has been almost constant for these 4 years.   When 10^5 cells are fused with 6×10^5 chick embyro cells and cultured with an agar overlay, almost equal numbers of infective centers, around 100, are obtainable.

In addition, quantitative studies using anti-HVJ antibodies, which are known to enhance cell fusion efficiency particularly at an antigen excess zone in HVJ-anti-HVJ immune reaction (*18, 19*), showed the quite parallel enhancement of the number of infective centers after the cell fusion reaction of SR-C3H-2127 cells and chick embryo cells.   The time course kinetic studies at different temperatures, 4°C and 37°C, also showed the requirement of energenesis, not only in cell fusion reactions but also in the increasing production of infective centers (*36*).   These findings lead us to the proposal that the rescue of the viral genome in SR-RSV-induced mammalian tumor cells should be through such a particular cell fusion reaction with permissive chicken cells, but not through the mere contact or aggregation of two kinds of cells.   Similar conclusions were also drawn by other investigators (*13, 23–25, 32*).

More recently, Yamaguchi made an interesting experiment on the effect of excess thymidine on the SR-RSV production from these fused cells (*34*).   No difference in the production of infective centers was observed even after 0–12 or 0–48 hr treatment with 20 mM thymidine (*15*) after the fusion reaction.   Although the true mode of existence of viral genome awaits further investigations, the data might support Temin's provirus theory (*28*) of possible integration of the SR-RSV genome with the host cell DNA, to which one becomes much more amenable since the recent discovery of RNA-DNA and DNA-DNA polymerases in the virion of RNA tumor viruses (*2, 29*).

Characteristics of the Virus Produced by SR-C3H-2127 Cells

The incorporation of ^{3}H-uridine into 2127 viruses was first studied by the isopycnic centrifugation procedure described by Robinson *et al.* (*21*), with minor modifications.   Ammonium sulfate was added to culture fluids from 5 to 10×10^6 cells previously exposed to 100 μCi of ^{3}H-uridine for 48 hr.   The resulting precipitates were centrifuged in preformed linear gradients of 15–60% sucrose in a Spinco SW 41 rotor tube at 40,000 rpm for 90 min.   As shown in Fig. 3a, the 2127

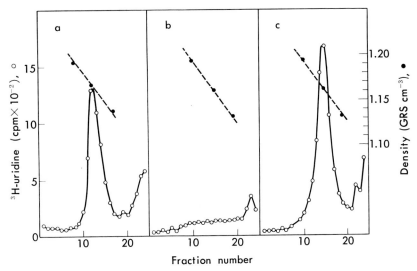

Fig. 3. Sucrose gradient profiles of ammonium sulfate-treated culture fluids from 5 to 10×10^6 cells exposed to 100 μCi of ^{3}H-uridine for 48 hr from (a) SR-C3H-2127 cells, (b) C/O chick embryo cells after infection with SR-C3H-2127 virus, and (c) C/O chick embryo cells after fusion reaction with gamma ray-irradiated SR-C3H-2127 cells.

virus appeared to belong to an RNA-type virus with a buoyant density of 1.16–1.18 g/cm³, of very similar value to C-type RNA virus.   C/O-type RAV (Rous associated virus), RIF (Resistance inducing factor)-free chick embryo cells, inoculated with this virus preparation, transferred twice and exposed to ^{3}H-uridine, failed to produce the progeny virus (Fig. 3b); but when the 2127 cells, previously irradiated with gamma rays from ^{60}Co, were fused with C/O-type chick embryo cells with the aid of UV-irradiated HVJ and once transferred, the incorporation of ^{3}H-uridine into the virus band was clearly observed at the buoyant density of 1.16 g/cm³ (Fig. 3c).   These experiments strongly suggested that the two viruses differed from one another, the former being the 2127 virus and the latter, SR-RSV.

Since C-type RNA tumor viruses are characterized by a species-specific group-reactive internal virus antigen (gs antigen) (33), the possible preparation of rabbit antisera reactive with the murine gs antigen in the COMUL test (complement fixation test for murine leukemia virus) (22) was then investigated using a purified 2127 virus preparation.   The 2127 virus contained in 5 to 10 liters of pooled cell culture fluids was first cleared by low centrifugation, salted out with 50% ammonium sulfate saturation, and then sedimented through 20% sucrose to a cushion of 60% sucrose in Spinco 25–2 rotor tubes at 25,000 rpm for 120 min.   After one more cycle of salting out and sedimentation, the virus concentrate was subjected to isopycnic centrifugation in a preformed linear density gradients of 15–60% sucrose in Spinco 41 rotor tubes at 40,000 rpm for 90 min.   The procedure of virus purification mentioned above followed that of Duesberg et al. (5) with some modifications. The purified virus preparation in 1 : 1,000 to 1 : 2,000 volumes of original stock was finally treated with 1% sodium dodecyl sulfate (SDS) at room temperature for

TABLE 1.   Varies Existence of Murine and Avian gs Antigens in Tissues and Cells

Test antigens[a]	Murine gs	Avian gs[c]
Normal mouse spleen	25[b]	
Normal C3H/He spleen	12.5	
Normal C3H/He embryo	50	
SR-DDD ascites sarcoma	< 4	64
SR-C3H/He ascites sarcoma Th62A	4	16
SR-C3H-2127 cell	600	< 6
„ purified virus	800	
„ SDS treated virus	> 6,400	
FLV-infected DDD spleen	1,600	
AKR thymic tumor	1,600	
AKR serum	200	
MLV-induced rat thymic tumor	> 6,400	
Spontaneous DDD lymphoma L28	25	
„ L32	50	
„ L48	50	
„ L82	200	
„ L83	400	

[a] All the antigens were prepared from a 50% emulsion of tissues or cells, centrifuged at 3,000 rpm for 20 min.

[b] Complement fixing titer reciprocals with 4 units of antiserum.

[c] Pooled sera of SR-RSV-induced, tumor-bearing hamsters were used.

10 min.   Potassium chloride was added, and then it was chilled and centrifuged. The supernatant was dialyzed and used as antigen.   Two doses of 0.5 ml of antigen mixed with complete Freund adjuvant were injected into the foot pads of rabbits at 3 weeks interval; 3 weeks after the last injection a booster injection of 0.5 ml antigen was given intravenously.   The rabbits were bled a week later.   A detailed description of the properties of the antibodies will be made in another paper (8). By this method highly specific anti-murine gs antisera were obtained.   They have no anti-Forssman and no anti-mouse serum proteins, and no anti-avian gs antibodies. Table 1 shows the summarized results of complement fixation test in a microplate procedure undertaken at the same time.   Anti-2127 virion-inner-protein rabbit sera react very well with Friend leukemia virus (FLV)-infected DDD mouse spleen, AKR mouse thymus tumor, Moloney leukemia virus (MLV)-induced rat thymus tumor and even several spontaneous lymphomas of DDD mice.   Thus the sera proved to contain anti-murine gs antibodies with high specificity.   As also indicated in Table 1, anti-avian gs antigen hamster sera reacted fairly well with SR-DDD ascites sarcoma, another strain of SR-RSV-induced ascites sarcoma of DDD mouse, and the abovementioned SR-C3H/He ascites sarcoma Th62A strain, a mother strain comparable to the SR-C3H-2127 cell line.   They hardly reacted at all with the 2127 cell line, which, on the contrary, reacted very highly with anti-murine gs antibodies.   Thus the conclusion may be made that the virus produced by the SR-C3H-2127 cells is a kind of murine C-type RNA virus.

DISCUSSION

In this paper we have demonstrated a particular cell culture line, SR-C3H-2127 on the one hand maintaining the whole genome of SR-RSV and on the other producing a considerable quantity of murine C-type RNA virus, while an allied *in vivo* tumor cell line, Th62A ascites sarcoma, of the same origin does not show such a virus production. Similar observations were also given by other investigators. Valentine and Bader (*31*) observed that the virus particles were morphologically more similar to the murine leukemia virus in RSV-transformed rat embryo cells, in which, however, no infectious RSV was demonstrable. More recently, Gelderblom *et al.* (*6*) have demonstrated the existence of virus particles quite resembling typical leukemia virus in a Prague strain of RSV-induced C57BL mouse tumor RVP$_3$. The tumor strain was first established by Bubenik *et al.* (*4*) and, unaccountably enough, contained only RSV-induced tumor-specific transplantation antigen(s) (*3*). Neither avian gs antigen nor RSV genome could be demonstrated (*3*), but later, murine gs antigen was shown by Schäfer and Seifert (*22*). The SR-C3H-2127 cell line has a strong resemblance to RVP$_3$ but differs from it in the existence of the RSV genome, although a more sensitive assay method is used in the former case. A relevant question at present would be why the avian gs antigen, one of the most reliable expressions of the existing RSV genome, becomes undetectable in SR-C3H-2127 cells, while an allied *in vivo* tumor cell line, Th62A ascites sarcoma, possesses the antigen.

Existence of such a particular cell line might remind us of the unitary hypothesis recently described by Huebner and Todaro (*9*). Since some C3H/He mouse embryos in our colony were actually shown to possess the murine gs antigen as was indicated in Table 1, there had been a fair chance for the mother strain of the SR-C3H-2127 cells to receive the genome of murine C-type RNA virus in a so-called " switch-off " state, which in due time during long-term cultivation *in vitro* became " switch-on " so as to produce the mature virus in the case of SR-C3H-2127, while still remaining in the " switch-off " state in the Th62A ascites sarcoma. However, if one applies the unitary hypothesis extensively, the existing SR-RSV genome, exogenously introduced into a cell possessing another kind of " oncogene " in a form that can be rescued, should have had nothing but a trigger effect on inherited murine virus " oncogene " and " virogene " successively so as to make the cell malignant on the one hand and produce murine tumor virus on the other. Another explanation could also be made, provided that the " virogene " alone could be switched-on independent of the murine " virus oncogene " or the latter could be replaced by the term " cellular oncogene." Then the exixsting SR-RSV genome, probably localized near the cellular oncogene locus, would have played a role to activate or derepress the cellular oncogene so as to maintain the malignant nature of the SR-C3H-2127 cells and hence, in such a derepressed state of the tumor cells, a kind of murine C-type RNA virus, the 2127 virus, could be produced. These two possibilities are rather comically illustrated in Fig. 4. In search of the more proximate phenotypic expression of SR-RSV oncogene further studies are in progress.

The oncogenicity of so-called murine leukemia viruses such as those newly

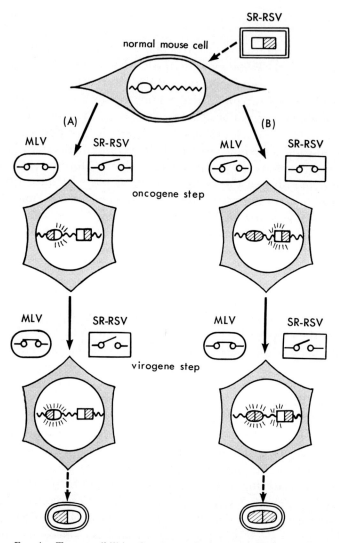

Fig. 4. Two possibilities for the producing mechanism of SR-C3H-2127 virus. (A) According to the Huebner-Todaro hypothesis, (B) According to our speculation.

detected from many kinds of cultured cells (*1*) has not been fully proved. Search for the possible leukemogenicity of the 2127 virus is yet under way. In this connection, the recent reports concerning the heterogeneity and/or variability of avian leucosis-sarcoma virus complex viruses are much more suggestive. Non transforming reproducing mutants or segregants such as NT(γ) from SR-RSV (*7*) and NT-B77 from the B77 strain of avian sarcoma virus (*30*) were isolated, reconfirming the limited localization of oncogene in the virus genome. Natural occurrence of leukemogenic and non leukemogenic viruses with just the same antigenicity was found even in the stock of the avian erythroblastosis virus strain R (*10*). A similar finding was also made in an avian myeloblastosis virus with a particular helper function (*14*). We have also made observations on the variability of some strains of subgroup A SR-RSV (*11*). On the other hand according to Odaka's recent observations (*16*), possible separation of target cells for infection and oncogenesis by Friend leukemia virus would be expected. More circumspect approaches would be required for elucidating oncogenic C-type RNA viruses.

REFERENCE

1. Aaronson, S. A., Hartley, J. W., and Todaro, G. J. Mouse Leukemia Virus: " Spontaneous " Release by Mouse Embryo Cells after Long-term *in vitro* Culture. Proc. N.A.S., *64*: 87–94, 1969.
2. Baltimore, D. RNA-dependent DNA Polymerase in Virion of RNA Tumor Viruses. Nature, *226*: 1209–1211, 1970.
3. Bubenik, J., and Bauer, H. Antigenic Characteristics of the Interaction between Rous Sarcoma Virus and Mammalian Cells. Complement-fixing and Transplantation Antigens. Virology. *31*: 489–497, 1967.
4. Bubenik, J., Koldovský, P., Svoboda, J., Klement, V., and Dvořák, R. Induction of Tumours in Mice with Three Variants of Rous Sarcoma Virus and Studies on the Immunology of These Tumours. Folia boli., *13*: 29–39, 1967.
5. Duesberg, P. H., Robinson, H. V., Robinson, W. S., Huebner, R. J., and Turner, H. C. Proteins of Rous Sarcoma Virus. Virology, *36*: 73–86, 1968.
6. Gelderblom, H., Bauer, H., and Frank, H. Investigations on Virus Production in RSV Mammalian Tumors. J. gen. Virol., *7*: 33–45, 1970.
7. Goldé, A. Radio-induced Mutants of the Schmidt-Ruppin Strain of Rous Sarcoma Virus. Virology, *40*: 1022–1029, 1970.
8. Hino, S., Yamaguchi, N., and Yamamoto T. Characteristics of a Virus Found in a Rous Mouse Cell Line. Japan. J. exp. Med., to be submitted.
9. Huebner, R. J., and Todaro, G. T. Oncogensis of RNA Tumor Viruses as Determinants of Cancer. Proc. N.A.S., *64*: 1087–1094, 1969.
10. Ishizaki, R., and Shimizu, T. Heterogeneity of Leukemogenesis with the Avian Erythroblastosis Virus Strain R. Xth ICC Abstract: 145, 1970.
11. Kawai, S., and Yamamoto, T. Isolation of Different Kinds of Non-Virus Producing Chick Cells Transformed by Schmidt-Ruppin Strain (subgroup A) of Rous Sarcoma Virus. Japan. J. exp. Med., *40*: 243–256, 1970.
12. Kumanishi, T. Brain Tumors Induced with Rous Sarcoma Virus, Schmidt-Ruppin Strain. I. Induction of Brain Tumors in Adult Mice with Rous Chicken Sarcoma Cells. Japan. J. exp. Med., *37*: 461–474, 1967.
13. Machala, O., Donner, L., and Svoboda, J. A Full Expression of the Genome of Rous Sarcoma Virus in Heterokaryons Formed after Fusion of Virogenic Mammalian Cells and Chicken Fibroblasts. J. gen. Virol., *8*: 219–229, 1970.
14. Moscovici, C., and Zanetti, M. Studies on Single Foci of Hematopoietic Cells Transformed by Avian Myeloblastosis Virus. Virology, *42*: 61–67, 1970.
15. Nakata, Y., and Bader, J. P. Studies on the Fixation and Development of Cellular Transformation by Rous Sarcoma Virus. Virology, *36*: 401–410, 1968.
16. Odaka, T. Inheritance of Susceptibility to Friend Mouse Leukemia Virus. VII. Establishment of a Resistant Strain. Int. J. Cancer, *6*: 18–23, 1970.
17. Okada, Y. Analysis of Giant Polynuclear Cell Formation Caused by HVJ Virus from Ehrlich's Ascites Tumor Cells. I. Microscopic Observation of Giant Poly-

nuclear Cell Formation.   Exp. Cell Res., *26*: 98–107, 1962.

18. Okada, Y., and Maruyama, F.   Fusion of Cells by HVJ: Requirement of Concentration of Virus Particles at the Site of Contact of Two Cells for Fusion.   Exp. Cell Res., *52*: 34–42, 1968.

19. Okada, Y., Yamada, K., and Tadokoro, J.   Effect of Antiserum on the Cell Fusion Reaction Caused by HVJ.   Virology, *22*: 397–409, 1964.

20. Puck, T. T., Marcus, P. I., and Cieciuca, S. J.   Clonal Growth of Mammalian Cells *in vitro*.   Growth Characteristics of Colonies from Single Hela Cells with and without a Feeder Layer, J. exp. Med., *103*: 273–284, 1956.

21. Robinson, W. S., Pitkanen, A., and Rubin, H.   The Nucleic Acid of the Bryan Strain of Rous Sarcoma Virus: Purification of the Virus and Isolation of the Nucleic Acid.   Proc. N.A.S., *54*: 134–144, 1965.

22. Schäfer, W., and Seifert, E.   Production of a Potent Complement-fixing Murine Leukemia Virus Antiserum from the Rabbit and Its Reactions with Various Types Tissue Culture Cells.   Virology, *35*: 323–328, 1968.

23. Svoboda, J., and Dourmashkin, R.   Rescue of Rous Sarcoma Virus from Virogenic Mammalian Cells Associated with Chicken Cells and Treated with Sendai Virus.   J. gen. Virol., *4*: 523–529, 1969.

24. Svoboda, J., Hložánek, T., and Machala, O.   Rescue of Rous Sarcoma Virus in Mixed Cultures of Virogenic Mammalian and Chick Cells, Treated and Untreated with Sendai Virus and Detected by Focus Assay.   J. gen. Virol., *2*: 461–465, 1968.

25. Svoboda, J., Machala, O., and Hozánek, I.   Influence of Sendai Virus on RSV Formation in Mixed Culture of Virogenic Mammalian Cells and Chicken Fibroblasts.   Folia biol., *13*: 155–157, 1967.

26. Takeuchi, M., Hino, S., and Yamamoto, T.   Studies on Rous Sarcoma Virus in Mice.   II. Clonal Analysis of Cell Populations of SR-RSV-induced Mouse Ascites Sarcoma (SR-3H/He ascites).   Japan. J. exp. Med., *37*: 107–120, 1967.

27. Takeuchi, M., Hino, S., and Yamamoto, T.   Studies on Rous Sarcoma Virus in Mice.   III. Three Lines of SR-RSV-induced Mouse Ascites Sarcomas.   Japan. J. exp. Med., *39*: 239–251, 1969.

28. Temin, H. M.   Carcinogenesis by Avian Sarcoma Viruses.   Cancer Res., *28*: 1835–1838, 1968.

29. Temin, H. M., and Mizutani, S.   RNA Dependent DNA Polymerase in Virion of Rous Sarcoma Virus.   Nature, 226:   1211–1213, 1970.

30. Toyoshima, K., Friis, R. R., and Vogt, P. K.   The Reproductive and Cell-transforming Capacity of Avian Sarcoma Virus B77:   Inactivation with UV Light.   Virology, *42*: 163–170, 1970.

31. Valentine, A. F., and Bader, J. P.   Production of Virus by Mammalian Cells Transformed by Schmidt-Ruppin Strain of Rous Sarcoma and Murine Sarcoma Viruses.   J. Virol., *2*: 224–237, 1968.

32. Vigier, P.   Persistence du Génome du Virus de Rous Dans les Cellules du Hamster Converties *in vitro* e Action du Virus Sendai Inactivé sur sa Transmission aux Cellules de Poule.   C. R. Acad. Sci. (Paris), *264*: 422–425, 1967.

33. Vogt, P. K.   Avian Tumor Viruses.   *In* Smith, K. H. and Laufer, M. A. (ed), Adv. in Virus Res., *11*: 293–385, 1965.

34. Yamaguchi, N., Hino, S., Takeuchi, M., and Yamamoto, T.   Recovery of Rous Sarcoma Virus from Non-Virus-Producing Rous Sarcoma Cells.   *In* Yamamoto, T. and Sugano, H. (ed), Experimental Leukemia.   GANN Monograph, *12*: 1971, in press.

35. Yamaguchi, N., Takeuchi, M., and Yamamoto, T.   Rous Sarcoma Virus Production in Mixed Culture of Mouse Tumor Cells and Chicken Embryo Fibroblasts by the Addition of UV-Irradiated HVJ.   Japan. J. exp. Med., *37*: 83–86, 1967.

36. Yamaguchi, N., Takeuchi, M., and Yamamoto, T.   Rous Sarcoma Virus Production in Mixed Cultures of Mammalian Rous Sarcoma Cells and Chick Embryo Cells.   Int. J. Cancer, *4*: 678–689, 1969.

37. Yamamoto, T.   A Study of Viral Tumor.   Igaku no Ayumi, *53*: 139–146, 1965. (in Japanese)

38. Yamamoto, T., and Takeuchi, M.   Studies on Rous Sarcoma Virus in Mice.   I. Establishment of an Ascites Sarcoma Induced by Schmidt-Ruppin Strain of Rous Sarcoma Virus in C3H/He Mouse.   Japan. J. exp. Med., *37*: 35–50, 1967.

Discussion of Papers by Drs. Rauscher, Ito, Moloney, and Yamamoto

DR. IDA: I have some comments on Dr. Moloney's lecture. Recently we obtained a potent MSV, a murine sarcoma virus from mice bearing a congenital sarcoma. The virus was obtained from a mother double-infected with MSV and MLV during her pregnancy. Of course, this came from Dr. Moloney's virus. This Moloney sarcoma subline virus could induce not only sarcoma but also bone tumor and brain tumor in rats. Brain tumor developed in mice also, when the virus was inoculated intracranially at birth. One of the rat brain tumors, which was astrocytoma, glioma, was grown as a pure culture in the media. From the biological study, it was evident that the cultured tumor astrocyte contained the virus. The astrocytoma cells were transplantable not only in the brain tissue but also in the subcutaneous tissue of the homogenic hosts. Thus, we learned that MSV could induce malignant tumor both in mesenchymal tissue and ectodermal tissue. And, what is more, the tumor from the ectodermal cells produced the sarcoma virus, so that there is some speculation of there being a similar phenomenon in human beings.

DR. AOKI: Concerning the helper virus and the C-type particles, we did some experiments in collaboration with Drs. Dixon and Oldstrong at Scripps Institute. We found this special phenomenon in NZW and NZB strain mice infected with LCM virus. In blood circulation, Gross soluble antigen remarkably increased after infection with this virus. At the same time, *in vitro*, we found an increase in Gross soluble antigen, type specific Gross antigen. This suggests two possibilities. One is that the LCM virus may activate the viral genome to produce cell surface type specific G antigen. Another possibility is that it may cause some special activity like a helper virus. If this is the case, different families of virus may react like a helper virus. It will be interesting if this can be applied to human problems.

DR. RAUSCHER: If you don't have any further questions, I am going to continue with some thoughts connected with my paper that I could not get in this morning. Let me ask you a question. I think one of the most important elements of progress in tumor virology in the past couple of years has been what you might call the elimination of the hit-and-run phenomenon. You remember four or five years ago, this dictum stated that many viruses, while having the capacity for inducing a malignant lesion, then disappeared absolutely completely from the lesion, so that no particulates or what we now call fingerprints could be picked up. It was a concept that I think was somewhat deleterious because I believe it prevented or discouraged many competent people from getting into the field. For instance, it is very likely that the latent period between infection, if you will, and the appearance of the neoplasm in primate systems, including man, is probably very long, and consequently, it seems that even if viruses were involved in the induction of the lesion, it would be difficult or impossible to demonstrate it, because the infection occurred many years ago and the agent had completely disappeared. But now, to my knowledge, there is not a single system left either of the DNA or RNA variety in which one cannot at least cook them up to make particles of the original virus or, if not, then some fingerprints, some code, some information that could only have come from the virus. This is exceedingly speculative, I think. Dr. Ito's work is a good example of this. Using the Shope papilloma system where there was not enough virus to be detectable by conventional and unsophisticated bioassay and extraction, he found that there was enough nucleic acid present that its information could be recovered. So may I pose a question. Does anyone know of a single system in which it is not possible to show that a particular virus induced a particular lesion using a homology technique with gs antigen detection? An excellent example of this technique is the recent work done by zur Hausen with Henle on the EB virus, in which it was shown that Raji and another line from Burkitt's lymphoma (and I suppose from many other systems as well) in which you can detect no virion and no antigen of the Henle type (reported by Henle several years ago, not the early antigens we are talking about now), do contain viral information. Does anybody know of any system today in which you cannot detect either the particulates or the information carried in by the virus and have thereby been unable to say with some confidence that this virus caused that cancer? Because if you get to man this is probably the only thing you are going to be able to do. What about the other rabbit carcinomas that have been carried so long and which seem to have lost their ability to make papillomas? Do you know of any such system?

DR. ITO: No.

DR. RAUSCHER: Well, I think there are none as no one seems to know of any. One other comment I would like to make so long as I know of no such systems, is sort of a take-off from this. I think the most important element of discussion and a very important one at this meeting for all of us in viral oncology is to try to define the criteria that a virus has to have in order to be a major candidate for oncogenicity in man. What does tumor virus do that other viruses don't do? The one direct experiment that one can use to demonstrate this is of course not open to it. We can't inoculate babies with RSV to prove a point, and this is going to make it exceedingly difficult, except by the back door or via a seroepidemiological approach, to show that any virus is oncogenic in man. With the herpes-type virus, or rather EBV (I am trying to be a bit provocative here to get you to say something), it seems to me that all of the criteria that are attainable by us, that are available to us, that are now at hand, is to find a role of oncogenicity for this virus in man. Take a look at the data. What you really need is a kind of serologic piece of information that shows a very high prevalence or association of virus and the antibody to the disease. This has been magnificently studied by so many of you in nasopharyngeal carcinoma and certainly with Burkitt's lymphoma.

Secondly, it has been shown very clearly, I think, by the Henles and others that it is possible for infectious mononucleosis. Here is a disease which, at least for a time, has a very rapid and uncontrolled proliferative state of the same series of cells which could be, or are, involved in leukemia. Then, there are two other points, and I would like to pose this as a question too. It seems to me tumor viruses do two things that all of the viruses not known to be oncogenic do not do. First, they transform cells. This has recently been easily measured *in vitro* but has not been measured entirely *in vivo* as well. EBV apparently has this capacity of inducing the lymphoblastoid transformation of peripheral leukocytes in tissue culture. Without the viruses, in fact, it appears you will not be able to grow most of the cells from peripheral blood in the sense of the kind of thing that the Drs. Henle have done before. By adding the viruses, by exposing normal cells from people having antibody to EBV viruses, the cells grow. Secondly, if you assign or assume an oncogenic role for any virus, you have to assume that it has the potential of incorporating and, therefore, modifying the cellular genome of the normal cell. Cancer is a heritable disease, and, therefore, any inducer must do something to the cellular genetics. They must change it in such a way that it can be incorporated and expressed time after time, and I think one of the best criteria showing that EBV has this capacity is that it has the ability, in a heritable way, to command a cell to make an antigen apparently not associated with the virus now, the so-called neoantigen or cellular antigen, that it would not have made before exposure. This finding, I think, is an inheritable firm incorporation. As far as I know, the viruses that do not induce tumor don't have this capacity. The influenzas, the polios, what have you. Is this an accurate function? And if it is, since we cannot prove this directly, what else can you do in order to say that this virus causes that cancer? Are we not paying enough attention to data already at hand? What other data can be sought to try to add to our confidence in calling this a tumor virus? First of all, does anybody know of a virus that is now known to be oncogenic in some system that has the capacity for a cellular incorporation of a modifying cellular genome? By the expression of a new antigen perhaps; Dr. Henle and I have talked about this many times. What else can you do there for virus like this? Dr. Epstein, what other kind of information do you need to say this virus causes cancer in man? Perhaps not as a sole factor, I understand this, but as a factor indispensably associated with the cancer. You are responsible for this, you found the virus first.

DR. EPSTEIN: I have talked about this before and I am sure lots of people heard all this. I think that anything you can do is the same thing as the tobacco smoking story. You know, we think that there is a statistical relationship between smoking tobacco cigarettes and getting carcinoma of the lung. You can't really prove this in any way because it is a very complex situation. In this connection it is interesting to mention the experiments which have been taking place in the United Kingdom for the last seven years, in which a record is being kept of the smoking habits of all registered medical practitioners.   Each one makes a return every year of how much he smokes.   When one dies, the cause of death is noted.   Certain pertinent information is already coming in.   It seems that this is the only group in the country in which cigarette smoking is decreasing, and in which the incidence of carcinoma of the lung is likewise decreasing.   In fact we are at the moment saving the lives of those who are not smoking equivalent to the output of a whole medical school-year of students.   This has been taking place over the last five years.   I think this shows that if you remove the thing you suspect of being related to the causation of the tumor, and you influence the incidence of the tumor, you have some indication that there must be some kind of relationship, however complicated. I would suggest to Dr. Rauscher in this connection, therefore, that the way to set about this is perhaps to produce a vaccine, to do a trial vaccine project somewhere, a field trial in a limited area.   You have a very advantageous situation with Burkitt's lymphoma because the peak incidence we know to be six years of age and if you can influence the incidence of the disease by preventing children from getting it, it is alterable in its horizontal transmission.   I think you then have some indication that there must be a causal relationship, however complicated.   Is this what you wanted me to say?

DR. RAUSCHER: Thank you, Dr. Epstein, yes.   Has anybody else a comment on this?   There are lots of problems, of course, in preparing a vaccine; there are many technical problems; viruses grow very poorly in the kind of cells we need to grow them in to make an acceptable vaccine.   One of the other problems we all know about is that Burkitt's lymphoma in very young children is probably the most amenable to effective chemotherapy of all lesions known—about 70 per cent of these children go, we know, into at least 8 years of regression following a single shot of Cycrophonate.   So you have a sort of a model tag here if one should put any effort into developing and testing a vaccine to prove the principle of viral oncogenesis in people.   I think so in this case, or in some other system like nasopharyngeal carcinoma, perhaps.

DR. W. HENLE: I agree that it would be a very nice test to immunize children and see whether Burkitt's lymphoma would disappear from a certain area.   But there are, in my mind, some insurmountable problems at hand.   If you were thinking of a killed-virus vaccine, I don't think that anyone has produced a herpes-group virus vaccine from killed organisms.   Am I correct, or not, Dr. Roizman?   It could be pretty tough to get a good antibody response to killed herpes-simplex virus.   If one looks for an attenuated virus, we would be dealing with potentially oncogenic virus.   We would only favor this particular property by using attenuated virus. So, I'm somewhat uncertain about this and I look at the suggestion of a vaccine with considerable reservation at the present time.

DR. DE THÉ: I think, indeed, that you have been quite provocative.   We have not at all any proof that EBV is indeed oncogenic for man.   It " transforms " human lymphocytes; we don't know what this means but can tell that something happens in the cell and also in the host. We don't have any proof that these cells injected in man would or would not cause cancer to develop; this is, I think, something that must be borne in mind. The transformation *in vitro* may resemble the transformation of infectious mononucleosis, which we know is not, in 99 per cent of cases, a premalignant disease. I think that we have some way to look concerning what is going on in the human population and must try to learn by prospective study. As you know, it has been discussed many times that someone should try to do with Burkitt's lymphoma what the Henles have done for infectious mononucleosis and prospective study at Yale University. I think it is absolutely prohibitive to have any idea of trying vaccine, at least in the Burkitt's population, that is, in an African population. Certainly, vaccine can be tried in infectious mononucleosis in an American population but you cannot try the vaccine on a foreign population before it has been proved to the satisfaction of that government. Indeed something has to be shown between the virus and the induced tumor. I think that is quite important.

DR. RAUSCHER: I think the major point that you make is that we have no proof and that is exactly the point I made. You will never get that proof, and in lieu of not being able to do this, what other criteria do you use, saying, this is the best bet to go on?

DR. DE THÉ: Do you agree with the work in infectious mononucleosis?

DR. RAUSCHER: Yes, indeed.

DR. DE THÉ: If you do agree I don't know why this cannot be done in a human tumor with a short latent period, such as Burkitt's lymphoma. Now, just last week, we had a last meeting on the feasibility of prospective study in Africa, and Schneiderman himself came out and said, " More and more I tend to believe that this disease might indeed have a very short latent period." Therefore, I think it is feasible, and I don't see how and why there is so much doubt about this type of study which, by the way, is not too much more difficult than what has been done for infectious mononucleosis. The size and the cost are a little different but the consideration of cost is not the answer. This is my proposition.

DR. RAUSCHER: One other question again I am going to ask you. Gurtner is conducting a prospective study of the type de Thé is talking about and we are all planning on. Are we sure right now that we are measuring, that we would be measuring, the right antibody? There are so many. If we had done this two or three years ago, I suppose, we would have probably been measuring the wrong antibody.

DR. DE THÉ: I think the secret of the success of the Henles with infectious mononucleosis is the result of wonderful natural history study and wonderful planning of the prospective study at Yale University, without any particular purpose in mind at the time. In any case, the pre-tumor sera will probably be the most precious material because any kind of test can be done later on.

DR. EPSTEIN: I think that what Dr. de Thé is saying is a very good idea and it has to be done. It is most important because it is the area of darkness about which we do not know anything. What it could be, if it's going to be meaningful, if one set of things happens, is that catching the virus will be followed by getting the tumor very quickly. If it doesn't work like that, and it may well not work like that, it may be that you can catch the virus and have it sitting about like most of the other people but you have something else which together with it brings on the tumor. If that is the case, then the information isn't going to help one way or the other. I am not saying that the information shouldn't be got, but it must be borne in mind that there are two possible situations that we can imagine, there are possibly more, but there are at least two.

DR. W. HENLE: Well, I think we all pretty well agree that if the EB virus is involved in Burkitt's lymphoma, it doesn't go the whole way by itself and that another factor must be present at the same time. And so, you remember, one point will be, is EB virus etiologically involved with any other factor? This I think you can learn from the prospective study if you could detect it in the ten or so cases of Burkitt's lymphoma that might affect a group of ten thousand children. If you know that all of them a year or two years ago had no antibodies to EBV then we know they have developed lesions from infection. This will be one of the two possibilities. The other possibility would be that the children developing the tumor had a high antibody level one or two years before. If we find that there is a group of children in East Africa who have high antibody levels—persistently high antibody levels—perhaps indicating a high level of persisting infection, this itself may set the stage for the other hypothetical factor to convert it into a tumor. Of course, there is a third possibility that is unrelated to any antibody level and virus. But somehow we have two possibilities out of three. There is another thing, which I think is mentioned in the paper I am giving tomorrow. There has been one case recently published of a girl in California who was diagnosed with two ovarian Burkitt type tumors sixteen months after the onset of infectious mononucleosis. It was quite clear that the transformation must have occurred many months ahead of the diagnosis of the tumor, and so we come very close to the point of the relation between infection and transformation. Of course, we probably can say that it is equally true that this is entirely coincidental and, therefore, unrelated. It is a matter of looking for more cases like that, and if there should be a number found, in time I think we will get more confidence in the possible relationships. I think this is the direction to look in.

DR. HIRAYAMA: I think both the vaccination program and the follow-up study are necessary and, if possible, I would like the two projects to be discussed simultaneously. Dr. Henle pointed out that there are insurmountable problems but I think they are surmountable problems. Dr. Epstein said that in case of lung cancer prevention to cut down cigarette smoking is the best method. Well, this has already been shown, as he said, in England, but in this particular case what you should really do is to reduce the causative factor or agent in cigarette smoke, and data have already shown that filter cigarette smokers carry lower risk of lung cancer compared to smokers of the same number of unfiltered cigarettes. I think in order to move into the vaccination program we should have a definite program to clarify necessary points, as Dr. Rauscher pointed out. For instance, what kind of antigens should be used as a marker to show successful immunization? We should try to get such indices before we rule out that kind of program. But anyhow, we cannot wait for 30 years and if we wish to do something, we should do two programs simultaneously.

DR. RAUSCHER: I agree.

DR. ITO: I hate to push the discussion back. If you look into the program we will have plenty of time for EBV tomorrow and the day after tomorrow, so anyone who wants to can comment on some of the general concepts of the problem. If I may be allowed to bring up one point, Dr. Rauscher referred to chemical carcinogenesis versus viral carcinogenesis, and I see in the hall quite a few people who have been for many years working on chemical and also on viral carcinogenesis. May I hear some comments from the floor from the chemical carcinogenesis side? Dr. Nakahara.

DR. NAKAHARA: You know there are some hard-boiled pathologists who doubt the neoplastic nature of the virus tumor. Some people distinguish between virus tumors and real autonomous growth. Now, from that point of view, it is gratifying to see that in the first slide, Dr. Rauscher had recognized three types of carcinogens. That is, viral, chemical, and physical. And I think one way to look at things may be to consider the three categories of carcinogens on an equal footing. So you may catch a virus and you may remain free from tumor for the rest of your life, unless something happens, some carcinogenic agent in the form of a chemical substance or physical radiation affects you, added to what you got in the form of the virus. Virus plus something else may precipitate the formation of tumor. It might be, of course, that this is far from attacking the human tumor problem directly, but still, theoretically at least, it should be or could be supplying useful information of importance for the elucidation of our knowledge of the carcinogenic mechanism in general.

DR. ITO: Thank you very much, Dr. Nakahara. Dr. Ho?

DR. HO: I just want to add one more factor, that is, the human soil. It might be that the human soil also plays a part in addition to the three others which have been mentioned.

DR. RAUSCHER: You are quite right; I should have mentioned that in human carcinogenesis, human soil must admittedly be very important.

DR. SOUTHAM: May I direct a question to Dr. Henle?   After getting infectious mononucleosis, how many ultimately developed Burkitt's lymphoma?   I don't think it would be difficult to find out.

DR. W. HENLE: I didn't quite get the last point of your question.

DR. SOUTHAM: You mentioned a girl developing Burkitt's lymphoma sixteen months after infectious mononucleosis.   If you go through any pathology department, you would have data regarding a popping-out case.   And then you could chase down how many of them developed Burkitt's lymphoma afterwards.

DR. W. HENLE: Well, those data are not available, but I think that you might know that the army has good records of infectious mononucleosis.   This, of course, is not quite true; it is only the air force.   But one could probably find out what is the incidence of any type of malignancy among these men.

DR. RAUSCHER: If I might comment, this has been done and there is no apparent difference.   There is one other study which I think is fascinating.   The National Cancer Institute has a large program in the State of Connecticut in the United States, Connecticut being one of the only states that has the type of cancer registry from which you can get these kind of data.   It was reported first at the Houston meeting, and we are now getting follow-up information.

ADVANCES IN MOLECULAR VIROLOGY

Chairmen:

M. A. Epstein, Tadashi Yamamoto

Molecular and Submolecular Programming of Viral Oncogenesis

Maurice GREEN, Makoto ROKUTANDA, Kei FUJINAGA, Hinae ROKUTANDA, Corrado GURGO, Ranjit K. RAY, and J. Thomas PARSONS

Institute for Molecular Virology, St. Louis University, School of Medicine, St. Louis, Missouri, U.S.A.

Oncogenic DNA and RNA viruses provide some of the most promising experimental systems for analyzing the molecular mechanisms of neoplasia and growth control in mammalian cells and for evaluating the role of viruses in human cancer. Below we summarize our present understanding of the chemistry of oncogenic viruses, their mechanism of replication and of cell transformation, and discuss in detail some of our recent studies on RNA tumor viruses. Oncogenic DNA viruses will be briefly discussed and described more fully by Dr. Kei Fujinaga in his presentation on the transcription of viral and cellular genes in adenovirus transformed cells. The application of our knowledge of oncogenic viruses to the study of the role of viruses in human cancer will be also briefly presented.

The known oncogenic viruses listed in Table 1 are divided into DNA viruses, *i.e.*, those which contain DNA as a genome, and RNA viruses, *i.e.*, those which contain RNA as a genome (*15*). The DNA viruses studied in most detail, the polyoma and adenovirus groups, have provided much recent information that promises to elucidate the basic mechanism of cell transformation. The polyoma and adenovirus groups have not been shown to induce tumors in their natural hosts but several members of the herpes virus group, including those associated with Burkitt's lymphoma, Marek's disease, and Lucké carcinoma, most likely cause neoplasms in their natural host, as discussed in detail in this symposium. Unfortunately the herpes viruses associated with cancer have not been well studied with regard to their chemistry and the biochemical mechanism of virus replication and cell transformation.

The RNA tumor viruses include the avian and murine leukemia-sarcoma viruses, the murine mammary tumor viruses, and several recently discovered leukemia-sarcoma viruses of the cat, rat, hamster, and guinea pig. Until recently little bio-

Present Addresses: Institute for Virus Research, Kyoto University, Kyoto, Japan [M.R., H.R.]; On leave from Aichi Cancer Center Research Institute, Nagoya, Japan [K.F.]; Institut für Molekularbiologie, Universität Zurich, Switzerland [T.P.]

TABLE 1. Oncogenic Viruses

I. DNA Viruses (about 50 different viruses)
  A. Papilloma virus group
     Papilloma viruses of rabbit, man, dog, cows, and others
  B. Polyoma virus group
     1. Polyoma virus (murine) (Py)
     2. SV40 virus (simian)
  C. Adenoviruses
     1. Human adenoviruses—31 members; 12 members (at least) induce tumors in newborn animals and/or transform cells *in vitro*
     2. Simian adenoviruses (6 viruses)
     3. Avian adenoviruses (2 viruses)
     4. Bovine adenovirus
  D. Herpes viruses
     1. Burkitt's lymphoma[a] (human)
     2. Lucké carcinoma[a] (frog)
     3. Marek's disease[a] (chicken)
II. RNA Viruses (about 100)
  A. Avian leukemia-sarcoma viruses (20 or more viruses)
  B. Murine leukemia-sarcoma viruses (several hundred isolates have been reported but the number of different types is not well established.
  C. Murine mammary tumor virus (3 types)
  D. Leukemia-sarcoma viruses of cat, hamster, rat, and guinea pig.

---

[a] Recent evidence, not yet conclusive, associates these diseases with new members of the herpes virus group. Taken from Green (*15*).

TABLE 2. RNA Leukemia-Sarcoma Viruses—Current Biochemical Knowledge (1970)

A. Chemistry of virion, poorly understood.
  1. *Structure*, particles 100 mμ in diameter with the viral RNA-containing nucleoid enclosed within several envelopes.
  2. *Viral genome*, 70S RNA of unknown size and configuration—irreversibly denatured to 36S RNA species.
  3. *Protein components*, 3 to 8 polypeptides by polyacrylamide gel electrophoresis of the disrupted virion
B. DNA replication, Unique requirement early after infection both for virus replication and for cell transformation. Probable explanation is RNA dependent DNA polymerase of virion which copies viral RNA to DNA.
C. RNA transcription, Uniquely required at all times after infection. Probable explanation is transcription of viral DNA to progeny viral RNA.
D. Mechanism of synthesis of viral RNA, unknown.
  1. Viral 70S RNA not detected in cells replicating RNA tumor viruses. Probable explanation is that intracellular RNA is present in a different size species.
  2. Possible presence of complementary viral RNA($-$) not yet established.
E. Cellular DNA contains large amount of base sequences and functions of unknown nature which hybridize with viral RNA. Possible explanations are:
  1. Viral genetic information is part of the normal cellular genome and possibly its expression is involved in cancer (Huebner's hypothesis)?
  2. Cellular DNA plays an active role in virus replication?
  3. Certain redundant cell DNA sequences also occur by chance in viral RNA?

---

chemical information was available on RNA tumor virus structure, replication, and cell transformation (15). But the exciting studies of the past six months on the RNA-dependent DNA polymerase of these RNA tumor viruses have changed our understanding of these viruses. The present knowledge and major problems of RNA tumor viruses are listed in Table 2 and briefly summarized here.

(a) The structure of the virus-specific 70S RNA genome and the polypeptide components of the virion are poorly understood.

(b) DNA synthesis is required early after infection both for virus replication and cell transformation, a requirement not exhibited by other RNA animal and bacterial viruses.

(c) Actinomycin D inhibits RNA tumor virus replication at all times after infection but not that of other RNA-containing animal viruses and bacteriophages, suggesting the continuous requirement for RNA transcription. Both (b) and (c) can be explained by the recently discovered enzyme of RNA tumor viruses, the RNA-dependent DNA polymerase which utilizes endogenous viral RNA as a template (1, 16, 20, 33, 36) and synthesizes DNA sequences complementary to those of viral RNA (31, 33).

(d) The mechanism of synthesis of viral RNA is unknown. RNA complementary to viral RNA has been reported to be present in the nucleus of rat cells transformed by the Moloney sarcoma virus (4), suggesting that viral RNA is made in much the same way as is viral RNA in other RNA animal viruses and RNA bacteriophage, i.e., complementary viral RNA minus strands (−) are copied on a viral RNA template (+). However, the discovery of an RNA-dependent DNA polymerase changes the options and suggests that viral RNA is probably made on a viral DNA template.

(e) Mammalian cells possess DNA base sequences which hybridize with the RNA of leukemia and sarcoma viruses, an observation reported initially by Harel et al. (18) and subsequently by others [see (15) and (29)]. Whether cells transformed by RNA tumor viruses possess more sequences complementary to viral RNA than do normal cells has not yet been established. Up to 20,000 DNA gene copies per cell complementary to murine sarcoma virus RNA have been detected in several mammalian cells (29). But the significance of these observations is not clear and several possible interpretations are listed in Table 2.

RNA Tumor Virus DNA Polymerase Activities—Mechanism of Action and Possible Functions

Ten RNA tumor viruses including the murine leukemia virus (MLV), murine sarcoma virus (MSV), Rous sarcoma virus (RSV), Rous-associated virus (RAV), mammary tumor virus (MTV), avian myeloblastosis virus (AMV), feline leukemia virus (FLV), feline sarcoma virus (FSV), hamster leukemia virus and the viper C-type particle have been reported recently to possess RNA-dependent DNA polymerase activity. In addition to these endogenous RNA dependent DNA polymerase activities, MSV, RSV, AMV, and MTV also have been shown to possess DNA-dependent DNA polymerase activity (10, 26, 34) demonstrated by the stimulated incorporation of deoxynucleoside triphosphates into an acid-insoluble form in the

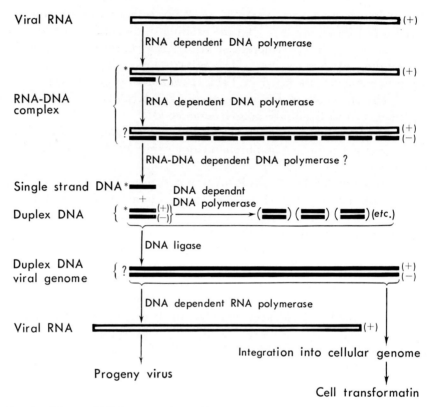

FIG. 1.   Scheme of RNA tumor virus DNA polymerase activities and possible functions of DNA product.   *Intermediate isolated.

presence of added template DNA.   In most cases, only fragmentary data have been reported on the kinetics of DNA synthesis and the properties of the DNA intermediates and products.   To compare in detail the viral enzyme of three widely different animal species we studied the DNA polymerase of FSV, AMV, and MSV under the same experimental conditions.   Before presenting these results, we briefly describe below the present stage of knowledge of the mechanism of DNA synthesis by RNA tumor viruses and the role of the reversibly transcribed viral DNA in virus replication and in cell transformation (Fig. 1).   The initial product of the viral enzyme is a RNA-DNA hybrid consisting of 70S viral RNA $(+)$ complexed with a small DNA strand $(-)$ of approximate molecular weight 150,000 daltons.   Subsequently single- and double-stranded DNA molecules of the same molecular length are generated free of a viral RNA template.   Duesberg reports (personal communication) that most of the RSV RNA genome copies DNA and, similarly, we have found that at least 85% of MSV RNA copies DNA *in vitro*.   Although the further fate of the viral DNA fragments is not known, possibly they are joined end to end to form a duplex DNA copy of the entire RNA viral genome.   The entire viral DNA genome may be incorporated into the cell chromosome providing integrated viral genetic information for cell transformation.   Also the viral DNA genome may be transcribed to viral RNA progeny for the replication of both leukemia and sarcoma viruses.

Properties of MSV, AMV, and FSV DNA Polymerase

The DNA polymerase activities of purified MSV, AMV, and FSV are similar in their requirements for all four deoxyribonucleoside triphosphates, Mg^{2+} or Mn^{2+}, and for activation by nonionic detergents. The initial MSV DNA product is an

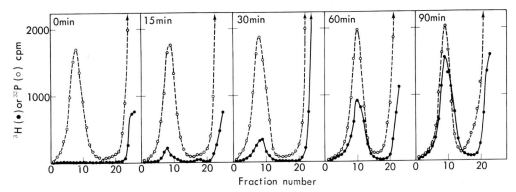

Fig. 2. Zone sedimentation of the product of the MSV DNA polymerase reaction with ^{32}P-labeled MSV(M) and ^{3}H-labeled DNA product.

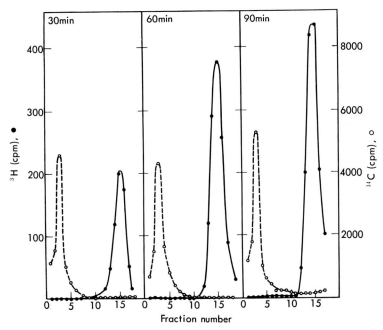

Fig. 3. Zone sedimentation of ^{3}H-DNA from RNA-^{3}H-DNA hybrids in alkaline sucrose density gradients.

RNA-DNA hybrid detected as ³H-DNA which co-sediments with viral ³²P-RNA in pre labeled virus after 30, 60, and 90 min of DNA synthesis (Fig. 2).   MSV ³H-DNA isolated from RNA-DNA hybrids sediments in alkaline sucrose gradients at 5–7S (based on the 34S adenovirus DNA marker), corresponding to a molecular weight of about 150,000 daltons (Fig. 3).

Careful kinetic analysis of DNA synthesis at early times by AMV and FSV polymerase shows several similarities.   ³H-dTTP (deoxythimidine triphosphate) incorporation appears to be biphasic—an initial rapid rate for about 4 min followed by a slower rate, reaching a plateau at about 20 to 60 min (Fig. 4, *e.g.* AMV).   DNA-RNA hybrids are detected within 30 sec as shown by equilibrium centrifugation in Cs_2SO_4 density gradients (*i.e.*, ³H-DNA is shifted to the position of the RNA marker).   Free DNA is formed subsequently (³H-DNA at densities slightly higher than that of the adenovirus DNA marker) (Fig. 5), and most of the four min and later DNA product consists of DNA free of RNA template.   In the AMV and

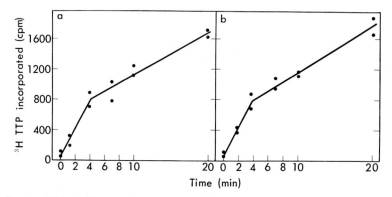

FIG. 4.   Biphasic kinetics in the AMV DNA polymerase reaction.

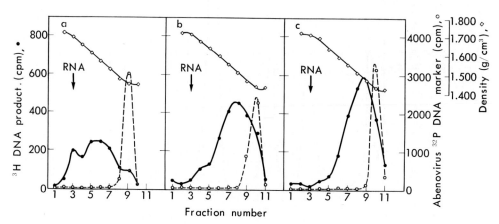

FIG. 5.   Equilibrium sedimentation of AMV DNA in Cs_2SO_4 density gradients.   a, expt. 1 (30 sec); b, expt. 1 (7 min); c, expt. (60 min).

FSV DNA polymerase reaction, the RNA-DNA hybrid is rapidly converted to free DNA. But MSV DNA polymerase forms mainly a DNA-RNA hybrid, probably reflecting differences either in the preparation of the enzyme or the degree of disruption of the virion by detergent. The kinetics of early DNA synthesis have not been reported in detail for other RNA tumor viruses.

The MSV, AMV, and FSV DNA products formed from 30 sec to 60 min after the initiation of DNA synthesis sediment in alkaline sucrose gradients with S values of 5–7S, corresponding to a molecular weight of approximately 150,000 daltons (9, 10, 31). The rate of chain growth, estimated from the 30 sec S value, is 10–20 nucleotides per sec, similar to the rate of DNA replication of mammalian cells *in vivo* (22).

The formation of short DNA fragments suggests that the mechanism of DNA polymerase may involve the recognition of multiple initiation and termination signals at discrete sites on viral RNA. If viral DNA fragments are assembled to larger molecules within the cell, other factors such as cellular, viral, or virus-induced ligase enzymes must be involved.

The denatured MSV, AMV, and FSV DNA products form very broad bands in CsCl density gradients, reflecting their small size and expected heterogeneity in base composition since DNA fragments are copied from different portions of viral RNA (14). The average buoyant density of the denatured MSV DNA product is 1.735, AMV is 1.721, and FSV is 1.725, consistent with the product of the viral polymerase being DNA.

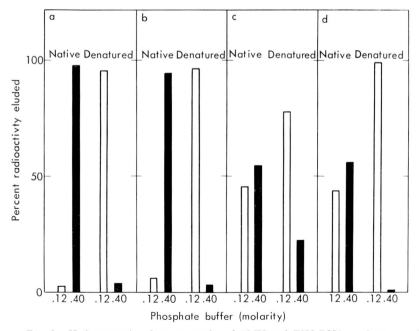

FIG. 6. Hydroxyapatite chromatography of AMV and FSV DNA products. a, adenovirus DNA; b, adenovirus-transformed cell DNA; c, avian myeloblastosis virus DNA (60 min); d, feline sarcoma DNA (60 min).

The relative amount of single-stranded and duplex DNA molecules in the AMV and FSV DNA products, formed late after the beginning of DNA synthesis, was analyzed by hydroxyapatite chromatography (Fig. 6). Control experiments utilizing adenovirus and transformed cell ^{3}H-DNA show that 0.12 M phosphate buffer (PB) eluted 98% of single-stranded DNA and less than 2% of duplex DNA, while 0.4 M PB eluted 98% of duplex DNA and 2% of single-stranded DNA (Fig. 6). Since 45% of the native FSV ^{3}H-DNA elutes with 0.12 M PB and 55% with 0.4 M PB (Fig. 6), we conclude that 55% of the FSV DNA product is duplex. The FSV DNA product, after denaturation, is eluted quantitatively by 0.12 M PB as expected of single-stranded DNA. These results agree with the studies with exonuclease III, an enzyme which degrades single-stranded DNA from the 3′–OH end (9, 10). The AMV DNA product also contains about 50% duplex structures, but, unexpectedly, about one-third of the DNA product retains duplex properties even after denaturation (Fig. 6), suggesting that some of the AMV DNA product may be selfcomplementary, possessing a hairpin structure. In contrast, RSV DNA polymerase was reported to synthesize only duplex DNA (12). Whether single-stranded DNA is a true intermediate or the result of nuclease action on the RNA-DNA hybrid is not known.

Specific Inhibitors of the RNA- and DNA-dependent Polymerase Activities of RNA Tumor Viruses

Compounds which block the RNA-dependent DNA polymerase of the leukemia-sarcoma viruses can help analyze its possible role in neoplasia and also might be useful for therapy of leukemia and cancer. We have found that the RNA-dependent DNA polymerase of RNA tumor viruses is inhibited specifically by several rifampicin derivatives with modified aminopiperazine side chains, including 4-N-demethyl rifampicin, 2,5-dimethyl-4-N-benzyl demethyl rifampicin (AF/ABDMP), 4-N-benzyl demethyl rifampicin (AF/ABP) but not by several aminopiperazines (Fig. 7). Rifampicin derivatives, prepared by condensing 3-formyl rifampicin SV (AF) with the appropriate aminopiperazines, were supplied by Gruppo Lepetit, Milano, Italy. Rifampicin drugs inhibit bacterial and mitochondrial RNA polymerase and also the replication of poxviruses (3, 21, 25, 27, 28, 35, 38), adenovirus (35), and focus formation by RSV (6). Rifampicin inhibits vaccinia virus by blocking the cleavage of a polypeptide precursor of an internal protein of vaccinia virus (24), not by its effect on an RNA polymerase.

As shown in Fig. 8, 400 μg/ml of rifampicin has no effect on the MSV DNA polymerase, but 50–100 μg/ml of AF/ABDMP, AF/ABP, and demethyl rifampicin inhibits MSV DNA polymerase over 50%. The most effective inhibitor is AF/ABDMP which at 100 μg/ml reproducibly inhibits dTTP incorporation into DNA 95% to 100%. The aminopiperazines AP4, AP5, and AP8, shown by Thiry and Lancini (37) to inhibit vaccinia virus and herpes virus, did not inhibit MSV DNA polymerase.

AF/ABDMP (Fig. 9) and AF/ABP block DNA polymerase activity, not only of MSV, but also of FLV and AMV. These findings indicate that the DNA poly-

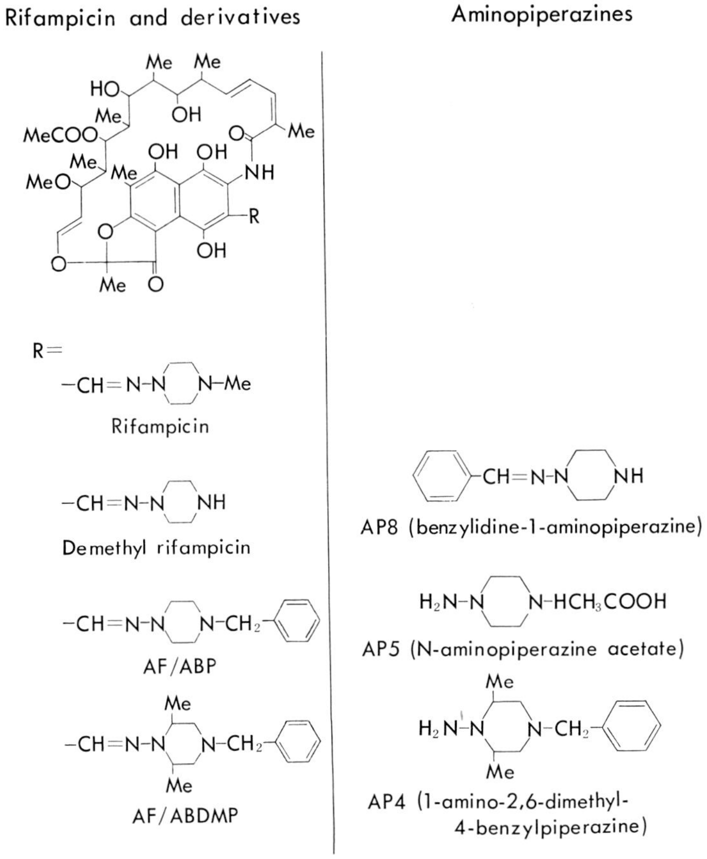

Rifampicin and derivatives   Aminopiperazines

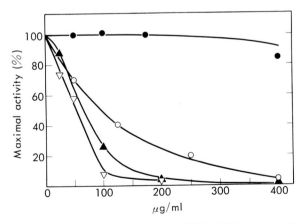

FIG. 7.   Structure of rifampicin and derivatives.

FIG. 8.   Effect of AF/ABDMP, AF/ABP, N-demethyl rifampicin, and rifampicin on the MSV DNA polymerase reaction.   ●, rifampicin; ○, N-demethyl rifampicin; ▲, AF/ABP; △, AF/ABDMP.

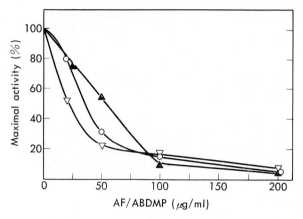

Fig. 9.   Inhibition of MSV, FLV, and AMV DNA polymerase by AF/ABDMP.   ▲, MSV; ○, FeLV; △, AMV.

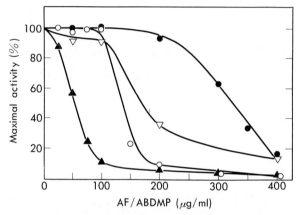

Fig. 10.   Effect of AF/ABDMP on the RNA- and DNA-dependent DNA-polymerase activities of MSV, the *E. coli* DNA polymerase, and the KB cell DNA polymerase.   ●, KB cell DNA polymerase; △, *E. coli* DNA polymerase; ○, MSV DNA polymerase+native DNA; ▲, MSV DNA polymelase.

merase of at least three RNA tumor viruses possesses common structural features recognized by certain rifampicin derivatives.

Most interesting, levels of AF/ABDMP that inhibit MSV RNA-dependent DNA polymerase activity (endogenous activity) over 90% show little inhibition of the DNA polymerase of the KB cell (established human cell line), *Escherichia coli* (Fig. 10), and MSV (Fig. 10, +native DNA), although higher levels of AF/ABDMP will inhibit these enzyme activities.

Actionomycin D (Act D) is known to block transcription by the DNA-dependent RNA polymerase by binding to the duplex DNA template.   High levels of Act D block also the DNA polymerase of KB cell and *E. coli* DNA over 90% (Fig. 11), most likely by binding to the denatured DNA template, but inhibit the MSV DNA polymerase (endogenous RNA template) a maximum of only 50–70%.   Evidence that Act D inhibits the MSV DNA-dependent DNA polymerase while AF/ABDMP

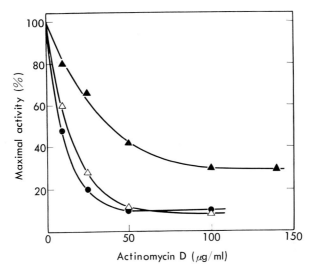

F$_{IG}$. 11.   Effect of Actinomycin D on the MSV, KB cell, and *E. coli* DNA polymerase.   ▲, MSV DNA polymerase;   △, KB cell DNA polymerase;   ●, *E. coli* DNA polymerase.

TABLE 3.   Effect of Actionomycin D and AF/ABDMP on MSV RNA- and DNA-dependent Polymerase Activities

Treatment	^{3}H-TTP incorporated (cpm)[a]	
	− DNA	+ DNA
None	12,300	89,400
+Act D (100 μg/ml)	5,670	8,600
+AF/ABDMP (100 μg/ml)	1,900	113,000
+Act D+AF/ABDMP	1,300	9,300

[a] Average of duplicate enzyme assays.

(at 100 μg/ml) inhibits the MSV RNA-dependent DNA polymerase activity is given in Table 3.   In the absence of added template (column 1, Table 3), Act D inhibits MSV DNA polymerase activity only 50%, while AF/ABDMP inhibits 90%. But when template DNA is present (column 2, Table 3), Act D inhibited 90%, while AF/ABDMP has no inhibitory activity.

In conclusion, the two DNA polymerase activities of RNA tumor viruses can be inhibited independently.   Rifampicin itself has no anti-polymerase activity but the removal of the 4-methyl group on the aminopiperazine side chain or its substitution by a benzyl group produces an effective inhibitor.   The macrocyclic ring of rifampicin is required for anti-polymerase activity.   Perhaps further modification of the aminopiperazine side chain or the macrocyclic ring will provide a more potent inhibitor of RNA tumor virus polymerase.   Based on the studies with bacterial RNA polymerase one expects a direct interaction between viral DNA polymerase and rifampicin derivatives (*7, 13, 19, 32*).   Our preliminary results indicate that this is so (*17*).   The inhibition of viral polymerase by molecules that interact with bacterial polymerase is both exciting and reassuring, for it shows that basic findings on the molecular biology of normal and virus infected cells do provide the basis for understanding the mechanism of animal virus infection and carcinogenesis and for developing a rational chemotherapy.

Detection, Localization, and Quantitation of Virus-specific RNA in MSV-transformed Cells

Attempts to detect the 70S viral RNA in cells replicating RNA tumor viruses have been mainly unsuccessful (2, 15, 30), suggesting that less than 0.01% of the cell's RNA is of viral origin, perhaps resulting from the rapid incorporation of viral RNA into virions which are released rapidly into the medium. But we show below that MSV-transformed rat and mouse cells contain large quantities of virus-specific RNA detected readily by hybridization with the ³H-DNA product of MSV DNA polymerase. Furthermore, MSV hamster cells cryptically transformed by MSV, which contain no detectable virus, do synthesize virus-specific RNA.

Highly radioactive MSV ³H-DNA, prepared by incorporation of ³H-TTP into purified MSV, was annealed with RNA isolated from the nucleus and cytoplasm (S30 fraction) of virus-producing MSV(M)-transformed rat cells and MSV(H)-transformed mouse cells. DNA-RNA hybrid formation was measured both by

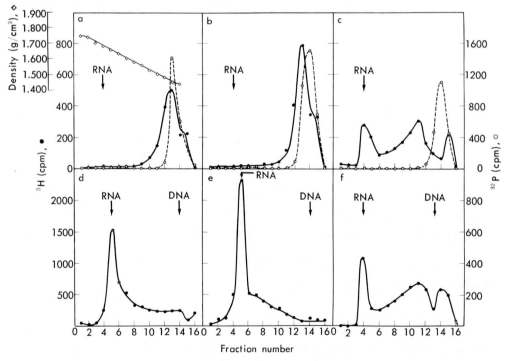

FIG. 12.   Detection of viral RNA in MSV transformed cell nuclei by hybrid formation with MSV ³H-DNA product. a, KB cells (50 μg); b, adenovirus-type 2-transformed rat cells (50 μg); c, MSV(H)-transformed mouse cells (2 μg, treated with NP 40); d, MSV(H)-transformed mouse cells (50 μg); e, MSV(M)-transformed rat cells (50 μg); f, MSV(H)-transformed mouse cells (2 μg, treated with DOC+tween 40). ○, adenovirus ³²P-DNA; ●, ³H-MSV(H) DNA.

sedimentation in Cs_2SO_4 density gradients and by hydroxyapatite chromatography. As shown in Fig. 12, annealing MSV ³H-DNA with 50 μg of RNA from the nucleus of MSV(H) or MSV(M) transformed cells converts most of the RNA to an RNA-DNA hybrid, as shown by the shift of ³H-DNA to the RNA regions of the gradient. RNA from KB cells or adenovirus-type 2-transformed rat cells did not hybridize with MSV ³H-DNA.

The amount of viral RNA in the cell can be estimated quantitatively by hydroxyapatite chromatography as shown in Fig. 13.   A constant amount of the MSV ³H-DNA product was annealed with increasing amounts of cell RNA or viral RNA. Unhybridized ³H-DNA product is eluted with 0.12 M phosphate buffer (PB) and the hybrid is eluted with 0.4 M PB.   Annealing 0.01 to 0.04 μg of viral RNA with ³H-DNA yielded 10 to 40% hybrid (Table 4, Fig. 13) and provides a standard for evaluating the relationship between the viral RNA content and degree of hybrid formation.   From these calibrations and the data in Table 4 on the per cent hybrid formation with different amounts of nuclear and cytoplasmic RNA from MSV(M)-transformed rat cells annealed with MSV ³H-DNA, we estimate that nuclear and cytoplasmic RNA contain 5 and 1% virus-specific RNA sequences, respectively. But since the cytoplasm contains 10–20 times more RNA than the nucleus (14), the total amount of virus-specific RNA in the cytoplasm is about twice that of the cytoplasm.

It was of interest to determine whether hamster tumor cells cryptically transformed by MSV [hamster (MSV)], i.e., synthesizing neither infectious virus nor gs antigen (23), contain virus-specific RNA.   As shown in Table 5, viral RNA is

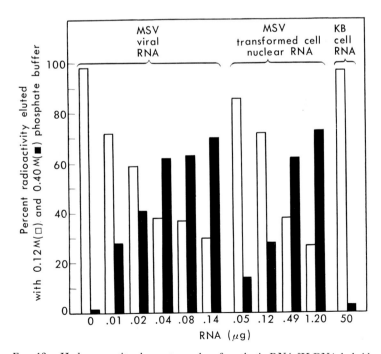

Fig. 13.   Hydroxyapatite chromatography of synthetic RNA-³H-DNA hybrids.

TABLE 4. Hybrid Formation between MSV(H) ³H-DNA and RNA from MSV(M)-transformed Rat Cells (78A1)

Source of RNA	Amount μg	Hybrid Formation			
		Hydroxyapatite		Cesium sulfate	
		cpm recovered	% RNA-DNA hybrid	cpm recovered	% RNA-DNA hybrid
Nuclei	50			4646	73
	10	1447	68	3939	62
	5	1496	53	2801	57
	0.94	1740	70	1293	45
	0.20	1716	34	1744	20
	0.19	2766	22		
	0.20	2659	26		
	0.10	2014	13		
Cytoplasm (S30)	50			4539	63
	10	1632	48	2942	33
	5	1455	32	3486	24
	1.02	1784	30	1236	17
	0.5	1763	16	978	16
	0.5	1008	16		

TABLE 5. Hybrid Formation between MSV(H) ³H-DNA and RNA from Cryptic Hamster (MSV) Cell Line

Source of RNA	Amount μg	% RNA-DNA hybrid
Nuclei	2	5
	5	16
	10	32
Nuclei (detergent washed)	2	12
	5	26
Nuclear detergent wash	7.8	14
	19.6	31
Cytoplasm (S30)	2.4	3
	6.1	7
	12.2	13
	24.4	15

detected in the nucleus and cytoplasm.   But much larger amounts of cell RNA from hamster (MSV) are required to form hybrids.   From the data in Fig. 13 and Table 5, we estimate that hamster (MSV) contains about 1/50th to 1/100th as much virus-specific RNA as does the MSV(M)- and MSV(H)-transformed rat and mouse cell lines which replicate virus.   Further studies will determine whether RNA(+) or RNA(−) are formed in transformed cells and whether all viral genome sequences are present.

RNA-dependent DNA Polymerase Activity in Human Neoplasia

The properties of the RNA-dependent DNA polymerase of RNA tumor viruses has suggested studies on the role of this enzyme in human disease.   Gallo *et al.* (*11*) and Spiegelman *et al.* (personal communication) have detected DNA polymerase activity in human leukemia cells which is stimulated by liver RNA or by a synthetic RNA-DNA hybrid.   However, further studies are needed to substantiate these exciting reports and to determine whether these enzyme activities are unique to malignant cells.

Mechanism of Oncogenesis by DNA Tumor Viruses and Tests for Viral Gene Sequences in Human Tumors

Table 6 lists the properties of cells transformed by DNA tumor viruses, which form the basis for understanding the mechanism of oncogenesis by DNA viruses. The molecular basis for understanding oncogenesis by DNA viruses will be discussed in detail by Dr. Kei Fujinaga in the following paper.   (a) Transformed cells permanently acquire new properties and are no longer subject to normal cellular growth controls.   (b) There are multiple viral gene copies in a noninfectious state present in cells transformed by human adenovirus A, B, and C, polyoma, and SV40 virus. Although the entire viral genome is present in some SV40 transformed cells, as demonstrated by the rescue of infectious virus after fusion with permissive cells, similar experiments have failed to rescue virus in cells transformed by polyoma and adenoviruses.   (c) Cells transformed by at least five different classes of oncogenic DNA viruses, including polyoma, SV40, and the three human adenovirus groups, transcribe viral RNA sequences.   Although viral genes are transcribed more frequently than the average cellular gene, only specific viral gene sequences are synthesized and the nature of the transcriptional controls is unknown.   (d) Some virus-specific RNA sequences most likely form a code for viral protein(s) which regulate the growth of the transformed cell, but the major unsolved problem is the nature and function of these viral coded proteins.   Only two new proteins are known, the T antigen and the transplantation antigen, but their role, if any, in cell transformation is not known.   It seems likely that these or other viral proteins function somehow in the synthesis and regulation of cellular macromolecules.   But, unfortunately, the mechanism of DNA replication and RNA transcription and translation in mammalian cells is poorly understood and we extrapolate mainly from studies on bacteria and bacteriophage.   Thus a satisfactory explanation of the mechanism of oncogenesis by DNA viruses in molecular terms will require further studies on the synthesis and regulation of macromolecules in mammalian cells.   But we may be optimistic since

TABLE 6.   Characteristics of Cells Transformed by DNA Viruses

1.   Hereditary change in morphology, physiology, and antigenic composition.
2.   Multiple copies of viral genes.
3.   Synthesis of virus-specific mRNA.
    a.   Transcription of viral genes in preference to cellular genes.
    b.   Selective transcription of certain viral genes.
4.   Presence of nuclear virus-specific T antigen(s).
5.   Presence of cell surface virus-specific transplantation antigen(s).

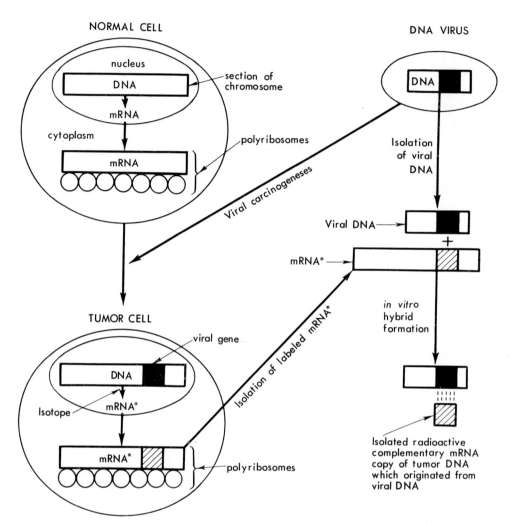

FIG. 14. Tests for viral genes in cancer cells. This scheme depicts the incorporation of viral genes in cells neoplastically transformed by virus infection. Viral mRNA synthesized in the cell nucleus is subsequently transported to the cytoplasm to form viral polyribosomes. Transformed cells are grown in media containing radioactive precursors of RNA and labeled RNA is isolated from the nucleus and polyribosomes and annealed with viral DNA. The formation of viral DNA-labeled RNA hybrids provides direct evidence for the presence of functioning viral genes in the cancer cell.

only several viral gene functions are involved in cells transformed by oncogenic DNA viruses.

The transcription of viral genes in cells transformed by ten human adenoviruses has suggested a method for testing adenoviruses as etiological agents of human cancer, namely the annealing of human cancer RNA with adenovirus DNA to detect the possible presence of viral RNA sequences (Fig. 14). This procedure has successfully detected virus-specific RNA in primary hamster tumors induced by human

TABLE 7. Hybridization-inhibition Test for Viral Genetic Information in Human Cancer

Step 1

Viral DNA+human cancer RNA $\xrightarrow[20\ hr]{66°C}$ DNA-RNA hybrid

Step 2

+virus-specific RNA[a] $\xrightarrow[20\ hr]{66°C}$ DNA-RNA hybrid[a]

[a] Radioactive molecules. Positive reaction, inhibition of radioactive hybrid formation. Negative reaction, no inhibition of radioactive hybrid formation.

adenoviruses (8) and virus-specific RNA in virus-free Lucké summer frog tumors (5). Unfortunately, the direct hybridization of labeled RNA from human tumors with viral DNA is not feasible because human tissues do not incorporate ³H-uridine adequately *in vitro*. Therefore we have developed a sensitive two-step DNA-RNA hybridization-inhibition test (Table 7) which utilizes unlabeled human cancer RNA. In step 1, 0.1 μg of adenovirus DNA immobilized on a nitrocellulose membrane was annealed with 1–2 mg of RNA isolated from human cancer tissue. In step 2, the human cancer RNA was removed and viral DNA was annealed further with highly radioactive virus-specific RNA isolated from adenovirus-transformed cells. Adenovirus specific RNA sequences, if present in the human cancer RNA, should hybridize with viral DNA and block the hybridization with radioactive virus-specific RNA in step 2. Inhibition of hybridization would mean that adenovirus-specific RNA may be present in the cancer specimen. Normal infection with an adenovirus could be ruled out by characterizing the species of adenovirus-specific mRNA in the specimen.

We have tested over 200 human cancer RNA specimens by the hybridization-inhibition test and some sample data are given in Table 8. Unlabeled virus-specific RNA, the positive control in all hybridization-inhibition tests, inhibited hybridization to 20–30% of the control value. The human cancer RNA specimens did not reduce the levels to below 70% of control values. Table 9 lists the numbers of human tumors by organs thus far analyzed with negative results for RNA specific for adenovirus types 2, 7, and 12, members of groups C, B, and A, respectively. Since members within each group share base sequences, our tests include the 13 human adenoviruses of groups A, B, and C.

These negative results probably do not exclude a role for adenoviruses in human neoplasia because of the limited sensitivity of these measurements. From hybridization-saturation measurements, about 10,000 viral mRNA molecules are present in an adenovirus-transformed cell grown in culture. Our hybridization-inhibition tests may detect one-tenth this amount of virus-specific RNA, *i.e.*, about 1,000 virus-specific RNA molecules per cancer cell. But human cancers may possess far fewer virus-specific RNA molecules than do adenovirus-transformed cells in culture. We are developing a test which utilizes highly radioactive adenovirus complementary RNA made *in vitro* with the *E. coli* RNA polymerase which should be 10 to 100 times more sensitive. This may permit the detection of as little as ten

TABLE 8. Hybridization-inhibition Analysis of Human Tumor RNA for Adenovirus-specific RNA

Unlabeled RNA	Virus tested	μg competing RNA	Input cpm ×10⁶	cpm bound above background		Background cpm	Percent of control		Comments
Ad 12 RNA	Ad 12	150	1.31	81,	80	36	26,	26	Ad 12
KB RNA (control)	Ad 12	300	1.31	310,	364	31	99,	116	controls
Ad 7 RNA	Ad 7	150	5.69	50,	42	20	15,	12	Ad 7
KB RNA (control)	Ad 7	300	5.69	366,	340	19	108,	101	controls
Ad 2 RNA	Ad 2	150	5.39	91,	93	74	36,	37	Ad 2
KB RNA (control)	Ad 2	300	5.39	252,	271	65	99,	107	controls
Oral cavity,	Ad 12	150	1.31	335,	354	17	107,	113	Negative
Epid. Ca (1)	Ad 7	194	5.69	360,	316	11	106,	93	,,
	Ad 2	201	5.39	246,	269	57	97,	106	,,
Parotid	Ad 12	265	1.31	345,	323	16	110,	103	,,
(Worthim) (1)	Ad 7	234	5.69	331,	371	14	98,	109	,,
	Ad 2	301	5.39	249,	236	27	98,	93	,,
Bowel, Ca (2)	Ad 12	170	1.31	338,	318	14	108,	101	,,
	Ad 7	161	5.69	324,	320	25	96,	94	,,
	Ad 2	197	5.39	253,	276	29	99,	108	,,
Colon (2)	Ad 12	123	1.31	354,	353	23	113,	112	,,
	Ad 7	131	5.69	334,	326	8	99,	96	,,
	Ad 2	132	5.39	258,	232	47	101,	91	,,
Liver (2)	Ad 12	143	1.31	323,	291	26	103,	93	,,
	Ad 7	122	5.69	330,	346	10	97,	102	,,
	Ad 2	195	5.39	277,	275	28	109,	108	,,
Sigmoid, Ca (2)	Ad 12	255	1.31	311,	333	17	99,	106	,,
	Ad 7	272	5.69	330,	332	10	97,	98	,,
	Ad 2	300	5.39	231,	261	45	91,	103	,,
Larynx, epid.	Ad 12	523	1.31	323,	295	20	103,	94	,,
Ca (3)	Ad 7	469	5.69	353,	353	18	104,	104	,,
	Ad 2	144	5.39	237,	261	40	93,	103	,,
Breast (4)	Ad 12	188	1.31	339,	360	10	108,	114	,,
	Ad 7	180	5.69	355,	343	11	105,	101	,,
	Ad 2	205	5.39	280,	237	34	110,	93	,,
Breast, metaductal	Ad 12	123	1.31	332,	329	20	106,	105	,,
Ca (4)	Ad 7	110	5.69	352,	350	9	104,	103	,,
	Ad 2	162	5.39	242,	224	54	95,	88	,,
Prostate, adeno-	Ad 12	241	1.31	351,	354	7	116,	113	,,
sarcoma (5)	Ad 7	227	5.69	346,	294	10	102,	87	,,
	Ad 2	304	5.39	239,	260	34	94,	102	,,
Uterus (5)	Ad 12	104	1.31	312,	291	40	99,	93	,,
	Ad 7	102	5.69	358,	344	17	106,	102	,,
	Ad 2	117	5.39	232,	224	37	91,	88	,,
Brain (8)	Ad 12	157	1.31	317,	298	17	101,	95	,,
	Ad 7	163	5.69	335,	360	10	99,	106	,,
	Ad 2	192	5.39	249,	280	39	98,	110	,,

Continued . . .

TABLE 8. Hybridization-inhibition Analysis of Human Tumor RNA for Adenovirus-specific RNA

Unlabeled RNA	Virus tested	μg com-peting RNA	Input cpm ×10⁶	cpm bound above background		Back-ground cpm	Percent of control		Comments
Brain (8)	Ad 12	297	1.31	340,	355	13	108,	113	,,
	Ad 7	240	5.69	364,	342	12	107,	101	,,
	Ad 2	329	5.39	253,	229	25	99,	90	,,
Thyroid, adenoma (9)	Ad 12	240	1.31	374,	370	8	119,	118	,,
	Ad 7	223	5.69	356,	328	10	105,	97	,,
	Ad 2	245	5.39	227,	255	41	89,	100	,,
Liposarcoma (11)	Ad 12	87	1.31	267,	346	24	85,	110	,,
	Ad 7	65	5.69	320,	297	19	94,	88	,,
	Ad 2	114	5.39	235,	249	39	92,	98	,,

TABLE 9. Distribution of Tumors Tested for Adenovirus RNA by Hybridization-inhibition

Site of origin	Labeled RNA from cells transformed by:		
	Ad 12	Ad 7	Ad 2
1) Buccal cavity, pharynx, and salivary glands	11	10	11
2) Digestive organs	54	50	54
3) Respiratory system	24	22	24
4) Breast	7	7	7
5) Genital organs	23	23	23
6) Urinary organs	9	8	8
7) Skin	8	8	8
8) Brain and nervous system	15	15	15
9) Endocrine glands	12	12	12
10) Bone	0	0	0
11) Mesenchymal tissue	18	18	18
12) Lymph nodes and reticuloendothelial system	10	9	10
13) Miscellaneous	16	16	16
Total	207	198	206

virus-specific RNA molecules per cancer cell and thus detect or decisively eliminate adenoviruses as a causative agent of human cancer.

SUMMARY

Both DNA and RNA tumor viruses may transform cells as a result of the integration into cellular chromosomes of viral DNA sequences. Viral DNA sequences may be transcribed into RNA molecules coding for proteins which function to perpetuate the transformed properties of the cell. Direct evidence for this mechanism is available for DNA tumor viruses. The properties of the viral RNA and DNA-dependent polymerase activities present in RNA tumor viruses suggest that similar mechanisms operate in transformation by these viruses.

The viruses of several leukemias and sarcomas possess an enzyme thus far unique—a DNA polymerase which utilizes endogenous viral RNA as template, and synthesizes DNA sequences complementary to those of viral RNA. We have studied the RNA- and DNA-dependent DNA polymerase activities of two murine sarcoma viruses (MSV), avian myeloblastosis virus (strain BAI) (AMV), and feline sarcoma virus (FSV).   In the absence of added template the DNA polymerase of AMV and FSV exhibits two phase kinetics—an initial rapid reaction for four min followed by a slower reaction for 20–60 min.   Equilibrium sedimentation in Cs_2SO_4 density gradients show the rapid formation of RNA-DNA complexes composed of 70S RNA with small DNA strands (molecular weight 150,000), followed by the formation of DNA free of an RNA template; about half the final DNA product is double-stranded.   The denatured DNA product of the MSV, FSV, and AMV DNA polymerase sediments at 6 S, has a molecular weight of 150,000 daltons, and bands in CsCl gradients at $\rho=1.721$ to 1.735.

The RNA-dependent DNA polymerase activity of MSV, feline leukemia virus (FLV), and AMV is inhibited by several rifampicin derivatives but not by rifampicin itself, while the DNA-dependent DNA polymerase activities of these viruses is inhibited by actinomycin D.   Mammalian cell and *E. coli* DNA-dependent DNA polymerases are not inhibited by comparable amounts of rifampicin derivatives.

Molecular hybridization between the highly radioactive MSV DNA product and RNA from the nucleus and cytoplasm of MSV-transformed cells was performed to detect and quantitate viral RNA in these organelles.   A large fraction of the nuclear RNA ($\sim 5\%$) and cytoplasmic RNA ($\sim 1\%$) is virus-specific in MSV-transformed cells which replicate virus.   A much smaller fraction of RNA is virus-specific in MSV-transformed cells which are cryptic, *i.e.*, they do not replicate virus.

Molecular hybridization was used to examine over 200 human cancers for the presence of viral RNA specific for 13 oncogenic human adenoviruses.   Hybridization-competition with labeled adenovirus-specific RNA gave no evidence for functioning adenovirus genetic information in human cancers.

This investigation was supported by USPHS grant AI-01725, research contract PH43–64–928 from the National Institute of Allergy and Infectious Disease, Infectious Disease Branch, National Institutes of Health, and research contract PH43–67–692 from the National Cancer Institute, USPHS, Viral Carcinogenesis Branch, Etiology Area, National Institutes of Health, Bethesda, Maryland.   Maurice Green is a Research Career Awardee (5-K6-AI-4739), National Institutes of Health, Bethesda, Maryland, U.S.A.   J. Thomas Parsons is a postdoctoral fellow of the American Cancer Society (PF-500).

REFERENCES

1. Baltimore, D.   Viral RNA-dependent DNA Polymerase.   Nature, *226*: 1209–1211, 1970.
2. Baluda, M. A., and Nayak, D. P.   Sym.   Biology Large RNA Viruses, 1969, Cambridge, England, in press, 1970.
3. Ben-Ishai, Z., Heller, E., Goldblum, N., and Becker, Y.   Rifampicin Poxvirus and Trachoma Agent.   Nature, *224*: 29–32, 1969.
4. Biswal, N., and Benyesh-Melnick, M.   Complementary Nuclear RNA's of Murine Sarcoma-leukemia Virus Complex in Transformed Cells.   Proc. Nat. Acad. Sci. U.S. *64*: 1372–1379, 1969.

5. Collard, W., Thornton, H., Mizell, M., and Green, M. In manuscript.

6. Diggelman, H., and Weissmann, C. Rifampicin Inhibits Focus Formation in Chick Fibroblasts Infected with Rous Sarcoma Virus. Nature, *224*: 1277–1279, 1969.

7. diMauro, E., Snyder, L., Marino, P., Lamberti, A., Coppo, A., and Tocchini-Valentini, G. P. Rifampicin Sensitivity of the Components of DNA-dependent RNA Polymerase. Nature, *222*: 533–537, 1969.

8. Fujinaga, K., and Green, M. The Mechanism of Viral Carcinogenesis by DNA Mammalian Viruses. I. Viral-specific RNA in Polyribosomes of Adenovirus Tumor and Transformed Cells. Proc. Nat. Acad. Sci. U.S. *55*: 1567–1574, 1966.

9. Fujinaga, K., and Green, M. Mechanism of Carcinogenesis by RNA Tumor Viruses. V. The RNA and DNA Dependent DNA Polymerase Activities of Feline Sarcoma Virus. J. gen. Virol., in press.

10. Fujinaga, K., Parsons, J. T., Beard, J., Beard, D., and Green, M. Mechanism of Carcinogenesis by RNA Tumor Viruses. III. Formation of RNA-DNA Complex and Duplex DNA Molecules by the DNA Polymerase(s) of Avian Myeloblastosis Virus. Proc. Nat. Acad. Sci, U.S., *67*: 1432–1439, 1970.

11. Gallo, R. C., Yang, S. S. and Ting, R. C. RNA Dependent DNA Polymerase of Human Acute Leukaemic Cells. Nature, *228*: 927–929, 1970.

12. Garapin, A. C., McDonnell, J. P., Levinson, W., Quintrell, N., Fanshier, L., and Bishop, J. M. Deoxyribonucleic Acid Polymerase Associated with Rous Sarcoma Virus and Avian Myeloblastosis Virus: Properties of the Enzyme and its Product. J. Virol., *6*: 589–598, 1970.

13. Geiduschek, E. P., and Sklar, J. Continual Requirement for a Host RNA Polymerase Component in a Bacteriophage Development. Nature, *221*: 833–836, 1969.

14. Green, M. Unpublished data.

15. Green, M. Oncogenic Viruses. Ann. Rev. Biochem., *39*: 701–756, 1970.

16. Green, M., Rokutanda, M., Fujinaga, K., Ray, R. K., Rokutanda, H., and Gurgo, C. Mechanism of Carcinogenesis by RNA Tumor Viruses. I. An RNA-Dependent DNA Polymerase in Murine Sarcoma Viruses. Proc. Nat. Acad. Sci. U.S.A., *67*: 385–393, 1970.

17. Gurgo, C., Ray, R. K., and Green, M. Unpublished data.

18. Harel, L., Harel, J., Lacour, F., and Huppert, J. Cancerologie—Homologie Entre Genome du Virus de la Myeloblastose Aviaire (AMV) et Genome Cellulaire. C.R. Acad. Sci., Paris, *263*: 616–619, 1966.

19. Haselkorn, R., Vogel, M., and Brown, R. D. Conservation of the Rifampicin Sensitivity of Transcription During T4 Development. Nature, *221*, 836–838, 1969.

20. Hatanaka, M., Huebner, R. J., and Gilden, R. M. DNA Polymerase Activity Associated with RNA Tumor Viruses. Proc. Nat. Acad. Sci. U.S.A., *67*: 143–147, 1970.

21. Heller, E., Argaman, M., Levy, H., and Goldblum, N. Selective Inhibition of Vaccinia Virus by the Antibiotic Rifampicin. Nature, *222*: 273–274, 1969.

22. Huberman, J. A., and Riggs, A. D. On the Mechanism of DNA Replication in Mammalian Chromosomes. J. Mol. Biol., *32*: 327–341, 1968.

23. Huebner, R. J., Hartley, J. W., Rowe, W. P., Lane, W. T., and Capps, W. I. Rescue of the Defective Geome of Moloney Sarcoma Virus from a Noninfectious Hamster Tumor and the Production of Pseudotype Sarcoma Viruses with Various Murine Leukemia Viruses. Proc. Nat. Acad. Sci. U.S.A., *56*: 1164–1169, 1966.

24. Katz, E., and Moss, B. Formation of a Vaccinia Virus Structural Polypeptide from a Higher Molecular Weight Precursor: Inhibition by Rifampicin. Proc. Nat.

Acad. Sci. U.S.A., *66*: 677–684, 1970.

25. McAuslan, B. R. Rifampicin Inhibition of Vaccinia Replication. Biochem. Biophys. Res. Com., *37*: 289–295, 1969.

26. Mizutani, S., Boettiger, D., and Temin, H. M. A DNA-dependent DNA Polymerase and a DNA Endonuclease in Virions of Rous Sarcoma Virus. Nature, *228*: 424–427, 1970.

27. Moss, B., Rosenblum, E. N., Katz, E., and Grimley, P. M. Rifampicin: A Specific Inhibitor of Vaccinia Virus Assembly. Nature, *224*: 1280–1284, 1969.

28. Nagayama, A., Pogo, B.G.T., and Dales, S. Biogenesis of Vaccinia: Separation of Early Stages from Maturation by Means of Rifampicin. Virology, *40*: 1039–1051, 1970.

29. Rokutanda, H., Rokutanda, M., and Green, M. Unpublished data.

30. Rokutanda, M., Rokutanda, H., and Green, M., Unpublished data.

31. Rokutanda, M., Rokutanda, H., Green, M., Fujinaga, K., Ray, R. K., and Gurgo, C. Formation of Viral RNA-DNA Hybrid Molecules by the DNA Polymerase of Sarcoma-Leukemia Viruses. Nature, *227*: 1026–1028, 1970.

32. Sippel, A., and Hartmann, G. Mode of Action of Rifampicin on the RNA Polymerase Reaction. Biochem. Biophys. Acta, *157*: 218–219, 1968.

33. Spiegelman, S., Burny, A., Das, M. R., Keydar, J., Schlom, J., Travnicek, M., and Watson, K. Characterization of the Products of RNA-directed DNA Polymerases in Oncogenic RNA Viruses. Nature, *227*: 563–567, 1970.

34. Spiegelman, S., Burney, A., Das, M. R., Keydar, J., Schlom, J., Travnicek, M., and Watson, K. DNA-Directed DNA Polymerase Activity in Oncogenic RNA Viruses. Nature, *227*: 1029–1031, 1970.

35. Subak-Sharpe, J. H., Timbury, M. C., and Williams, J. F. Rifampicin Inhibits the Growth of Some Mammalian Viruses. Nature, *222*: 341–345, 1969.

36. Temin, H. M., and Mizutani, S. RNA-dependent DNA Polymerase in Virions of Rous Sarcoma Virus. Nature, *226*: 1211–1213, 1970.

37. Thiry, L., and Lancini, G. Unpublished data.

38. Zakay-Rones, Z., and Becker, Y. Anti-poxvirus Activity of Rifampicin Associated with Hydrazone Side Chain. Nature, *226*: 1162–1163, 1970.

Viral and Cellular Gene Expression in Cells Transformed by Human Adenoviruses

Kei Fujinaga, Maurice Green, Koichiro Shimada, Deane Tsuei, Kenji Sekikawa, and Yohei Ito

Aichi Cancer Center Research Institute, Nagoya, Japan [K. F., K. S., K. S., Y. I.] ; Institute for Molecular Virology, St. Louis University, St. Louis, Missouri, U.S.A. [M. G., D. T.]

The various members of the DNA-containing human adenoviruses (Ad) can productively infect cultured human cells, transform rodent cells in culture, and induce tumors in newborn rodents (*9, 13, 20*, Green, Pina, and Thornton, unpublished data), thus providing excellent systems for the study of viral oncogenesis. As shown in Table 1, oncogenic and transforming human adenoviruses can be divided into three groups: highly oncogenic group A, which includes Ad 12, 18, and

TABLE 1. Human Adenoviruses—Relationship among Viral DNA's, Oncogenicity and Transformation

Adenovirus		Oncogenicity	Viral DNA % G+C[a]	DNA-DNA homology % related
Group	Members			
A	Ad 12, 18, and 31	" Highly oncogenic "[b] in newborn hamsters	48–49	80–85[c]
B	Ad 3, 7, 11, 14, 16, and 21	" Weakly oncogenic "[b] in newborn hamsters (all but Ad 11)	49–52	70–100[d]
C	Ad 1[e], 2, 5, and 6	" Nononcogenic " in newborn hamsters but morphologically transformed rat embryo cells *in vitro*[f]	57–59	85–95[g]

[a] Pina and Green (*18*).

[b] Highly oncogenic adenoviruses induce tumors in a large proportion of newborn hamsters within two months after injection with purified virus ; " weakly oncogenic " in a small proportion after 4–18 months.

[c] Lacy and Green (*14*).

[d] Lacy and Green (*15*).

[e] Ad 1 produced tumors in newborn hamsters (Trentin, Hoosier, and Samper) (*19*).

[f] Freeman *et al.* (*1*).

[g] Fujinaga, Pina, and Green (*8*).

31; weakly oncogenic group B, which includes Ad 3, 7, 14, 16, and 21; and transforming group C, which includes Ad 1, 2, 5, and 6 (*11*).   Members of the same
group share 70–100% of their DNA base sequences while members of different
groups share 10–35% of their DNA base sequences.   Members of groups A and B
induce tumors in newborn hamsters and transform cells *in vitro*, while group C
viruses transform cells *in vitro* but do not induce tumors.   We present here studies
on the transcription of viral and cellular genes in cells transformed by members
of human adenovirus groups A, B, and C.

Transcription of Virus-specific RNA (vRAN) in Virus-free Transformed Cells

Virus-free tumor and transformed cells induced by human adenoviruses contain no infectious virus but possess functioning viral genes (*2*).   As shown in Table
2, labeled RNAs from whole cell polyribosomes, and nuclei from Ad 12-transformed
cells hybridize with Ad 12 DNA, demonstrating the presence of virus-specific mRNA
in virus-free transformed cells.   Pulse labeling experiments have shown that at least
2–5% of the labeled polyribosomal RNA is viral mRNA (*2*).

As shown in Table 3, virus-specific RNAs synthesized in cells transformed by
groups A, B, and C human adenoviruses hybridize only with DNA from members of
the same group, not with that of other groups (*2–5, 8*).   These results indicate that
three different classes of virus-specific RNAs are transcribed in adenovirus-transformed cells, one specific for group A, the second specific for group B, and the third
specific for group C.   Although viral DNAs from different groups share 10–35%

TABLE 2.   Hybridization of RNA from Polyribosomes, and Nuclei of Ad 12 Transformed Cells with Viral
DNA[a]

RNA from	Input RNA (cpm)	Ad 12 DNA μg/filter	Bound RNA (cpm)	Bound % (background not subtracted)
Polyribosomes[b]	52,400	3	146	0.28
,,		3	134	0.26
,,		None	2	0.004
Nuclei[b]	214,000	3	438	0.20
,,		3	423	0.20
,,		None	26	0.01
	42,500	3	97	0.23
,,		3	114	0.27
,,		None	12	0.03
Whole cell[b]	283,100	3	356	0.13
,,		3	406	0.14
,,		None	60	0.02
	59,600	3	113	0.19
,,		3	103	0.17
,,		None	14	0.02

[a] Fujinaga and Green (*2*).
[b] Labeled for 180 min with ^{3}H-uridine (μCi/ml).

TABLE 3. Relationship between Viral-specific RNA's in Tumor and Transformed Cells Induced by Group A, B, and C Human Adenoviruses[a]

RNA from	RNA bound (% relatedness[b])									
	RNA from tumor or tranformed cells induced by									
	Ad 12	Ad 18	Ad 31	Ad 3	Ad 7	Ad 14	Ad 16	Ad 2	Ad 5	Ad 6
Ad 12	100	29	62	15[c]	10[c]	10[c]	10[c]	10	10	20[c]
Ad 18	34	100	62	15[c]	10[c]	10[c]	10[c]	—	—	—
Ad 31	61	30	100	—	—	—	—	—	—	—
Ad 3	10	5[c]	10[c]	100	69	74	100	—	—	—
Ad 7	10[c]	5[c]	10[c]	100	100	88	81	10	10	20[c]
Ad 14	10[c]	5[c]	10[c]	100	69	100	89	—	—	—
Ad 21	10	5	10	100	78	93	92	—	—	—
Ad 1	—	—	—	—	—	—	—	102	105	110
Ad 2	10[c]	5[c]	10[c]	15[c]	10[c]	10[c]	10[c]	100	95	105
Ad 4	10[c]	5[c]	10[c]	17[c]	19	15[c]	18[c]	10[c]	10[c]	20[c]
Ad 5	—	—	—	—	—	—	—	94	100	101
Ad 6	—	—	—	—	—	—	—	100	104	100

[a] Fujinaga and Green (2–4), Fujinaga, Pina and Green (8).

[b] Average of duplicate hybridization experiments. Binding to homologous DNA was normalized to 100%.

[c] The % relatedness cannot be estimated since too few counts were bound (less than 25 cpm above that bound to a DNA-free membrane).

of their base sequences (11), the common DNA sequences are not transcribed significantly in adenovirus-transformed cells. Purified virus-specific RNA of these three different classes have similar guanine plus cytosine contents (G+C), 47–51% (5, 8). Group B virus-specific RNAs have a 2 to 5% lower G+C content, and group C virus-specific RNAs have a 7–8% lower G+C content than those of the corresponding viral DNAs. The results of both comparative hybridization experiments and base analysis of virus-specific RNAs strongly suggest that only a part of the viral genome is transcribed in adenovirus-transformed cells.

Fractions of Viral Genome Transcribed in Adenovirus-transformed Cells

The adenovirus DNA has a molecular weight of 23×10^6 daltons (12), containing sufficient information for 23 to 46 genes coding for proteins of average molecular weight 25,000 to 50,000. In cells productively infected with Ad 2 and 12, all or nearly all (80–100%) of these viral genes are transcribed (7, 17). The following results of hybridization competition experiments among " early," " late," and " transformed " virus-specific RNAs (6) were obtained using virus-specific RNA synthesized during infection as a standard for 100% viral gene transcripts (Fig. 1): (1) 8 to 20% of the viral genome (2–10 genes) is transcribed early after Ad 2 infection, before viral DNA synthesis begins at 6 hr after infection. (2) 4 to 10% of the viral genome (1–5 genes), half of the early genes, is transcribed in Ad 2-transformed cells. (3) Viral genes transcribed late after infection (18 hr after infection) are not transcribed detectably in Ad 2-transformed cells.

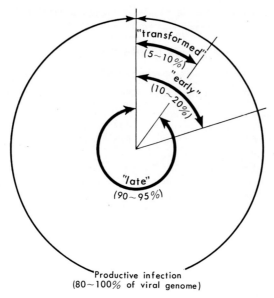

Fig. 1.   Diagram representing the fractions of the viral genome transcribed in Ad 2-infected and -transformed cells (6).

Viral DNA Sequences in Transformed Cell DNA—Control at the Transcription Level in Transformed Cells

Viral DNA sequences in transformed cell DNA were investigated by DNA-RNA hybridization between transformed cell DNA and complementary RNA (cRNA) synthesized on a viral DNA template by *E. coli* polymerase *in vitro*. As shown in Table 4, RNA hybridizes with chromosomal DNA from transformed cells to the same extent as that from nuclear DNA, indicating that viral DNA sequences are present in cellular chromosomes.   From reconstruction experiments, we estimate the following number of viral DNA copies present in adenovirus-transformed cells (Table 5): 58–61 copies in Ad 12-transformed hamster embryo, 21–23 in Ad 12-

TABLE 4.   Association of Ad 12 DNA with Chromosomes of Transformed Cells[a]

Source of Immobilized DNA	Ad 12 [³H] cRNA[b] 50 μg of DNA
Ad 12-transformed cell chromosomes	569
,,	613
Ad 12-transformed cell nuclei	666
,,	628
Ad 7-transformed cell nuclei	113
,,	122
NIL-2E (normal hamster cell) nuclei	79
,,	67

[a] Green *et al.* (*11*).

[b] Input is 100,000 cpm.   Background subtracted.

TABLE 5. Number of Viral DNA Copies in Adenovirus Tumor and Transformed Cells[a]

Cell lines	Ratio of cellular to viral DNA[b]		Viral DNA copies/cell[c]
Ad 12-transformed hamster embryo	7,100	7,500	58–61
Ad 12-induced hamster tumor	18,600	21,100	21–23
Ad 7-transformed hamster embryo	5,000	5,200	84–87
Ad 2-transformed rat embryo (8617)	15,400	17,200	25–28
Ad 2-transformed rat embryo (8629)	15,200	18,900	23–29

[a] Green (*10*); Green *et al.* (*11*).

[b] Determined by hybridization of transformed cell DNA with radioactive adenovirus complementary RNA.

[c] Calculated on the basis of 10^{13} daltons of DNA per cell and 23×10^6 daltons of DNA per adenovirion. One whole adenovirus genome per cell would represent one part of viral DNA per 435,000 parts of cell DNA.

induced hamster tumor, 84–87 in Ad 7-transformed hamster embryo, and 23–29 in Ad 2-transformed rat embryo cells.

Whether the whole viral genome is present in cellular chromosomes is not known. However, the following experiment shows that only a portion of the viral DNA sequences present in transformed cells is transcribed. "Early" and "late" RNAs

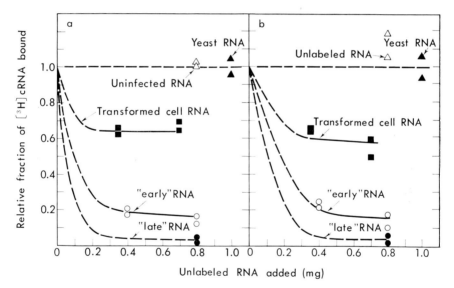

FIG. 2. Hybridization-inhibition between Ad 12-[³H]cRNA (synthetic complementary RNA) and (a) Ad 12-DNA or (b) Ad 12-transformed cell DNA. Each hybridization vessel contained two filters, a 6.5 mm filter containing 0.0024 μg of Ad 12-DNA and a 25 mm filter containing 50 μg of Ad 12-transformed cell DNA. In step 1, filters were incubated with different amounts of unlabeled RNA either from cells 10 hr after productive infection with Ad 12-(early RNA), or from cells 45 hr after productive infection with Ad 12 (late RNA), or from Ad 12-transformed hamster embryo cells, or from uninfected KB cells, or from yeast, in 4× SSC with 0.1% SDS for 20 hr at 66°C. Filters were rinsed once with 4× SSC and further incubated with 100,000 cpm of Ad 12-[³H] cRNA in 4× SSC with 0.1% SDS for 20 hr at 66°C. Filters were washed, treated with RNAase, washed, and counted. Counts bound to DNA filters incubated with 4× SSC 0.1% SDS instead of unlabeled RNA in step 1 were normalized to 1.0 (*10*).

from Ad 12-infected KB cells block almost completely RNA-DNA hybrid formation between Ad 12 cRNA and DNA from Ad 12-transformed cells, while RNA
from Ad 12-transformed cell RNA competes with only about 50% (Fig. 2b). Ad
12 cRNA contains mainly early gene transcipts as shown by the competition experiment with viral DNA using " early," " late," and transformed cell RNA (Fig. 2a).
" Early " RNA blocks almost completely the hybridization between Ad 12 cRNA
and viral DNA, and transformed cell RNA competes with 50% of labeled Ad 12
cRNA. These results suggest that most of early viral genes may be present in the
transformed cell but only part of these viral sequences are transcribed. The mechanism of control of transcription of the viral genome in transformed cells is of
great interest but is completely unknown.

Synthesis of Virus-specific RNA in the Cell Nucleus and Transport to the Cytoplasm

As suggested by the above experiments, virus-specific RNA is synthesized in
the cell nucleus and transported to the cytoplasm. Pulse labeling and chase experiments show the rapid synthesis of virus-specific RNA in the cell nucleus and its transport into the cytoplasm where it is degraded with a half-life of approximately 2 hr
(Shimada, Fujinaga, and Ito, unpublished data). Hybridization competition experiments with nuclear and cytoplasmic RNAs did not detect differences in base
sequences between nuclear and cytoplasmic virus-specific RNAs indicating that all
viral RNAs synthesized in the cell nucleus are transported to the cytoplsam (Shimada,
Fujinaga, and Ito, unpublished data).

Possible Existence of Hybrid Molecules Containing Both Cellular and Viral RNA Sequences

Since 4 to 10% of the viral genome is transcribed in Ad 2-transformed cells, at
most 1.1×10^6 daltons of RNA could be transcribed. Sedimentation on sucrose
density gradients shows that virus-specific RNA from Ad 2-transformed cell nuclei
is heterogeneous with sedimentation values ranging from 10 to 40 S, indicating the
presence of virus-specific RNA molecules larger that 1.1×10^6 daltons (Sekikawa,
Shimada, Fujinaga, and Ito, unpublished data). This suggests the presence of
polycistronic " viral-cell " RNA molecules in adenovirus-transformed cells, as suggested also for the virus-specific RNA from SV-40-transformed cells (*16*).

We have attempted to demonstrate the presence of viral-cell hybrid RNA molecules by DNA-RNA hybridization (Table 6). Virus-specific RNA was isolated and
purified from transformed cells by two or three cycles of DNA-RNA hybrid formation with viral DNA and elution without RNAase treatment. Purified virus-specific
RNA from Ad 7-transformed cells hybridized with Ad 7 DNA but also with normal
hamster cell (Nil 2E) DNA. Similarly, purified virus-specific RNA from Ad 2-
transformed rat embryo cells (8617) hybridized both with Ad 2 DNA and with normal rat embryo cell (9258) DNA. Virus-specific RNA isolated from cells infected
with adenovirus does not hybridize significantly with normal cell DNA (Table 7).
These results provide the experimental evidence for existence of hybrid RNA molecules containing both cellular and viral base sequences.

TABLE 6. Hybridization of Viral Specific RNA from Transformed Cells with Viral and Cellular DNA

RNA			DNA		Bound radioactivity[b]	
Source	Purification cycle	Input (cpm)	Source	μg/filter	cpm[b]	%
Ad 7 transformed hamster cells[a]	2	763	Ad 7	5	587	76.5
			normal hamster cells (Nil/ 2E)	50	182	24.0
			E. coli	50	28	3.6
			blank	0	12	1.5
Ad 7 transformed hamster cell nuclei[a]	3	860	Ad 7	5	532	62.0
			normal hamster cells (Nil/ 2E)	50	213	24.8
			blank	0	10	1.2
Ad 2 transformed rat cells[a]	2	1852	Ad 2	5	358	19.4
			normal rat cells (9258)	50	485	25.9
			E. coli	50	79	4.2
			blank	0	33	1.8

[a] RNA was isolated from transformed cells or nuclei, and purified through hybrid formation with viral DNA and elution from the hybrid.

[b] Average of duplicate hybridization reactions.

TABLE 7. Hybridization of Viral Specific RNA from Infected Cells with Viral and Cellular DNA

RNA		DNA		Bound radioactivity[b]	
Source	Input (cpm)	Source	μg/filter	cpm	%
Ad 7-infected cells[a]	14750	Ad 7	5	9,360	63.50
		KB	50	46	0.31
		Nil 2E	50	21	0.14
		Ad 2	5	2,617	17.85
		E. coli	5	38	0.25
		blank	0	38	0.35
Ad 2-infected cells[a]	1261	Ad 2	5	832	52.75
		KB	50	21	1.31
		KB	6	11	0.70
		9258	50	22	1.40
		E. coli	50	9	0.56
		Ad 7	5	83	6.60
		blank	0	12	0.76

[a] Virus-specific RNA was isolated from Ad 7- or Ad 2- infected KB cells and purified through one cycle of hybrid formation with viral DNA and elution from the hybrid.

[b] Average of duplicate hybridization reactions.

Cellular RNA Species Transcribed in Transformed Cells

Preliminary experiments show the presence of cellular RNA species in Ad 12-transformed cells which are not transcribed detectably in normal cells (Fujinaga, Sekikawa, Shimada, and Ito, unpublished data). As shown in Fig. 3, RNA from

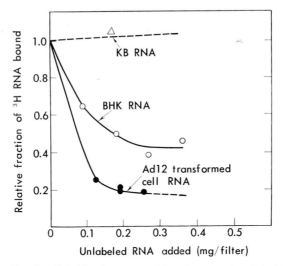

FIG. 3. Hybridization competition between labeled Ad 12-transformed cell RNA and unlabeled Ad 12-transformed cell RNA or normal hamster cell RNA (BHK. RNA). In step 1, filters containing 0.075 μg of BHK DNA were incubated for 20 hr at 66°C with different amounts of unlabeled RNA. The filters were incubated further for 20 hr at 66°C with 2×10^6 cpm/filter of [^{3}H]RNA from Ad 12-transformed cells labeled with 8 μCi/ml of [^{3}H] uridine for 6 hr. The filters were washed, treated with RNAase, and counted. Counts bound to DNA filters incubated with $2 \times$ SSC 0.1% SDS instead of unlabeled RNA in step 1 were normalized to 1.0 (Fujinaga, Sekikawa, Shimada and Ito, unpublished data).

normal hamster cells (baby hamster kidney cell, BHK) competed with only part of the labeled Ad 12-transformed hamster embryo cell RNA for sites on BHK DNA. Similar results were obtained when RNA from normal hamster embryo cells (Nil 2E) was employed in place of BHK cell RNA. The portion of the cellular genome which is transcribed in Ad 12-transformed cells, but not in normal cells, is not transcribed detectably in Ad 12-infected KB cells, as shown by additional hybridization competition experiments. These results suggest that some cellular genes may be activated by transformation with oncogenic human adenoviruses.

SUMMARY

Viral and cellular gene transcription in virus-free cells transformed by human adenoviruses was studied with the following results.

(1) Three different classes of virus-specific RNAs are synthesized in cells transformed by human adenoviruses (Ad), one specific for group A (Ad 12, 18, and 31), the second for group B (Ad 3, 7, 14, 16, and 21) and the third for group C (Ad 1, 2, 5, and 6). Only part of the viral genome (half of the early genes) is transcribed in transformed cells, while all or nearly all of the viral genome is transcribed in productively infected cells.

(2) Virus-free transformed cells contain viral DNA sequences associated with cellular chromosomal DNA. Only a part of the viral genome is transcribed in trans-

formed cells.   Most, if not all, of virus-specific RNA sequences synthesized in the cell nucleus is transported to the cytoplasm where it degrades with a half-life of approximately 2 hr.

(3) High molecular weight RNA molecules containing virus-specific sequences can be detected in the cell nucleus. Purified virus-specific RNA hybridizes with both cellular and viral DNA, providing evidence for hybrid RNA molecules containing both cellular and viral RNA sequences.

(4) Hybridization competition suggests the presence of cellular RNA species in Ad 12-transformed cells which are not transcribed detectably in normal cells.

REFERENCES

1. Freeman, A. E., Black, P. H., Vanderpool, E. A., Henry, P. H., Austin, J. B., and Huebner, R. J.   Transformation of Primary Rat Embryo Cells by Adenovirus Type 2. Proc. Natl. Acad. Sci. U.S., *58*: 1205–1212, 1967.

2. Fujinaga, K., and Green, M.   The Mechanism of Viral Carcinogenesis by DNA Mammalian Viruses.   I. Viral-specific RNA in Polyribosomes of Adenovirus Tumor and Transformed Cells. Proc. Natl. Acad. Sci. U.S., *55*: 1567–1574, 1966.

3. Fujinaga, K., and Green, M.   The Mechanism of Viral Carcinogenesis by DNA Mammalian Viruses.   II. Viral-specific RNA in Tumor Cells Induced by " Weakly " Oncogenic Human Adenoviruses. Proc. Natl. Acad. Sci. U.S., *57*: 806–812, 1967.

4. Fujinaga, K., and Green, M.   Mechanism of Viral Carcinogenesis by Deoxyribonucleic Acid Mammalian Viruses.   IV. Related Virus-specific Ribonucleic Acids in Tumor Cells Induced by " Highly " Oncogenic Adenovirus Type 12, 18, and 31.   J. Virol., *1*: 576–582, 1967.

5. Fujinaga, K., and Green, M.   Mechanism of Viral Carcinogenesis by DNA Mammalian Viruses.   V. Properties of Purified Viral-specific RNA from Human Adenovirus-induced Tumor Cells.   J. Mol. Biol., *31*: 63–73, 1968.

6. Fujinaga, K., and Green, M.   Mechanism of Viral Carcinogenesis by DNA Mammalian Viruses.   VII. Viral Genes Transcribed in Adenovirus Type 2 Infected and Transformed Cells. Proc. Natl. Acad. Sci. U.S., *65*: 375–382, 1970.

7. Fujinaga, K., Mak, S., and Green, M.   A Method for Determining the Fraction of the Viral Genome Transcribed during Infection and Its Application to Adenovirus-infected Cells. Proc. Natl. Acad. Sci. U.S., *60*: 959–966, 1968.

8. Fujinaga, K., Pina, M., and Green, M.   The Mechanism of Viral Carcinogenesis by DNA Mammalian Viruses, VI.   A New Class of Virus-specific RNA Molecules in Cells. Transformed by Group C Human Adenoviruses. Proc. Natl. Acad. Sci. U.S., *64*: 255–262, 1969.

9. Girardi, A. J., Hilleman, M. R., and Zwickey, R. E.   Tests in Hamsters for Oncogenic Quality of Ordinary Viruses Including Adenovirus Type 7.   Proc. Soc. Exptl. Biol. Med., *115*: 1141–1150, 1964.

10. Green, M.   Effect of Oncogenic DNA Viruses on Regulatory Mechanisms of Cells. Fed. Proc., *29*: 1265–1275, 1970.

11. Green, M., Parsons, J. T., Fujinaga, K., Caffier, H., and Landgraf-Leurs, I.   Transcription of Adenovirus Genes in Productively Infected and in Transformed Cells. Cold Spring Harbor Symp. Quant. Biol., XXXV,: 803–818, 1970.

12. Green, M., Pina, M., Kimes, R., Wensink, P. C., MacHattie, L. A., and Thomas,

Jr., C. A. Adenovirus DNA. I. Molecular Weight and Conformation. Proc. Natl. Acad. Sci. U.S., *57*: 1302–1309, 1967.

13. Huebner, R. J., Rowe, W. P., and Lane, W. T. Oncogenic Effects in Hamster of Human Adenovirus Type 12 and 18. Proc. Natl. Acad. Sci. U.S., *48*: 2051–2058, 1962.

14. Lacy, SR. S., and Green, M. Biochemical Studies on Adenovirus Multiplication. VII. Homology between DNA's of Tumorigenic and Nontumorigenic Human Adenoviruses. Proc. Natl. Acad. Sci. U.S., *52*: 1053–1059, 1964.

15. Lacy, SR. S., and Green, M. The Mechanism of Viral Carcinogenesis by DNA Mammalian Viruses: DNA–DNA Homology Relationships among the " Weakly " Oncogenic Human Adenoviruses. J. Gen. Virol., *1*: 413–418, 1967.

16. Lindberg, U., and Darnell, J. E. SV40-specific RNA in the Nucleus and Polyribosomes of Transformed Cells. Proc. Natl. Acad. Sci. U.S., *65*: 1089–1070.

17. Mak, S., and Green, M. Biochemical Studies on Adenovirus Multiplication. XIII. Synthesis of Virus-specific Ribonucleic Acid during Infection with Human Adenovirus Type 12. J. Virol., *2*: 1055–1063, 1968.

18. Pina, M., and Green, M. Biochemical Studies on Adenovirus Multiplication. IX. Chemical and Base Composition Analysis of 28 Human Adenoviruses. Proc. Natl. Acad. Sci. U.S., *54*: 547–551, 1965.

19. Trentin, J. J., Van Hoosier, Jr., G. L., and Samper, L. The Oncogenicity of Human Adenovirus in Hamster. Proc. Soc. Expl. Biol. Med., *127*: 683–689, 1968.

20. Trentin, J. J., Yabe, Y., and Taylor, G. The Quest for Human Cancer Viruses. Science, *137*: 835–841, 1962.

Changes in Permissiveness for Virus Infection in Cells Transformed by the SV40 Genome

Hiroto Shimojo

Department of Tumor Virus Research, Institute of Medical Science, University of Tokyo, Tokyo, Japan

Various heritable changes are induced in cells transformed by oncogenic viruses. Some of these changes, such as the synthesis of T antigen or virus-specific mRNA, are coded for by the viral genome. Some other changes, such as changes in the growth regulation, in morphology or in various macromolecular syntheses, result from changes in the gene expression of the cellular genome after the interaction of cellular and viral genomes, and are not coded for by the viral genome. The replication of a virus depends on the cell species employed. Some viruses, such as the herpes simplex virus, have a broad host range and can replicate in cells of various species. Some other viruses, such as the human adenovirus, have a narrow host range and can replicate in cells of only one species. After infection with a virus of a narrow host range, some cells permit the replication of the virus and some other cells do not. The former permissive cells may have necessary material and no inhibitor for viral replication. The latter non-permissive cells may lack in some materials necessary for viral replication or may have inhibitor(s) for viral replication.

These considerations lead to the examination whether or not changes in permissiveness for virus infection are induced in transformed cells. These changes have already been observed in hamster cells transformed by adenovirus 12 (*12, 15*) and in green monkey kidney cells (GMK) (*1, 11, 13, 14, 16*) or human cells (*8, 16*) transformed by simian virus 40 (SV40). The present report describes in some detail one of these reports (*14*), which was carried out in my laboratory, as an example of these changes and discusses the significance of these changes.

While GMK are permissive for SV40 infection, several investigators have reported the transformation of GMK by SV40 or adeno 7-SV40 hybrid virus (*4, 5, 8, 13, 14, 18*). Human adenoviruses do not usually replicate in GMK but coinfection with SV40 resulted in the efficient replication of human adenoviruses (*10*). It has been reported that GMK transformed by the SV40 genome supported the efficient replication of human adenoviruses (*11, 13, 14*). It has also been reported that GMK transformed by SV40 are resistant to superinfection (*8, 11, 16*), and that GMK transformed by hybrid virus are permissive to SV40 (*5, 13*). These changes in permissiveness for infection with human adenoviruses and SV40 were further clarified as follows.

Establishment of Cell Lines of GMK Transformed by the SV40 Genome

Since GMK are permissive for SV40 infection, transformed GMK were obtained by the use of ultraviolet (UV)-irradiated viruses. The following viruses were used.

1   Adeno 7-SV40 hybrid virus (E46), designated as hybrid virus; cell lines transformed by this virus were designated as H-lines.

2   T antigen-forming defective virions of SV40, designated as T fraction; cell lines transformed by this fraction were designated as T-lines. The T fraction was prepared by undiluted passages of SV40 in GMK as described by Uchida *et al.* (*17*) and purified by isopycnic centrifugation. Its density was 1.33 to 1.32. It had a 100 to 1,000 times higher titer in T antigen-forming units (TFU) (*17*) than in plaque-forming units (PFU).

3   Plaque-forming complete virions of SV40, designated as P virus; cell lines transformed by this virus were designated as P lines. Its density was 1.34. It had an equal titer in TFU and PFU.

One-fifth ml of hybrid virus, UV-irradiated for 20 or 40 min, was inoculated onto a semiconfluent monolayer of GMK in a 2 oz. bottle. After adsorption at 36°C for 2 hr, 5 ml of growth medium (Eagle's MEM, supplemented with 15% bovine serum) was added, and the cultures were incubated at 36°C for 48 hr. Then, cells were harvested, resuspended in the growth medium at a concentration of 5×10^4 cells/ml and subcultured at 36°C in 2 oz. bottles with rubber stoppers. Confluent monolayers were formed in 2 to 3 days and the medium was changed once a week. Small white foci became visible in the monolayers in 2 to 3 weeks and gradually grew in size. Microscopic examination revealed that a focus consisted of epitheloid cells densely piled up, while the other part of the culture consisted of elongated cells in a fairly oriented monolayers. No cytopathic effect (CPE) was observed in 4 weeks. Cells in foci were easily subcultured and 7 cell lines (H lines) were established. It was confirmed that all the cells in each H-line were SV40 T antigen-positive and SV 40 V antigen-negative. Neither SV40 nor adenovirus was detected in the culture fluid. Cells in a monolayer of normal morphology were randomly selected, subcultured and used as the control (C lines). Cells in the C lines were SV40 T antigen negative.

GMK transformed by T fraction, UV-irradiated for 40 min, were established similarly by subcultivation of cells in foci. Five cell lines thus established (T lines) were T antigen positive and two of them were V antigen-negative. However, 3 other lines contained a small number of V antigen-positive cells and a small amount of SV40 was detected in the culture fluid. These cells were recloned in media containing anti-SV40 serum (20 neutralizing units per ml). Cells in colonies formed in this medium were subcultured. Cell lines thus established from the colonies did not contain V antigen-positive cells and were SV40-free.

When GMK were infected with T fraction, UV-irradiated for 20 min and subcultured in a similar manner, confluent monolayers were formed in 2 to 3 days. However, CPE became visible in 10 to 14 days and the cell degeneration progressed to the whole culture in a few days. These cultures were further incubated at 36°C without changing medium. After incubation for 50 to 60 days, small colonies appeared in degenerated cell sheets. Cell lines, established from these surviving colonies, were T antigen-positive and one of them did not contain V antigen-positive cells. However, three lines contained a small number of V antigen-positive cells. These cells were recloned in media containing anti-SV40 serum, and cell lines, which were T antigen-positive and V antigen-negative, were established. Culture fluids of these lines were SV40-free.

Transformed foci of GMK could not be obtained with P virus UV-irradiated extensively (for 40 min or longer), since CPE became apparent in 2 weeks after subcultivation. However, surviving colonies appeared in degenerated cell sheets after incubation for a long period. Three cell lines were then obtained by subcultivation of surviving colonies. All P-lines contained a small number of V antigen-positive cells and the culture fluid contained SV40. By means of recloning in a medium containing anti-SV40 serum, P-lines free of SV40 were established. Established H-, T-, and P-lines are summarized in Table 1.

Cells in H-, T-, and P-lines were epitheloid in shape and grew well in Eagle's MEM with 15% bovine serum. After formation of confluent monolayers, cells continued to grow to form multilayers and then sloughed off the glass abruptly. These

TABLE 1. GMK Cell Lines Transformed by SV40 Genome (*14*).

Transforming virus	Cell lines from foci		Cell lines from survived colonies	
	SV40 (−)[a]	SV40 (+)[a]	SV40 (−)	SV40 (+)
Hybrid virus	H–1 H–9 H–2 H–16 H–3 H–19 H–5	—[b]	Hy-Tr GMK[d]	—
SV40 T-fraction	T–22 T–52	T–50–1, –4, –11[c] T–51–2, –4, –11 T–54–2, –5, 9	T–56	T–64–1, –2 T–65–1, –3 T–66
SV40 P rirus	—	—	—	P–55 P–58–1, –2 P–67–1, –2

[a] SV40 (−) means that the first subculture from a focus or a colony was SV40 free. SV40 (+) means that the first subculture from a focus or a colony contained SV40 and SV40-free cell lines were established by recloning cells in medium containing anti-SV40 serum.

[b] — means that transformed cell line could not be obtained under this condition.

[c] The third figure means the designation of a colony formed in media containing anti-SV40 serum. For instance, T–50, which was subcultured from a foci and initially SV40-positive, was recloned in media containing anti-SV40 serum and 10 colonies were subcultured. Of these subcultures, 3 cell lines (T–50–1, T–50–4, T–50–10) free from SV40 were established.

[d] cited from (*13*).

TABLE 2. Replication of Adenovirus 2, 7 and 12 in Transformed and Nontransformed GMK (*14*)[a]

Transformed by	Cell lines	Virus yields (log PFU/ml)					
		Ad 2		Ad 7		Ad 12	
		7 hr[b]	48 hr	7 hr	72 hr	7 hr	72 hr
Hybrid virus	H–1	3.0	7.2	1.0	7.2	1.0	6.5
	H–2	2.7	6.7	1.7	7.3	1.2	6.5
	H–3	3.2	7.7	2.0	7.5	1.0	6.5
	H–5	2.7	8.7	1.3	7.5	1.0	7.3
	H–9	3.0	7.3	3.3	7.5	1.0	7.3
	H–16	3.2	6.7	3.5	7.7	2.4	6.2
	H–19	3.0	8.7	3.3	8.3	1.0	7.0
SV40 T-fraction	T–22	3.5	8.7	3.7	7.7	1.0	7.7
	T–52	4.0	7.5	1.0	5.7	1.0	4.7
	T–50–4	2.7	7.5	2.7	6.5	1.0	4.7
	T–50–10	4.0	9.0	3.5	7.5	1.0	4.7
	T–51–2	4.0	7.7	3.7	7.7	1.0	4.7
	T–51–4	4.0	8.7	3.7	7.5	1.0	5.6
	T–54–2	4.0	8.7	3.5	7.6	1.0	6.7
	T–54–9	4.0	9.2	3.2	7.5	1.0	6.7
	T–56	4.0	8.7	2.7	7.7	n.d.	n.d.
	T–65–3	3.5	8.0	2.3	7.0	2.5	6.2
SV40 P virus	P–58–1	2.7	8.5	1.2	6.5	1.2	5.2
	P–58–2	2.0	7.7	1.2	6.5	1.7	5.7
	P–67–1	3.0	8.0	1.9	6.6	1.9	5.8
Nontransformed	C–7	2.7	3.3	1.7	2.0	1.0	1.0
	C–8	2.7	3.0	1.7	2.0	1.0	1.0
	C–10	3.2	3.7	n.d.	n.d.	1.7	2.0
	C–11	2.7	3.0	1.7	2.0	1.0	1.0
	C–14	2.7	2.7	2.2	2.0	1.0	1.0
	C–15	3.2	3.0	2.0	2.0	1.0	1.0
	C–24	3.2	3.5	2.0	2.0	1.0	1.0

[a] GMK, transformed or nontransformed, was infected with adenovirus 2, 7 or 12. After adsorption, and incubation, infected cells were harvested and the virus content in each harvest was titrated.

[b] Time of harvest after incubation. Titers 7 hr *p.i.*, show virus content before replication and those 48 or 72 hr *p.i.*, virus content after replication.

TABLE 3. Replication of SV40 in Transformed Cells Established from Foci, from Colonies, and

H-lines from foci	Virus yields		T-lines from foci	Virus yields		T-lines from colonies
	7 hr	72 hr		7 hr	72 hr	
H–1	2.0	5.7	T–22	3.0	7.4	T–56
H–2	2.2	5.7	T–52	4.5	7.5	T–64–1
H–3	2.4	7.0	T–50–4	4.2	7.5	T–64–2
H–5	2.7	7.0	T–51–2	3.0	7.5	T–65–1
H–9	2.5	6.5	T–54–9	4.5	7.3	T–65–3

[a] Replication of SV40 in transformed and nontransformed cells was examined and expressed as log PFU/ml.

cells were T antigen-positive and V antigen-negative. The size of the SV40 genome transcribed in transformed cells was estimated by DNA-RNA hybridization competition, in which hybridization of ^{3}H-labeled late SV40 mRNA with SV40 DNA competed with increasing amounts of cold RNA extracted from H-5, T-22, and P-58-1 lines. The portions of the SV40 genome transcribed were estimated as approximately 40% in H-5 and T-22 and 50% in P-58-1. SV40 could not be detected or rescued from all of these cells by cocultivation on GMK or cell-fusion with GMK by the use of UV-inactivated Sendai virus(6). Similar tests with SV40-transformed hamster cells, carried out simultaneously as controls, gave positive results.

Replication of Human Adenoviruses and SV40 in Transformed Cells

Replication of adenovirus 2, 7, and 12 in transformed cells was examined. All cell lines of transformed GMK (H-, T-, and P-lines) supported the efficient replication of adenovirus 2, 7, and 12; whereas, non-transformed GMK (C lines) did not (Table 2). Adenovirus 2, which had replicated once in transformed cells, did not become able to replicate in nontransformed GMK (C-14), although they did replicate in nontransformed GMK (C-14) when coinfected with SV40. These observations excluded the possibility that the efficient replication of human adenoviruses in transformed GMK may have resulted from contamination by enhancing factors such as SV40 or monkey cell-adapting component (MAC) (2).

Replication of SV40 in transformed cells was then examined. SV40 could replicate efficiently in all H- and T-lines established from foci. However, none of the P-lines nor any of the T-lines established from surviving colonies could support the replication of SV40 (Table 3). Then, transformed cell lines, nonpermissive for SV40, were infected with SV40 DNA and assayed for the replication of SV40 at 48 hr post infection (p.i.). These cells produced a small amount of SV40. However, the virus yield per cell was very low, compared to that in T-22 cells. One of the P-lines, P-58-2, did not produce any SV40 (Table 4).

Implication of Changes in Permissiveness for Virus Infection

The above study showed two types of selection of cells transformed by UV-irradiated virus. The first type was detected as a focus of transformed cells in normal GMK. No CPE was observed during incubation for focus-formation and trans-

Nontransformed GMK (14)[a]

Virus yields		P-lines from colonies	Virus yields		C-lines from nontransformed GMK	Virus yields	
7 hr	72 hr		7 hr	72 hr		7 hr	72 hr
4.7	4.9	P-58-1	4.0	3.7	C-7	2.2	6.7
4.6	5.0	P-58-2	4.6	4.3	C-10	2.4	6.3
4.0	4.6	P-67-1	4.7	4.9	C-14	2.0	6.6
4.3	4.8				C-15	2.2	6.7
4.3	4.8				C-24	2.2	6.7

TABLE 4.   Replication of SV40 in Transformed Cells after Infection with SV40 DNA (14)[a]

Transformed cells	Virus yields	
	log PFU/10^6 cells	PFU/cell
T–22	7.1	10
T–56	3.2	0.009
T–64–1	2.7	0.001
T–64–2	2.9	0.001
T–65–1	4.0	0.01
T–65–3	5.0	0.1
P–58–1	4.3	0.07
P–58–2	0	0
P–67–1	4.1	0.08

[a] Transformed cells in the table were infected with SV40 DNA by the method of McCutchan and Pagano (9). After incubation at 36°C for 48 hr, virus yields were examined and expressed as log PFU/10^6 cells and PFU per cell.

formed cell lines thus established were SV40 T antigen positive but SV40 could not be detected or rescued from these cells.   The second type was detected as a surviving colony in degenerated GMK.   The cells subcultured from surviving colonies were SV40 T antigen-positive and mostly V antigen-negative.

It has been reported that simian cells transformed by SV40 are resistant to superinfection with SV40 (1, 11, 16) and that SV40 replicates in these cells when the cells are infected with SV40 DNA (16).   Thus, Swetley et al. (16) excluded the existence of the repressor proposed by Cassingena and Tournier (3).   Most of the transformed cell lines belonging to the second type supported the inefficient replication of SV40, when cells were infected with SV40 DNA.   However, the virus yields were very low, showing an average burst size of 10^{-2} to 10^{-3} PFU per cell.   This value is near to those reported by Swetley et al. (16).   Kit et al. (7) reported similar results in SV40-transformed human cells and called these cells semipermissive.   Since the virus yield in permissive cells (T-22) after infection with SV40 DNA was 10 PFU per cell, it was calculated that cells of the second type may contain one permissive cell in 10^3 to 10^4 cells.   Thus, it is suggested that most of the cells of the second type may be nonpermissive for SV40, even when cells were infected with SV40 DNA.   This suggestion is supported by the finding that one of these cell lines, P-58-2, did not produce SV40, even when the cells were infected with SV40 DNA, indicating that P-58-2 cells contained no permissive cells.   Another evidence for this suggestion was obtained by immunofluorescent examination of transformed cells infected with SV40 DNA.   In this test, most cells of T-22 became V antigen-positive, whereas very few, if any, V antigen-positive cells were observed in T-58-1.   This suggestion made it difficult to exclude the existence of the repressor.   There may be two possibilities as to the origin of the transformed cells of the second type.   The one is that the existence of the SV40 genome may have modified the nature of the cells so that they are resistant to superinfection, perhaps by the formation of a repressor like that in lysogenic bacteria.   The other is that these cells have originated from a cell non-permissive for SV40, which may have existed originally in a GMK population.   Further studies on this problem will clarify the similarity or dissimilarity between transformed cells and lysogenic bacteria.

It was shown that all transformed cell lines supported the efficient replication of human adenoviruses, in contrast to that all nontransformed GMK cell lines (C-lines) did not.   It was clarified that GMK, originally nonpermissive for infection with human adenoviruses, became permissive after transformation.   Thus, it was established that the permissiveness for infection with human adenoviruses could be one of the markers of GMK transformed by the SV40 genome.   Hagura showed that hamster cells, originally nonpermissive for infection with polyoma virus, became permissive after transformation by SV40, although virions produced in transformed hamster cells were defective (personal communication).   This observation also suggests that the permissiveness for infection with polyoma virus may be one of the markers of hamster cells transformed by SV40.   These are changes from nonpermissive to permissive cells induced by transformation.   The reverse changes from permissive to nonpermissive cells were observed in transformed GMK from surviving colonies, when cells were infected with SV40.   It was reported that hamster cells supported the replication of adenovirus 2, whereas hamster tumor cells induced by adenovirus 12 were resistant to infection with adenovirus 2 (12, 15).   Thus, the reverse changes in permissiveness to virus infections may also be one of the markers of transformed cells.

Changes in permissiveness for virus infections may be not only markers of transformed cells but also useful clues for studying the nature of transformed cells.   The nonpermissiveness for superinfection described above may be one tool with which to examine the repressor.   The preliminary analysis of the replication of adenovirus 2 in transformed and nontransformed GMK revealed that adenovirus DNA replicated and a complete set of viral mRNA was transcribed in either kind of cells but capsid proteins were synthesized only in transformed GMK (Hashimoto and Shimojo, unpublished).   A factor(s) necessary for translation in adenovirus replication is lacking in GMK and supplemented by transformation with the SV40 genome.   Sekiya and Oda showed altered species of tRNA in cells transformed by SV40 (personal communication).   Thus, the analysis of this problem will provide a useful method for studying the mechanism of translation.

Finally, it must be mentioned that the examination of the permissiveness for virus infections of human cancer cells cultured *in vitro* should be a useful method with which to aproach the complex problems of human cancer.

REFERENCES

1.   Black, P. H.   The Oncogenic DNA Viruses : A Review of *in vitro* Transformation Studies.   Ann. Rev. Microbiol., *22* : 391–426, 1968.
2.   Butel, J., S., Rapp, F., Melnick, J. L., and Rubin, B. A.   Replication of Adenovirus Type 7 in Monkey Cells : A New Determinant and Its Transfer to Adenovirus Type 2.   Science, *154* : 671–673, 1966.
3.   Cassingena, R., and Tournier, P.   Mise en Évidence d'un " Represseur " Spécifique dans des Cellules D'espàces Differentes Transformées par le Virus SV40.   C. R. Acad. Sci., *267* (25) : 2251–2254, 1968.

4. Fernandes, M. Y., and Moorhead, P. S.   Transformation of African Green Monkey Kidney Cultures Infected with Simian Vacuolating Virus (SV40).   Texas Rep. Biol. Med., *23*: 242–258, 1965.

5. Jensen, F., and Defendi, V.   Transformation of African Green Monkey Cells by Irradiated Adenovirus 7-simian Virus 40 Hybrid.   J. Virol., *2*: 173–177, 1968.

6. Koprowski, H., Jensen, F. C., and Steplewski, Z.   Activation of Production of Infectious Tumor Virus SV40 in Heterokaryon Cultures.   Proc. Natl. Acad. Sci. U. S., *58*: 127–133, 1967.

7. Kit, S., Kurimura, T., Brown, M., and Dubbs, D. R.   Identification of the Simian Virus 40 which Replicates When Simian Virus 40-transformed Human Cells are Fused with Simian Virus 40-transformed Mouse Cells or Superinfected with Simian Virus 40 Deoxyribonucleic Acid.   J. Virol., *6*: 69–77, 1970.

8. Margalith, M., Volk-Fuchs, R., and Goldblum, N.   Transformation of BSC-1 Cells Following Chronic Infection with SV40.   J. Gen. Virol., *5*: 321–327, 1969.

9. McCutchan, J. H., and Pagano, J. S.   Enhancement of Infectivity of Simian Virus 40 Deoxyribonucleic Acid with Dimethylaminoethyl-dextran.   J. Nat. Cancer Inst., *41*: 351–357, 1968.

10. Rabson, A. S., O'Conor, G. T., Beregesky, I. K., and Paul, F. J.   Enhancement of Adenovirus Growth in African Green Monkey Kidney Cell Cultures by SV40.   Proc. Soc. Exp. Biol. Med., *116*: 187–190, 1964.

11. Rapp, F., and Trulock, S. C.   Susceptibility to Superinfection of Simian Cells Transformed by SV40.   Virology, *40*: 961–970, 1970.

12. Rouse, H. C., Strohl, W. A., and Schlesinger, R. W.   Properties of Cells Derived from Hamster Tumor by Long-term *in vitro* Cultivation I.   Clonal Stability of Three Biological Characteristics.   Virology, *24*: 633–644, 1966.

13. Shiroki, K., and Shimojo, H.   Replication of Human Adenoviruses in Green Monkey Kidney Cells Transformed by Adeno 7–SV40 Hybrid Virus.   Jap. J. Microbiol., *13*: 125–128, 1969.

14. Shiroki, K., and Shimojo, H.   Transformation of Green Monkey Kidney Cells by SV40 Genome : The Establishment of Transformed Cell Lines and the Replication of Human Adenoviruses and SV40 in Transformed Cells.   Virology, *45*: 163–171,. 1971.

15. Strohl, W. A., Rouse, H. C., and Schlesinger, R. W.   Properties of Cells Derived from Adenovirus-induced Hamster Tumors by Long Term *in vitro* Cultivation.   II. Nature of Restricted Response to Type 2 Adenovirus.   Virology, *28*: 645–658, 1966.

16. Swetley, P., Brodano, G. B., Knowles, B., and Koprowski, H.   Response of Simian Virus 40 Transformed Cell Lines and Cell Hybrids to Superinfection with Simian Virus 40 and Its Deoxyribonucleic Acid.   J. Virol., *4*: 343–355, 1969.

17. Uchida, S., Yoshiike, K., Watanabe, S., and Furuno, A.   Antigen-forming Defective Viruses of Simian Virus 40.   Virology, *24*: 1–8, 1968.

18. Wallace, R.   Viral Transformation of Monkey Kidney Cell Cultures.   Nature, *213*: 768–770, 1967.

Discussion of Papers by Drs. Green, Fujinaga, and Shimojo

DR. YANG: Dr. Shimojo, do you have information concerning the tumorigenicity of your transformed cell in hamsters or monkeys?

DR. SHIMOJO: I have not yet examined this. Of course, I don't think the transformed cell will cause tumors in humans or hamsters. In monkeys, I don't think tumors will be produced, since the monkey is not immunogenetically homogeneous.

DR. MURAMATSU: Dr. Green, I think it is very surprising that as much as 10% of the nuclear RNA transcribed in viral transformed cells is hybridizable with "viral DNA." So I would like to know the real entity of this RNA. It is messenger RNA transcribed on the viral gene of the cell or is it viral RNA itself? To solve this problem, you might extract RNA from the nucleus and then fractionate with a sucrose gradient and do DNA-RNA hybridization experiments on each fraction.

DR. GREEN: I am glad to be able to speak again to acknowledge my co-workers on this, Drs. H. Rokutanda and M. Rokutanda and K. Fujinaga, and also to say that the experiments you are suggesting are being done right now by Dr. Tsuchida from Tokyo. Precisely as you said, we are looking for nucleoplasmic or nucleolar RNA and fractionating by sucrose gradient; he just started it last week.

DR. MURAMATSU: Is it also important to see which strands, plus or minus strands, are being read?

DR. GREEN: We are looking mainly for the positive strand because this product has been known from 70S RNA. There could be negative strands, also; this is something we want to look for. I'll outline a research project for a new colleague.

DR. G. KLEIN: You found the enzyme in a lymphoblastoid leukemia line. Did you show that this was a DNA-dependent DNA polymerase or was it an RNA-dependent DNA polymerase?

DR. GREEN: Our procedure is to screen by looking for polymerase which will respond to poly-dAT, which will amplify the action of the purified enzyme. But DNA-dependent DNA polymerase will also respond to this. So once we separate from the column then we will go and use as a template viral RNA, 70S viral RNA; nobody has done this yet as far as I know. You get a response there. Now, whether this is really a true response, meaning that it is being copied, we are trying to find out right now. Dr. Gallo has used rat liver RNA which is a crude material and he gets an increase of thousands of counts; Dr. Spiegelman used poly-dCrG which he says he doesn't find normal cells responding to; however, I have received telephone calls from other people who have had difficulties with poly-dCrG, but Dr. Spiegelman has done extensive work on it. Obviously it is copying DNA.

DR. YAMAMOTO: I have one question for Dr. Green. We had done some experiments on the effect of rifampicin on cell transformation by Rous sarcoma virus (RSV) like Dr. Weismann. We used a non-defective subgroup A Schmidt-Ruppin strain of RSV, while Weismann's group used RSV(RAV-1) containing much greater amounts of helper virus. We observed all the same dose-response curves not only by cell transformation assay but also by virus multiplication assay. I thought at that time the effect would be on virus multiplication dependent on RNA–DNA polymerase and that the discrepancy in the results, between ours and theirs, would be caused by the total amount of input viruses. Now, are your rifampicin derivatives also effective on cell transformation? And do they affect the transformed cells, that is, can they be used for the therapy of such transformed cells?

DR. GREEN: Weismann reported that rifampicin would block transformation but not replication, and that rifampicin has no effect on the enzyme action of RNA-dependent DNA polymerase. Our work, testing these derivatives, is still preliminary as far as their effects on transformation is concerned. Dr. M. Rokutanda used some of the derivatives and they did block the transformation. We subsequently carried out work on several other derivatives and we found that they also blocked the transformation.

MECHANISM OF
HERPESVIRUS INFECTION

Chairmen:

Tadashi Yamamoto, M. A. Epstein

Biochemical Features of Herpesvirus-infected Cells

Bernard Roizman

Department of Microbiology, University of Chicago, Chicago, Illinois, U.S.A.

Nearly all of our information concerning the biochemistry of herpesviruses is derived from studies of infected cells grown *in vitro*. Analyses of tissue culture cells infected with a variety of herpesviruses have yielded a relatively uniform picture which may be summarized as follows:

(1) Once the cells become productively infected the process is irreversible; the sequence of events is rigidly controlled and reproducible. The cells act as if they were made to reproduce the virus.

(2) Viral macromolecules are made in the same compartments of the cell as host macromolecules. Thus, viral DNA is duplicated in the nucleus. Viral RNA is synthesized and processed in the nucleus, then transported to the cytoplasm. Viral proteins are made on free and bound polyribosomes in the cytoplasm. Some of the proteins are transported into the nucleus whereas others bind to the nuclear and cytoplasmic membranes.

(3) Viral nucleocapsids are assembled in the nucleus and become enveloped by a modified membrane of the cell. The egress of virus appears to take place by way of the endoplasmic reticulum.

(4) Coincidental with the synthesis of virus-specific proteins there occur several changes in the function, structure, and architecture of the infected cell. Thus, margination of chromatin and segregation of the nucleoli coincide with cessation of host macromolecular synthesis, whereas changes in the chemical composition of cellular membranes coincide with changes in cell permeability and in the interaction of cells among themselves.

The biochemical features of herpesvirus-infected cells of major interest to this Symposium concern the nature, extent, and mechanisms of modification of normal host functions following infection. My paper shall deal with two kinds of modification of the host. The first is modification of host macromolecular metabolism. The second is the modification of host membranes which manifest themselves in new surface antigens and in altered social behavior of infected cells.   I would like to close with a very brief consideration of the extent to which the description of events occurring in cells in culture is applicable and reflects events occurring in infected cells in multicellular organisms.

Inhibition of Host Macromolecular Synthesis

The inhibition of host macromolecular synthesis begins very shortly after the entry of virus into the cell and is nearly complete by 4 or 5 hr after infection.

DNA synthesis

The experiments performed in our laboratory (*33*; Sydiskis and Roizman, unpublished data; Schwartz and Roizman, unpublished data) were done on HEP-2 cells infected with herpes simplex virus and then pulse-labeled with ³H-thymidine at intervals after infection.   Immediately after the pulse the DNA was extracted and viral and cellular DNA were separated by isopycnic sedimentation in cesium chloride solutions.   The results, summarized in Fig. 1, show that inhibition of host DNA synthesis could be extrapolated to the time of entry of the virus into the cell and reached a maximum at 4 hr post infection.   Autoradiographic studies on cells which were labeled with thymidine before infection show that inhibition of host DNA synthesis is accompanied by extensive aggregation and displacement of chromosomes to the nuclear membrane (Fig. 2).   On the other hand, autoradiographic studies on cells pulse-labeled 4 hr post infection, *i.e.*, at a time when host DNA synthesis is almost completely inhibited, show that viral DNA is made in

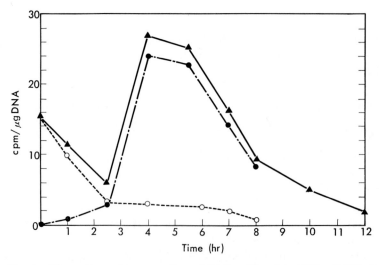

Fig. 1.   The pattern of incorporation of ³H-thymidine into DNA of HEp-2 cells infected with herpes simplex virus.   The cells were pulse-labeled for 15 min at different times after infection.   The DNA extracted after the pulse was centrifuged to equilibrium in cesium chloride density gradients (Sydiskis and Roizman, unpublished data).   ▲, total ;   ●, viral ;   ○, cellular.

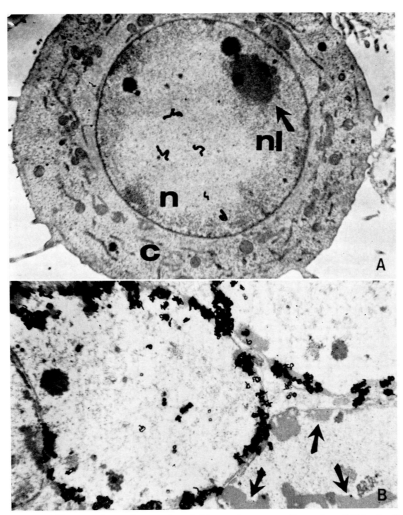

FIG. 2. Electron photomicrographs of thin section autoradiography of HEp-2 cells infected with herpes simplex virus. A, 4 hr-infected cells pulse-labeled for 15 min with thymidine-methyl ³H prior to fixation. B, portions of 3 nuclei of 18 hr-infected cells labeled with thy-midine-methyl ³H prior to infection. Unlabeled thymidine was present in the medium during and after infection. Arrows point to aggregated chromosomes in the cells which did not synthesize DNA during labeling. n, nucleus; c, cytoplasm; nl, nucleolus (Schwartz and Roizman, unpublished data).

the center of the nucleus, *i.e.*, in a space topologically different from that of the host DNA.

The mechanism by which pseudorabies virus inhibits rabbit kidney DNA synthesis has been studied extensively by Ben-Porat and Kaplan (*4*). Largely on the basis of the ability of puromycin to prevent the inhibition of host DNA synthesis by pseudorabies virus, Ben-Porat and Kaplan concluded that the inhibition of host DNA synthesis is a consequence of a product made in infected cells after infection. Newton's studies, on the other hand, as reported in 1968 (*16*), suggest that the inhibition of host DNA synthesis by herpes simplex virus is the consequence of the action of a structural component of the virus which remains active even after the infectious property of the virion is inactivated by ultraviolet light. Clearly, neither the factor responsible for the inhibition nor the mechanism by which it acts are presently known.

RNA synthesis

Most of the information currently available on the effect of herpesviruses on host RNA metabolism is derived from studies on HEp-2 cells infected with herpes simplex virus (*29, 50, 51*). The data show that this virus has three effects on host RNA metabolism. First, infection causes a general reduction in host RNA synthesis beginning shortly after infection (Fig. 3). Analysis of the inhibition of two species of RNA, namely ribosomal and 4S RNA, show that the rate of decline is to some extent multiplicity dependent (Fig. 4). Ultimately, however, the residual level of synthesis of these species of RNA was about the same at all multiplicities of infection (*50*).

The second effect of herpes simplex virus on RNA metabolism relates to the fact that in uninfected mammalian cells a large proportion of newly synthesized RNA must be processed, *i.e.*, it must be occasionally methylated and most often appropriately cleaved before it is utilized (*6*). Analyses of nuclear RNA synthesis

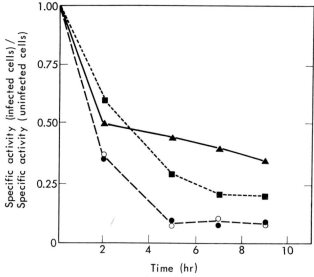

Fig. 3.　The synthesis of various classes of cytoplasmic RNA in herpesvirus infected HEp-2 cells. The cells were labeled with ³H-uridine for 30 min then incubated for an additional 2 hr in medium containing unlabeled uridine. The RNA was extracted and electrophoresed in acrylamide gels. The relative specific radioactivity of the ribosomal RNA and 4S RNA was computed from the absorbance at 260 nm and the radioactivity of RNA in acrylamide gels as compared with the values for the RNA from uninfected control cultures. The recovery of radioactivity of the polydisperse RNA was corrected for the recovery of ribosomal RNA in the corresponding cultures and was also compared to values of uninfected controls (*50*). ▲, polydisperse RNA <28S ; ■, 4S RNA ; ● and ○, ribosomal RNA.

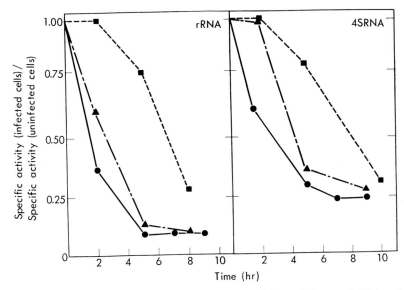

FIG. 4. Effect of multiplicity of infection on the inhibition of ribosomal RNA and 4S RNA synthesis in HEp-cells. At the time shown the cells were pulse-labeled for 20 min with ^{3}H-uridine and then incubated for 90 min in fresh medium containing 10^{-4}M unlabeled uridine. The cytoplasmic RNA was extracted and fractionated as described in the legend to Fig. 3. The relative specific activities of the ribosomal RNA (average of both 28S and 18S) and 4S RNA were also calculated as described by Wagner and Roizman (50). ■, 20 pfu ; ▲, 80 pfu ; ●, 200 pfu.

TABLE 1. The Relative Specific Activities of Nuclear and Cytoplasmic RNA Species in HEp-2 Cells Infected with Herpes Simplex Virus

RNA fraction	Distribution of RNA		Relative specific Activity [B/A]
	Per cent of total CPM [A]	Per cent of total viral CPM [B]	
Cytoplasmic			
FPS	24.7	1.04	0.04
FPP	8.2	19.6	2.39
EDTA	1.2	3.5	2.91
DOC	7.6	13.6	1.79
Nuclear			
NP	23.2	25.8	1.11
NS	34.6	36.6	1.06

Approximately 2×10^8 HEp-2 cells were labeled from 6–8 hr post infection with ^{3}H-uridine and fractionated into nuclear and cytoplasmic RNA species as described by Roizman et al. (29). These species were free cytoplasmic RNA (FPS), free polyribosomal RNA (FPP), RNA released from polyribosomes bound to membranes by EDTA (EDTA) and RNA released from membranes by desoxycholate (DOC). The nuclear RNA species were nuclear particulate RNA (NP) and nucleoplasmic RNA (NS). The RNA species extracted from the various fractions were measured with respect to radioactivity and with respect to ability to hybridize with viral DNA. All hybridizations were done under conditions such that the amount of CPM was proportional to input. The per cent of total CPM (column A) for each RNA species is the ratio of total CPM in the corresponding fraction over the total CPM in all fractions. The amount of viral RNA in each fraction was determined by multiplying the net bound CPM by the ratio of total CPM in fractions to input CPM in the hybridization tests. The basis for this calculation is that the amount of viral RNA used in hybridization is well below saturation levels. The per cent of total viral RNA was determined by dividing the total viral RNA in each fraction by the sum of total viral RNA in all 6 fractions. Data from Roizman et al. (29).

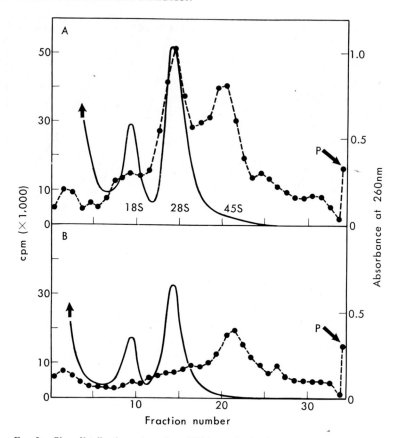

Fig. 5. Size distribution of nuclear RNA synthesized in HEp-2 cells infected with herpes simplex virus. Duplicate cultures of 3×10^7 HEp-2 cells were mock-infected (A) or infected with 100 PFU/cell (B). After 4.5 hr the cultures were incubated for 60 min in medium containing 5 μCi of ^{3}H-uridine per ml and then harvested. The nuclei of the cells were isolated with Nonidet P-40, and the nuclear RNA was extracted by the hot phenol-SDS method. The extracted nuclear RNA was precipitated with ethyl alcohol and centrifuged in an 0.5% SDS 15–30% (w/w) sucrose density gradient for 15 hr at 25°C and at 21,000 rpm in a Spinco SW 25.3 rotor. The 1 ml fractions were collected through a Gilford recording spectrophotometer. The RNA was precipitated with trichloroacetic acid and assayed for radioactivity. P marks the pellet at the bottom of the tube (*50*).

showed that the newly synthesized 45S ribosomal precursor RNA, made at reduced rates after infection was methylated. However, it was subsequently degraded rather than processed into 18s and 28S ribosomal RNA (Figs. 5 and 6). This finding indicates that the virus affects not only synthesis but also the processing of host RNA. It is noteworthy that the inhibition of synthesis and processing of ribosomal RNA coincides with the segregation of the nucleolus (Fig. 7).

The third effect of the virus is on the transport and utilization of host RNA. Recent studies in our laboratory (*29*) have shown (Table 1) that in cells pulse-labeled for 2 hr between 6 and 8 hr post infection, a substantial amount of labeled RNA accumulates free in the cytoplasm. Hybridization tests with viral DNA show

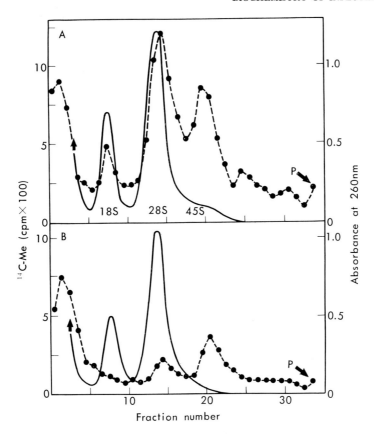

Fig. 6.   Methylation of 45S nuclear RNA synthesized in infected HEp-2 cells.   Duplicate cultures of 5×10^7 cells were either mock-infected (A) or infected with a multiplicity of 50 PFU/cell of herpesvirus (B).   The cells were incubated for 4 hr in EMEM containing 50% of the normal amount of methionine and then for 60 min in methionine-free EMEM containing 0.8 μCi of ^{14}C-methyl methionine per ml and 2×10^{-4}M unlabeled adenosine and guanosine.   The isolation of nuclei and the extraction and fractionation of nuclear RNA were the same as described in the legend to Fig. 5.   P marks material found as a pellet at the bottom of the tube (50).

that very little of this RNA is virus-specific.   By contrast, the amount of labeled RNA in free and in bound polyribosomes is relatively small but a very much higher proportion of this RNA is virus-specific.   Kinetic studies published elsewhere (29) have indicated that the host RNA which accumulates free in the cytoplasm is transported from the nucleus into the cytoplasm much faster than the RNA which ultimately finds its way into the free and bound polyribosomes.   These studies indicate that host RNA may be transported differently and is less able to function in protein synthesis than virus-specific RNA.

Protein synthesis

Electropherograms of total proteins from cells infected with herpesviruses show a gradual diminution in the number of bands of newly synthesized proteins, from

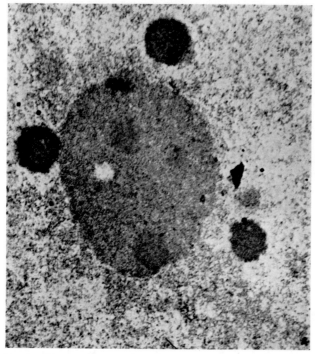

FIG. 7. Electron photomicrograph of thin section of HEp-2 cells 4 hr post infection with herpes simplex virus. Photomicrograph shows several components of disaggregated nucleolus (*38*).

too numerous to resolve at 0–2 hr post infection to some 10 or 12 bands corresponding both numerically and with respect to molecular weight to viral structural components at 8 hr post infection (*40*).   The mechanism of inhibition of host protein synthesis is uncertain.   The available data may be summarized as follows:

(i)   Amino acid incorporation into peptides takes place in the cytoplasm; entry of labeled proteins into the nucleus follows their synthesis by 2 to 3 hr (*9, 19, 45*).   These and other data indicate that the synthesis of viral proteins takes place in the cytoplasm.

(ii)   The rates of incorporation of labeled amino acids into acid precipitable peptides show an interval of initial decline lasting 2 to 3 hr, an interval of rapid increase in the rate of incorporation lasting approximately 2 to 4 hr, and, lastly, an interval of slow and irreversible decline lasting approximately 6 hr.   The pattern of initial reduction, subsequent stimulation and terminal, irreversible decline correlates well with the amounts of polyribosomes recovered from infected cells at different times after infection (*46, 47*).   The rate of decrease in the amounts of polyribosomes within the first 3 hr post infection is to some extent multiplicity dependent (Fig. 8) (*47*).   The sedimentation profiles of polyribosomes from cells infected with herpesviruses vary.   During the early decline in protein synthesis the sedimentation profiles are similar to those of uninfected cells.   Electropherograms show that both preexisting and new proteins are being synthesized during

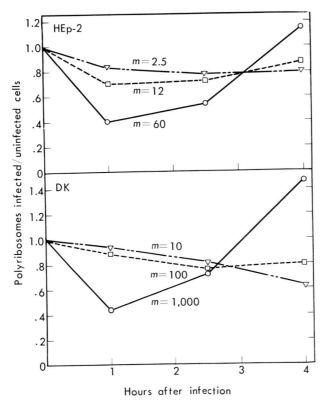

FIG. 8.   Effect of multiplicity of infection on the recovery of cytoplasmic polyribosomes at different times after infection of HEp-2 and DK (dog kidney) cells with MP strain of herpes simplex virus. *m*, multiplicity of infection.   Data from Sydiskis and Roizman (*46*).

this interval.   The polyribosomes extracted during the interval of stimulated protein synthesis are hydrodynamically larger and more homogeneous than those made in uninfected cells.   Electropherograms indicated that the proteins made during this interval are largely the structural components of the virus.   These data indicate that viral proteins are made on cytoplasmic polyribosomes, both free and bound.

(iii)   Recent studies of membrane proteins made after infection revealed that host membrane proteins are no longer made at 4 hr post infection (*39*).   Moreover, the proteins made before and very early after, infection are not glycosylated extensively, if at all, beginning 4 hr post infection (*41*).   We are not certain how long it takes for host membrane glycoproteins to become completely glycosylated.   As far as we can tell, viral glycoproteins take at least 2 hr and possibly longer.   These observations suggest that infection inhibits not only the synthesis but also the processing of host proteins.

These observations and the finding that viral RNA is selectively transported and associated with ribosomes in the cytoplasm (*29*), reported earlier in the text, indicate that the virus has three effects on the cell's protein metabolism.   First, the virus causes preexisting polyribosomes to disaggregate. Second, the virus precludes attachment of new host messenger RNA to ribosomes by modifying one or both components in the system. Lastly, the infection may also inhibit special aspects of protein metabolism, such as protein glycosylation.

Is inhibition of host macromolecular metabolism an essential feature of infection with herpesviruses?

In order to answer this question experimentally it must be rephrased. The experimentally definable question is whether it is possible for a cell to make both viral structural components including complete virions and its own macromolecules simultaneously. To date this has not been observed and thus the answer to the question is based on negative, and therefore inconclusive, findings. Nevertheless, it seems very likely that the failure to find cells which make both host and viral macromolecules simultaneously is meaningful, in that the inhibition of host functions is a necessary prerequisite to the biosynthesis of the structural components of the virus. This conclusion is based on studies carried out several years ago on the effect of multiplicity of infection on its outcome in productively and abortively infected cells. Specifically, in productively infected HEp-2 cells the outcome of infection—the production of the structural components of the virus and the death of the cells—is much less dependent on the multiplicity of infection than in dog kidney (DK) cells abortively infected with the same virus. As shown in Fig. 9, at high multiplicities of infection (100–1,000 p.f.u./cell), DK cells made viral DNA and proteins (2) which aggregated to form viral nucleocapsids (42). At relatively low multiplicities (0.1–100 p.f.u./cell) the cell made interferon and very few or no structural components of the virus (2). The remarkable aspect of these findings is

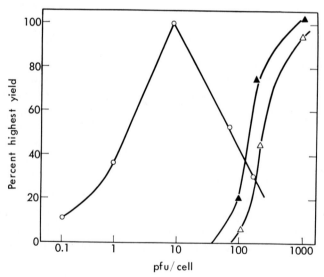

Fig. 9. The effect of multiplicity of infection on the outcome of infection in DK cells infected with MP strains of herpes simplex virus. Data from Aurelian and Roizman (2). O, interferon; ▲, DNA; △, antigen.

related to the fact that the physiologic states of the cells conducive for the synthesis of interferon, a host product, and of viral structural components, were mutually exclusive.   We subsequently learned that the production of interferon reflected the inability of the virus to shut off effectively host macromolecular synthesis in abortively infected cells and that in fact, as shown in Fig. 8, the inhibition of RNA and protein synthesis in abortively infected cells is far more multiplicity dependent than in productively infected cells (2, 47).   These data indicated that at least in the productive and abortive systems investigated to date (a) the synthesis of interferon directed by the cell and the synthesis of inhibitors directed by the virus are mutually competing events, (b) the outcome of infection depends on which of these events dominates, and (c) in productively infected cells the virus expresses its functions far more efficiently than in abortively infected cells, and consequently, the host is inhibited and only viral products are made.   On the basis of these findings it seems reasonable to expect that if a virus is capable of inducing interferon in a particular cell, rapid inhibition of host macromolecular synthesis would be an essential prerequisite for an abundant virus yield.

Modification of Host Membranes

Current studies indicate that cellular membranes become structurally and functionally altered between 3 and 7 hr post infection.   It is convenient to subdivide the membranes of the cells into two groups, i.e., internal membranes involved in virus multiplication and the external membranes which mediate changes in the interaction of cells among themselves.

Internal membranes

Electron microscopic studies indicate that internal membranes perform two functions in viral multiplication; i.e., they envelope the nucleocapsid and second, they assist in the egress of the enveloped nucleocapsids from infected cells.

Electron microscopic studies rely on the presence of partially enveloped nucleocapsids lined in apposition to membranes as evidence for the site and mechanism of envelopment.   This line of evidence (17, 25, 38) indicates that early in infection most herpesviruses are enveloped by the inner lamellae of the nuclear membrane, whereas, late in infection, envelopment takes place at all membranes of the cell. Three apparent exceptions to this rule have been reported to date.   First, the genital strain of herpes simplex has been reported to be enveloped by both the nuclear and cytoplasmic membranes not only late but also early in infection (37).   Second, Stackpole (43) published electron microscopic data which he interpreted as indicating that the herpesviruses associated with Lucké adenocarcinoma migrate from the nucleus into the cytoplasm by being successively enveloped and unenveloped by the inner and outer lamellae of the nuclear membrane respectively.   According to this scheme, the nucleocapsid is then enveloped by the internal cytoplasmic membranes of the frog kidney cell.   The third apparent exception is that of Marek's disease herpesvirus whose envelope is derived from the lamellae of the nuclear membrane and becomes further modified in a cytoplasmic inclusion (15).

The kinetics and molecular basis of envelopment are not known. Available information may be summarized as follows. (i) There is suggestive evidence that in order to become enveloped, the nucleocapsid must acquire on its surface a structural component designated as the inner envelope and containing lipids. The evidence for the existence of this component is based on three observations (*35*). First, an electron translucent shell with an ordered strucuure can be seen surrounding nucleocapsids in apposition to the nuclear membrane. Second, infectious virus particles from the nuclei of infected cells sediment in sucrose density gradients more rapidly than naked nucleocapsids, but more slowly than enveloped nucleocapsids from extracellular fluid and the cytoplasm of infected cells. The increase in the hydrodynamic size of infectious nuclear particles is too small to account for a complete envelope similar to that present on cytoplasmic and extracellular particles. Lastly, whereas both the nuclear and cytoplasmic infectious particles are rapidly inactivated by lipases and lipid solvents, the nuclear particles are far less stable in cesium chloride solutions than the cytoplasmic particles. (ii) Several observations suggest that envelopment takes place in two steps. The first step is a generalized modification of all of the membranes involved in envelopment. The evidence for

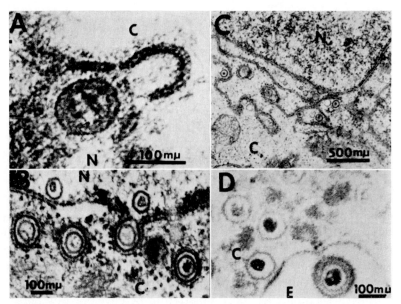

Fig. 10. HEp-2 membranes and herpes simplex virus envelopment. Electron microscopic studies. A, nucleocapsid (F strain) in apposition to the inner lamella of the nuclear membrane; the photomicrograph shows details of a structure surrounding the nucleocapsid. B, enveloped, unenveloped, and partially enveloped nucleocapsids (F strain). The nucleocapsids in the cytoplasm are enveloped and, moreover, they are surrounded by an additional membrane. The unenveloped nucleocapsids are in the nucleus. One nucleocapsid is partially enveloped by a thickened membrane continuous with the inner lamella of the nuclear membrane. C, unenveloped nucleocapsids in the cytoplasm of cells infected with G strain. Note that the nucleocapsids are in apposition to the endoplasmic reticulum. D, unenveloped nucleocapsids in apposition to the thickened cytoplasmic membrane of cells infected with G strain (*35, 37, 38*). c, cytoplasm; n, nucleus; e, extracellular fluid.

this step is based largely on the observation by Nii *et al.* (*17, 18*) who reported that virus-specific antigens line all internal membranes of the cells. The second step is a secondary, topologically limited modification of the membrane directly involved in envelopment; it occurs at the time the nucleocapsid comes in apposition to the membranes. The nuclear membrane at this stage manifests two changes, *i.e.*, first, the inner and outer lamellae dissociate and segments of the inner lamellae become thicker and exhibit a greater affinity for heavy metal stains (*37*). In general three lines of evidence suggest that the second step does in fact take place. First, the modification takes place only at the site of attachment of particles to membranes; distant sites do not become altered. The modified region resembles in structure and affinity for heavy matal stain the appearance of the envelope of the extracellular and cytoplasmic virus. Second, similar or identical modifications take place at the site of nucleocapsid envelopment at all of the membranes of the cell (Fig. 10). Lastly, in DK cells abortively infected with herpes simplex virus the nucleocapsids do not come in apposition to the nuclear membranes, the nuclear membrane does not become altered, and envelopment does not ensue (*42*). The molecular nature of the alterations is not known. It is conceivable that the modification reflects the change in membrane structure resulting from the expulsion of host membrane proteins.

The enveloped particles accumulate between the inner and outer lamellae of the nuclear membrane and in the tubules and vesicles of the endoplasmic reticulum (Fig. 11). There is suggestive evidence that the internal cytoplasmic membranes function as a special compartment which shields the virus from degradation in the cytoplasm—the site of initial uncoating immediately after infection—and transports the virus from the site of envelopment to the extracellular fluid (*25,26, 37*). The evidence is based on two observations. First, enveloped virions are usually found inside a tubule or vesicle (Fig. 11) and only very rarely are they free in the cytoplasm (*14, 37, 38*, and Felluga, 1963 cited in *37*, and *38*). Second, enveloped particles

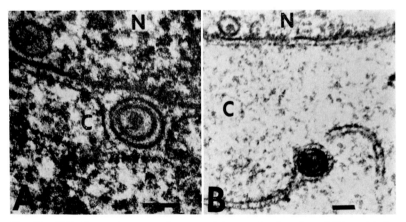

FIG. 11. HEp-2 membranes and egress of herpes simplex virus (MP strain) from HEp-2 cells. Electron microscopic studies. A, enveloped nucleocapsid between two lamella of the nuclear membrane at the point of ORIGIN of the endoplasmic reticulum in cells 8 hr post infection. B, enveloped nucleocapsid in the cytoplasmic tubule 12 hr post infection. c, cytoplasm ; n, nucleus ; e, extracellular fluid. Scale marker=100 mμ (*37*).

begin to accumulate in the extracellular fluid as early as 5–6 hr post infection, *i.e.*, long before the death and dissolution of the cells. Opinion varies as to whether egress is by way of tubules of the endoplasmic reticulum which communicate with extracellular fluid (*37*), or by way of vacuoles which break off from the endoplasmic reticulum and transport the virus to the plasma membrane (*14*).

External membranes

There is no specific evidence indicating that external membranes play a defined, unique role in virus multiplication other than to maintain the integrity of the cell. Nevertheless, there is considerable evidence that herpesvirus infection causes extensive structural, functional, and immunological modification of the plasma membrane and that at least some, if not all, of these alterations are due to virus-specific products incorporated into the membranes. The evidence dealing specifically with the external membranes may be summarized as follows:

(i) At least two laboratories have reported that infected cells leak macromolecules (*11, 50*). The leakage of macromolecules is intensified after the onset of viral DNA and structural protein synthesis. It seems very likely that the increased permeability of the membranes is responsible for the ultimate cessation of all macromolecular synthesis in the infected cells and that the phenomenon is due to an alteration in the structure and function of the plasma membrane.

(ii) A characteristic of herpesvirus infection of cells in culture is that the interaction of cells among themselves becomes altered. The nature of the change in the interaction—henceforth designated as the social behavior of cells—varies depending on the virus strain. Some strains cause the cells to form clumps of various dimensions and adhesiveness. Other strains cause cells to fuse (Fig. 12). The changes in the social behavior of cells require, at least in our hands, macromolecular synthesis corresponding in time to the onset of synthesis of structural components of the virus (*23, 24*). In general, the type of social behavior induced by a particular variant is reproducible and readily differentiated from that produced by another variant. The alteration of the social behavior of cells is therefore genetically determined by the virus.

(iii) The change in the social behavior of cells in necessarily mediated by a change in the structure of the plasma membrane. To paraphrase, any change in the function of the cytoplasmic membrane should necessarily be reflected in a change in its structure and, hence, in its immunologic specificity. The evidence that infected cells acquire a new immunologic specificity was obtained with the aid of a test designed to measure immune injury of somatic cells by antibody and complement. The test is based on the observation that infected cells fail to form plaques when seeded on monolayers of uninfected cells, if they had been previously treated with antibody and complement (*30*). The sensitivity of the test stems from the fact that very few cells are needed because nearly every infected cell produces a plaque. The plaque assay is simple and reproducible. The experiments, designed to test whether cells exhibiting an altered social behavior also manifest an altered immunologic specificity, where done with 24 and 48 hr-infected cells and rabbit sera prepared against infected cells (*22, 23*). The results showed that

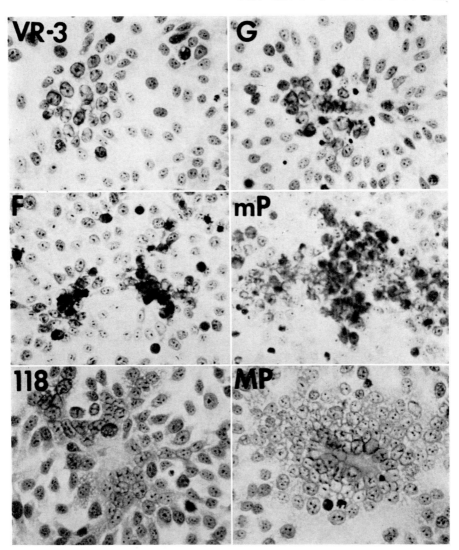

Fig. 12. The social behavior of HEp-2 cells infected with herpes simplex variants. VR-3 virus, rounding but little or no clumping of cells; G virus, loose clumps of rounded cells; mP virus, tight large clumps of rounded cells; 118 virus, small polykaryocytes which tend to fragment; MP, large polykaryocytes. HEp-2 cells were infected at a multiplicity of 1 PFU/ 1,000 cells and stained with giemsa 24 hr after infection. Photomicrographs were taken and printed at the same magnification. The size of clumps, polykaryocytes, etc., is representative except for that produced by MP virus, which is the smallest found in that culture.

complement and unabsorbed anti-infected cell serum preclude the formation of plaques by cells infected for 2, 24, and 48 hr. However, complement and anti-infected cell serum absorbed with uninfected cells were active only against 24 and 48 hr-infected cells; two hr-infected cells were unaffected. Clearly, the 24 and 48 hr-infected cells contained on their surface one or more antigens not present on the surface of uninfected cells. The basic conclusion presented here, namely, that the membranes of infected cells become altered with respect to structure and immunologic specificity was corroborated by Watkins (52). It is now clear that not only cells infected by herpes simplex virus but also cells infected with the virus associated with Burkitt's lymphoma (21), also exhibit new determinant antigens.

(iv)   Several lines of evidence indicate that the antigen on the surface of cells exhibiting an altered social behavior is a structural component of the envelope of the herpes virion. First, absorption of anti-infected cell serum with partially purified virus depletes the cytolytic activity of the serum (32). Second, as indicated earlier in the text, DK cells infected with the macroplaque strain of herpes simplex produce nucleocapsids which are not enveloped. Anti-sera made in rabbits against infected DK cells have very low cytolytic and virus neutralizing titers (42). In cell lysis-competition tests it has been established that infected DK cells compete very poorly with infected HEp-2 cells for cytolytic antibody. In these series of experiments the absence of envelopment correlated well with the absence of surface antigens and with the inability of infected DK cell lysates to induce both cytolytic and neutralizing antibody in rabbits (34, 42). The third line of evidence relating the surface antigen to a structural component of the virus is based on the correlation between neutralizing and cytolytic titers of various sera. We have produced anti-sera against a variety of viral preparations treated with reagents designed to degrade the virion. The potencies of the antisera in neutralization and in cytolytic tests vary considerably. However, there was a very good correlation between the neutralizing and cytolytic titers and of various antisera (34).

(v)   On the basis of the evidence that (a) the social behavior of infected cells varies depending on the virus strain and (b) the cells acquire on their surface a new determinant antigen similar or identical to that on the surface of the virion, it could be predicted that strains differing with respect to their effect on the social behavior of cells should also differ with respect to properties and characteristics related to their envelopes. This is precisely what was found. Extensive studies in our laboratory (7, 28, 31, 32, 49) have shown that herpesviruses differing with respect to their effects on the social behavior of cells also differ with respect to immunologic specificity, elution profiles from Brushite columns, stability at 40°C, and other properties related to their surface. These studies led to the conclusion that in the course of virus multiplication one or more structural components of the envelope of the herpes virion binds to the plasma membrane and that this component is responsible for the structural and functional modification of the membranes.

The chemical nature of the membrane macromolecules specified by herpesviruses

The preceding section enumerated the evidence indicating that both internal and external membranes of the infected cells become modified after infection by the addition of new antigenic determinants. The objectives of the experiments described in this section were to determine the nature of the virus specific components present in the envelope of the herpesviruses and in the membranes of infected cells. It should be pointed out here that the experimental objectives required membranes free of virus particles and conversely enveloped virus particles free of membranes. The procedures for the isolation and purification of the membranes and of the virus were designed to meet these requirements. It is convenient to present the results of these experiments in three sections dealing respectively with viral envelopes, membranes, and with the chemical nature of the changes in the membranes underlying the social behavior of infected cells.

(i) *Purification and analysis of viral envelopes*—We have purified enveloped and unenveloped nucleocapsids by the following procedure. The infected cells were Dounce homogenized in saline buffered with 0.05 M tris at pH 7.2 and then centrifuged at low speed to remove large debris. The cell sap was then centrifuged on a 10–50% w/w sucrose density gradient for approximately 45–60 min at 20,000 rpm in an SW25.3 rotor. On centrifugation, virus particles formed three bands designated from the top as No. 1, 2, and 3 and containing largely, but not exclusively, empty nucleocapsids, full nucleocapsids, and enveloped full nucleocapsids respectively (Fig. 13). In general the naked nucleocapsids (band 2) were by electron microscopic and other criteria quite pure. Band 1 was heavily contaminated by

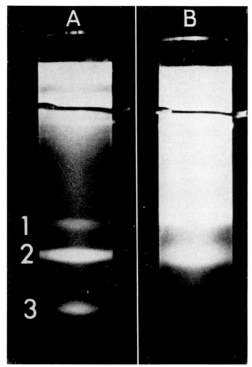

FIG. 13. Banding of herpes simplex virus particles extracted from the cytoplasm of 18 hr infected HEp-2 cells. Cytoplasmic extract was prepared by homogenization of infected cells in a Dounce homogenizer in 0.15 M NaCl, 0.05 M tris buffer, pH 7.2. The nuclei were removed by centrifugation at 2,000 rpm for 5 min. The non-ionic detergent Nonidet P-40 (Shell Oil Co.) was added to approximately one-half of the cytoplasmic extract in sufficient amounts to make 0.5%. The treated and untreated extracts were centrifuged on a linear 10–50% sucrose density gradient at 20,000 rpm for 40 min in the SW 25.3 rotor. Band 1 contained predominantly unenveloped empty nucleocapsids. Band 2 contained predominantly unenveloped full nucleocapsids. A, untreated; B, NP40-treated.

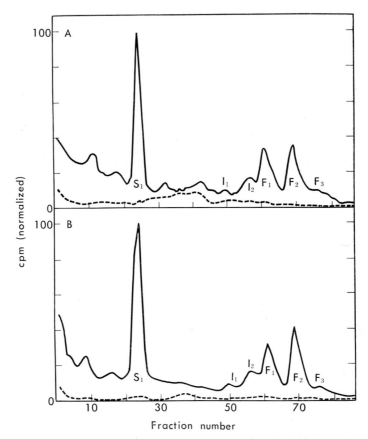

Fig. 14. Electropherograms of proteins in band 2 (Nonidet treated and untreated) of Fig. 13. The cells were labeled with ^{3}H-amino acids and ^{14}C-glucosamine. The nucleocapsids were solubilized in 0.1% SDS, 0.5 M urea, 0.01% β-mercaptoethanol at 37°C for 2 hr prior to electrophoresis (39). The data were normalized as follows: The amino acid counts were normalized with respect to the amino acid content of protein S_1. The glucosamine was normalized with respect to the glucosamine content in fully enveloped particles.

A, untreated ; B, NP40-treated.   ———, ^{3}H-Leu, Ile, Val ; ······, ^{14}C-glucosamine.

soluble proteins and was not purified further.   Band 3 was contaminated by membranes.   A higher degree of purification of enveloped particles in band 3 was obtained in the third step.   The material in band 3 was rendered 45% w/w with respect to sucrose, layered on the bottom of the tube, overlayed by a 20–35% w/w sucrose density gradient, then centrifuged to equilibrium.   Enveloped particles floated to form a band above the 35–45% sucrose interphase.   It should be pointed out that although this band contained fewer impurities than band 3, free membranes and unenveloped or partially enveloped particles were still present.

The electrophoretic analyses in acrylamide gels were done on viral proteins labeled with ^{3}H amino acids (Leu, Ile, Val) and ^{14}C glucosamine.   The electropherograms of proteins contained in naked nucleocapsids of strain MP (band 2 of sucrose density gradients shown in Fig. 14) revealed 6 bands.   Similar bands were obtained from virions treated with Nonidet P-40 which strips the envelope

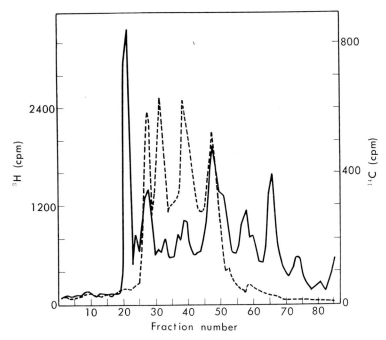

FIG. 15.   Electropherograms of enveloped nucleocapsids prepared from HEp-2 cells labeled between 4 and 18 hr post infection with ¹⁴C-amino acids and ³H-glucosamine. The enveloped nucleocapsids were prepared by isopycnic flotation of band 4 of sucrose density gradient centrifugation of cytoplasmic extracts.   ———, ¹⁴C-Leu, Ile, Val ; ······, ³H-glucosamine.

leaving the nucleocapsid intact.   The proteins contained in the 6 bands were not glycoylated extensively, if at all; this conclusion is based on the fact that the amounts of glucosamine which migrated with these bands was very much less than that present in the proteins extracted from the purified enveloped virus shown in Fig. 15. The difference between electrophoretic profiles of the intact virions and naked nucleocapsids which must be attributed to the envelope consist of 4 major and one minor band of highly glycosylated proteins.   Preliminary evidence, furthermore, suggests that one of the bands contains at least two glycoproteins.

(ii)   *Purification and analysis of protein membranes of infected cells*—In these experiments we employed the procedure described by Bosmann *et al.* (*3*) for the extraction and purification of cellular membranes.   The products obtained by this procedure satisfied the rigorous requirement that the purified cellular membranes be free of both naked and enveloped nucleocapsids.   The most important step in this procedure is equilibrium flotation of the membranes through a discontinuous sucrose density gradient from a sample layer containing 45% w/w sucrose.   This step separates membranes according to buoyant density rather than cellular topology and yields 4 bands.   Of these bands, No. 2 consistently contained smooth membranes free of virus, ribosomes, soluble proteins, and the other constituents of the cell.   Analysis of the membranes extracted from infected and uninfected cells revealed the following: (a) The electrophoretic profiles of glycoproteins made after

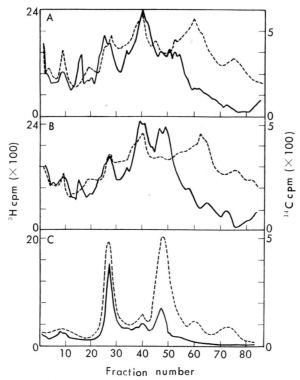

Fig. 16. Electropherograms of labeled membrane proteins and glycoproteins in infected and uninfected HEp-2 cells labeled with ³H-glucosamine and ¹⁴C-leucine, isoleucine, and valine of equal specific activities. A: Electropherograms of membrane proteins of infected cells; B: Electropherograms of membrane proteins extracted from cells labeled 12–23 hr before infection, then infected and inactivated for an additional 23–26 hr in a medium containing unlabeled precursor; C: Electropherograms of membrane proteins extracted from cells labeled after infection. The details concerning the solubilization and acrylamide gel electrophoresis of proteins, scintillation counting of acrylamide gel slices, etc., were the same as described by Spear and Roizman (40). The smooth membranes were prepared according to the procedures of Bosmann et al. (3) as described by Spear et al. (39). In this and other electropherograms the migration of proteins is from left to right; ———, ¹⁴C-glucosamine; ······, ³H-amino acid.

infection and extracted from membranes of infected cells revealed two major and several minor bands. The electrophoretic profiles of membrane glycoproteins from infected cells were consistently different from those of uninfected cells which contained too many bands to be resolved in acrylamide gels (Fig. 16). This finding is consistent with the observation that the virus inhibits not only the synthesis of host proteins but also further glycosylation of the proteins following infection. (b) The binding of the new glycoproteins to membranes is sufficiently strong to withstand considerable hydrodynamic stress. Thus, exposure of the membranes to anti-infected cell antibody increases their density and precludes the membrane floating to the top of the sucrose density gradient (Fig. 17). (c) To date incomplete analyses of the sugars present in membrane glycoproteins have revealed the presence of galactosamine, mannose, fucose and galactose in addition to glucosamine. Of

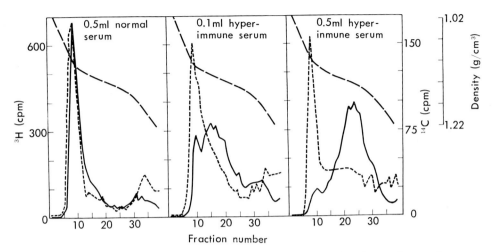

Fig. 17. Flotation of mixtures of infected and uninfected cell membranes in sucrose density gradients after incubation for 4 hr with normal rabbit serum or with varying amounts of hyperimmune serum. The incubation mixtures were made 45% (w/w) with respect to sucrose, overlayed with linear gradients of 10–35% (w/w) sucrose and then 3 ml saline and centrifuged for 20 hr at 25,000 rpm in a Spinco SW 27 rotor. The top of the tube is at the left. ——, infected cell membranes labeled with ^{3}H-glucosamine; ······, uninfected cell membranes labeled with ^{14}C-glucosamine; ----, density.

these sugars, fucose is quantitatively incorporated into the membranes as fucose. Most of the glucosamine is incorporated into the glycoproteins as glucosamine and galactosamine (Keller, unpublished observations). (d) Experiments designed to determine the site of glycosylation of these proteins have shown that the glucosamine is not incorporated into nascent peptides on polyribosomes, that glucosamine is incorporated into acid-insoluble material in the presence of puromycin, and, finally, that membrane proteins are largely glycosylated in the membranes. Concurrently with glycosylation, membrane proteins show an increase in apparent molecular weight in that they migrate more slowly in acrylamide gels (41).

(iii) *Membrane glycoproteins and the social behavior of infected cells*—As enumerated in the preceding section, there is considerable evidence indicating a correlation between the surface properties of infectious herpes simplex virions and the social behavior of infected cells. It was also shown that herpes virions have on their surface an envelope containing several glycoproteins. It could be predicted therefore that, if the glycoproteins are the macromolecular species involved in determination of the antigenic specificity of the virus and of the surface properties of the virion, viruses differing with respect to their effects on the social behavior of cells would specify (a) different membrane glycoproteins and (b) different envelope glycoproteins. In general, two lines of evidence indicate that this prediction is correct. First, and directly to the point, herpes simplex virus strains differing with respect to their effects on the social behavior of cells also differ with respect to the membrane and envelope glycoproteins they specify. As shown in Fig. 18, strains MP and G specify not only different viral envelope glycoproteins but also different smooth

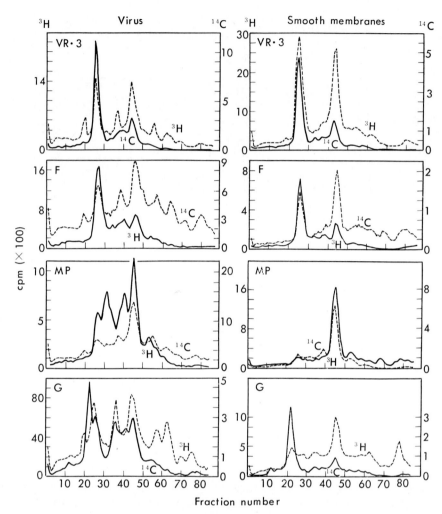

FIG. 18. Electropherograms of membrane and viral proteins prepared from HEp-2 cells labeled simultaneously with glucosamine and a mixture of amino acids (leucine, isoleucine and valine). The smooth membranes and partially purified virus were prepared from the same batch of infected cells. Solid line-profile of labeled glucosamine incorporated into glycoproteins. Dashed line-profile of labeled amino acids incorporated into proteins. Radioactive markers are as shown. The cells were labeled between 4 and 22 hr post infection with the strain of virus indicated. Data from Keller *et al.* (*12*).

membrane glycoproteins. Parenthetically, a very interesting observation which emerged from this study is that the binding of glycoproteins to membranes is ordered and not random. This emerges from the fact that in cells infected with the MP and G strains, the envelope glycoproteins differ from those associated with smooth membranes of the cells. This observation is particularly significant for the macroplaque strain which becomes enveloped at the nuclear membrane. The data suggest that the glycoproteins binding to the nuclear membrane—the site of envelopment—are different from those binding to smooth cytoplasmic membranes.

The second observation deals specifically with the significance of the apparent correlation between membrane and envelope glycoproteins, and the social behavior of infected cells. Several years ago, we reported that in cells infected with F and macroplaque strains, both viruses multiplied equally well, but the doubly-infected cells exhibited the social behavior of the cells infected with F strain alone. Although we concluded that the F strain was dominant over the macroplaque strain, the significance of this observation remained obscure. Recent analyses of the envelope and membrane glycoproteins specified by herpesviruses in singly and doubly-infected cells, revealed that, as would be predicted from the social behavior of

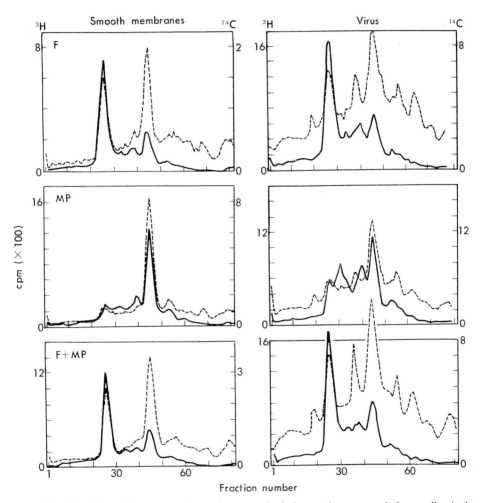

FIG. 19. Electropherograms of membrane and viral proteins prepared from cells singly and doubly-infected with virus strains differing with respect to their effect on the social behavior of cells. The doubly-infected cells were infected with F and MP strains at identical multiplicities of infection. All infected cells were labeled between 1 and 22 hr post infection in medium containing ^{14}C-amino acid mixtures (leucine, isoleucine and valine) and ^{3}H-glucosamine (Keller *et al.*, unpublished studies). ······, ^{14}C-amino acid mixtures ; ——— ^{3}H-glucosamine.

doubly-infected cells, both membrane and envelope glycoprotein profiles in acrylamide gels were those of the dominant F mutant (Fig. 19). The data indicated that the F strain was dominant and specified both the social behavior of cells and the composition of virus-specific glycoproteins binding to cellular membranes.

It should be pointed out that these studies are not yet complete. One of the questions that remains to be answered relates to the fact that the membrane studies to date were done on smooth membranes of the cell which are characterized by density rather than cellular topology. Since social behavior of cells is specifically mediated by the plasma membrane, it remains to be shown that viruses differing with respect to the social behavior of cells also differ with respect to the plasma membrane glycoproteins they specify. Studies designed to answer this question are in progress.

CONCLUSIONS

In the preceding sections we have outlined the evidence that productive infection with herpesviruses inhibits host macromolecular synthesis, modifies the membranes of the cell, and irreversibly leads to cell death. Obviously, we have a problem in that the behavior of this virus appears inconsistent with that of an oncogenic virus. In this conclusion I would like to develop the argument that the inconsistency is deceptive, and that the infection of cells in culture is not a faithful reproduction of the events occurring in multicellular animals. For the sake of simplicity and clarity I would like to present two arguments. The first deals with the comparison of cellular and viral functions expressed in cells grown in culture with those expressed in multicellular organisms. The second deals with the expression of viral functions in multicellular organisms.

Differentiation between cellular and viral functions in cells in culture and in multicellular organisms

There is considerable indirect and perhaps tenuous evidence suggesting that infections of cells grown in culture and in multicellular organisms probably do not follow an identical course. The argument may be summarized as follows:

(i) There is considerable difference in the function of animal cells in the artificial *in vitro* environment of the cell culture and in the whole animal. In principle, cultured cells act as single entities competing independently for survival. In the animal they are dependent components of a multicellular organism, perhaps readily expendable if they constitute a threat to the life of the animal. In evolution, the selective processes operate only at the level of the entire animal, whereas in cultures they operate at the level of the single cell. It is also very likely that regulatory pressures on cells in a multicellular organism and in culture are entirely different. This argument cannot be readily tested experimentally and perhaps it is trivial. The unavoidable conclusion is, however, that cells grown in culture and those in multicellular organisms may not react in the same fashion to the physiological stresses of infection.

(ii)   Cells *in vivo* do not become infected under the same conditions as cells in culture.   One of the requirements of biochemical studies is that cells in culture be infected synchronously or at least para-synchronously.   This requirement is easily satisfied by infecting cells at relatively high multiplicities.   As indicated in the studies presented in this paper, multiplicity of infection plays a role in its outcome and is more pronounced in cells which are non-permissive or at least which reproduce the virus very poorly than in cells which are entirely permissive and reproduce the virus very well.   In general, the measurements of the multiplicity of infection are misleading, because for every infectious virus particle there can be many hundreds, and sometimes thousands, of noninfectious particles which also enter the cell.   It is very likely that the multiplicity of infection of cells in multicellular organisms under natural conditions is probably no greater than one virus particle per cell and not just one infectious unit per cell.   On the basis of the data presented in this paper we could predict that at very low multiplicities inhibition of cellular metabolism would occur much more slowly and that, if indeed the cell is able to react to the presence of the virus, the outcome of infection would be completely unpredictable.

(iii)   It is very unlikely that the virus expresses all of its genetic information in infected cells in culture.   The arguments are based on the fact that most laboratory strains were recovered at one time or another from sick individuals.   Prior to infection of cells *in vitro* the information content of the virus was shaped and molded for many millenia for better survival in the complex multicellular organisms it normally infects.   Unlike the small DNA or RNA viruses, herpesviruses have established in the course of evolution a unique relationship with the host they usually infect.   The main feature of this relationship is that following primary infection, herpesviruses survive asymptomatically in some specific tissue for the life span of the host and only rarely do specific and predictable stimuli provoke the cell harboring the virus to reproduce it.   The significant aspect of this relationship, which is pertinent here, is that the capacity of the virus to survive in the host is not an indication that it is not capable of inflicting injury: herpesviruses frequently cause death or even severe illness in species other than their natural host.   Thus, herpes simplex virus infection of man is usually inapparent, and frequently serious, and rarely fatal; in the rabbit, the viruses cause severe damage to the central nervous system.   Pseudorabies is a mild disease of pigs resembling herpes simplex in man but fatal in sheep and cattle.   Herpes B virus causes an innocuous disease of monkeys; as many virologists have discovered too late, it is a very severe and frequently fatal disease of man.   In the light of these unique features of the natural history of herpesviruses, it seems reasonable to postulate that herpesviruses express their genetic potentialities more fully and effectively in the host in which they coexist than in the one they destroy.   Simple calculations in fact show that the virus contains sufficient genetic information for nearly 150 proteins of 50,000 daltons each. Present data indicate that no more than 10% of this genetic information specifies the structural proteins of the virus.   The functions specified by the rest of the genetic information are not clear.   In view of the complex behavior of the virus *in vivo* and the rather simplistic lytic cycle in cells cultured *in vitro* it cannot be excluded that the virus expresses more genetic information in multicellular organisms than in cells in culture.

It seems clear from the foregoing considerations that, while the biochemical features of productive infection of cells in culture are likely to reveal the minimum genetic information required to reproduce the virus, they do not reflect the full genetic potential of viruses in this group.

The expression of viral functions in cells of multicellular organisms

Attempts to reconstruct the events occurring in infected cells in multicellular organisms are beset by two problems. First, there is a clear difference between the response of animals naturally infected with herpesviruses native to them and the reaction of animals experimentally infected with herpesviruses native to a different species. The difficulty arises from the fact that these " natural experiments " are neither predictable nor easy to control; yet they are the ones in which we are obviously most interested. The second problem emerges from the fact that it is very difficult to study in a multicellular organism the events occurring in a single cell. Nevertheless some information, ideas, and surmises have emerged. These may be summarized as follows:

(i) The infected cell engaged in the synthesis and assembly of virions undergoes functional and structural modifications very similar to those which occur in the infected cell in culture. This conclusion is based on the fact that electron photomicrographs of cells producing virions in biopsy materials show nuclear and cytoplasmic changes identical to those seen in infected cells in culture (*13, 20, 44*). These changes are so drastic as to preclude any possibility that the cell might recover.

(ii) There is evidence that herpesviruses can survive in some cells without reproducing and possibly without killing it. The evidence is based on studies of recurrent infection with herpes simplex virus in man. In general, most individuals infected with this disease can predict very accurately the onset of recrudescences. The lesions usually recur at a particular site. In wrestlers and in patients vaccinated with live virus both the primary lesion and the recurrent ones often occur at the site of innoculation. These facts strongly support the argument that the recurrent lesions are due to an endogenous virus which survives in the tissue of the host. Moreover, extensive studies by numerous investigators have failed to reveal the presence of infectious virus at the site of recurrent lesions in the interim between recrudescences, suggesting that the virus is not multiplying at the site of recurrent lesions (*1, 5, 8, 10, 36*). Parenthetically, only a small proportion of Burkitt's lymphoma cells produce viral structural components and fail to multiply. Yet cloning experiments seem to indicate that all of the cells carry the virus.

(iii) Numerous observations, but particularly the data cited above, have indicated that following primary infection some cells reproduce the virus, whereas others retain the virus for intervals spanning the life of the host (see reviews by Roizman *24, 27*; Terni *48*). To paraphrase, herpesviruses naturally infecting a multicellular organism encounter two populations of cells. One population is directly permissive, reproduces the virus, and perishes in the process. The second population is conditionally restricted in that it retains the virus but does not reproduce it at that particular time. These observations raise three obvious questions, *i.e.*, what determines the status of the cell, what induces the conditionally restricted cells to become permissive, and lastly, what viral functions could be expressed in the conditionally restricted cells.

To restate the facts in a more elegant fashion, it could be predicted that in conditionally permissive cells the expression of genetic information for the synthesis of structural components and for the inhibition of the host is not expressed, and that induction of the permissive state terminates the repression of the genome. It could also be argued that at least some viral genes are transcribed in the conditionally restricted host and that the product of these genes is responsible for all of the immunologic, karyologic, and putative neoplastic properties of the cell harboring the virus. Some of the problems concerning the permissive and restricted cells have been dealt with elsewhere (*24, 27*). Fundamentally, however, the answers to these questions are not known. They are in fact key questions which must be answered if we are to understand the biology of this group of viruses. In reference to the topic of the Symposium it is clear that the biochemical features described in this paper are those of cells committed to make virus, and therefore not even potentially malignant.

These studies were aided by grants from the Whitehall Foundation, the U.S. Public Health Service (CA 08494), the American Cancer Society (E 314F) and the Leukemia Research Foundation, Inc. I am indebted to one of my colleagues, Professor J. W. Moulder, for pointing out to me the relatively low multiplicity of infection of cells in man and multicellular organisms in nature.

REFERENCES

1. Antonelli, A., and Vignali, C. Ricerche Sulla Localizzazione Del Virus Dell'Herpes Simplex Dopo Guarigione Delle Recidive Cutanee. Coltivazione Di Cellule Della Zona Colpita Da Eruzione Recidivante. Riv. 1st Sieroter. Italiano, *43* : 43–51, 1968.
2. Aurelian, L., and Roizman, B. Abortive Infection of Canine Cells by Herpes Simplex Virus. II. The Alternative Suppression of Synthesis of Interferon and Viral Constituents. J. Mol. Biol., *11* : 539–548, 1965.
3. Bosmann, H. B., Hagopian, A., and Eylar, E. H. Cellular Membranes: The Isolation and Characterization of the Plasma and Smooth Membranes of HeLa Cells. Arch. Biochem. Biophy., *128* : 51–69, 1968.
4. Ben-Porat, T., and Kaplan, A. S. Mechanism of Inhibition of Cellular DNA Synthesis by Pseudorabies Virus. Virology, *25* : 22–29, 1965.
5. Coriell, L. L. Discussion of the paper by B. Roizman. *In* Viruses, Nucleic Acids and Cancer. Williams and Wilkins Co., Baltimore, p. 241, 1963.
6. Darnell, J. E., Jr. Ribonucleic Acids from Animal Cells. Bact. Reviews, *32* : 262–290, 1968.
7. Ejercito, P. M., Kieff, E. D., and Roizman, B. Characterization of Herpes Simplex Virus Strains Differing in Their Effect on the Social Behavior of Infected Cells. J. Gen. Virology, *3* : 357–364, 1968.
8. Falchi, G. Herpes Sperimentale Recidivante Nell'uomo. Nota Riassuntiva. Boll. Soc. Med. Chirurg. Pavia, *37* : 885, 1925.

9. Fujiwara, S., and Kaplan, A. S. Site of Protein Synthesis in Cells Infected with Pseudorabies Virus. Virology, *32*: 60–68, 1967.

10. Findlay, G. M., and MacCallum, F. O. Recurrent Traumatic Herpes. Lancet, *238*: 259–261, 1940.

11. Kamiya, T., Ben-Porat, T., and Kaplan, A. S. Control of Certain Aspects of the Infective Process by Progeny Viral DNA. Virology, *26*: 577–589, 1965.

12. Keller, J. M., Spear, P. G., and Roizman, B. The Proteins Specified by Herpes Simplex Virus. III. Viruses Differing in Their Effects on the Social Behavior of Infected Cells Specify Different Membrane Glycoproteins. Proc. Nat. Acad. Sci., *65*: 865–871, 1970.

13. Luse, S. A., and Smith M. G. Electron Microscope Studies of Cells Infected with the Salivary Gland Viruses. Annals of the New York Acad. Sci., *81*: 133–144, 1959.

14. Morgan, C., Rose, H. M., Holden, M., and Jones, E. P. Electron Microscopic Observations on the Development of Herpes Simplex Virus. J. Extl. Med., *110*: 643–656, 1959.

15. Nazerian, K., and Witter, R. L. Cell Free Transmission and *in vivo* Replication of Marek's Disease Virus. J. Virology, *5*: 388–397, 1970.

16. Newton, A. A. Report of A. A. Newton's Paper by Cohen and Joklik. International Virology 1, J. L. Melnick Ed., S. Karger Basel, New York, pp. 65 and 253, 1969.

17. Nii, S., Morgan, C., and Rose, H. M. Electron Microscopy of Herpes Simplex Virus. II. Sequence of Development. J. Virology, *2*: 517–536, 1968a.

18. Nii, S., Morgan, C., Rose, H. M., and Hsu, K. C. Electron Microscopy of Herpes Simplex Virus. IV. Studies with Ferritin-conjugated Antibodies. J. Virology, *2*: 1172–1184, 1968b.

19. Olshevsky, U., Levitt, J. and Becker, Y. Studies on the Synthesis of Herpes Simplex Virions. Virology, *33*: 323–334, 1967.

20. Patrizi, G. Human Cytomegalovirus: Electron Microscopy of a Primary Viral Isolate. J. Lab. Clin. Med., *65*: 825–838, 1965.

21. Pearson, G., Dewey, F., Klein, G., Henle, G., and Henle, W. Correlation between Antibodies to Epstein-Barr Virus (DEBV—Induced Membrane Antigens and Neutralization of EBV Infectivity. J. Nat. Cancer Inst., *45*: 989, 1970.

22. Roane, P. R., Jr., and Roizman, B. Studies of the Determinant Antigens of Viable Cells. II. Demonstration of Altered Antigenic Reactivity of HEp-2 Cells Infected with Herpes Simplex Virus. Virology, *22*: 1–8, 1964.

23. Roizman, B. Polykaryocytosis. *In* Cold Spring Harbor Symp. on Quant. Biol., *27*: 327–342, 1962.

24. Roizman, B. An Inquiry into the Mechanisms of Recurrent Herpes Infections of Man. *In* Perspectives in Virology IV. M. Pollard, Ed., Harper Row Publishers, Hoeber Medical Division, pp. 283–304, 1965.

25. Roizman, B. The Herpesviruses—A Biochemical Definition of the Group. *In* Current Topics in Microbiology and Immunology, *49*: 1–79, Spinger-Verlag, Hidelberg, 1969.

26. Roizman, B. Herpesviruses, Membranes and the Social Behavior of Infected Cells. Proc. of the 3rd International Symposium on Applied and Medical Virology. Fort Lauderdale, Florida, Warren Green Publishers, St. Louis, Mo., pp. 37–72, 1970.

27. Roizman, B. Herpesviruses, Man and Cancer or the Persistence of the Viruses of

Love. *In* Of Microbes and Life, Columbia University Press, E. Borek and J. Monod Eds., in press, 1971.

28. Roizman, B., and Aurelian, L.   Abortive Infection of Canine Cells by Herpes Simplex Virus.   I. Characterization of Viral Progeny from Cooperative Infection with Mutants Differing in Ability to Multiply in Canine Cells.   J. Mol. Biol., *11*: 528–538, 1965.

29. Roizman, B., Bachenheimer, S. L., Wagner, E. K., and Savage, T.   Synthesis and Transport of RNA in Herpesvirus Infected Mammalian Cells.   *In* Cold Spring Harbor Symp. on Quant. Biol., *35*, 753–771, 1970.

30. Roizman, B., and Roane, P. R., Jr.   Studies of the Determinant Antigens of Viable Cells.   I. A Method and Its Application in Tissue Culture Studies, for Enumeration of Killed Cells, Based on the Failure of Virus Multiplication Following Injury by Cytotoxic Antibody and Complement.   J. Immunol., *87*: 714–727, 1961a.

31. Roizman, B., and Roane, P. R., Jr.   A Physical Difference between Two Strains of Herpes Simplex Virus Apparent on Sedimentation in Cesium Chloride.   Virology, *15*: 75–79, 1961b.

32. Roizman, B., and Roane, P. R., Jr.   Demonstration of a Surface Difference between Virions of Two Strains of Herpes Simplex Virus.   Virology, *19*: 198–204, 1963.

33. Roizman, B., and Roane, P. R., Jr.   The Multiplication of Herpes Simplex Virus.   II. The Relation between Protein Synthesis and the Duplication of Viral DNA in Infected HEp-2 Cells.   Virology, *22*: 262–269, 1964.

34. Roizman, B., and Spring, S. B.   Alteration in Immunologic Specificity of Cells Infected with Cytolytic Viruses.   Proc. Conference on Cross Reacting Antigens and Neoantigens, J. J. Trentin Ed., Williams & Wilkins Co., Baltimore, pp. 85–96, 1967.

35. Roizman, B., Spring, S. B., and Schwartz, J.   The Herpesvirion and its Precursors Made in Productively and in Abortively Infected Cells.   Symp. on Viral Defectiveness, Federation Proceedings, *28*: 1890–1898, 1969.

36. Rustigian, R., Smulow, J. B., Tye, M., Gibson, W. A., and Shindell, E.   Studies on Latent Infection of Skin and Oral Mucosa in Individuals with Recurrent Herpes Simplex J.   Investigative Dermatology, *47*: 218–221, 1966.

37. Schwartz, J., and Roizman, B.   Concerning the Egress of Herpes Simplex Virus from Infected Cells : Electron Microscope Observations.   Virology, 38 : 42–49, 1969a.

38. Schwartz, J., and Roizman, B.   Similarities and Differences in the Development of Laboratory Strains and Freshly Isolated Strains of Herpes Simplex Virus in HEp-2 Cells : Electron Microscopy.   J. Virology, *4*: 879–889, 1969b.

39. Spear, P. G., Keller, J. M., and Roizman, B.   The Proteins Specified by Herpes Simplex Virus.   II. Viral Glycoproteins Associated with Cellular Membranes.   J. Virology, *5*: 123–131, 1970.

40. Spear, P. G. and Roizman, B.   The Proteins Specified by Herpes Simplex Virus.   I. Time of Synthesis, Transfer into Nuclei, and Proteins Made in Productively Infected Cells.   Virology, *36*: 545–555, 1968.

41. Spear, P. G., and Roizman, B.   The Proteins Specified by Herpes Simplex Virus.   IV. ₁The Site of Glycosylation and Accumulation of Viral Membrane Proteins.   Proc. Nat. Acad. Sci., *66*: 730–737, 1970.

42. Spring, S. B., Roizman, B., and Schwartz, J.   Herpes Simplex Virus Products in Productive and Abortive Infection.   II. Electron Microscopic and Immunological Evidence for Failure of Virus Envelopment as a Cause of Abortive Infection.   J. Virology, *2*: 384–392, 1968.

43. Stackpole, C. W. Herpes-Type Virus of the Frog Renal Adenocarcinoma. I. Virus Development in Tumor Transplants Maintained at Low Temperature. J. Virology, *4*: 75–93, 1969.

44. Swanson, J. L., Craighead, J. E., and Reynolds, E. S. Electron Microscopic Observations on Herpes Virus Hominis (Herpes Simplex Virus) Encephalitis in Man. Laboratory Investigation, *15*: 1966–1981, 1966.

45 Sydiskis, R. J., and Roizman, B. Polysomes and Protein Synthesis in Cell Infected with a DNA Virus. Science, *153*: 76–78, 1966.

46. Sydiskis, R. J., and Roizman, B. The Disaggregation of Host Polyribosomes in Productive and Abortive Infection with Herpes Simplex Virus. Virology, *32*: 678–686, 1967.

47. Sydiskis, R. J., and Roizman, B. The Sedimentation Profiles of Cytoplasmic Polyribosomes in Mammalian Cells Productively and Abortively Infected with Herpes Simplex Virus. Virology, *34*: 562–565, 1968.

48. Terni, M. L'Infezione Erpetica Recidivante: Conoscenze E Problemi. L'Arcispedale S. Anna di Ferrara, *18*: 515–532, 1965.

49. Terni, M., and Roizman, B. Variability of Herpes Simplex Virus: Isolation of Two Variants from Simulatneous Eruptions at Different Sites. J. Infectious Dis., *121*: 212–216, 1970.

50. Wagner, E. K., and Roizman, B. RNA Synthesis in Cells Infected with Herpes Simplex Virus. I. The Patterns of RNA Synthesis in Productively Infected Cells. J. Virology, *4*: 36–46, 1969a.

51. Wagner, E. K., and Roizman, B. RNA Synthesis in Cells Infected with Herpes Simplex Virus. II. Evidence That a Class of Viral mRNA is Derived from a High Molecular Weight Precursor Synthesized in the Nucleus. Proc. Nat. Acad. Sci., *64*: 626–633, 1969b.

52. Watkins, J. F. Adsorption of Sensitized Sheep Erythrocytes to HeLa Cells Infected with Herpes Simplex Virus. Nature, *202*: 1364–1365, 1964.

Membrane Changes of Cells Infected with Herpes Simplex Virus

Kozaburo Hayashi

Department of Pathology, Institute of Medical Science, University of Tokyo, Tokyo, Japan

A number of papers have appeared which dealt with the alteration of the cell membrane due to infection by herpes simplex virus (HSV). These alterations include cell fusion or polykaryocytosis (*4, 34*), paralysis of cells (*14, 33, 42*), and a specific change of cell surface detectable by the adsorption of sensitized sheep erythrocytes (*46, 47*). The hemadsorption phenomenon of HeLa cells with sensitized sheep erythrocytes was first reported by Watkins in 1964 (*43*), who established that sheep erythrocytes sensitized with rabbit anti-sheep erythrocyte serum adhered to infected HeLa cells in an early phase. However, what actually is responsible for the phenomenon and what biological meaning it has remain yet to be understood.

In Watkins's report, he discussed the analogy between this phenomenon and the malignant transformation of cells induced by DNA viruses. He said " If a transformed cell is defined as a cell which has been infected with a virus, has undergone a change in the properties of its surface, and yields no infections virus when disintegrated, then for a period from about 6 hr after infection to the end of the latent phase, HeLa cells infected with herpes simplex virus can formally considered as transformed cells " (*44*).

The purpose of the present study is to follow Watkins's experience with the specific aim of elucidating the mechanism of the phenomenon and to examine its possible relationship to viral transformation.

MATERIALS AND METHODS

Virus

The HF strain of HSV was grown in HeLa cells. Infected cells and tissue culture fluid [Eagle's minimum essential medium (MEM) with 10% calf serum] were harvested when the maximum cytopathic effect appeared, pooled together, and frozen and thawed for three or four cycles. After centrifugation at 2,000 rpm for 10 min, the supernatant was removed, and was stored in separate ampules at $-90°C$ for use throughout the experiments. The titer of this preparation was approximately 10^8 $TCID_{50}$ per ml.

The Takaichi strain of HSV, which had been isolated in tissue culture from a patient of herpetic keratitis, was grown in HeLa cells and stored as mentioned above. The UW 268 strain and 196–2 strain (herpes virus type 2) were obtained through the courtesy of Dr. Wen-Tsuo Chiang, Department of Obstetrics and Gynecology, National Taiwan University Hospital, Taipei, Taiwan. These were passaged in HeLa cell cultures and stored. The Ska strain is an HSV highly attenuated for newborn mice (48). It was a gift from Dr. Kamesaburo Yoshino, Department of Virology, Institute of Medical Science, University of Tokyo, Tokyo, Japan.

Inoculation of cell cultures with HSV

Monolayer cultures of HeLa cells were grown in Eagle's MEM, supplemented with 10% calf serum on the coverslips of Leighton tubes. Two or three-day old cultures of HeLa cells in Leighton tubes were inoculated with approximately 10^7 $TCID_{50}$ of virus. By the time of inoculation, the cells usually formed almost complete monolayer sheets. Control tubes of uninoculated cell cultures were included in all cases. Cultures were incubated at 37°C for 12–16 hr and then tested for hemadsorption.

Antibodies and sera

Anti-HSV antibody was prepared in this laboratory with the following schedule. Rabbits were inoculated in their bilateral corneas with the Takaichi strain (0.05 ml, $10^{6.8}TCID_{50}$ per ml) after scraping the corneal epithelium with a 1/4 gauge needle. After 3 weeks, the rabbits were bled.

The immune sera thus obtained were subjected to fractionation by Sephadex G200 column chromatography to separate 19S and 7S antibodies. The specificity and reactivity were examined by immunoelectrophoresis and the complement fixation test (18). Rabbit anti-sheep erythrocyte serum was kindly supplied by Dr. Kusuya Nishioka, Virology Division, National Cancer Center Research Institute, Tokyo, Japan.

This serum was obtained by the immunization of rabbits with multiple intravenous and subcutaneous injections of Forssman's antigen of sheep erythrocyte. The 19S and 7S fractions were separated by Sephadex G200 gel filtration and DEAE cellulose chromatography. Antisera to human γ, μ, and α globulins were obtained by immunization of rabbits with pooled human IgG, IgM, and IgA myeloma protein mixed with Freund's complete adjuvant (Difco) (41). They were adsorbed by immunoadsorbent using Avrameas's method (3), and the specificities of these antisera were confirmed by immunoelectrophoresis. Anti-BJK (kappa), anti-BJL (lambda), and anti-Fab antibody were obtained from Dr. Morinobu Takahashi, Department of Molecular Immunology, Kanazawa University, Kanazawa, Japan.

Normal human IgG was obtained from the pooled sera of healthy staff members of this Institute. The gamma globulin fraction was prepared by precipitation with one-third saturated ammonium sulfate. Normal rabbit IgG was obtained from the pooled sera of healthy rabbits in the same manner as normal human IgG.

Hemadsorption

A suspension of sheep erythrocytes (5×10^8 cells/ml) in veronal buffered saline containing gelatine, $MgCl_2$ and $CaCl_2$ (GVB^{2+})(*18*) was mixed with an equal volume of antibody (antisheep erythrocyte 7S antibody) at a suitable dilution and incubated at 37°C for 60 min with gentle agitation.

The hemadsorption of sensitized sheep erythrocytes was performed on covers lips in Leighton tubes with cell cultures infected by virus.   These cultured cells were washed once with GVB^{2+}, to which was added 0.5 ml of sensitized sheep erythrocytes. The tubes were left at 37°C for 60 min or at room temperature for 120 min and unadsorbed erythrocytes were removed by washing the cells with GVB^{2+}.   The degree of hemadsorption was determined microscopically (*21*).

HSV-infected cell cultures were incubated with various dilutions of antibodies, chemical agents and sugars at room temperature for 120 min, which was followed by the addition of sensitized sheep erythrocytes.

Coverslip cultures of HeLa cells were infected with virus and incubated in an incubator at 37°C for a desired period.   Then, the infectivity and hemadsorbing ability were examined.

For a quantitative study of hemadsorbing ability, sheep erythrocytes were labeled with ^{51}Cr (*40*) and the CPM of hemadsorbing cells was measured by an Automatic gamma counter (Nuclear-Chicago Co.).

Treatment of culture cells with chemical agents and sugars

Infected cells and uninfected control cells were washed with GVB^{2+} and pretreated with chemicals in GVB^{2+} at room temperature for 60 or 120 min.   Following this step, the cells were again incubated in GVB^{2+} containing sensitized sheep erythrocytes as described above.   For treatment with sugars, the cells were incubated in GVB^{2+} containing sensitized sheep erythrocytes and test sugars.   The degree of hemadsorption was determined microscopically after a 60–90 min incubation at 37°C.

Of the enzymes used for the treatment of infected cell cultures, trypsin and phospholipase C were products of the Sigma Chemical Co., St. Louis, Mo., U.S.A.

Test for the agglutinability of cells using plant agglutinins

Wheat germ lipase and concanavalin-A were purchased from the Calbiochemicals Co.   Wheat germ lipase (100 mg) was dissolved in 5 ml of phosphate buffered saline (PBS), heated in a 63°C water bath for 15 min, and then centrifuged at 3,000 rpm for 10 min (*1, 7*).   The supernatant was serially diluted and mixed with an equal volume (0.05 ml) of infected HeLa cell suspension (5×10^6 cells/ml) which had been prepared by dispersing the cells with Na-versenate in PBS.   Concanavalin-A was also dissolved in PBS, diluted serially and mixed with dispersed HeLa cells in a hole glass (*16*).   Agglutination of cells was observed under a light microscope and the concentrations of agglutinins and the time required for agglutination were recorded.

Fluorescent labeled antibody techniques

Anti-HSV 19S and 7S antibodies were labeled with FITC (B.B.L.) (*22*). The 19S antibody (2mg/ml) was mixed with FITC at a weight ratio of 1/50 and incubated at 9°C for 4 hr with gentle stirring. Free dye was removed by gel filtration through Sephadex G25 and then fractionated by DEAE cellulose column chromatography to obtain a fraction with the F/P molar ratio of 5. The staining titer was 1:2. The 7S antibody (2% protein solution) was mixed with FITC at a weight ratio of 1/100 and incubated at 7°C for 4 hr with gentle stirring. Free dye was removed as above to obtain a fraction with the F/P molar ratio 1.04. The staining titer of the labeled 7S antibody was 1:128.

Coverslip cultures of HeLa cells were infected with the HF strain of HSV and placed in an incubator at 37°C. After an appropriate period, culture fluid was removed and washed with PBS. Then, one set of the culture cells in the Leighton tubes were pretreated with acetone at room temperature for 10 min and stained with labeled antibodies, while another set of the cells were stained with labeled antibodies, omitting the step of acetone treatment. The staining was carried out at 37°C for 60 min or at 4°C overnight. The stain was washed off by gentle agitation with PBS for 15 min. The preparations were then mounted with buffered glycerol and examined under a Tiyoda's fluorescent microscope (*22*).

Immunoelectron microscopic technique with enzyme-labeled antibodies (28, 29, 45)

Anti-HSV 19S and 7S antibodies were labeled with horseradish peroxidase (*2*), purchased from the Boehringer & Sohne Co. The 19S and 7S antibodies were mixed with the peroxidase at the weight ratio of 1:2 and 1:1, respectively. Then, they were coupled with 0.05 ml/ml of protein of 1% glutaraldehyde for chemical coupling and reacted for 2 hr at room temperature with gentle agitation. Free enzyme was removed off by salting out with ammonium sulfate and purified by gel filtration through a Sephadex G200 column.

Monolayers of infected HeLa cells were fixed *in situ* for 1 hr at 4°C with 1.25% glutaraldehyde and +2% formaldehyde (prepared from paraformaldehyde) (*20*) in 0.05M phosphate buffer at pH 7.2. After fixation, the cells were incubated at 4°C overnight with phosphate buffer, containing sucrose, with several changes. Then, the cells were scraped off from the glass bottom with a rubber policeman. After thorough rinsing with 0.05M phosphate buffer, the cells were incubated with horseradish peroxidase labeled antibody for 12 hr at 4°C with gentle agitation. The antibody was decanted and the cells were thoroughly washed with several changes of cold buffer at 4°C during a period of 12 hr. The cells were then treated with 2% glutaraldehyde for 1 hr at 4°C, and washed with phosphate buffered sucrose at 4°C with several changes overnight. The cells were placed in Karnovsky's solution without peroxide at 4°C for one hr, then incubated in complete Karnovsky's solution (*11, 19*) at room temperature for 30 min. On completion of the cytochemical reaction, the cells were washed with distilled water and exposed to 1% OsO_4 in Millonig's buffer for 1 hr, dehydrated in ethanol, and embedded in Epon. Polymerization was performed at 45°C for 24 hr and thereafter at 60°C for 48 hr.

To ascertain background peroxidase activity, some cells were reacted cytochemically for peroxidase without exposure to conjugated antibody. The embedded materials were sectioned on a Porter-Blum ultramicrotome MT-1. One group of sections was stained with uranyl acetate and lead, while another was left unstained and examined in a Hitachi HU-11D electron microscope.

RESULTS

Kinetics of virus growth and the development of hemadsorbing ability in HeLa cells infected with HSV

A one step growth experiment of HSV was carried out in Hela cells. For this purpose, confluent monolayers of HeLa cells in Leighton tubes (10^5 cells) were infected with the HF strain of HSV at a multiplicity of 10 $TCID_{50}$ per cell. At appropriate intervals, culture tubes were taken out and the total amount of virus was assayed after the freezing and thawing of the cells and culture fluid. To determine the hemadsorbing ability of cells in parallel, Leighton tubes were taken out and ^{51}Cr-labeled sheep erythrocytes sensitized with anti-sheep erythrocyte 7S antibody were added as described in Materials and Methods.

The results are illustrated in Fig. 1. The dotted line shows the infectivity and the straight line, the hemadsorbing ability expressed by the quantity of sensitized sheep erythrocytes labeled with ^{51}Cr. There was an increase of infectivity ($TCID_{50}$) from 4 to 24 hr after infection. On the other hand, an increase of hemadsorbing cells was observed for the first time 5 hr after infection; an exponential rise occurred thereafter, the maximum being reached at 12 hr after infection, following which a gradual decrease occurred. Thus, there was an apparent dissociation between the time courses of the hemadsorbing ability and the infectivity. A quantitative analysis of the number of ^{51}Cr-labeled sheep erythrocytes showed a perfect coincidence with that of hemadsorbing cells counted by a light microscope. Figure 2 demonstrates the hemadsorption pattern of HeLa cells infected with HSV, 12 hr after infection. The

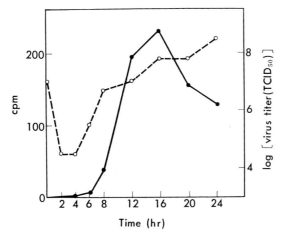

FIG. 1.   Kinetics of virus growth and the development of hemadsorption in HeLa cells infected with HSV.   ●, hemadsorption ; ○, virus growth.

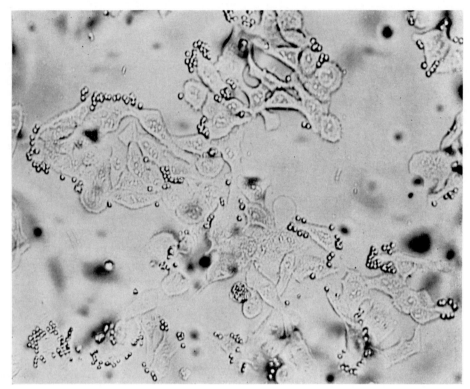

Fig. 2.   Hemadsorption of HeLa cells infected with herpes simplex virus.   Twelve hours after infection.

area adsorbing sensitized sheep erythrocytes did not cover the whole surface of the infected cell membrane, but was seen rather as a part of a distended cytoplasmic membrane in an early phase of infection.   Later, the entire surface of infected cells was surrounded by sensitized sheep erythrocytes, although some cells with uncovered surface were observed even in cases when the majority of cells revealed hemadsorption.   In contrast, hemagglutination of culture fluid and purified virus particle could not be observed.   The above mentioned hemadsorption experiments were made using sheep erythrocytes sensitized with anti-sheep erythrocyte 7S antibody.   When sheep erythrocytes sensitized with 19S antibody were used it was hardly possible to observe any hemadsorption in the infected cell membrane.

Effect of various physicochemical agents on hemadsorption

Table 1 presents results of experiments which tested the effects of various physicochemical agents on this HSV directed hemadsorption.   The cells used for this experiment had been infected for 12 hr.   They were treated with various chemical agents dissolved in PBS at room temperature for 120 min.   These treated cells then received sensitized sheep erythrocytes as in the preceding experiment.   Acetone, as well as phenol, iodoacetamide, dithiothreitol, mercaptoethanol, ethanol, ferricyanide, and, formalin, had the effect of abolishing the development of the hemadsorb-

TABLE 1.   Hemadsorption with Sensitized Sheep Erythrocytes

Treatment	Hemadsorption		
Acetone	₶5%	−20%	−50%
Phenol	₶1.25%	+2.5%	−5%
Iodoacetamide	₶5 mm	+10 mm	
Dithiothreitol	₶1×	−4×	
2-Mercaptoethanol	+0.2 m	+0.4 m	
Ethanol	₶5%	+20%	
Ferricyanide	+0.1 m		
Phospholipase C	−0.2%		
Trypsin	₶		
Formalin	−1%	−5%	−10%
Glutaraldeyde	₶2%		
Heating 56°C for 30 min	−		

Effect of treatment of HSV-infected HeLa cells with various chemical agents.

ing property of infected cell cultures to various degrees.   Phospholipase C also inhibited hemadsorption but conclusive evaluation of the result was rather difficult because of the equivocal purity of the enzyme used.   Trypsin was employed only at low concentrations so as not to cause detachment of cells; therefore, the evaluation of hemadsorption by cultures treated with trypsin was inconclusive.   Heating at 56°C for 30 min also abolished the hemadsorption property.

Effect of various sugars on the hemadsorption

Table 2 shows the results of experiments testing the effects of various sugars on hemadsorption.   The cells used for this experiment were at 12 hr post infection, as in the above experiments on the effects of chemical agents.   The infected cells received a suspension of sensitized sheep erythrocytes containing various sugars and were left at room temperature for 120 min.   Another set of the infected HeLa cell tubes was pretreated with GVB^{2+} containing the same concentration of the sugars or periodic acid at room temperature for 120 min and then received a suspension of sensitized sheep erythrocytes.   As shown in Table 2, periodic acid abolished the hemadsorption.   This may indicate participation of some sugar as the chemical structure of the receptor of this hemadsorption.   Fucose, N-acetyl-glucosamine,

TABLE 2.   Hemadsorption with Sensitized Sheep Erythrocytes

Periodic acid	±1.25%	−2.5%	−5%
Fucose	₶2.5 mm	₶5 mm	−10 mm
Galactose	₶2.5 mm	₶5 mm	+10 mm
N-acetylgalactosamine	₶2.5 mm	₶5 mm	₶10 mm
N-acetylglucosamine	₶2.5 mm	+5 mm	+10 mm
Glucosamine	₶2.5 mm	₶5 mm	₶10 mm
Mannosamine	₶1.25 mm	+25 mm	±5 mm
Mannite	₶2.5 mm	₶5 mm	+10 mm
Sialic acid	₶2.5 mm	₶5 mm	₶10 mm
Sialidase	₶		

Effect of treatment of HSV infected HeLa cells with various sugars.

mannosamine, and mannite showed weak inhibitory effects but evaluation of the effects of those sugars was inconclusive owing to their weak reactivity.

The relationship between the hemadsorption phenomenon and the agglutination of the cells by plant agglutinins

As described in the Introduction, Watkins discussed the similarlity of the phenomenon of hemadsorption and viral transformation. Hence, the next experiments aimed at determining whether this phenomenon shared some nature common to all viral transformations. Figure 3 summarizes the changes in the agglutinability of HeLa cells after infection with various strains of HSV. The upper half shows the agglutinability of concanavalin-A, and the lower half, that of wheat germ agglutinin. A HeLa cell suspension (about 5×10^6 cells/ml) harvested at various times after infection was mixed with agglutinin of various concentrations in hole glass and agitated gently 5 min at room temperature. The maximum dilution of agglutinin which agglutinated the cells is plotted in the graph. It was evident that the agglutinability of cells infected with various strains of HSV did not increase, but rather, decreased, during the process. These results show that the membrane changes detectable with these agglutinins did not occur on the membrane of HSV-infected HeLa cells. In other words, the agglutinability and the hemadsorption phenomenon are different

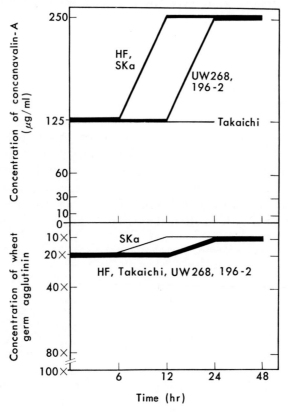

Fig. 3. Agglutination of HeLa cells after infection with various strains of HSV.

modifications of the cell membrane.   These results also coincided with those of the above sugar inhibition tests.

Effects of various antibodies on the hemadsorption

Effects of various antibodies on the hemadsorption of HSV-infected cells were examined, using HeLa cells infected with HSV for 12 hr, and, as a control, uninfected cells.   They were treated with serially diluted antibodies in GVB^{2+} at room temperature for 120 min.   After washing three times with GVB^{2+}, these treated cells received 0.5ml of sensitized sheep erythrocytes and were incubated at 37°C for 60 min.   The results obtained are compared in Table 3.   Rabbit antibodies against human γ, μ, and α clearly blocked the hemadsorption and anti-human kappa and lambda chain antibodies showed a weak inhibitory effect, whereas anti-human Fab antibody, normal human IgG, and normal rabbit IgG showed no inhibitory effect.   These results may indicate the participation of an antigenic determinant common to these human immunoglobulins in causing the phenomenon. Of course, there is a possibility that the results were due to a cross reaction caused by host components or calf serum gamma globulin molecules which were a constituent of the growth medium of HeLa cells.   In agreement with Watkins (*44*), rabbit anti-HSV 7S antibody was capable of inhibiting the adsorption of sensitized sheep erythrocytes, but 19S antibody did not inhibit it effectively.

TABLE 3.   Hemadsorption with Sensitized Sheep Erythrocytes

Treatment	Hemadsorption		
Anti HSV 7S Ab.	$+100\times$	$-50\times$	$-10\times$
Anti HSV 19S Ab.	$\text{卌}2\times$	$\text{卌}1\times$	
Anti human γ Ab.	$+8\times$	$-4\times$	$-2\times$
Anti human μ Ab.	$+8\times$	$-4\times$	$-2\times$
Anti human α Ab.	$+8\times$	$-4\times$	$-2\times$
Anti human κ Ab.	$\text{卌}4\times$	$\text{卌}2\times$	
Anti human λ Ab.	$\text{卌}4\times$	$\text{卌}2\times$	
Anti human $F_{ab}(I_gG)$ Ab.	$\text{卌}4\times$	$\text{卌}2\times$	
Normal human I_gG	卌		
Normal rabbit I_gG	卌		

Effect of treatment of HSV-infected HeLa cells with various antibodies.

Immunofluorescent study of HSV-infected cells

In connection with the inhibitory effect of anti-HSV serum, an immunofluorescent study of HSV-infected HeLa cells was performed.   After 3–4 hr incubation of HSV-infected HeLa cells, a weak fluorescence appeared in the cytoplasm near the nuclear membrane when reacted with an anti-HSV 19S antibody.   Figure 4 shows the antigen detected with anti-HSV 19S antibody.   Figure 5 shows the fine granular fluorescence corresponding to anti-HSV 7S antibody;   this appeared also in the cytoplasm, about 1 hr later than that corresponding to 19S antibody and spread gradually thereafter in the cytoplasm, increasing the intensity of the fluorescence. Fig. 6 shows the fluorescence of the cytoplasm 8 hr after infection as detected by staining with anti-HSV 7S antibody.

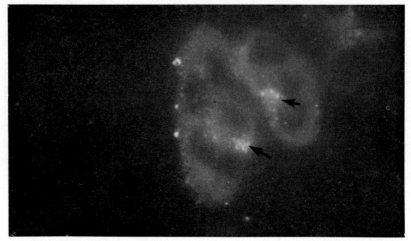

FIG. 4.　HeLa cells infected with HSV stained with anti-HSV 19S antibody (nonacetone treated).　Three hr after infection.　The arrows show the weak fluorescence near the nuclear membrane.

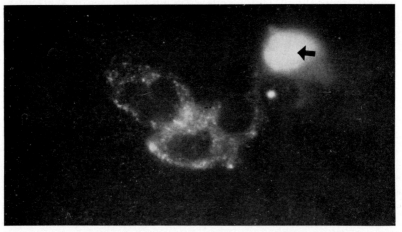

FIG. 5.　HeLa cells 5 hr after infection strained with anti-HSV 7S antibody (nonacetone treated).　The arrow shows the nonspecific autofluorescence of dust.

　　By 8 to 10 hr after infection, a specific fluorescence also appeared in the cytoplasmic membrane.　Figures 7, and 8 show the fluorescence of cells 12 and 16 hr after infection, stained with anti-HSV 19S and 7S antibody, respectively.　The cell surface membrane and cytoplasm fluoresced strongly.　This time corresponds to the stage of the maximal hemadsorbing ability of cells.　It is important that the fluorescence of acetone treated cells is different from that of the nontreated cells.　Fluorescence of the cytoplasmic membrane diminished to a considerable degree in acetone-treated cells.　This fact, taken together with the inhibitory effect of acetone on the hemadsorption of HeLa cells, may suggest that a substance of the receptor site responsible for combination with the Fc side of hemolysin is extracted or destroyed by acetone.

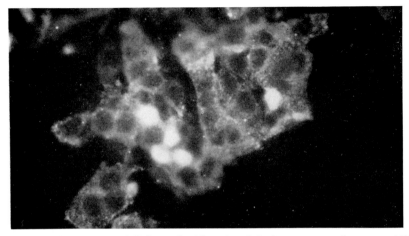

Fig. 6. Fluorescence of HeLa cells 8 hr after infection corresponding to anti-HSV 7S antibody (nonacetone treated).

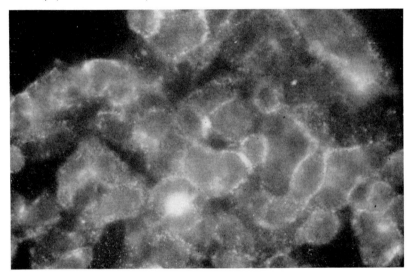

Fig. 7. HeLa cell 12 hr after infection stained with anti-HSV 19S antibody (nonacetone treated).

Immunoelectron microscopic study of infected HeLa cells

An immunoelectron microscopic study of infected HeLa cells was conducted as described in Materials and Methods. Peroxidase-labeled anti-HSV 7S and 19S antibodies were added separately to infected HeLa cells. Figure 9 shows cells 4 hr after infection, after reaction with labeled 7S antibody. In this early stage, specific reaction products are seen on the nuclear membrane (see arrow). Thereafter, after the 8th hr post-infection, the specific reaction products were also seen on the rough endoplasmic reticulum (ER), cytoplasmic free ribosomes, inner nuclear membrane, and cytoplasmic membrane. These patterns correspond well to the findings of the immunofluorescent study. Figures 10 and 11 show cells 12 hr after infection, after reaction with labeled 7S and 19S antibody, respectively.

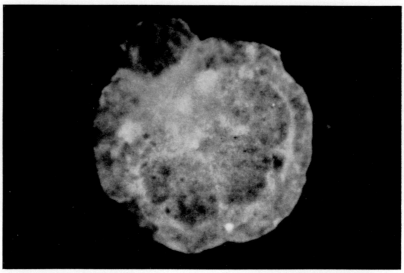

Fig. 8. HeLa cell 16 hr after infection stained with anti-HSV 7S antibody (acetone-treated).

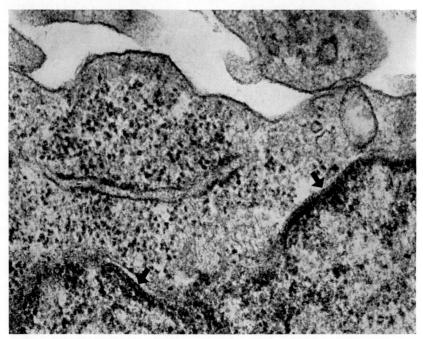

Fig. 9. HeLa cell infected with HSV after reaction with peroxidase labeled anti-HSV 7S antibody. Four hours after infection. The arrows show the positive reaction products.

The specific reaction products are seen on the rough ER and cytoplasmic membrane (see arrow). As described above, the earliest appearance of hemadsorption was at 5 hr after infection (Fig. 1). At this time, the viral antigen could not be detected either by immunofluorescence or by the immunoelectron microscopic method in the cytoplasmic membrane of cells.

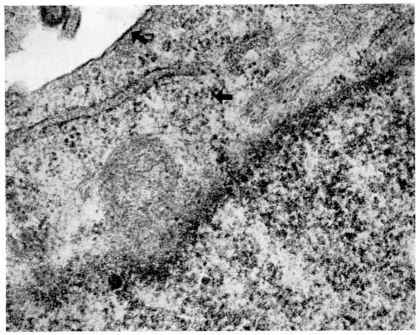

FIG. 10. HeLa cell 12 hr after infection of HSV after reaction with peroxidase labeled anti-HSV 7S antibody (no electron staining). The arrows show the positive reaction products in the cytoplasmic membrane and rough ER.

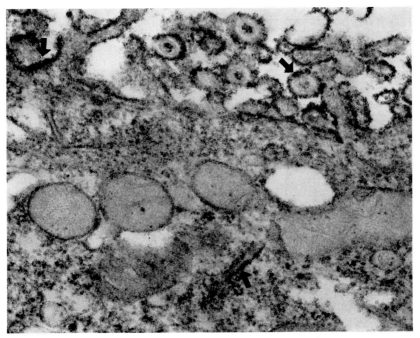

FIG. 11. HeLa cell 12 hr, after infection of HSV, stained with peroxidase-labeled anti-HSV 19S antibody (no electron staining). The arrows show the positive reaction products.

DISCUSSION

The present experiments have confirmed the report of Watkins concerning the adsorption to HSV-infected cell cultures of sheep erythrocytes sensitized with rabbit anti-sheep erythrocytes 7S antibody (43, 44, 47). The kinetics of virus growth and the development of the hemadsorbing ability in infected HeLa cells herein described were quite similar to the reported results (35, 44).

The early appearance of the hemadsorbing ability in advance of the rise of the infective virus titer was also confirmed.

The quantitation of hemadsorption using sensitized sheep erythrocyte labeled with ^{51}Cr was quite useful, the results coinciding well with the counts of hemadsorbing cells under a light microscope. This made feasible the performance of an extensive quantitative study on the inhibition of hemadsorption by a number of physicochemical agents, sugars, and antibodies, permitting an approach to the precise estimation of the binding force of erythrocytes to the infected cell membrane and the nature of the receptor site responsible for it.

It may be worthwhile to compare the physicochemical properties of the cell site responsible for this hemadsorption with those of the cytophilic antibody receptor site (IgG receptor) of macrophages found by Sorkins, and Howard and Benacerraf (15, 36). Chemicals which characteristically react with sulfhydryl groups, such as iodoacetamide, and those which react with free amino groups, such a formalin, both showed inhibitory effects on the activity of the IgG receptor of macrophages; whereas treatment with reducing agents, such as mercaptoethanol or inhibitors of the respiratory system, such as ferricyanide, did not cause such inhibition (15, 26, 35, 36). In contrast, the present experiments indicated various degrees of inhibition of the HSV directed hemadsorption by mercaptoethanol and ferricyanide. Therefore, these two phenomena may utilize different receptor sites.

Another difference, which is more important, is that acetone inhibits the HSV directed hemadsorption but not the activity of the cytophilic antibody receptor of macrophages. A finding of importance relevant to this was that the membrane fluorescence of HSV-infected HeLa cells diminished to a considerable degree after the acetone treatment. It can be assumed, therefore, that the substances functioning as the receptor sites for the Fc side of immunoglobulin and hemolysin may be identical or equally extracted or destroyed by acetone. Yasuda and Milgrom (47) and Shimizu (35) also discussed the similarity between this phenomenon and the cytophilic antibody receptor of macrophages. Recently, Gelderman (9) reported that cytomegalovirus infected cells acquired the property to engulf Toxoplasma gondii into their cytoplasm. Since cells infected with the other human herpes viruses, cytomegalo and varicella-zoster, failed to show the hemadsorbing ability in my experiments (not described in the Results), the modification of cell membrane activity may be evoked specifically by infection with a certain virus. Thus, the difference and similarity between the receptor responsible for the hemadsorption phenomenon and the cytophilic antibody receptor on the surface of macrophages must be open to further studies.

Phospholipase C inhibits hemadsorption, and the effect of this enzyme may be attributed to the destruction of the integrity of the cell membrane structure (*47*); in other words, some lipid components of the cell membrane may participate in the receptor site of this phenomenon. However, since the enzyme used was of doubtful purity, evaluation of the effect of its enzyme is inconclusive.

On the other hand, periodic acid abolished hemadsorption, which may indicate the participation of some sugars in the chemical nature of the receptor of the hemadsorption phenomenon. Recently, Roizman *et al.* reported that new glycoproteins are synthesized on the smooth cytoplasmic membrane between 4 and 22 hr after HSV infection (*23, 37–39*). The relationship of these glycoproteins to the chemical nature of the receptor site for hemadsorption must be further studied.

The experiments on the agglutinability of infected HeLa cells by plant agglutinins aimed at determining whether this hemadsorption phenomenon shared a feature common to all viral transformation as suggested by Watkins (*44*). It has been suggested that a certain cell surface carbohydrate may play a role in determining the specificity of intercellular interaction by forming a recognition site on the cell surface, and that the malignant transformation of cells may be the result of a change in such a recognition site on the cell surface (*6, 7, 13, 27, 32*).

This idea has supported by the presence of a specific carbohydrate on the surface of transformed cells (*12, 13*). In 1963, Aub (*1*) discovered that cancer cells were agglutinated strongly and selectively by wheat germ agglutinin and the receptor site responsible for this agglutination was an N-acetyl-glucosamine of the transformed cell membrane (*5*). Inbar and Sachs (*16, 17*) reported that concanavalin-A also has similar effects on transformed cells, and that the chemical nature of this receptor site was a-methyl-D-glucopyranoside (*10, 17, 46*). Hence, it was attempted to discover whether cell membrane changes detectable by these plant agglutinins also occurred in HSV-infected cells, and whether there was any correlation between the hemadsorption phenomenon and such agglutinability with plant agglutinins. However, membrane changes detectable by these agglutinins did not occur on the membrane of HSV-infected cells. Therefore, agglutinability and the hemadsorption phenomenon are different kinds of modification of the cell membrane. These results also coincided with those of the inhibition test of sugars, since N-acetyl-glucosamine did not inhibit this phenomenon so effectively.

The results of the inhibition test using anti-human immunoglobulin antibodies are very interesting. These rabbit antibodies against human γ, μ, and a antibodies clearly blocked hemadsorption, and anti-human kappa and lambda antibodies showed a weak inhibitory effect. On the other hand, anti-human Fab antibody, normal human IgG, and normal rabbit IgG showed no inhibitory effect. These results may indicate that an antigenic determinant common to these human immunoglobulins may participate in the present phenomenon, and that the inhibitory effects of anti-human antibodies were due to a cross reaction of such host components. But it is difficult to suppose the possible existence of components causing a cross reaction between the HeLa cell membrane and human immunoglobulin heavy chains. It is well known that the Fc side of hemolysin is responsible for this phenomenon (*35*), and, as reported by Yasuda and Milgrom (*47*), the hemadsorption was mediated not only by anti-sheep erythrocyte sera but also by anti-human γ and anti-human IgM sera, strongly positive results being obtained with the latter. Therefore, the positive inhibitory effects of anti-human immunoglobulin heavy chain antibodies may be attributable to the occupying of substances which commonly exist on the Fc side of heavy chains of human immunoglobulins and that Fc side of antibodies used for the sensitization.

But it is surprising, and difficult to explain, that such substances are newly produced or exposed by HSV infection, and there remains another possibility to account for this phenomenon, *e.g.*, cross reaction due to calf serum globulin which was a constituent of the growth medium of HeLa cells, or the impurity of the antibodies. As originally reported by Watkins, anti-HSV 7S antibody of rabbits was capable of inhibiting the adsorption of sensitized sheep erythrocytes, but 19S antibody did not inhibit it effectively. These results may indicate that the receptor site has some of the specificities induced by the virus on the cell membrane or the specific antigenic structure related to the virus, but on the other hand, a steric hindrance effect of antibodies combining with the cell surface must be considered, especially in view of the inhibitory effects produced by various anti-human immunoglobulin antibodies. In other words, the present experiments suggest that the receptor site may carry an antigenic specificity related to the virus, but some alternative explanation may be possible. Anti-HSV 19S antibody could not inhibit hemadsorption effectively, nor could sheep erythrocytes sensitized with 19S hemolysin adhere to the infected HeLa cells under the same conditions. Some explanation may be possible to account for this phenomenon, namely, that the structure of the 19S antibody molecule itself does not permit its Fc side to adhere to the receptor site of cells; or that the efficiency of adsorption of 19S antibody is different from that of 7S antibody requiring a greater number of molecules and a stronger intermolecular force for adherence. What is the true explanation is not known at the present stage of investigation.

The immunofluorescent and immunoelectron microscopic studies examined the antigenic site of infected HeLa cells (*8, 19, 24, 25, 30*). The earliest appearence of hemadsorption was at 5 hr after infection. At that time no viral antigens were detectable on the cytoplasmic membrane of cells.

Although there is a technical limitation in drawing a decisive conclusion, the development of hemadsorbing ability seems to appear before the increase of viral antigens, detectable by immuno-histochemical methods, on the cytoplasmic membrane. It is further suggested that a steric hindrance effect of anti-HSV antibodies combining with the cell surface may be the main cause of the inhibitory effect of anti-HSV 7S antibody. The precise localization of the receptor site and its relationship to the viral antigens must be further pursued as an extension of the present study.

Recently, Nishioka (*31*) discovered that lymphoid cells derived from Burkitt's lymphoma also adsorb sensitized sheep erythrocytes, the characteristics of this phenomenon being similar to those of the HSV directed hemadsorption.

This may predict that events similar to those of early stages of HSV infection also occur in EB virus infection, leading to a similar modification of the cell membrane as that evoked by HSV infection. The problem of whether this phenomenon occurred as a result of the unmasking of a normally hidden host genome or by the aquisition of a new substance directed by the virus is left for further studies.

SUMMARY

HeLa cells infected with HSV adsorb sheep erythrocytes sensitized by rabbit anti-sheep erythrocyte 7S antibody in agreement with the previous study of Watkins.

Quantitative study of hemadsorbing ability using ^{51}Cr-labeled sheep erythrocyte showed the early appearance of the phenomenon in advance of the rise of the infective virus titer.   It was demonstrated that the properties of hemadsorption, examined by using various physicochemical agents, were somewhat different from those of the cytophilic antibody receptor of macrophages, especially when the infected cell were treated with acetone.   The pretreatment with sugars did not affect the hemadsorption, but some sugars may participate in the chemical nature of the receptor of the hemadsorption since periodic acid abolished the phenomenon.

The experiment on the agglutinability of infected HeLa cells using wheat germ agglutinin and concanavalin-A was aimed at determining whether this phenomenon shared a feature common to all viral transformations, as suggested by Watkins.

The agglutinability of the cells infected with various strains of HSV decreased during the time procession even at the stage of the maximal hemadsorbing ability of cells.   Therefore, hemadsorption and agglutinability are different kinds of modifications of the cell membrane.

Hemadsorption could be inhibited by anti-human immunoglobulin heavy chain antibodies but not inhibited effectively by antisera to light chains and Fab fragment.   Some possible explanations of these phenomenon were discussed.

Hemadsorption could also be inhibited by anti-HSV 7S antibody but not so effectively by 19S antibody.

In connection with these inhibitory effects of anti-HSV serum, immunofluorescent and immunoelectron microscopic studies were performed.

After a comparison of the fluorescence of the cell membrane of acetone treated and nontreated cells, and taken together with the inhibitory effect of acetone on the hemadsorption of HeLa cells, the possibility of the extraction by acetone of a substance responsible for the receptor site of hemadsorption was suggested.

On the basis of the results obtained by these immuno-histochemical methods, localization of the viral antigens and their its relationship to the receptor site of hemadsorption was discussed.

I should like to thank Dr. Kamesaburo Yoshino, Department of Virology, Institute of Medical Science, University of Tokyo, for his very helpful comment and discussion. I am indebted to Dr. Kusuya Nishioka, Virology Division, National Cancer Center Research Institute, Tokyo, for his invaluable advice on the preparation of antisera and for performing inhibition tests for hemadsorption.

I am grateful to Dr. Satoru Shimizu, Laboratory of Ultrastructure Research, Aichi Cancer Center Research Institute, Nagoya, for his advice on the preparation of agglutinins and the test for agglutinability.

I am also grateful to Dr. Atushi Gotoh, my co-worker for the immunofluorescent study, and to Dr. Hai-Chi Chen, Department of Pathology, The National Taiwan University, Taipei, Dr. Ikuo Suzuki and Dr. Munemitsu Hoshino, Laboratory of Ultrastructure Research, Aichi Cancer Center Research Institute, for their help in performing the immunoelectron microscopic study.

REFERENCES

1. Aub, J. C., Tieslau, C., and Lankester, A.   Reactions of Normal and Tumor Cell Surfaces to Enzymes.   I. Wheat Germ Lipase and Associated Mucopolysaccharides. Proc. Nat. Acad. Sci., U.S.A., *50*: 613–619, 1963.
2. Avrameas, S.   Coupling of Enzymes to Proteins with Glutaraldehyde.   Use of the Conjugates for the Detection of Antigens and Antibodies Immunochemistry, *6*: 43–52, 1969.
3. Avrameas, S., and Ternynck, T.   The Cross Linking of Proteins with Glutaraldehyde and Its Use for the Preparation of Immunoadsorbents.   Immunochemistry, *6*: 53–66, 1969.
4. Burgay, C. and Watkins, J. F.   Observations on Polykaryocytosis in HeLa Cells Infected with Herpes Simplex Virus.   Brit. J. Exp. Path., *45*: 48–55, 1964.
5. Burger, M. M., and Goldberg, A. R.   Identification of a Tumor-specific Determination on Neoplastic Cell Surfaces.   Proc. Nat. Acad. Sci., U.S.A., *57*: 359–366, 1967.
6. Burger, M. M.   Isolation of a Receptor Complex for a Tumor Specific Agglutinin from the Neoplastic Cell Surface.   Nature, *219*: 499–500, 1968.
7. Burger, M. M.   A Difference in the Architecture of the Surface Membrane of Normal and Virally Transformed Cells.   Proc. Nat. Acad. Sci., U.S.A., *62*: 994–1001, 1969.
8. Géder, L., and Váczi, L.   Localization of Nuclear and Cytoplasmic Herpes Simplex Antigens in Infected Cells by Immunofluorescence.   Acta Virol., *12*: 97–105, 1968.
9. Geldermen, A. H., Grimley, P. M., Lunde, M. N., and Rabson, A. S.   Toxoplasma Gondii and Cytomegalovirus: Mixed Infection by a Parasite and a Virus.   Science, *160*: 1130–1132, 1968.
10. Goldstein, I. J., Hollerman, C. E., and Amith E. E.   Protein-carbohydrate Interaction.   II. Inhibition Studies on the Interaction of Concanavalin A with Polysaccharides.   Biochemistry, *4*: 876–883, 1965.
11. Graham, R. C., and Karnovsky, M. J.   The Early Stage of Absorption of Injected Horseradish Peroxidase in the Proximal Tubulus of Mouse Kidney; Ultrastructural Cytochemistry by a New Technique.   J. Histochem. Cytochem., *14*: 291, 1966.
12. Hakomori, S. I., and Murakami, W. I.   Glycolipids of Hamster Fibroblasts and Derived Malignant Transformed Cell Lines.   Proc. Nat. Acad. Sci., U.S.A., *59*: 254–261, 1968.
13. Hakomori, S. I., Teather, C., and Andrews, H.   Organizational Difference of Cell Surface " Hematoside " in Normal and Virally Transformed Cells.   Biophys. Res. Comm., *33*: 563–568, 1968.
14. Hampar, B., and Ellison, S. A.   Infection of MCH Chinese Hamster Cells with Herpes Simples Virus.   Relation of Cell Killing to Time of Division.   Virology, *24*: 654–659, 1964.
15. Howard, J. G., and Benacerraf, B.   Properties of Macrophage Receptors for Cytophilic Antibodies.   Brit. J. Exptl. Path., *47*: 193–200, 1966.

16. Inbar, M., and Sachs, Leo.   Interaction of the Carbohydrate-binding Protein Con-canavalin a with Normal and Transformed Cells.   Proc. Nat. Acad. Sci., U.S.A., *63*: 1418–1425, 1969.

17. Inbar, M., and Sachs, Leo.   Structural Differece in Sites on the Surface Membrane of Normal and Transformed Cells.   Nature, *223*: 710–712, 1969.

18. Kabat, E. A., and Meyer, M. M.   Experimental Immunochemistry.   2nd Ed. Charles, C. Thomas Publisher.   Springfield, Illinois, 1961.

19. Karnovsky, M. J.   Vesicular Transport of Exogenous Peroxidase Across Capillary Endothelium into the Transport System of Muscle.   J. Cell Biol., *27*: 49A, 1965.

20. Karnovsky, M. J.   A Formaldehyde-glutaraldehyde Fixative of High Osmolarity for Use in Electron Microscopy.   J. Cell Biol., *27*; 137A, 1965.

21. Kashiwazaki, H., Homma, M., and Ishida, N.   Assay of Sendai Virus by Immuno-fluorescence and Hemadsorbed Cell-counting Procedures.   Proc. Soc. Expt. Biol. and Med., *120*: 134–139, 1965.

22. Kawamura, A., Jr.   Fluorescent Antibody Techniques and Their Applications. University of Tokyo Press, Tokyo, 1969.

23. Keller, J. M., Spear, G., and Roizman, B.   The Proteins Specified by Herpes Simples Virus.   III. Viruses Differing in Their Effects on the Social Behavior of Infected Cells Specify Different Membrane Glycoproteins.   Proc. Nat. Acad. Sci., U.S.A., *65*: 865–871, 1970.

24. Lebrun, J.   Cellular Localization of Herpes Simplex Virus by Means of Fluorescent Antibody.   Virology, *2*: 496–510, 1956.

25. Lesso, J., and Szántó, J.   Reproduction of Herpes Simplex Virus in HeLa Cells Studiec by Immunofluorescence and Cytochemical Methods.   Acta Virol, *13*: 278–284, 1969.

26. LoBuglio, A. F., Cotran, R. S., and Jandl., J. H.   Red Cells Coated with Immuno-globulin G.:   Binding and Sphering by Mononuclear Cells in Man.   Science, *158*: 1582–1585, 1967.

27. Meezan, E., Wu, H.-C., Black, P. H., and Robbins, P. W.   Comparative Studies on the Carbohydrate-containing Membrane Components of Normal and Virus-trans-formed Mouse Fibroblast.   II: Separation of Glycoproteins and Glycopeptides by Sephadex Chromatography.   Biochemistry, *8*: 2518–2524, 1969.

28. Nakane, P. K., and Pierce, G. B., Jr.   Enzyme-labeled Antibodies.   Preparation and Application for the Localization of Antigens.   J. Histochem. Cytochem., *14*: 929–931, 1966.

29. Nakane, P. K., and Pierce, G. B., Jr.   Enzyme-labeled Antibodies: For the Light and Electron Microscopic Localization of Tissue antigens.   J. Cell Biol., *33*: 307–318, 1967.

30. Nii, S., Morgan, C., Rose, H. M., and HSU, K. C.   Electron Microscopy of Herpes Simplex Virus.   J. Virology, *2*: 1172–1184, 1968.

31. Nishioka, K., Tachibana, T., Sekine, T., Inoue, M., Hirayama, T., Sugano, H., Yoshida, T. O., Takada, M., Kawamura, A., Jr., and Wang, C.-H.   Immunocyto-logical Studies on Cultured Cells Derived from Nasopharyngeal Carcinoma and Burkitt's Lymphoma and an Improved Method of Immunoadherence Reaction. Gann Monograph, *11*: (in press).

32. Pollack, R. E., and Burger, M. M.   Surface-specific Characteristics of a Contact-inhibited Cell Line Containing the SV40 Viral Genome.   Proc. Nat. Acad. Sci., U.S.A., *62*: 1074–1076, 1969.

33. Roane, P. R., Jr., and Roizman, B.   Studies of the Determinant Antigen of Viable

Cells.   II. Demonstration of Altered Antigenic Reactivity of Hep-2 Cells Infected with Herpes Simplex Virus.   Virology, *22*: 1–8, 1964.

34.   Roizman, B.   Cold Spring Harbor Symp. Quant. Biol.   " Polykaryocytosis," *27*: 327–340, 1962.

35.   Shimizu, Y.   A Modification of Host Cell Membrane after Herpes Simplex Virus Infection (in press).

36.   Sorkin, E.   On the Cellular Fixation of Cytophilic Antibody.   Int. Arch. Allergy, *25*: 129–144, 1964.

37.   Spear, P. G. and Roizman, B.   The Proteins Specified by Herpes Simplex Virus. Time of Synthesis, Transfer into Nuclei, and Properties of Proteins Mad in Productively Infected Cells.   Virology, *36*: 545–555, 1968.

38.   Spear, P. G., Keller, J. M., and Roizman, B., Proteins Specified by Herpes Simplex Virus: II. Viral Glycoproteins Associated with Cellular Membranes.   J. Virol., *5*: 123–131, 1970.

39.   Spear, P. G., and Roizman, B.   Proteins Specified by Herpes Simplex Virus.   IV. Site of Glycosylation and Accumulation of Viral Membrane Proteins.   Proc. Nat. Acad. Sci., U.S.A., *66*: 730–737, 1970.

40.   Strumia, M. M., Yaylor, L. Sample, A. B., Colewell, L. S., and Dugan, A.   Uses and Limitations of Survival Studies of Erythrocytes Tagged with ^{51}Cr.   Blood, *10*: 429, 1955.

41.   Takahashi, M., Yagi, Y., and Pressman, D.   Preparation of Fluorescent Antibody Reagents Monospecific to Heavy Chains of Human Immunoglobulin.   J. Immunol., *100*: 1160–1175, 1968.

42.   Watkins, J. F., Inhibition of Spreading of HeLa Cells after Infection with Herpes Simplex Virus.   Virology, *23*: 436–438, 1964.

43.   Watkins, J. F.   Adsorption of Sensitized Sheep Erythrocytes to HeLa Cells Infected with Herpes Simplex Virus.   Nature, *202*: 1364–1365, 1964.

44.   Watkins, J. F.   The Relationship of the Herpes Simplex Hemadsorption Phenomenon to the Virus Growth Cycle, Virology, *26*: 746–753, 1965.

45.   Wicker, R., and Avrameas, S.   Localization of Virus Antigens by Enzyme-labeled Antibodies.   J. gen. Virol., *4*: 465–471, 1969.

46.   Yariv, J. A., Kalb, J., and Levitzki, A.   The Interaction of Concanavalin A with Methyl-alpha-D-glucopyranoside.   Biochem. Biophys. Acta, *165*: 303–305, 1968.

47.   Yasuda, J., and Milgrom, F.   Hemadsorption by Herpes Simplex-infected Cell cultures.   Int. Arch. Allergy, *33*: 151–170, 1968.

48.   Yoshino, K., and Taniguchi, S.   Isolation of a Clone of Herpes Simplex Virus Highly Attenuated for Newborn Mice and Hamster.   Jap. J. Exp. Med., *39*: 223–233, 1969.

Discussion of Papers by Drs. Roizman, and Hayashi

DR. HINUMA: Dr. Roizman, do you have any test for inhibition of glycoprotein synthesis in infected cells by cytosine arabinoside or FUDR? In other words, is synthesis of viral DNA necessary for formation of specific glycoprotein?

DR. ROIZMAN: Yes, as a matter of fact, we do have information on this. We have two observations. Cytosine arabinoside will inhibit the synthesis of membrane-specific glycoprotein. We do not know whether FUDR inhibits or not. IUDR does inhibit, but the effect is strange. If you wait for another 4 or 5 hr beyond the normal time of synthesis of glycoprotein, they will ultimately show up. But cytosine arabinoside, on the other hand, does inhibit glycoprotein and the effect is more than a delay, because we don't see it 24 hr later.

DR. G. KLEIN: I have a question for Dr. Hayashi, whether his hemadsorption phenomenon is easy to change in the sense that it appears in the presence of DNA inhibitors. As I recall from Watkins' paper, he studied IUDR, and, as I recall it, the change did appear. In relation to what Dr. Roizman just said, is it possible to say that the time of appearance or the inhibitability of the membrane change as studied in Dr. Hayashi's system is similar to the glycoprotein changes studied by Dr. Roizman? This is one question. The second point is that I did not quite follow the steric hindrance argument of Dr. Hayashi. Did I understand correctly that the anti-herpes simplex antiserum did inhibit the hemadsorption phenomenon, and that you nevertheless thought that the hemadsorption receptor was distinct from the virally induced membrane receptor and the cross reactivity of inhibition of this effect is due to steric hindrance? If so, what is the reason that you think so?

DR. HAYASHI: I don't think that there are no cross reactions but I do think that the steric hindrance effect may be the main component of the anti-herpes 7S inhibitory effect, because membrane fluorescence does not appear so early as 5 hr after infection. As to the effect of DNA inhibitor on the hemadsorption effect, I did not investigate it.

DR. NISHIOKA: Watkins showed inhibition by actinomycin D, but not by 5-iodo, 2-deoxyuridine, and in that way he described how inhibition of DNA-dependent RNA synthesis inhibited the appearance of the phenomenon of the adherence of sheep erythrocytes sensitized by rabbit 7S-antibody.

DR. W. HENLE: I would like to ask Dr. Hayashi whether antibodies to sheep erythrocytes can block the hemadsorption phenomenon. In another words, if the serum is used to treat the infected HeLa cells, would this block the hemadsorption? As the second part, can you get indirect immunofluorescent responses in infected HeLa cells with antiserum to sheep erythrocytes?

DR. HAYASHI: Anti-erythrocyte 7S-antibody is attached to erythrocytes and reacts to HeLa cells infected with herpes simplex virus. I have not yet tried it but anti-sheep erythrocyte antibody, if added at higher concentrations, causes sheep erythrocytes to agglutinate and the pattern cannot be observed. Anti-sheep erythrocyte 7S-antibody did not cause the infected HeLa cells to fluoresce.

DR. NISHIOKA: When HSV-infected HeLa cells were first treated with anti-sheep erythrocyte antibody and then sheep erythrocyte-IgG complex was added, inhibition occurred. Therefore, you can exclude the possibility of the cross reaction of anti-erythrocyte here and the receptor of HeLa cells infected with herpes simplex virus.

DR. DE THÉ: Dr. Roizman, you showed that in the F strain the virus had the same glycoprotein as the cellular membrane, but in the MPMG strain, the virus has a different glycoprotein from the cellular membrane. Now, in electron microscopy, do you find a difference in the virus between the nucleus and the extracellular space, because we have to have some reason why the envelope of the virus is different in these two strains, when it is on the envelope by other cytoplasmic channel of cell membrane in the different strains.

DR. ROIZMAN: This question is likely to open a hornet's nest because we have looked at this question very carefully. We find there is a difference between F or type 1 and type 2 early in infection, but possibly not very late in infection. There are a lot of unenveloped particles in the cytoplasm. They are attached to all sorts of membranes; they look partially enveloped or partially unenveloped, and it's difficult to tell what's going on. But we looked at cells 4, 8, 10 hr after infection, and the cell is still intact, and there are very clear differences between the two strains. The F strain has no unenveloped particles in the cytoplasm, the only unenveloped particles are in the nucleus. The only enveloped particles are either in the endoplasmic reticulum or in the space between the two lamellae of the nuclear membrane and the development is clearly on the nuclear membrane. For the genital virus, the enveloped and unenveloped particles are noted all over the place and both in nucleus and cytoplasm.

PROBLEMS IN
TISSUE CULTURE STUDY

Chairmen:

M. A. Epstein, Tadashi Yamamoto

A New Virus in Cultures of Human Nasopharyngeal Carcinoma

M. A. Epstein, B. G. Achong, and P. W. A. Mansell

Department of Pathology, University of Bristol Medical School, University Walk, Bristol, England

In recent years the Epstein-Barr virus (EBV) (7) has been found to be associated in some way with nasopharyngeal carcinoma. Thus, Old, Boyse, and their collaborators (19) had already shown four years ago that patients with anaplastic carcinoma of the postnasal space had a high incidence of precipitating antibodies to an antigen—apparently EBV—separable from cultured Burkitt's lymphoma cells. Following this, investigations using direct or indirect immunofluorescence tests (13) demonstrated by these further techniques, and on a wider scale, that all patients with nasopharyngeal carcinoma have antibodies to EBV capsid antigens, mostly at high titer, and usually also to other EBV related antigens. In addition, using a quite different approach, De Thé and his associates (4) have found that monolayers grown from biopsy samples of nasopharyngeal carcinoma frequently ultimately undergo " transformation " to give cultures of free-floating single cells which contain a virus morphologically indistinguishable from EBV. By present methods this virus is also immunologically indistinguishable from EBV. On the other hand, the importance of these results has been somewhat decreased by the further finding that control material from normal adenoids and from head and neck tumors other than nasopharyngeal carcinoma behaves in a comparable way to give floating cells likewise containing the virus (5).

In view of these observations connecting EBV with nasopharyngeal carcinoma, studies have been undertaken in this laboratory to investigate the nature of the relationship. Since EBV is known to be present in a high proportion of normal individuals throughout the world (9–11, 18, 20) and, like most herpes viruses, to be an agent which lurks for long periods in appropriate cells within the infected organism, it seemed important to establish whether the links between EBV and nasopharyngeal carcinoma were of an etiological nature or merely epiphenomena manifested by a " passenger " virus latent in infected individuals who happen to develop the tumor. Certainly, in the case of nasopharyngeal carcinoma the evidence for an etiological role for EBV is so far less striking than with Burkitt's lymphoma (see 12).

Material was therefore obtained from histologically authenticated cases of nasopharyngeal carcinoma from East Africa for a variety of virological and other investigations.

MATERIALS AND METHODS

Tissue culture studies

Biopsy samples were removed, through the kindness of Mr. Peter Clifford at the Kenyatta National Hospital, Nairobi, from East African cases of nasopharyngeal carcinoma and were flown overnight to London at aircraft cabin temperature in a transit fluid consisting of 50% human serum in Hanks saline solution. All the samples were set up in culture in Bristol within 24 hr. For this procedure, teased-

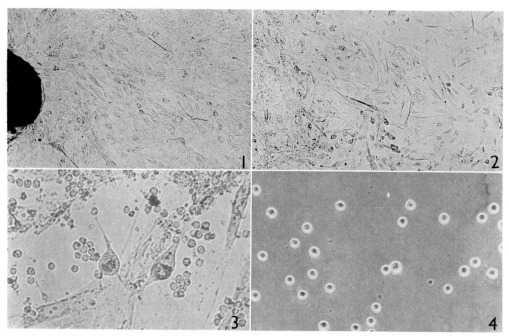

FIG. 1. Phase contrast photomicrograph of primary culture of nasopharyngeal carcinoma after 17 days *in vitro*. A fragment of biopsy material lies on the left surrounded by a monolayer outgrowth of cells of epithelial type. × 100.

FIG. 2. Same culture as that in Fig. 1, but showing the edge of the monolayer outgrowth. Epithelial cells are present on the left, nearest to the explanted tumor fragment, with fibroblasts on the right where the outgrowth ends. These latter cells subsequently rapidly overgrew the whole culture. Phase contrast photomicrograph. × 100.

FIG. 3. Same culture as foregoing but after 105 days *in vitro*. The fibroblasts, which have for many weeks apparently been the only cells present, are now accompanied by numerous small round cells of the lymphoblastoid type. Phase contrast photomicrograph. × 256.

FIG. 4. Lymphoblastoid cells from the culture shown in Fig. 3 after independent growth in suspension. Phase contrast photomicrograph. × 256.

out tumor fragments were placed in 4 oz flat glass bottles containing Eagle's minimal essential medium with non-essential amino acids, 20% human serum, and penicillin and streptomycin added.

First set of experiments—Of 21 biopsy samples from undoubted cases of naso-pharyngeal carcinoma, 20 gave rise to monolayer cultures; for the first two to three weeks, cells of epithelial appearance surrounded the explant (Fig. 1), but at the edge of the outgrowth some fibroblasts were also present (Fig. 2). The fibroblasts subsequently overgrew other cells and most cultures thereafter remained fibroblastic in nature. However, two cultures subsequently underwent " transformation " after about 100 days *in vitro* and released free-floating round cells into the medium (Fig. 3) which were found to grow independently in suspension (Fig. 4).

Second set of experiments—Further samples have been obtained from histologically confirmed cases of nasopharyngeal carcinoma and have been set up in culture as before. These cultures have not as yet been under observation for a prolonged period of time and the experiments are continuing.

Electron microscopy

Cells from monolayer cultures were scraped from the glass into suspension in a small volume of culture fluid. Samples of free-floating cells from suspension cultures were likewise collected in a small volume of culture fluid. In each case the cells were then fixed in suspension in glutaraldehyde followed by osmium tetroxide, pelleted, dehydrated, embedded in epoxy resin, sectioned, and stained in the section with uranyl acetate; the methods used have been described in full elsewhere (6). All the sections were examined in a Philips EM 300 electron microscope.

Discovery of the Virus

Virus was found only in the lymphoblastoid cells released after 105 days *in vitro* from monolayers grown from one of the two biopsy samples whose cultures showed this change. No virus was observed in any of the samples taken from monolayers before " transformation," nor in any of the round dying cells which were shed into suspension in the first few days after tumor fragments were explanted; these dying cells appear to have been derived from the epithelial elements of the tumor. In addition, although all the tumor biopsy samples were examined directly by electron microscopy, no virus was detected in any of them.

Structure of the virus

The virus particles were seen in about 10% of intact cells and more profusely in cell debris.

Immature virus—The immature virus appears as a spherical particle about 45 mμ in diameter with an electron opaque outer zone and an electron lucent center (Figs. 5 and 6). These particles were found only in the cytoplasm, either singly and in small groups (Fig. 5), or in large dense plaques. Immature particles were also often found in close relationship with an elaborate system of membrane-bounded flattened cytoplasmic cisternae (Fig. 6). It is interesting to note that where such

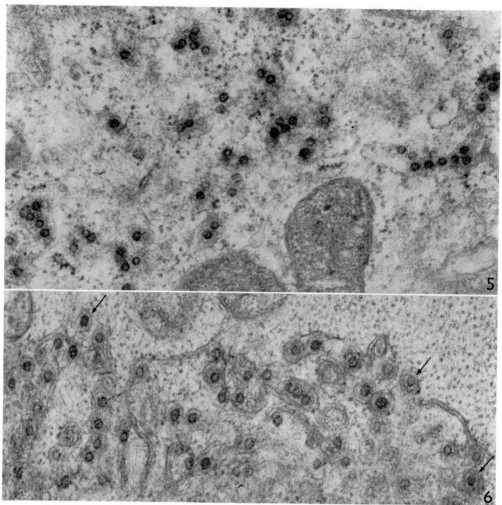

FIG. 5. Electron micrograph of an area of the cytoplasm of a lymphoblastoid cell from the culture shown in Fig. 4. Numerous spherical immature virus particles, 45 mμ in diameter, lie scattered between ribosomes, mitochondria, and other organelles. × 77,000.

FIG. 6. Cytoplasm from a virus-bearing lymphoblast. Numerous immature particles are present in close relation with masses of flattened cisternae bounded by smooth membranes. Where the cisternae curve closely around the particles and have been sectioned in certain planes the virus appears to be enclosed by an additional membrane (arrows). This membrane belongs, of course, to the cisternae but can be misinterpreted as being an extra viral envelope. Electron micrograph. × 75,000.

ring-shaped immature particles were sectioned beside the cisternae in certain planes, the cisternal membrane lay around the naked particle in such a way as to suggest at first glance that there was an additional outer viral coat (Fig. 6). If the true relationship of the immature particle to the cisternal membranes is understood, the latter cannot be confused with extra-viral envelopes, and errors of interpretation can be avoided.

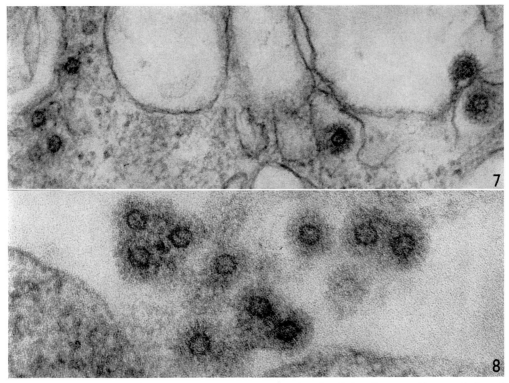

FIG. 7.   Area [of lymphoblast cytoplasm showig virus-induced cytopathic vacuolation of cisternae with immature particles near the cisternal membrane on the left, and budding through the membrane on the right.   The membrane overlying the viral buds is covered by striking radiating spines and comes to envelope the matured particle as it passes through. Electron micrograph.   × 125,000.

FIG. 8.   Electron micrograph of mature particles lying just outside a lymphoblast whose cell membrane is visible at the bottom and on the left of the field.   The mature virus has budded out from the cell membrane and lies in the extra-cellular space enveloped by an additional cell-derived membrane covered by radiating spines.   × 192,000.

Maturation of virus—Immature virus particles were regularly observed both around cytoplasmic vacuoles and below the cell membrane.   At these sites, the immature particles pass through the membranes by budding, the portion of the membrane forming the bud being covered by a striking radial array of spines (Fig. 7). Because of the sites at which budding took place, mature virus was released either into the cytoplasmic vacuoles (Fig. 7) or into the extracellular space (Fig. 8).

Mature virus—Mature particles were present in profusion at the sites where budding occurred and consisted of the spherical immature component in the center, surrounded by an outer coat of cell-derived membrane covered by a striking array of evenly spaced spines radiating uniformly over the entire surface (Figs. 7 and 8).   The overall dimension of the particle, including the spines, was found to be about 110 mμ and the diameter of the immature component within was the same as when it was seen free in the cytoplasm (45 mμ).   The surface spines measured 13 mμ in length, with a tip-to-tip spacing between adjacent spines of 13 mμ.

Cytopathic effects

Besides inducing the accumulation of quantities of membrane-bounded flattended cisternae in association with immature virus (Fig. 6), virus maturation led to the formation of large cytoplasmic vacuoles (Fig. 7), and to characteristic changes on the cell surface. Thus, where cells were close together, the thickening of the plasmalemma and the development of radiating spines at the site of viral budding were followed by the attachment of one surface membrane to that of a neighbouring cell. Multiple development of this " spot welding " progressed to the formation of intercellular bridges and, ultimately, to frank syncytia.

DISCUSSION

The cultures in which the new virus was found were maintained at all times in medium supplemented only with human serum, thus excluding the possibility that a virus of animal origin could have been inadvertently introduced along with animal serum. It seems, therefore, that the present virus is undoubtedly of human origin and it would appear likely that it was derived from the original nasopharyngeal carcinoma biopsy sample removed in East Africa.

From the morphological point of view this virus has several peculiar features which seem to make it unique as a human agent. In recent months indistinguishable viruses, likewise causing the formation of syncytia *in vitro*, have been isolated from bovine lymphosarcomas (*1, 14*) and a feline fibrosarcoma (*15*), although in one case the authors have confused the structure of the virus they describe by misinterpreting the closely applied smooth cytoplasmic membranes as being part of the viral envelope (*1*) (c.f. Fig. 6). In addition, evidence has newly been obtained showing that monkey foamy virus is also morphologically identical (*3*).

These animal viruses, together with the new human virus reported here, do not fit into any currently recognised structural group, and pose difficulties in classification.

At first sight, this group of viruses have certain superficial resemblances to the mouse mammary tumor virus (*8, 16, 17*) and the new virus grown recently from a monkey mammary carcinoma (*2*). However, when all the characteristics of these agents are carefully considered, it becomes evident that there are major differences. Thus, although all consist of naked immature cytoplasmic particles (similar to type "A") which mature by budding through membranes to form a " B " type particle, the immature forms of the mouse and monkey mammary carcinoma viruses are considerably larger than those from human nasopharyngeal carcinoma, from the bovine lymphoscarcomas, from the feline fibrosarcoma, and from the simian foamy virus. Secondly, " B " particles of the last four viruses are covered with striking spines so that, although their overall diameter, including the spines, is much the same as the " B " particle of mouse and monkey mammary tumors, the size of the particle itself without the spines is, again, smaller.

Thirdly, the " B " particle of mouse and monkey mammary tumors undergoes further maturation consisting of the condensation of the nucleoid into a dense structure, whereas maturation of this type has not been reported with the viruses of nasopharyngeal carcinoma, bovine lymphosarcomas, feline fibrosarcoma, or simian foamy virus. A final morphological difference lies in the fact that, in addition to preformed "A" type particles entering membranous buds during maturation, as happens with all the viruses under consideration, in the case of mouse mammary tumor virus budding may also consist of a *de novo* condensation of dense crescentic material at the site of the bud which enters the bud to form the core of the " B " particle; this mechanism has never been seen with the present nasopharyngeal carcinoma virus or reported for the viruses of bovine lymphosarcomas, feline fibrosarcoma, or monkey foamy virus.

In addition to these morphological differences, there also seem to be biological differences. The mouse and monkey mammary tumor viruses can be readily seen by electron microscopy of the original tumor, whereas the new viruses from nasopharyngeal carcinoma, bovine lymphosarcomas, and feline fibrosarcoma have not been found in the tumor material from which they grew out *in vitro;* similarly, simian foamy virus has never been reported in biopsies of monkey kidneys from whose cells it can readily be grown in tissue culture. As well as this, all four viruses in the nasopharyngeal carcinoma group induce syncytia in cultured infected cells, presumably as a result of some function of spine formation in the cell membrane at the sites where the particles bud out. The mouse and monkey mammary tumor viruses, on the other hand, covered only by a short fringe of projections, do not appear to have this property. It would seem, therefore, that for purposes of classification the viruses from nasopharyngeal carcinoma and bovine lymphosarcomas, feline fibrosarcoma, and simian foamy virus require to be placed in a new group different from, but with some resemblances to, mouse and monkey mammary tumor viruses.

As regards the significance of the present agent to human nasopharyngeal carcinoma, further studies are currently in progress to establish whether it can be isolated from other examples of this tumor, what its immunological relationships may be to the disease, and whether it is present merely as a passenger or perhaps in some more important role. In any event, it is considered of interest that a new human agent has been defined for fine structure, and found to be morphologically indistinguishable from certain new animal viruses whose position as regards classification was hitherto obscure. With this definition it has now been possible to propose the recognition of a new morphological group of viral agents from vertebrates.

SUMMARY

A new human virus, unassignable to any known morphological group, has been observed in cultures of a nasopharyngeal carcinoma from Kenya. The virus was only found in suspension cultures of lymphoblastoid cells released from the original monolayer after 105 days *in vitro*. In its morphology, the virus closely resembles three recently described viruses from animals; although having some features of the mouse mammary tumor agent, it differs in several respects. The nature and possible significance of this virus is discussed. It is considered that a new virus group will be required to classify this virus and the related animal viruses.

REFERENCES

1. Boothe, A. D., Van Der Maaten, M. J., and Malmquist, W. A. Morphological Variation of a Syncytial Virus from Lymphosarcomatous and Apparently Normal Cattle. Arch. Ges. Virusforsch, *31* : 373–384, 1970.
2. Chopra, H. C., and Mason, M. M. A New Virus in a Spontaneous Mammary Tumor of a Rhesus Monkey. Cancer Res., *30* : 2081–2086, 1970.
3. Clarke, J. K., Attridge, J. T., and Gay, F. W. The Morphogenesis of Simian Foamy Agents. J. Gen. Virol., *4*: 183–188, 1969.
4. De-Thé, G., Ambrosioni, J. C., Ho, H.-C., and Kwan, H. C. Lymphoblastoid Transformation and Presence of Herpes-Type Viral Particles in a Chinese Nasopharyngeal Tumour Cultured *in vitro*. Nature, *221*: 770–771, 1969.
5. De-Thé, G., Ho, H.-C., Kwan, H. C., Desgranges, C., and Favre, M. C. Nasopharyngeal Carcinoma (NPC). 1. Types of Cultures Derived from Tumor Biopsies and Non-tumerous Tissues of Chinese Patients with Special Reference to Lymphoblastoid Transformation. Int. J. Cancer, *6*: 189–206, 1970.
6. Epstein, M. A., and Achong, B. G. Fine Structural Organization of Human Lymphoblasts of a Tissue Culture Strain (EB1) from Burkitt's Lymphoma. J. Nat. Cancer Inst., *34*: 241–253, 1965.
7. Epstein, M. A., Achong, B. G., and Barr, Y. M. Virus Particles in Cultured Lymphoblasts from Burkitt's Lymphoma. Lancet, *1*: 702–703, 1964.
8. Goldfeder, A., Gelber, D., and Moore, D. H. An Electron Microscope Study of Spontaneous Mammary Carcinomas in a Subline of Strain DBA Mice. J. Nat. Cancer Inst., *25*: 827–845, 1960.
9. Goldman, M., Reisher, J. I., and Bushar, H. F. Serum-Antibodies to Burkitt Cell Virus. Lancet, *1*: 1156, 1968.
10. Henle, G., and Henle, W. Studies on Cell Lines Derived from Burkitt's Lymphoma. Trans. N.Y. Acad. Sci., *29*: 71–79, 1966.
11. Henle, G., and Henle, W. Immunofluorescence, Interference, and Complement Fixation Technics in the Detection of the Herpes-type Virus in Burkitt Tumor Cell Lines. Cancer Res., *27*: 2442–2446, 1967.
12. Henle, W. Evidence for a Relation of EBV to Burkitt's Lymphoma and Nasopharyngeal Carcinoma. Proceedings of the 1st International Symposium of the Princess Takamatsu Cancer Research Fund. pp. 361, University of Tokyo Press, Tokyo, Japan, 1971.
13. Henle, W., Henle, G., Ho, H.-C., Burtin, P., Cachin, Y., Clifford, P., De Schryver, A., De-Thé, G., Diehl, V., and Klein, G. Antibodies to Epstein-Barr Virus in Nasopharyngeal Carcinoma, Other Head and Neck Neoplasms, and Control Groups. J. Nat. Cancer Inst., *44*: 225–231, 1970.
14. Malmquist, W. A., Van Der Maaten, M. J., and Boothe, A. D. Isolation, Immunodiffusion, Immunofluorescence, and Electron Microscopy of Syncytial Virus of Lymphosarcomatous and Apparently Normal Cattle. Cancer Res., *29*: 188–200, 1969.

15. McKissick, G. E., and Lamont, P. H.   Characteristics of a Virus Isolated from a Feline Fibrosarcoma.   J. Virol., *5*: 247–257, 1970.

16. Moore, D. H.   The Milk Agent.   *In* A. J. Dalton and F. Haguenau (Eds.), Tumors Induced by Viruses: Ultrastructural Studies, pp. 113–150.   New York and London: Academic Press Inc., 1962.

17. Moore, D. H., Charney, J., Lasfargues, E. Y., Sarkar, N. H., Rubin, R. C., and Ames, R. P.   Mammary Tumor Virus (MTV) Virions in a Transplantable Ependymoblastoma.   Proc. Soc. Exp. Biol. Med., *132*: 125–127, 1969.

18. Moore, G. E., Grace, J. T., Citron, P., Gerner, R., and Burns, A.   Leukocyte Cultures of Patients with Leukemia and Lymphomas.   N.Y. State J. Med., *66*: 2757–2764, 1966.

19. Old, L. J., Boyse, E. A., Oettgen, H. F., de Harven, E., Geering, G., Williamson, B., and Clifford, P.   Precipitating Antibody in Human Serum to an Antigen Present in Cultured Burkitt's Lymphoma Cells.   Proc. Nat. Acad. Sci., *56*: 1699–1704, 1966.

20. Svedmyr, A., and Demissie, A.   Age Distribution of Antibodies to Burkitt Cells.   Acta Path. Microbiol. Scandinav., *73*: 653–654, 1968.

Discussion of Paper by Dr. Epstein

DR. YAMAMOTO: Let's begin our discussion now on Dr. Epstein's paper. As you have just heard, he proposes that a new virus, other than the EB virus, has been found in nasopharyngeal carcinoma.

DR. EPSTEIN: We cannot say how often it occurs in the tumors, because we only had two lymphoblastoid transformations in our first series of experiments. In the cultures, the virus is present in something of the order of 10–15% of the cells.

DR. HINUMA: Have you any data about immunofluorescent staining of cells with human sera?

DR. EPSTEIN: We have done nothing about this yet immunologically. It is obviously the next thing that we have to do.

DR. HINUMA: Is this particular cell line very similar, morphologically, to the lymphoid cells which have been derived from Burkitt's lymphoma?

DR. EPSTEIN: Yes, I think that these cells belong to the same family.

DR. G. KLEIN: I want to know whether the cells carrying the new virus also carries EBV, and whether EBV and the new virus co-exist in the same cell?

DR. EPSTEIN: The answer to that is, yes. Both viruses are present in the cultures but not in the same cell.

DR. G. KLEIN: Thank you. The other question I had is, did you even see EBV and/or the new virus in the monolayer type of culture or in the fibroblast culture.

DR. EPSTEIN: No, never.

DR. NAKAHARA: I would like to ask Dr. Epstein whether do you find this new type of virus in all the cells in your culture or only in some particular type of cells?

DR. EPSTEIN: In about 10%.

DR. NAKAHARA: Then, you find virus-containing and nonvirus-containing cells in the same cultures.   Do you think that the two types of cell come from the same strain?

DR. EPSTEIN: Well, I wouldn't be prepared to say that there are nonvirus containing cells.   All one can say is that at a given microsecond when one takes a sample and looks, some have visible virion and some do not.   We don't know how many contain virus genome.   We don't really know what's going on.   We can only tell you that at that moment some can be seen be producing virus particles.

DR. NAKAHARA: Correct.   Now, at the symposium we had last spring at Shima, where Dr. Epstein was unfortunately not present, I suggested the importance of using cell clones in making a cell culture studies, because when you say lymphoid or lymphoblastoid cells, you think it is one type of cell, but, they could come from different types of cell, originally.   To start with, you have a mixed cell population, and what you eventually get from them may be quite unknown, unless you do the clone cultures.   Am I asking too much?

DR. EPSTEIN: I absolutely agree with you, and this is why I think this term lymphoblastoid transformation is such a bad one, it is really saying something on which we have no evidence whatsoever.   I wish we could get it out of the literature. It came in six years ago and it still tends to be used.   I think it is a very bad term and I quite agree with you.   It's convenient to call the cells lymphoblastoid cells since this is what they look like, but where they come from, goodness only knows.

DR. NAKAHARA: Then the thing to do is to chase down the origin of lymphoblastoid cells?

DR. EPSTEIN: Of course, cloning would be another way of finding out whether all of the cells are infected or just some of them as you ask.

DR. AOKI: I was interested in the particle.   I would like to ask you about its characteristics.   Have you examined this particle by negative staining?

DR. EPSTEIN: This is being done at the moment.

DR. AOKI: I see.   From our experience with the Friend leukemia virus system where there is budding of mature virus particles, these sometimes reacted with immunoglobulin which exists in the tissue culture medium.   In such a case, very similar spikes, different from the spikes of B-type viruses, could be seen.   At another point, you said mature particles like naked A-particles, were present.   But my impression was that thery were a little bit different from A-particles.   So I look forward to seeing in the near future your results on negative staining to compare these with B-type particles and/or Friend virus coated with immunoglobulin.

DR. EPSTEIN: Yes, I absolutely agree with you. The virus belongs in a completely separate group from the A-type mammary tumor virus, although it seems to be superficially similar and to behave in the same kind of way. But I absolutely agree they are different. With regard to spikes, I don't think that your immunoglobulin is going to appear in this way. It will appear more as a uniform fuzz around the viruses where as here we get spikes not only on the particles themselves, but, as I showed you, actually on the cell membrane as it begins to form the bud; I think this is rather unusual. This is not the image we have ever seen with immunoglobulin deposited on EB virus for instance.

DR. AOKI: Yes, in our case in some established culture lines from BBS2 which are induced by Friend virus especially when we use some special serum, there are always carriers of such a spike just after starting the budding. In addition, the naked A-particles always shows common antigenicity to B-particle. So, we thought that a naked A-particle might be a premature type of B-particle, not a C-particle. It is also an interesting point for future study.

DR. EPSTEIN: Yes, I think that is very interesting, thank you. There is just one other point argumented by analogy. We haven't done PTA on our virus but it has been done on the monkey-foamy virus and there you see a very long spike. So, I am hoping again to find the same thing on our agent and not a fringe such as you get on the mammary tumor virus.

DR. DE THÉ: This is a fine example of electron microscopy and I have to congratulate Dr. Epstein for his beautiful pictures. I think that there is absolutely no doubt from the electron microscope point of view that this virus does not resemble any known RNA-type enveloped particle that we are used to seeing. The second point, I think, as Dr. Aoki stressed, that there is no need to discuss the classification of virus A, naked, enveloped A, etc. I would say that this agent here is completely new and we should make a new class " E " to describe the type. We have A, B, C, D, and then the next letter is E. The next point is the tissue culture point. If you have used only human serum in your tissue cultures, is it pooled serum or not?

DR. EPSTEIN: Yes, human serum from British donors. We have not pooled their sera. We have tested out each one before use because some, as you know, inhibit growth.

DR. DE THÉ: The last point is that all the three syncytial viruses cause syncytia. Do you find syncytia in these lymphoblastoid lines?

DR. EPSTEIN: Yes, this was shown in my last slide.

DR. DE THÉ: It was visible, in the electron microscope, but how about in the light microscope?

DR. EPSTEIN: This was very difficult because, as you know, the cells are not usually in clumps and it is the only when was contact actually made that syncytium sometimes takes place. I think it is bad to call it syncytium formation where two cells become a polykaryon.

DR. DE THÉ: In our quite long experience with 35 cell lines originating from a number of Chinese and a few of African nasopharyngeal carcinoma, we have never seen such pictures. It may be that the conditions of culture are different. Did you modify the temperature?

DR. EPSTEIN: No, but I do hope I stressed that I am not suggesting that this is connected particularly with nasopharyngeal carcinoma. I am just saying it came out of one. It could be a quite casual passenger phenomenon.

EB Virus as a Biologically Active Agent

J. H. Pope, W. Scott, B. M. Reedman, and M. K. Walters

The Queensland Institute of Medical Research, Herston Road, Brisbane, Australia

The etiological role of the EB virus (*7*) in one lymphoproliferative disease (infectious mononucleosis) (*11, 20*) alone warrants investigation of its biological properties, but such studies are made even more important by the serological evidence of an association of EB virus with Burkitt's lymphoma (*10*) and postnasal carcinoma (*13, 21*). Two fundamental approaches to the investigation of the biological properties of EB virus are possible, determining its causal role in various diseases and examining its behaviour in *in vitro* systems. Direct examination of the effects of EB virus in man is not practicable because of the potential hazards; research into the possible etiological roles of EB virus must necessarily be indirect. Experimental *in vitro* systems have an advantage in being direct but it may be difficult to equate *in vitro* functions with disease processes *in vivo*.

So far, two effective *in vitro* systems have been developed for the study of the biological properties of EB virus. In one system, EB virus can be shown to induce continuous proliferation in human leucocytes which would otherwise die (*9, 12, 18, 24, 25*). This phenomenon is referred to as transformation, the term being used for the present in a sense similar to that in the tumor virus field (*1*), as distinct from the sense in which it describes a transient blast response of lymphocytes to nonspecific mitogens or specific antigens (*16*). In the second system, EB virus-free leucocyte cell lines infected with EB virus may respond by the induction of newly-recognized EB viral antigens or cell death (*14, 15*). It is proposed to deal only with transformation by EB virus in the present paper. The results presented are an extension of earlier reports (*24–26*).

MATERIALS AND METHODS

Virus pools

Cultures of the QIMR-WIL line containing EB virus (*22*) were grown in either Eagle's basal medium (5) or Eagle's minimum essential medium F15 (Grand Island Biological Co., N.Y.), containing 10% inactivated foetal calf serum.   Cells were harvested and resuspended at a concentration of 1×10^7 to 2×10^7 cells/ml in modified Eagle's medium (24) or Roswell Park Memorial Institute (R.P.M.I.) medium 1640 (19), with 16% foetal calf serum.   The suspension was frozen and thawed twice, centrifuged at $1,200 \times g$ for 20 min and $5,000 \times g$ for 5 min. and filtered through a millipore membrane (Millipore Corporation, Bedford, Mass.) with an average pore diameter of 300 mμ. Aliquots of approximately 1 ml were stored at 60°C.

Foetal leucocyte cultures

Fresh foetuses obtained at miscarriage were the source of the leucocytes for culture.   The long bones were split longitudinally and the bone marrow was scraped out into the growth medium.   Thymic leucocytes were teased directly into the medium.   The cells were washed twice and suspended to give a final concentration of 5×10^6 cells/ml.   The volume of inoculum was 0.2 ml and the final culture volume was 1 ml in flat bottomed vials (24).   The cultures were maintained at 36°C in a humid atmosphere of 5% CO_2 in air by changing 30% of the medium twice weekly.

Growth medium was either the modified Eagle's medium or R.P.M.I. medium 1640, containing 16% inactivated foetal calf serum.

Adult peripheral leucocyte cultures

Blood was collected in heparin or citrate; the plasma containing leucocytes was separated either by light centrifugation or by layering on a mixture of methylcellulose (Dow Chemical Co.) and sodium diatrizoate (Wintrop Laboratories) (17). Leucocytes were washed and cultured as described for foetal leucocytes except that a lower cell concentration was generally used, as indicated in the text.

Incorporation of tritiated thymidine

Cultures to be examined for uptake of tritiated thymidine received 0.5 μCi/ml [Thymidine (methyl-T), 23.5 Ci/mM, Radiochemical Centre, Amersham] and after incubation for 6 hr, the cultures were placed on ice.   The cultures were stirred briefly on a Vortex-Genie stirrer (Scientific Industries Inc., Mass.) and, using Whatman GF/C filters, the free cells were collected and washed with phosphate buffered saline (40 ml), 10% trichloracetic acid (40 ml) and methanol (20 ml). The filters were dried overnight at 37°C, scintillator added (5.0 g PPO and 0.3 g dimethyl POPOP in 1 liter of toluene), and counts made in a Beckman LS-100 liquid scintillation system.   In earlier work, dried filters were treated with hyamine for 24 hr and then held in the dark for 24 hr after the addition of scintillator before counting.

Immunodiffusion

Soluble antigens were prepared from leucocyte suspensions by freezing, thawing, and light sonication followed by centrifugation at $12,000 \times g$ for 15 min and at $1000,000 \times g$ for 1 hr.   Immunodiffusion tests were conducted in 0.7% agarose.

RESULTS

Transformation of foetal leucocytes

The essential characteristics of foetal leucocyte cultures transformed by EB virus have been described in detail previously (*24*).   In brief, outgrowth of transformed cells usually became microscopically evident in infected cultures at 19–21 days, while cultures which received control inocula failed to become established. Transformed leucocyte lines consistently grew in suspension as irregular blast cells with a tendency to aggregate.

Further experience has amply confirmed this general pattern of transformation of foetal leucocytes by EB virus.   To date, leucocytes from 16 foetuses have been utilized in transformation experiments.   Cell lines were consistently established from leucocytes from each foetus when EB virus was inoculated but on no occasion was a leucocyte line established from control cultures which were either uninoculated or had received a filtrate prepared from the virus-free Raji line (*6, 27*).

Titration of EB virus in foetal leucocytes

Foetal leucocyte cultures inoculated with EB virus from QIMR-WIL cells began proliferating much sooner than those inoculated with virus from the QIMR-GOR line (*23*); this observation aroused our interest in the effect of the dose of EB virus on the transformation process.   Consequently, foetal bone marrow cultures were inoculated with a series of two-fold dilutions (from 1/10 to 1/10, 240) of a pool of EB virus from QIMR-WIL cells, two cultures being used per dilution.

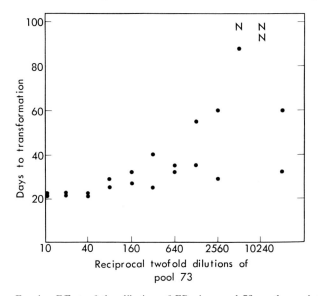

FIG. 1.   Effect of the dilution of EB virus pool 73 on the period before the transformation of foetal leucocytes was detected microscopically.   Each point represents an individual culture.   N, not transformed.

The results (Fig. 1) showed that transforming activity was detectable after considerable dilution of the virus pool.   Up to a dilution of 1/40, the time at which proliferation began remained constant (22 days).   Further dilution, however, resulted in a gradual increase in the period elapsing before proliferation, so that at higher dilutions several cultures did not transform until 2 months, and one was as late as 3 months.   With the lower dilutions of EB virus, transformation appeared to involve many leucocytes, as was indicated by the concurrent outgrowth of many aggregates of leucocytes. However, in cultures receiving higher dilutions and showing delayed proliferation, it was evident that only a small number of leucocytes was involved.   Sometimes the initial stages of late proliferation were observed as apparently single foci, consisting of very few leucocytes overlying the residual fibroblasts.   The leucocytes in the first stages of proliferation were usually round, but became characteristically irregular once growth was well advanced and aggregates formed.

Once proliferation was initiated, it proceeded in characteristic fashion and yielded typical cell lines.   Control cultures remained negative throughout the observation period.

Delayed inoculation of foetal bone marrow cultures

Cultures were normally inoculated immediately after preparation and it was important to determine whether this was necessary.   To investigate this point, a series of cultures of foetal bone marrow leucocytes were prepared.   Some were inoculated immediately, while others were inoculated at intervals up to 15 days later. A fresh ampoule of the same stored EB virus pool was used for each inoculation and each group consisted of two cultures.   Control cultures inoculated at the time of preparation were negative.

The results are represented in Fig. 2.   They show that foetal bone marrow cultures inoculated up to 15 days after preparation (the longest period tested) remained susceptible to transformation by EB virus.   No dramatic effect of delayed inoculation on the period before proliferation was noted.   The earliest onset of proliferation was recorded in the cultures inoculated at 12 days, but the number of cultures available in this experiment was insufficient for statistical analysis.   Further investigation of this phenomenon is warranted.

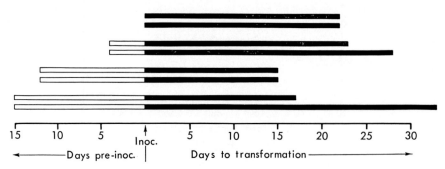

FIG. 2.   Effect of inoculation of cultured foetal leucocytes with EB virus at various intervals.   Each bar represents one culture.

General studies of the transformation of leucocytes from adult peripheral blood

Although leucocytes from human foetuses provided an extremely useful and reliable system for studying the transformation by EB virus, the irregularity of the supply of foetuses prompted a search for an alternative and more readily available system.   Leucocytes from children without antibody to EB virus could not be obtained routinely and the incidence of EB antibody in adults in Brisbane is such that no staff members were found free of antibody.   An investigation was therefore made of the practical value of leucocytes from persons with low level antibody to EB virus for studies of EB virus-transformation.   Although it has been established that leucocyte cell lines may be established from the leucocytes of normal persons with antibody to EB virus (*3, 8, 19*), our previous experience had indicated that, in practice, small scale cultures failed to yield cell lines.   Subsequently, it was found that such leucocyte cultures were indeed quite satisfactory for transformation studies.   Cells from three donors were used, with similar results.

Small cultures (1 ml) of peripheral leucocytes were set up using a cell concentration of 2×10^5 to 2×10^6/ml.   Some variation occurred in the appearance of uninoculated cultures during the first few weeks; this appeared to be largely dependent upon the initial cell concentration.   With smaller numbers of cells, there was little attachment of leucocytes to the glass, small clumps of leucocytes were formed, and the cultures degenerated relatively quickly (1–2 weeks).   Higher cell concentrations resulted in the better survival of leucocytes and the attachment of some cells in a predominantly focal distribution.   These foci appeared to consist of macrophages and a few fibroblastic cells to which were attached leucocytes which were usually in definite aggregates.   The number of macrophages appeared to increase gradually, possibly arising from the scattered smaller leucocytes present.   The aggregates of leucocytes remained largely unchanged in appearance for several weeks and later slowly degenerated.

Inoculation of such cultures with EB virus from QIMR-WIL cells resulted in proliferation which was detectable microscopically at about 19–21 days.   At this stage, in cultures set up with a small number of cells, the majority of leucocytes were dead and proliferation began in some of the small aggregated of surviving leucocytes, the number of active foci being dependent on the initial cell number.   By 3 weeks there was usually a clear distinction between the EB virus-transfromed cultures with their actively proliferating clumps of cells and the control cultures (inoculated with Raji filtrate, or uninoculated) which contained few or no live cells.   Cultures initially containing more cells transformed similarly when inoculated with EB virus but the contrast with the controls at three weeks was not so distinct because of the better survival of the latter.

The addition of phytohaemagglutinin (PHA-M, Difco) to adult leucocyte cultures (0.01 ml per ml) was found to enhance the transformation by EB virus when the modified Eagle's medium was used.   Cultures inoculated with both PHA and EB virus showed a typical blast response due to PHA followed by the death of most of these cells and outgrowth of some of the surviving aggregates.   Enhancement of viral transformation was indicated by an increased number of active proliferating aggregates of leucocytes in the PHA cultures compared with the controls receiving EB virus only, but proliferation began at a similar time in each group.   Addition of EB virus to PHA-treated cultures immediately or up to 3 days later resulted in successful transformation, while cultures inoculated with PHA alone invariably died. When a different growth medium (R.P.M.I. 1640) was used, the addition of PHA was not found to enhance EB virus-transformation, but this may possibly have been due to difficulty in pH control resulting from active response to PHA.

Thus, the general features of transformation of adult peripheral leucocytes by EB virus (whether or not PHA was used) and the cultural characteristics of the established cell lines bore a close resemblance to those described in experiments with foetal leucocytes.

Kinetics of transformation by EB virus

It has been noted that with active preparations of EB virus microscopic evidence of transformation may be seen at 19–21 days.   However, it was of interest to attempt to follow the pattern of proliferation; for this purpose techniques employing the incorporation of tritiated thymidine into DNA were used.   In preliminary unpublished autoradiographic experiments inoculation of human foetal bone marrow

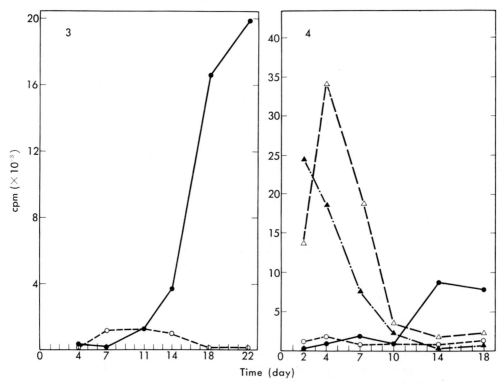

FIGS. 3 and 4.   Incorporation of tritiated thymidine into cultured peripheral leucocytes inoculated with filtrates of QIMR–WIL (EB virus) or Raji (control) cells, or with PHA. Each point represents the geometric mean of triplicate cultures.   ●, QIMR–WIL ; ○, Raji ;   ▲, PHA ;   △, PHA+QIMR–WIL.

leucocytes with EB virus resulted in an increase in the proportion of labelled cells at 8–10 days, while the proportion in the controls continued to decline. This detection of proliferation well before it became evident microscopically encouraged further investigation, and attention was turned to the study of the transformation of adult leucocytes using liquid scintillation counting instead of autoradio graphy.

During the first 10 days there was little difference between the uptake of tritiated thymidine by adult leucocyte cultures inoculated with either QIMR-WIL (EB virus) or Raji filtrates. However, at between 10 and 14 days a dramatic increase in uptake occurred in the EB virus-inoculated cultures while the control Raji cultures remained at the lower level. This pattern (Fig. 3) occurred in two transformation experiments.

In uninoculated cultures, the uptake was low for the first five days, then rose to a level similar to that of the cultures inoculated with Raji filtrate. Addition of PHA to cultures resulted in a characteristic vigorous response at 2–3 days followed by a rapid decrease in activity (Fig. 4). It was clear that the presence of EB virus did not interfere with the response to PHA (although it appeared to delay it), that EB virus was not able to induce the majority of PHA-transformed cells to continue proliferation and that, under these particular experimental conditions, EB virus transformation proceeded more satisfactorily in the absence of PHA (Fig. 4).

Soluble complement fixing (CF) antigen related to EB virus infection of man

Several transformed cell lines were shown to contain EB virus-related CF antigen in spite of a low level of EB viral fluorescence (*24*), and CF antigen was demonstrated in transformed lines derived from leucocytes of a human foetal thymus initially free of antigen (unpublished). Interest was thus aroused as to the significance of EB viral CF antigen in transformed cell lines.

Recently, we drew attention to the existence in certain human leucocyte cell lines of a soluble CF antigen which was associated with EB virus. This antigen was detectable by means of reactive human sera, as antibody to the soluble antigen is produced in man during infection with EB virus (*26*). It was most interesting that not only was soluble antigen present in cell lines carrying EB virus, but a related antigen was present in the Raji line, which was free of detectable EB virus. We discussed the possibility that the soluble antigens might be equivalent to the virus-induced " tumor " antigens of other viral transformation systems (*26*).

Although CF tests indicated a relationship between the soluble antigens of the QIMR-WIL and Raji lines, it remained unknown whether or not the antigens of the two cell lines were indentical. Immunodiffusion studies were made to investigate this problem. All human sera reacting in immunodiffusion with the QIMR-WIL soluble antigen showed one strong precipitation line, while with some sera an additional faint line occurred. These sera did not react with a control antigen prepared from neonatal human thymus. Sera containing precipitins had high titers of CF antibody to EB virus, but sera without EB antibody or with low titers failed to give lines. A group of reactive sera tested against QIMR-WIL antigen showed identity of both the major and minor lines, when present. Finally, when individual reactive sera were tested against QIMR-WIL and Raji antigens, the

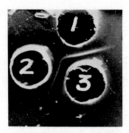

FIG. 5.   Immunodiffusion test showing identity of the soluble antigens of the QIMR–WIL and Raji cell lines.   Well 1, QIMR–WIL ; well 2, Raji ; well 3, human serum.

resulting lines showed reactions of identity (Fig. 5).   This applied particularly to the major line and these results demonstrated the presence in QIMRWIL and Raji lines of at least one common and identical soluble antigen.

DISCUSSION

Farlier observations on the transformation of human leucocytes by EB virus were confirmed in the present study and were extended in several ways.   First, the series of foetuses studied was extended to 16 with results similar to those previously reported (24, 25), i.e., cell lines were established only from cultures inoculated with EB virus. As the evidence so far (4, 9, 12, 24, 25) associates EB virus with the establishment of leucocyte cell lines, it was concluded that EB virus was either absent or below detectable levels in the leucocytes of the foetuses examined.   It would be of considerable interest for foetuses from other localities to be studied in a similar way.

Extension of the latent period before proliferation from the usual 3 weeks to 2–3 months by the dilution of the EB virus inoculum was an important new finding. It suggests that the difference in the latent period between QIMR-WIL and QIMR-GOR filtrates was due to a lower level of EB virus in the latter; this was supported by the lower level of EB viral fluorescence in the QIMR-GOR line (25).   Involvement of EB virus-transformation in the establishment of many leucocyte cell lines has already been suggested (24), and the effect of dilution described here may provide an explanation of the different times of proliferation recorded in primary leucocyte cultures, those initially containing less virus taking longer to begin proliferation.

It is not clear at the moment whether delayed proliferation results from a genuine delayed response of cells infected at the time of inoculation, from a belated infection of the responsive cells, or from continual proliferation at a low level during the latent period.   Whatever the explanation, it is evident that the capacity to induce a delayed proliferation of leucocytes in vitro is a basic biological property of EB virus.   Another point of interest in this experiment was that the time before proliferation showed a minimum which was independent of increased viral inoculum.

An unexpected finding concerning transformation was that foetal bone marrow leucocytes inoculated with EB virus up to 15 days later still showed characteristic transformation.   These observation suggest that the transformed cell lines arose from a population of cells surviving well in vitro and, more important, that the usual delay of about 3 weeks before proliferation was related to processes associated with viral infection rather than to factors involved in the adaptation of leucocytes to culture.

EB virus may persist in leucocytes after primary infection and leucocyte lines may be established from some normal persons (3, 8, 19). However, this was not found to prohibit the use of peripheral leucocytes from certain donors with low level EB antibody in EB virus-transformation studies. The failure of control cultures of small numbers of peripheral leucocytes to transform was probably due to a low incidence of EB virus-infected cells in the peripheral blood at the time, but it is possible that the culture system used was unsuitable for the expression of the proliferative effects of any EB virus-infected cells present. So far, peripheral leucocytes from donors with a high antibody level have not been studied by this culture method. The results of the inoculation of EB virus into peripheral leucocytes were similar to those seen with foetal leucocytes and only those cultures inoculated with EB virus were transformed. The similarity in cultural characteristics and morphology of transformed peripheral and foetal cells indicates that the observed transformation process is an expression of a constant biological property of the EB virus.

Incorporation of tritiated thymidine proved to be useful for the study of cell proliferation in cultures transformed by EB virus. By this method, the onset of continuous proliferation was detectable in the second week of culture, but was not detectable microscopically until about a week later. The response occurred later than that due to PHA, specific antigen, or the mixed leucocyte reaction (16).

Knowledge of the EB virus-associated soluble CF antigen(s) of leucocyte cell lines was extended by the demonstration of identity by the immunodiffusion of antigens present in the QIMR-WIL and Raji lines. This finding is compatible with virus induction of the soluble antigen. A similar antigen is present in at least one cell line transformed by EB virus (unpublished) and, as previously suggested (26), the antigen may prove to be an indicator of the presence of the EB viral genome in a manner similar to the virus-induced antigens of classical tumor viruses (28). This interpretation of the significance of soluble EB virus-related CF antigen (26) is supported by the recent report of the detection of the EB viral genome in the Raji cell line (30).

The virus-cell relationship in leucocyte lines carrying EB virus is poorly understood, but even less is known about the events leading to the transformation of normal leucocytes by EB virus. Several possible mechanisms may be considered. Thus, EB, virus-transformation may be due to persistence in the cells of the viral genome, either as virion or in another form such as one integrated with cellular DNA, as is the case with SV 40 virus (29). The evidence suggesting that the persistence of the EB viral genome may be associated with transformation and proliferation has already been discussed. A second possibility is that the EB virus induces the transformation of leucocytes by a mechanism similar to that occurring in blast transformation by nonspecific mitogens such as PHA. An important difference between transformation by EB virus and by PHA is that the latter does not normally result in the establishment of cell lines. In this regard, it should be noted that in a recent report concerning the role of PHA in the establishment of leucocyte cell lines (2), a contributing role for the EB virus was not excluded.   Third, EB virus-transformation could conceivably be immunological in nature, a response of sensitive cells to a specific antigen, which in this case would be an EB viral antigen.   Against this possibility is the lack of evidence that lymphoid cells stimulated by specific antigen yield cell lines, and in the fact that EB virus transforms leucocytes from both foetuses (25) and children without antibody to EB virus (4).   Obviously, further critical work is required before the mechanism of EB virus transformation can be clarified.

SUMMARY

Leucocytes from 16 foetuses were transformed by EB virus (i.e. cell lines established) but no cell lines were established from control cultures.   Dilution of an EB virus pool increased the period before the onset of proliferation of foetal leucocytes from 22 days to 60–88 days, a phenomenon which may explain the delayed outgrowth of some primary leucocyte cultures.   Foetal leucocytes cultured up to 15 days before inoculation with EB virus showed typical transformation after a similar incubation period, suggesting that the usual delay before proliferation is virus-dependent rather than a reflection of the adaptation of cells to culture.   Under conditions suboptimal for the establishment of cell lines, leucocytes from adults with a low titer of antibody to EB virus failed to yield cell lines unless inoculated with EB virus, after which transformation similar to that of foetal cells occurred.   Radioisotope studies showed that increased proliferation occurred 10–14 days after inoculation with EB virus.   Soluble EB virus-associated complement fixing antigens of the virus-carrying QIMR-WIL line and the virus-free Raji line were shown by immunodiffusion to contain identical components, providing further evidence that the EB viral genome is present in the Raji line.

REFERENCES

1.   Black, P. H.   The Oncogenic DNA Viruses: A Review of in Vitro Transformation Studies.   Ann. Rev. Microbiol., 22: 391–426, 1968.
2.   Broder, S. W., Glade, P. R., and Hirschhorn, K.   Establishment of Long-term Lines from Small Aliquots of Normal Lymphocytes.   Blood, 35: 539–542, 1970.
3.   Diehl, V., Henle, G., Henle, W., and Kohn, G.   Demonstration of a Herpes Group Virus in Cultures of Peripheral Leukocytes from Patients with Infectious Mononucleosis.   J. Virol., 2: 663–669, 1968.
4.   Diehl, V., Henle, G., Henle, W., and Kohn, G.   Effect of a Herpes Group Virus (EBV) on Growth of Peripheral Leukocyte Cultures.   Hemic Cells in Vitro, in Vitro, 4: 92–99, 1969.
5.   Eagle, H.   Nutrition Needs of Mammalian Cells in Tissue Culture.   Science, 122: 501–504, 1955.
6.   Epstein, M. A., Achong, B. G., Barr, Y. M., Zajac, B., Henle, G., and Henle, W.   Morphological and Virological Investigations on Cultured Burkitt Tumor Lymphoblasts (Strain Raji).   J. Natl. Cancer Inst., 37: 547–559, 1966.
7.   Epstein, M. A., Achong, B. G., and Barr, Y. M.   Virus Particles in Cultured Lymphoblasts from Burkitt's Lymphoma.   Lancet, 1: 702–704, 1964.

8. Gerber, P., and Monroe, J. H.   Studies on Leukocytes Growing in Continuous Culture Derived from Normal Human Donors.   J. Natl. Cancer Inst., *40*: 855–866, 1968.

9. Gerber, P., Whang-Peng, J., and Monroe, J. H.   Transformation and Chromosome Changes Induced by Epstein-Barr Virus in Normal Human Leukocyte Cultures. Proc. Natl. Acad. Sci. U.S., *63*: 740–748, 1969.

10. Henle, G., Henle, W., Clifford, P., Diehl, V., Kafuko, G. W., Kirya, B. G., Klein, G., Morrow, R. H., Munube, G. M. R., Pike, P., Tukei, P. M., and Ziegler, J. L.   Antibodies to Epstein-Barr Virus in Burkitt's Lymphoma and Control Groups.   J. Natl. Cancer Inst., *43*: 1147–1157, 1969.

11. Henle, G., Henle, W., and Diehl, V.   Relation of Burkitt's Tumor-associated Herpes-type Virus to Infectious Mononucleosis.   Proc. Natl. Acad. Sci. U.S., *59*: 94–101, 1968.

12. Henle, W., Diehl, V., Kohn, G., zur Hausen, H., and Henle, G.   Herpes-Type Virus and Chromosome Marker in Normal Leukocytes after Growth with Irradiated Burkitt Cells.   Science, *157*: 1064–1065, 1967.

13. Henle, W., Henle G., Ho, H.-C., Burtin, P., Cachin, Y., Clifford, P., de Schryver, A., de Thé, G., Diehl, V., and Klein, G.   Antibodies to Epstein-Barr Virus in Nasopharyngeal Carcinoma, Other Head and Neck Neoplasms and Control Groups.   J. Natl. Cancer Inst., *44*: 225–231, 1970.

14. Henle, W., Henle, G., Zajac, B. A., Pearson, G., Waubke, R., and Scriba, M.   Differential Reactivity of Human Serums with Early Antigens Induced by Epstein-Barr Virus.   Science, *169*: 188–190, 1970.

15. Horoszewizc, J. S.   *In* Virus-induced Immunopathology.   Perspectives in Virology, *6*: 123–124, 1968.

16. Ling, N. R.   Lymphocyte Stimulation.   North-Holland Publishing Company, Amsterdam, 1968.

17. Main, R. K., and Jones, M. J.   Mixed Leucocyte Interaction Involving Mouse Strains of Strong and Weak Allogeneic Specificities.   Nature, *218*: 1251–1252, 1968.

18. Miller, G., Enders, J. F., Lisco, H., and Kohn, H. I.   Establishment of Lines from Normal Human Blood Leukocytes by Co-cultivation with a Leukocyte Line Derived from a Leukemic Child.   Proc. Soc. Exptl. Biol. Med., *132*: 247–252, 1969.

19. Moore, G. E., Gerner, R. E., and Franklin, H. A.   Culture of Normal Human Leukocytes.   J. Am. Med. Assoc., *199*: 519–524, 1967.

20. Niederman, J. C., McCollum, R. W., Henle, G., and Henle, W.   Infectious Mononucleosis.   Clinical Manifestations in Relation to EB Virus Antibodies.   J. Am. Med. Assoc., *203*: 205–209, 1968.

21. Old, L. J., Boyse, E. A., Oettgen, H. F., de Harven, E., Geering, G., Williamson, B., and Clifford, P.   Precipitating Antibody in Human Serum to an Antigen Present in Cultured Burkitt's Lymphoma Cells.   Proc. Natl. Acad. Sci. U.S., *56*: 1699–1704, 1966.

22. Pope, J. H.   Establishment of Cell Lines from Australian Leukaemic Patients: Presence of a Herpes-like Virus.   Australian J. Exptl. Biol. Med. Sci., *46*: 643–645, 1968.

23. Pope, J. H., Achong, B. G., Epstein, M. A., and Biddulph, J.   Burkitt Lymphoma in New Guinea: Establishment of a Line of Lymphoblasts *in Vitro* and Description of their Fine Structure.   J. Natl. Cancer Inst., *39*: 933–945, 1967.

24. Pope, J. H., Horne, M. K., and Scott, W.   Transformation of Foetal Human Leukocytes *in Vitro* by Filtrates of a Human Leukaemic Cell Line Containing Herpes-like

Virus. Intern. J. Cancer, *3*: 857–866, 1968.

25. Pope, J. H., Horne, M. K., and Scott, W. Identification of the Filtrable Leukocyte-transforming Factor of QIMR–WIL Cells as Herpes-like Virus. Intern. J. Cancer, *4*: 255–260, 1969.

26. Pope, J. H., Horne, M. K., and Wetters, E. J. Significance of a Complement-Fixing Antigen Associated with Herpes-Like Virus and Detected in the Raji Cell Line. Nature, *222*: 186–187, 1969.

27. Pulvertaft, R. J. V. A Study of Malignant Tumors in Nigeria by Short-term Tissue Culture. J. Clin. Pathol., *18*: 261–273, 1965.

28. Rowe, W. P. Virus-Specific Antigens in Viral Tumors. *In* J. J. Trentin (ed.), Cross-reacting Antigens and Neoantigens (with Implications for Autoimmunity and Cancer Immunity), pp. 74–84. The Williams & Wilkins Company, Baltimore, 1967.

29. Sambrook, J., Westphal, H., Srinivasan, P. R., and Dulbecco, R. The Integrated State of Viral DNA in SV40-transformed Cells. Proc. Natl. Acad. Sci. U.S., *60*: 1288–1295, 1968.

30. zur Hausen, H., and Schulte-Holthausen, H. Presence of EB Virus Nucleic Acid Homology in a " Virus-free " Line of Burkitt Tumour Cells. Nature, *227*: 245–248, 1970.

Biological Activities of Herpes-type Virus Derived from Nasopharyngeal Carcinoma and Burkitt's Lymphoma

Mitsuru TAKADA, Akiyoshi KAWAMURA, Jr., and Haruo SUGANO

Department of Virology, The Kitasato Institute, Tokyo, Japan [M. T.] ; *Department of Immunology, Institute of Medical Science, University of Tokyo, Tokyo, Japan [A. K.]* ; *Department of Pathology, Cancer Institute, Tokyo, Japan [H. S.]*

In 1964, Epstein *et al.* (*6*) first demonstrated the presence of a herpes-type virus (Epstein-Barr virus: EBV) in cultured cells derived from Burkit's lymphoma (BL). Since then morphologically similar particles have been found in the other cell lines derived from BL (*7, 13, 25, 28, 29, 33*), nasopharyngeal carcinoma (NPC) (*30, 31*), other diseases (*2, 14*) and normal healthy subjects as well (*22*).

EBV has been classified morphologically as a member of the herpes virus group (*32, 34*), EBV-associated antigens have been demonstrated by immunofluorescence (FA) tests (*11, 17, 30*), complement fixation (CF) tests (*1, 8*), and agar immunogel diffusion tests (*19, 24*). Prepared rabbit anti-EBV sera showed a specific reaction in the FA test (*4, 5*), and in the immunogel diffusion test (*19*) with EBV-associated BL cell antigen. It is well documented that EBV is antigenically distinct from the other known herpes group viruses (*16*). However, most of the biological activities of EBV remain to be elucidated.

In 1967, Henle *et al.* (*10*) reported that co-cultivation of leucocytes with irradiated BL cells gave suggestive evidence of a growth stimulatory effect of the latter. More recently, Pope *et al.* (*26, 27*) and Gerber *et al.* (*9*) demonstrated the transformation of human leucocytes *in vitro* by the inoculation of extracts of EBV-carrying cells. It is conceivable that EBV may possibly have a transforming activity in human leucocytes.

The activity of thymidine kinase has been shown to increase in cells infected with a variety of DNA virus. With herpes simplex virus, the increase in thymidine kinase after infection is thought to be due to the synthesis of a new virus-specific enzyme, since it occurs in infected thymidine kinase-deficient mouse fibroblasts (*3*) and BHK 21 cells (*18*). So far, virus-specific thymidine kinase is not known to be increased by EBV, which is morphologically similar to the herpes virus group.

The present study was undertaken to demonstrate the infectivity and transforming ability of EBV derived from NPC (*30*) and BL (*12*) cells against the NPC cul-

189

tured cell sheets (*30*) (non-leucocyte cells).   Increased activity of the kinase induced by the EBV-containing extracts is also reported.

MATERIALS AND METHODS

Cell sheets derived from NPC

Cell sheets (*30*) were obtained from the tenth and seventh passage-levels of cultured cells, derived from the biopsy materials of NPC patients No. 12 and No. 27., respectively.   The presence of EBV particles and their antigenically distinct nature were not detected in these cells either with electron microscopy or with immuno-fluorescent staining before being infected and transformed.   After the cell sheets were fully formed, one half of the spent medium was replaced with fresh medium (Eagle's minimum essential medium (MEM) containing 10% fetal calf serum) once a week.   They were alternately maintained at 35°C and 37°C, with a pH below 7.0 for more than four weeks.   Under such conditions, they formed cell sheets which appeared to consist of multiple cell layers.

Preparation of cell free extracts (containing EBV) from the P3HR-1 and NPC-204 cells

Two cell lines, P3HR-1 (*12*) derived from BL and NPC-204 (*30*) derived from NPC, were grown in MEM or RPMI 1640 medium congaining 20 % fetal calf serum, 10 unit/ml of penicillin, 100γ/ml of streptomycin, and 5 unit/ml of my-costatin.   These cultured cells contained variable numbers of EBV.   The medium was changed at 4 to 5 day intervals, and the culture medium was adjusted to main-tain a cell density of about 5×10^5 cells/ml.   After the cell density reached about 1 to 2×10^6 cells/ml, the culture was incubated for 7 days at 32°C without changing the medium.   Each cell suspension, containing about 8×10^7 cells/80 ml was centrifuged at 1,200 rpm for 10 min at 4°C, and the packed cells were resuspended in 10 ml of spent medium.   They were subjected to quick freezing and thawing two times.   All the cell debris was removed by centrifugation at 3,000 rpm for 20 min at 4°C, and the supernatant fluid was filtered through a 0.3 μ millipore filter membrane.   The filtrates were used as a cell-free extract containing EBV.

Inoculation and maintenance of NPC cell sheets

The cell sheets (in 4 ounce bottles), maintained at pH 7.0 or below as described above, were inoculated with 10 ml of cell extracts, and were incubated at 35°C for 5 days, then at 37°C.   One-half of the culture fluid was replaced every 5 days with RPMI 1640 medium containing 20% fetal calf serum.   Untreated cultures served as controls.

Immunofluorescent staining

The indirect method established by Henle and Henle (*11*) was employed with a slight modification (*16*).   Acetone-fixed transformed cells were treated with serum from an NPC patient containing high titer of anti-EBV antibody.   Subsequently, fluorescein isothiocyanate (FITC)-labeled anti-human IgG-rabbit antibody at an optimal dilution was added to the preparation.   The stained preparations were examined under UV-illumination (Tiyoda FM-200B fluorescence microscope equipped with an Osrum HBO 200 high-pressure mercury lamp).

Electron microscopy

The transformed cells were fixed for 30 min with 4.2% glutaraldehyde buffered with cacodylate (pH 7.2). The fixed cells were then treated with 2% OsO_4 in the same buffer for 30 min, dehydrated with a series of gradated alcohol solutions, and embedded in an Epon 812-Araldite mixture, according to Mollenhauer (*21*). Ultra-thin sections were prepared with a Porter-blum MT-2 Ultratome. Then, they were doubly stained with saturated uranyl acetate and Karnovsky's lead solution (*15*). A Hitachi electron microscope (Hu-11B) was used for observation.

Cells and preparation for inducing an increase in thymidine kinase activity

NPC No. 115 cell sheets derived from NPC (*30*) and human embryo kidney (HEK) cells (a generous gift from Dr. F. Taguchi, School of Hygienic Sciences, Kitasato University) were used for the induction of thymidine kinase. Both cell sheets were obtained from the twelfth passage of the primary culture. They were grown in MEM containing 10% calf serum. Monolayer cells (in 4 ounce bottles) were inoculated with 5 ml of cell extracts, containing EBV and culture medium, instead of extracts, as the control. After the cells were exposed to the extract for 2–3 hr at 37°C, 5 ml of fresh medium was added, and the cells were reincubated. At different intervals after inoculation, the medium was discarded and the monolayer cells were washed 3 times with phosphate buffered saline (PBS). The cells were collected from the culture bottles, dispersed with a mixture of 0.05% trypsin and 0.05% disodium ethylenediamine tetraacetate (EDTA), centrifuged at 1,000 rpm for 5 min at 4°C, and the cells were again washed with PBS twice.

Preparation of extracts from HEK and NPC 115 cells

Approximately 4×10^5 to 4×10^6 cells were suspended in 0.5 ml distilled water and were disrupted. To prepare extracts for determining thymidine kinase activity, the disrupted cell suspension was centrifuged at 9,000 rpm for 15 min at 4°C. The supernatant from this centrifugation was collected for use in the assay of thymidine kinase. Preparation of unexposed cell extracts was carried out in a similar manner.

Assay of thymidine kinase activity

The assay of the enzyme was employed was the same as that described for BHK 21 cells infected with herpes simplex virus (*18*) with a slight modification. The reaction mixtures (total volume 0.25 ml) contained supernatant from extracts, together with 0.1 μ Ci thymidine-2-^{14}C (specific activity 50.0 m Ci/mM), 5 m MATP, 2.5 mM MgCl$_2$, and 0.05 M Tris-HCl (pH 8.0).

The reaction mixture was incubated for 7 to 10 min at 37°C, then heated for 2 min at 100°C, and cooled quickly in ice water. Denatured protein was removed by centrifugation for 20 min at 3,000 rpm and 0.1 ml of the supernatant was applied to 2.5 cm-wide strips of DEAE-cellulose paper. Free labeled thymidine was removed

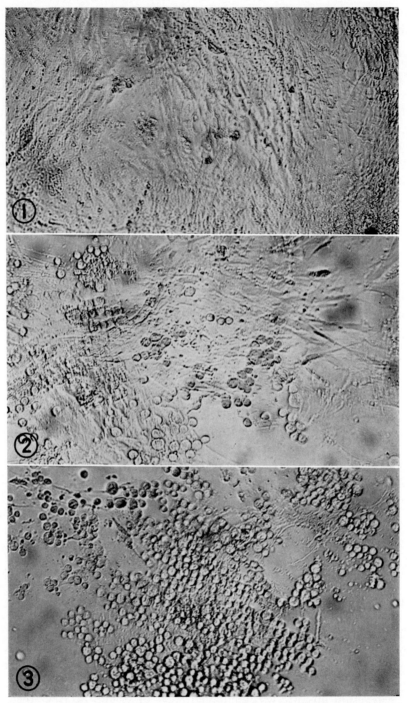

Fig. 1. Control culture NPC–12–(10) cell sheet on the 66th day after the 10th passage.
Fig. 2. Transformed round cells on the cell sheet 22 days after inoculation with P3HR–1 cell-free extract (N12T–1).
Fig. 3. Fifty-two days after inoculation with P3HR-1 cell-free extract (N12T-1).

by descending chromatography for 2 hr in 1.0 mM ammonium chloride.   These strips of paper were dried at room temperature and placed in vials containing 10 ml toluene and scintillator (3 g 2, 5-diphenyloxazole and 100 mg 1,4-bis-2-(4-methyl-5-phenyloxazolyl)-benzene per liter) for measurement of the radioactivity in a liquid scintillation counter.

RESULTS

Transformation of NPC cell sheets

In NPC No. 12, at its 10th passage level (Fig. 1), each culture was exposed to 10 ml of P3HR-1 cell extract and its filtrate.   Each 4 ounce flat glass bottle contained 10 ml of culture.   After inoculation, cell sheets were incubated at 35°C for 5 days, then at 37°C.   Round cells appeared on the cell sheets on the 22nd day of inoculation (Fig. 2).   Round cells continued to increase in number (Fig. 3) during cultivation and became floating in the fluid, but the culture exposed to the filtrate, instead of the cell extract, was lost accidentally, due to fungus contamination, three weeks after inoculation.

In NPC No. 12-(10) and NPC No. 27-(7) (Fig. 4) culture cell sheets were exposed to the filtrate of NPC-240 cell extract.   Round cells were detected in the cul-

TABLE 1.   Transformation of Host Cells by Extracts or Filtrates of the P3HR-1 and NPC 204 Cell Lines

NPC culture cell sheets		Type of cell extracts	Days of transforma-tion	Immunofluorescent staining of cells in culture fluid	
	Days after passage			Days after inoc.[a]	Per cent[b]
12-(10)	42	P3HR-1 unfiltered supernatant	22	7	0.0
				14	0.0
				22	0.6
				35	2.2
				41	8.9
12-(10)	42	— (control)		7	0.0
				22	0.0
				41	0.0
12-(10)	99	NPC204 300 mμ filtrate	18	7	0.0
				14	0.0
				28	8.1
				35	7.7
12-(10)	99	— (control)		7	0.0
				28	0.0
27-(7)	88	NPC204 300 mμ filtrate	107	7	0.0
				35	0.0
				112	13.5
27-(7)	88	— (control)		7	0.0
				35	0.0
				112	0.0

[a] Days after inoculation.
[b] Fluorescent positive cells.
( ) No. of passage.

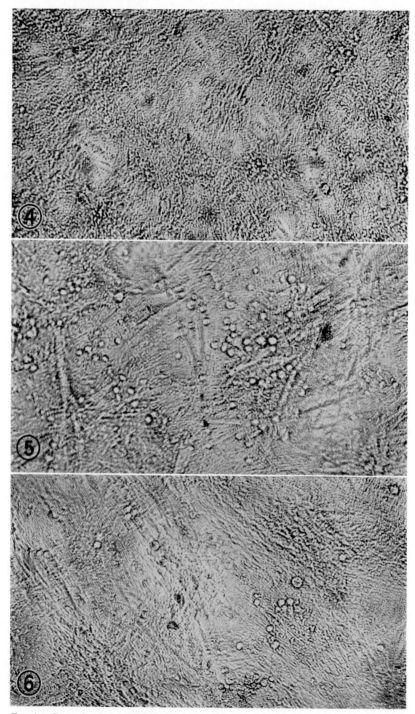

Fig. 4.   Control culture NPC-27-(7) cell sheet on the 196th day after the 7th passage.
Fig. 5.   Transformed round cells on the cell sheet 20 days after inoculation with the filtrate from the NPC-204 cell-free extract (N12T-3).
Fig. 6.   Transformed round cells on the cell sheet 108 days after inoculation with the filtrate from NPC-204 cell-free extract (N27T-4).

tures 18 (Fig. 5) and 107 days (Fig. 6) after exposure, respectively, and they also became floating. At the early stage of transformation, transformed floating cells were observed in smears with Wright stain.

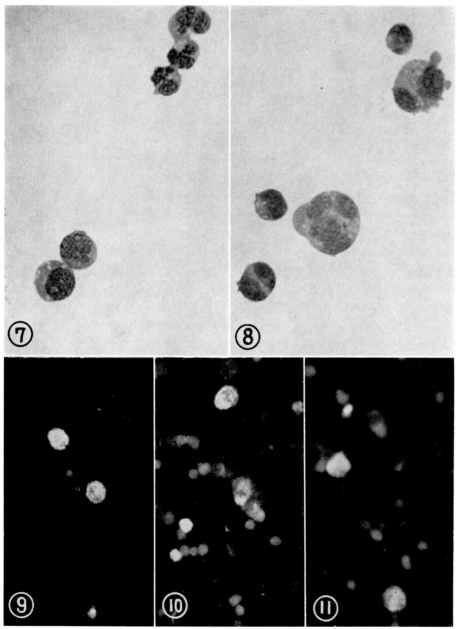

FIG. 7. Large nucleus and sparse cytoplasm.
FIG. 8. Multinucleated giant cell.
FIG. 9. Indirect immunofluorescent staining of N12T-1 cells.
FIG. 10. Indirect immunofluorescent staining of N12T-3 cells.
FIG. 11. Indirect immunofluorescent staining of N27T-4 cells.

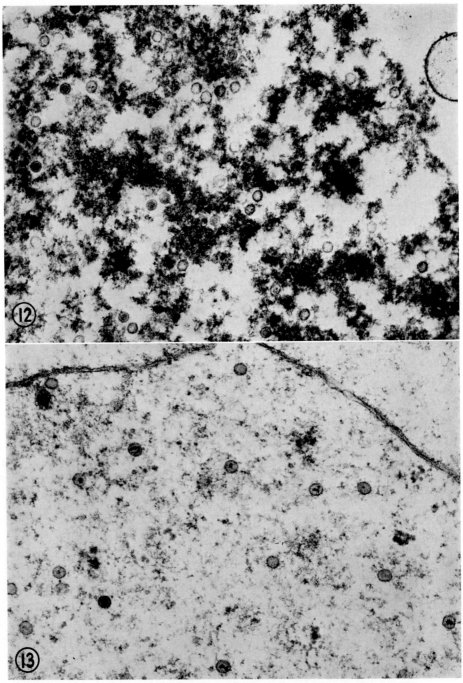

Figs. 12 and 13. Electron micrographs of a thin section of transformed cells. Herpes-type virus particles are demonstrated in the nucleus of the degenerating cell.

In the transformed floating cell population, there were two types of cells.   Approximately 5% of the cells were multinucleated giant cells, and 95% were cells with a large round nucleus and sparse cytoplasm (Figs. 7, and 8).   Cultures of transformed floating cells were free from mycoplasma.

NPC No. 12 (10) cultured cells, transformed by the inoculation of P3HR-1 cell extract, were designated as the N12T-1 line.   NPC No. 12-(10) and NPC No. 27-(7) cultured cells, transformed with NPC-204 cell extract, were designated N12T-3 and N27T-4, respectively, as shown in Table 1.   The three cell lines were established *in vitro* by transformation.

Immunofluorescent staining of transformed cells

Transformed N12T-1, N-12T-3, and N27T-4 cells were shown to be fluorescent positive (Figs. 9, 10, and 11) by direct and indirect immunofluorescent staining against NPC patient serum containing a high titer of anti-EBV antibody.   These transformed floating cells failed to react with FITC-labeled anti-human IgG. Fluorescent positive cells were not detected until round floating cells appeared on the cell sheets.   Control cell sheets without exposure gave negative results.

Presence of EB virus

In these three cell lines, herpes-type virus particles were observed in the nuclei

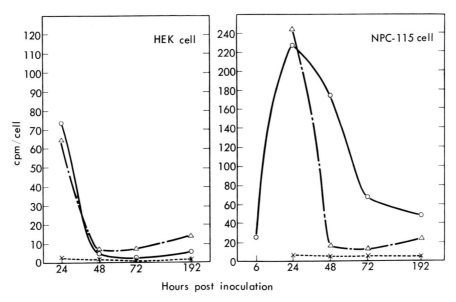

Fig. 14.   Activity of thymidine kinase in cells exposed to EBV-containing extracts.   Samples were taken at intervals for the determination of thymidine kinase activity.   Cell extracts were assayed for the determination of thymidine kinase.   Enzyme activity was measured at pH 8.0 reaction mixtures were contained in a final volume of 0.25 ml, 0.1 μCi thymidine-2-^{14}C (specific activity 50.0 mCi/mM), 5 mM ATP, 2.5 mM MgCl$_2$, 0.05 M Tris-HCl (pH 8.0), and Supernatant (from extracts). $\bigcirc$, P3HR-1 cells extract-exposed; $\triangle$, N12T3 cell extract-exposed cells; $\times$, MEM-exposed cells.

of transformed cells in a degenerating state (Fig. 12), but transformed cells in an intact state were also observed to be producing virus (Fig. 13).

Thymidine kinase activity in cells exposed to EBV containing extracts

Figure 14 shows the activities of thymidine kinase in HEK and NPC-115 cultured cell sheets exposed to an extract of P3HR-1 and N12T-3 cells.

The activity of thymidine kinase was increased within 24 hr of exposure to both extracts. The enzyme, 24 hr after exposure, was at a level about 21 to 33 times higher than in the control cells. The enzyme activity was measured at 6 hr in the cells exposed to P3HR-1 extract.

DISCUSSION

Pope *et al.* (*25, 27*) and Gerber *et al.* (*8,9*) demonstrated the transformation of human leucocytes *in vitro* by infection with EBV. Therefore, it can be seen that certain human cells are permissive hosts for *in vitro* cell transformation by EBV. BL and NPC have many similar aspects in epidemiological pictures. It seems likely that EBV is a causative agent for both human neoplasms. If EBV is able to transform normal lymphoid cells to lymphoma cells *in vivo* in the case of BL, EBV might possiblly be a causative agent for BL.

From the experimental results of an *in vitro* transformation of human cells derived from the nasopharynx by infection with a cultured cell extract (containing EBV) from NPC and BL, it is conceivable that NPC might also be induced by infection with EBV. So far, many investigators have failed to demonstrate the infection and transformation of monolayer cells by EBV *in vitro*. However, EBV has been shown to infect human leucocytes (*9, 26, 27*). In this study, cultured cell sheets derived from the nasopharynx were also demonstrated to be infected and transformed by EBV. Therefore, it is suggested that EBV has a certain susceptible host cell range.

Thymidine kinase activity was shown to increase in cells exposed to EBV-containing cell extracts. Increased activity of the enzyme in the early stage of infection, as seen in experiments with other DNA viruses, suggests the occurrence of a synthesis of virus-specific enzyme following EBV infection.

There is a difference between the levels of enzyme activities induced by HEK cells and NPC-115 cells derived from NPC. It was noted that the level in terms of activity per cell induced by the latter is 3.1–3.8 times higher than the former. The difference might be due to differences in cellular susceptibility to viruses, or to the presence of some favorable characteristics for EBV infection in the cell sheets derived from NPC patients. If infection, which is not present in normal cells of EBV, is affected by the character of these cells, it may well be that our host cells, derived from NPC and maintained in the conditions described above, have better affinity for EBV.

Some new supporting evidence about the infectivity of EBV was reported by Nishioka *et al.* (*23*) in this symposium. They found a new biological activity of EBV. It takes the form of an adherence of EA(IgG) cells (*23*) to transformed cells (N12T-1, N12T-3, and N27T-4), whose mother cells before infection by EBV-containing cell extracts did not show any sign of floating or spontaneous transformation and negative adherence with EA(IgG) cells. Therefore, they suggested that the adherence of EA(IgG) cells to cells transformed by EBV containing extracts is a manifestation of the viral genome (in a state of persistent infection) of EBV contained in NPC-204 or P3HR-1 cell extracts.

SUMMARY

Inoculation of cell-free extracts containing EBV into NPC cultured sheets led to morphologically distinct cell transformation *in vitro*. A long term culture of floating cells became possible.

In NPC No. 12, at the 10th passage level, cultures were exposed to P3HR-1 cell extract. Round transformed cells appeared on the cell sheets on the 22nd day of inoculation. In the NPC No. 12-(10) and NPC No. 27-(7) cultures, cell sheets were exposed to the filtrate of the NPC-204 cell extract. Round transformed cells were detected in the culture 18 days and 107 days after exposure, respectively, and they also became floating.

These transformed floating cells were shown to be fluorescent positive by direct and indirect immunofluorescent staining against NPC patient serum containing a high antibody titer to EBV. Control cell sheets without exposure gave negative results. EBV particles were demonstrated in these transformed cells.

Thymidine kinase increased within 24 hr, in NPC-derived cells and HEK cells exposed to EBV containing cell extracts. The enzyme, 24 hr after exposure, was present in quantities 21 to 33 times higher than the amount in the control cells. The enzyme activity from exposed NPC-115 cells was 3.1 to 3.8 times higher than that in exposed HEK cells.

These results possibly indicate that the EBV in the cell extracts from the P3HR-1 and NPC-204 cultured cells is an infectious agent to cells derived from the nasopharynx of NPC patients and is a factor responsible for making the NPC derived cell sheets floating *in vitro*.

The authors are indebted to Dr. Y. Saito, the Kitasato Institute, for his help and advice. This work was supported by grants from the Ministry of Health and Welfare, the Princess Takamatsu Fund for Cancer Research, and the Society for Promotion of Cancer Research.

REFERENCES

1. Armstrong, D., Henle, G., and Henle, W. Complement-fixation Tests with Cell Lines Derived from Burkitt's Lymphoma and Acute Leukemias. J. Bact, *91*: 1257–1262, 1966.

2. Diehl, V., Henle, G., Henle, W., and Kohn, G. Demonstration of a Herpes Group Virus in Cultures of Peripheral Leukocytes from Patients with Infectious Mononucleosis. J. Virol., *2*: 663–669, 1968.

3. Duffs, D. R., and Kit, S. Mutant Strains of Herpes Simplex Deficient in Thymidine Kinase-inducing Activity. Virology, *22*: 493–502, 1964.

4. Epstein, M. A., and Achong, B. G. Observations on the Nature of the Herpes-type

Virus in Cultured Burkitt Lymphoblasts, Using a Specific Immunofluorescence Test. J. Nat. Cancer Inst., *40*: 609–621, 1968.

5. Epstein, M. A., and Achong, B. G. Specific Immunofluorescence Test for the Herpes-type EB Virus of Burkitt Lymphoblasts, Authenticated by Electron Microscopy. J. Nat. Cancer Inst., *40*: 593–607, 1968.

6. Epstein, M. A., Achong, B. G., and Barr, Y. M. Virus Particles in Cultured Lymphoblasts from Burkitts Lymphoma. Lancet, *1*: 702–703, 1964.

7. Epstein, M. A., Achong, B. G., and Pope, J. H. Virus in Cultured Lymphoblasts from a New Guinea Burkitts' Lymphoma. Brit. Med. J., *2*: 290–291, 1967.

8. Gerber, P., and Birch, S. M. Complement-fixing Antibodies in Sera of Human and Nonhuman Primates to Viral Antigen Derived from Burkitt's Lymphoma Cells. Proc. Nat. Acad. Sci., U.S.A., *58*: 478–484, 1967.

9. Gerber, P., Whang-Peng, J., Monroe, J. H. Transformation and Chromosome Changes Induced by Epstein-Barr Virus in Normal Human Leukocyte Cultures. Proc. Nat. Acad. Sci., U.S.A., *63*: 740–747, 1969.

10. Henle, W., Diehl, V., Kohn, G., zur Hausen, H., and Henle, G. Herpes-type Virus and Chromosome Marker in Normal Leukocytes after Growth with Irradiated Burkitt Cells. Science, *157*: 1064–1065, 1967.

11. Henle, G., and Henle, W. Immunofluorescence in Cells Derived from Burkitt's Lymphoma. J. Bact., *91*: 1248–1256, 1966.

12. Hinuma, Y., and Grace, J. T., Jr. Cloning of Immunoglobulin-producing Human Leukemic and Lymphoma Cells in Long Term Cultures. Proc. Soc. Exp. Biol. Med., *124*: 107–111, 1967.

13. Hummeler, K., Henle, G., and Henle, W. Fine Structure of a Virus in Cultured Lymphoblasts from Burkitt Lymphoma. J. Bact., *91*: 1366–1368, 1966.

14. Iwakata, S., and Grace, J. T., Jr. Cultivation *in vitro* of Myeloblasts from Human Leukemia. New York State J. Med., *64*: 2279–2282, 1964.

15. Karnovsky, M. J. Simple Methods for " Staining with Lead " at High pH in Electron Microscopy. J. Biophys. Biochem. Cytol., *11*: 729–732, 1961.

16. Kawamura, A., Jr., Takada, M., Gotoh, A., Hamajima, K., Sanpe, T., Murata, M., Ito, Y., Takahashi, T., Yoshida, O. T., Hirayama, T., Tu, S.-M., Liu, C.-H., Yang, C.-S., and Wang, C.-H. Seroepidemiological Studies on Nasopharyngeal Carcinoma by Fluorescent Antibody Techniques with Cultured Burkitt Lymphoma Cell. GANN, *61*: 55–71, 1970.

17. Klein, G., Clifford, P., Klein, E., and Stjernsward, J. Search for Tumor-specific Immune Reaction in Burkitt Lymphoma Patients by the Membrane Immunofluorescence Reaction. Proc. Nat. Acad. Sci., U.S.A., *55*: 1628–1635, 1966.

18. Klemperer, H. G., Haynes, G. R., Shedden, W. I. H., and Watson, D. H. A Virus-specific Thymidine Kinase in BHK 21 Cells Infected with Herpes Simplex Virus. Virology, *31*: 120–128, 1967.

19. Konn, M., Yohn, D. S., Hinuma, Y., Yamaguchi, J., and Grace, J. T., Jr. Immuno-gel Diffusion Studies with the Herpes Type Virus (HTV) Associated with Burkitt's Lymphoma. Cancer, *23*: 990–997, 1969.

20. Levy, J. A., and Henle, G. Indirect Immunofluorescence Tests with Sera from African Children and Cultured Burkitt Lymphoma Cells. J. Bact., *92*: 275–276, 1966.

21. Mollenhauer, H. H. Plastic Embedding Mixtures for Use in Electron Microscopy. Stain Tech., *89*: 111–114, 1964.

22. Moore, G. E., Gerner, R. E., and Franklin, H. A. Culture of Normal Human Leukocytes. J.A.M.A., *199*: 519–524, 1967.

23. Nishioka, K., Tachibana, T., Hirayama, T., de Thé, G. Klein, G., Takada, M., and Kawamura, A., Jr. Immunological Studies on the Cell Membrane Receptors of Cultured Cells Derived from Nasopharyngeal Cancer, Burkitt's Lymphoma and Ifectious Mononucleosis. pp. 401, Proceedings of the 1st International Symposium of the Princess Takamatsu Cancer Research Fund, University of Tokyo Press, Tokyo, 1971.

24. Old, J., Boyse, E. A., Oettegen, H. F., de Harven, F., Geering, G., Williamson, B., and Clifford, P. Precipitating Antibody in Human Serum to an Antigen Present in Cultured Burkitt Cells. Proc. Nat. Acad. Sci., U.S.A., 56: 1699–1704, 1966.

25. Pope, J. H., Achong, B. G., Epstein, M. A., and Biddulph, J. Burkitt Lymphoma in New Guinea: Establishment of a Line of Lymphoblasts in vitro and Description of Their Fine Structure. J. Nat. Cancer Inst., 39: 933–945, 1967.

26. Pope, J. H., Horne, M. K., and Scott, W. Identification of the Filtrable Leukocyte-transforming Factor of QIMR-W1L Cells as Herpes-like Virus. Int. J. Cancer, 4: 255–260, 1969.

27. Pope, J. H., Horne, M. K., and Scott, W. Transformation of Foetal Human Leukocytes in vitro by Filtrate of a Human Leukaemic Cell Line Containing Herpes-like Virus. Int. J. Cancer, 3: 857–866, 1968.

28. Rabson, A. S., O'conor, G. T., Baron, S., Whang, J. J., and Legallais, F. Y. Morphologic, Cytogenetic and Virologic Studies in vitro of a Malignant Lymphoma from an African Child. Int. J. Cancer, 1: 89–106, 1966.

29. Stewart, S. E., Lovelace, E., Whang, J. J., and Ngu, V. A. Burkitt Tumor: Tissue Culture, Cytogenetic and Virus Studies. J. Nat. Cancer Inst., 34: 319–327, 1965.

30. Takada, M., Lin, T.-C., Shiratori, O., Sugano, H., Yang. C.-S., Hsu, M.-M., Lin, T.-C., Tu, S.-M., Chen, H.-C., Hamajima, K., Murata, M., Gotoh, A., Kawamura, A., Jr., Yoshida, O. T., Osato, T., and Ito, Y. Cultivation in vitro of Cells Derived from Nasopharyngeal Carcinoma. GANN Monograph, 10: 149–161, 1971.

31. de Thé, G., Ambrosioni, J. C., Ho, H.-C., and Kwan, H.-C. Lymphoblastoid Transformation and Presence of Herpes-type Viral Particles in a Chinese Nasopharyngeal Tumor or Cultured in vitro. Nature, 221: 770–771, 1969.

32. Toplin, I., and Schidlovsky, G. Partial Purification and Electron Microscopy of Virus in the EB-3 Cell Line Derived from a Burkitt Lymphoma. Science, 152: 1084–1085, 1966.

33. Toshima, S., Takagi, N., Minowada, J., Moore, G. E., and Sandberg, A. A. Electron Microscopic and Cytogenetic Studies of Cells Derived from Burkitt's Lymphoma. Cancer Res., 27: 753–771, 1967.

34. Yamaguchi, J., Hinuma, Y., and Grace, J. T., Jr. Structure of Virus Particles Extracted from a Burkitt Lymphoma Cell Line. J. Virol., 1: 640–642, 1967.

Discussion of Papers by Drs. Pope, and Takada

DR. EPSTEIN: Are there any questios or commens on the last reports?

DR. HAYASHI: I would like to make some comments about Dr. Takada's report. First, the examination was performed in connection with the agglutinability of the EB virus-carrying cells, using concanavalin A and wheat germ agglutinin. The results of the experiment with the cell line of EB virus-carrying cells, P3HR-1 from Burkitt's lymphoma, NPC 323-3 from NPC, LY-B from infectious mononucleosis and LY-6 from normal tonsils but carrying EB virus, show similar patterns to those reported by Inbar and Sachs (Inbar, M., and Leo Sachs, Interaction of the carbohydrate-binding protein concanavalin A with normal and transformed cells. Proc. Nat. Acad. Sci. *63*, 1418–1425, 1969) concerning the agglutinability of the cells transformed by various chemical carcinogens, SV40 virus, or X-rays, using concanavalin A. But the control experiments are insufficient and the malignancy of EB virus-carrying cells is inconclusive from these data alone. Second, the agglutinability of HeLa cells after infection with EB virus (inoculation of the extract of EB virus-carrying cells), as in Dr. Takada's report, was examined using concanavalin A and wheat germ agglutinin. From 12 to 96 hr after infection, HeLa cells did not show an increase in agglutinability. Third, the agglutinability of EB virus-carrying cells which were infected with herpes simplex virus was examined. Twelve hr after infection, a slight increase in agglutinability was observed, but the meaning of this increase is unclear.

DR. TAKAHASHI: Dr. Pope, we know there are plenty of human lymphoid cell lines derived from normal donors, general patients, and from Burkitt's lymphoma; I think there are more than 600 such lines and about 30% of these cell lines contain EB-like particles. Experiments performed by Moore and his associates, and also by Gerber and his associates, clearly showed that such lymphoid cells can be established without addition of EB virus preparation. I would like to know the relevance of their experiments to your experiment. The second question is, I would like to know whether cell-free extracts from lymphoid lines can or cannot cause lymphoid proliferation.

DR. POPE: If I understand you correctly, you have asked for comments on the meaning of Dr. Moore's experiments in establishing cell lines from normal persons. My interpretation of this, is, I think, completely opposite to Dr. Moore's. In my experience it means to me that some of his cultures had EB virus in them, which led to the establishment of cell lines. I know Dr. Moore does not believe this, however. In any case, this is my opinion at this time.

DR. EPSTEIN: Am I allowed to say something, because I think I quite agree with Dr. Pope on this point? The thing is that when his first line was established there was no information on how widespread the infection was. This was just about the time Dr. and Mrs. Henle were beginning to do the antibody studies. This was in early '66, or '65 so what he was probably doing was collecting from normal donors, most of whom were antibody positive, that is to say, carrying the virus. So he was putting into the culture, cells which were already infected. Pope's work was presumably done with antibody negative donors who, therefore, were not carrying the virus. I don't think there is any difficulty in his interpretation. Wouldn't you agree with that?

DR. G. HENLE: Dr. Moore starts out with a very large amount of blood, something like 500 cc, from adults. This has been done by Dr. Pope. Dr. Ogata and ourselves, starting out with only 10 cc of blood. This is quite a different situation. Dr. Moore and several other people in the United States use from very large volumes to very small volumes. So the environment in the two sets of experiments is different.

DR. TAKAHASHI: Do you think cell-free extracts from such lymphoid cells derived from normal donors can also induce lymphoid proliferation?

DR. POPE: We have known the EB virus titer of the normal person from whom the cell line was derived. There is also a technical factor: just the mere presence of EB virus does not mean transforming activity. It is necessary to have a sophisticated virus to get a successful transformation. You can have EB virus present and still have an ineffective preparation.

DR. SOUTHAM: Going back to the same question, I rather share the opinion that George Moore's studies indicate the lack of the necessity for EB virus. You assume that the line established by George Moore from normal sources actually carried EB virus and that this was the reason for the successful establishment of the culture. Then we are assuming that the EB virus need not persist once the cell line is established and need not persist in any form whatsoever. However, we do know that Dr. Pope's experiment failed to show any evidence of a transforming effect in the Raji line. In Raji there is neither morphological evidence for a virus particle nor is there serological evidence.

DR. EPSTEIN: No, the viral genome is present, the DNA homology experiment shows that there are one to six genomes per cell.

DR. Southam: But the capacity to transform is not present in spite of this.

DR. EPSTEIN: That argument is with regard to infectious particles. Complete intectious particle has not been found.

DR. SOUTHAM: Then, the last point that puzzles me is, in the Dr. Takada's report, the monolayer was from nasopharyngeal carcinoma. This is an established line. Did it contain EB virus particles to start with? If not, had they disappeared?

DR. TAKADA: We thought cultured fibroblastic cells derived from the non-tumorous tissue of NPC were genetically more susceptible to the infection of EB virus. We selected these cells as the target. The possibility that spontaneous floating, due to pre-existing EBV-carrying cells in the starting fibroblastic cell mixtures, could be excluded, as will be shown in Dr. Nishioka's presentation tomorrow.

RESEARCH ON NASOPHARYNGEAL CANCER: A REVIEW

Chairmen:

Tadashi Yamamoto, M. A. Epstein

Present Status of Studies on Nasopharyngeal Carcinoma

Akiyoshi KAWAMURA, Jr.

Department of Immunology, Institute of Medical Science, University of Tokyo, Tokyo, Japan

The presence of herpes-type virus (HTV) or Epstein-Barr virus (EBV) has been confirmed in a number of cultured cells derived from Burkitt's lymphoma (BL). Meanwhile, many cultured cell lines derived from nasopharyngeal carcinoma tumor tissues has shown the presence of HTV. In NPC patient sera, a high antibody titer reacting with HTV antigens and/or HTV-related antigens of the cells carrying HTV was observed, as well as in BL patient sera. These findings are compatible with the hypothesis on the viral etiology of these tumor cells.

As shown in Table 1, BL and NPC showed strikingly different epidemiological pictures with regard to geographical distribution, race, sex, age, clinical manifestation, and histopathological picture, as well as susceptibility to chemotherapeutics. It is necessary to differentiate these two disease entities by virological and immunological methods in order to explain the essential difference between them.

In order to clarify the role of HTV in the etiology of NPC, a task force composed of Japanese and Taiwanese researchers of different specialities was organized

TABLE 1. Comparison of Epidemiological Pictures of Burkitt's Lymphoma and Nasopharyngeal Carcinoma

	Burkitt's lymphoma (BL)	Nasopharyngeal carcinoma (NPC)
Geographical distribution	Africa	South China
Race	African	Chinese
Sex (M/F)	1	2–3
Age	Children	about 40
Susceptibility to chemotherapeutics	+	?
Clinical manifestations	tumor of jaw	headache, tinnitus,
	paraplegia	hearing disturbance,
		nasal obstruction,
		nasal bleeding
Histopathological pictures	lymphoma	epitherial carcinoma anaplastic

TABLE 2. Study Organization of the Japan-China Cooperative Study on Nasopharyngeal Carcinoma

	China	Japan
Clinical subgroup		
(Otorhinolaryngology)	Shih-Mien Tu, Ti Shieh	
	Mow-Ming Hsu, Tsong-Chou Lynn	
(Internal medicine)	Chen-Hui Liu, Chiu-Hwa Wang	
Pathological subgroup	Shu Yeh, Hai-Chin Chen	Haruo Sugano
Epidemiological subgroup	Kung-Pei Chen, Tong-Ming Lin	Takeshi Hirayama
Virological and	Czau-Siung Yang, Yuan-Chuan Lin	Yohei Ito, Akiyoshi Kawamura, Jr.
Immunological subgroup	Shen-Wu Ho, Shiow-Hua Shieh,	Kusuya Nishioka, Yorio Hinuma
	Chien-Ts Chu	Takehiko Tachibana, Takato O. Yoshida
		Toyoro Osato, Rei Hatano
		Masaharu Inoue, Osamu Shiratori
		Akinori Ishimoto, Ikuo Kimura
		Mitsuru Takada, Kozaburo Hayashi
		Takeshi Hosokawa, Michisato Murata
		Kenji Hamajima, Atusi Gotoh
		Tsuneo Sanpe, Ming-Nan Huang

Chairman: Dr. Shu Yeh
Moderators: Drs. Chen-Hui Liu and Yohei Ito

in November, 1968, in Taipei. Table 2 shows the study organization of the Japan-China cooperative study on NPC. The chairman is Dr. Shu Yeh, the moderator of the Chinese side is Dr. Chen-Hui Liu and the moderator of the Japanese side is Dr. Yohei Ito. The following is an explanation of the main points of the present status of our studies.

Clinical study

As shown in Table 3, during the five year period from 1965 to 1969, more than 1,000 patients visited the National Taiwan University Hospital with signs and symptoms suggestive of NPC. The diagnosis was histopathologically verified by nasopharyngeal biopsy in 850 of these patients: 839 carcinoma and 11 sarcoma. For the 839 cases of NPC, age and sex incidence, yearly incidence, and symptomatology were studied. A record linkage system was established assembling clinical, immunological, and pathological data.

Pathological study

The results of systematic histological and cytological classification of NPC in

TABLE 3. Clinical Study (1965–1969)

Number of NPC patients	more than 1,000
Confirmed by histopathology	850
carcinoma	839
sarcoma	11

National Taiwan University Hospital

TABLE 4.   Epidemiological Study

Morbidity survey	Male	Female
Phase I Descriptive epidemiology (1968)		
Annual incidence rate/100,000	5.26	2.17
Peak age group	60–64	60–64
(Incidence rate)	(20.19)	(8.50)
Phase II Serological case control studies (1969–1970)		
Phase III Population prospective study (1970–)		

80 Chinese patients were compared with immunological data for the patients. Virus-like particles were observed in the cancer cells from 4 patients who possessed high titers of antibody against HTV in their sera.

Epidemiological study

The first phase—As shown in Table 4, the frequency of NPC in Taiwan was studied in 1968 by conducting a morbidity survey covering the whole country.   The annual incidence rate per 100,000 was calculated as 5.26 for males and 2.17 for females. At the peak age group of 60–64, the rates were 20.19 and 8.50, respectively.

The second phase—Based on our standard method of fluorescent antibody technique, serological case control studies were done in 1969 to 1970 for NPC patients, and family and neighbourhood controls in both northern and southern Taiwan. The results will be described by Dr. Lin *et al.* in this symposium.   A large scale follow up of the general population group is now planned as the third phase of the study based on these results.

Virological study

The tissue culture and electron microscope group found virus particles identified as HTV in eight cell culture lines derived from NPC patients.   They confirmed that the cultured cells belong to the reticular cell group from their morphological pictures and from the existence of an immune adherence (IA) receptor reacting with 19S antibody sensitized sheep erythrocytes combined complement components [EA(IgM)C43 cells], on the cell membrane as Dr. Nishioka *et al.* reported

TABLE 5.   Comparison of Characteristics of Floating Cultured Cells Derived from Burkitt's Lymphoma, Nasopharyngeal Carcinoma, Infectious Mononucleosis, and Normal Healthy Subjects

	Burkitt's lymphoma	Nasopharyngeal carcinoma	Infectious mononucleosis	Normal healthy subjects
Anti-HTV antibody titer	high	high	moderate	low
Detection of HTV in biopsy materials	−?	+	−	−
Floating cultured cells derived from	+	+	+	+
Detection of HTV in cultured cells	+	+	+	+
Morphological figures of cultured cells	lymphoblastoid	reticular	reticular	reticular
IA receptor	−	+	+	+
Hemadsorption of EA (IgG)	+	−	−	−
Agglutination by wheat germ agglutinin or concanavalin A	+	+		

in this symposium.   On the other hand, we did not observe adherence of EA(IgM) C43 cells on the membrane of BL cultured cells, which belong to the lymphoblastoid cell group, as shown in Table 5.   Although the HTV-carrying BL cell lines showed adherence of 7S antibody-sensitized sheep erythrocytes [EA(IgG)cells], the NPC cell lines did not demonstrate such hemadsorption.   Table 5 shows other characteristics of floating cultured cells derived from BL, NPC, infectious mononucleosis, and normal healthy subjects.

As Dr. Takada *et al.* reported in this symposium, inoculation of HTV into NPC cultured HTV-free cell sheets led to morphologically distinct cell transformation *in vitro* and long term culture of floating cells carrying HTV became possible. These cell lines showed adherence of EA(IgG)cells, but not EA(IgM)C43 cells.

Immunological study
    Our standard method of anti-HTV measurement—Table 6 shows the standard for

TABLE 6.   Our Standard Measurement of Anti-HTV Antibody Titer by Indirect Fluorescent Antibody Technique

Antigen :	Burkitt's lymphoma cultured cell line (P3HR–1) viability of cells —— 40–60%			
Antibodies :	Primary —— diluted test serum into 1 : 40, 1 : 160, 1 : 640, 1 : 2,560, and 1 : 5,120			
	Secondary —— fluorescein isothiocyanate conjugated anti-human IgG rabbit-IgG			
Dilution of positive control serum (NPC No. 137 patient)	1 : 40	1 : 160	1 : 640	1 : 2,560
Degree of positive	4+	3+	2+	1+
Percent of positive cells/total cells	> 10%	5–10%	2–5%	Ca 1%

The standard for the determination of the results of the immunofluorescence reaction was set in reference to the ratio of fluorescence-positive cells over the total cells as 4+, 3+, 2+, 1+ and 0.   The preparation of over 1+ was considered as positive.

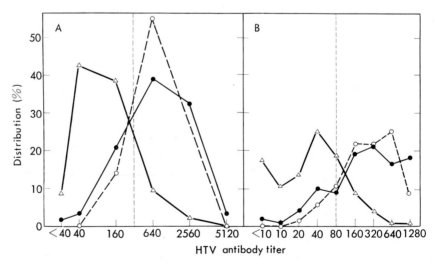

FIG. 1.   Percentile distribution of anti-HTV antibody titers among Burkitt's lymphoma patients, nasopharyngeal carcinoma patients, and normal subjects.   A, Japan-Taiwan Co-operative study ;   B, Henle *et al.* ;   ○, Burkitt's lymphoma ;   ●, nasopharyngeal carcinoma ; △, normal subjects.

the determination of the results of the immunofluorescence reaction. It was set in reference to the ratio of fluorescence-positive cells over the total cells on the following scale: 4+, 3+, 2+, 1+, and 0. The preparation of over 1+ was considered as positive (*1*).

The boundary of positive reaction—From close observation of the frequency distribution of anti-HTV antibody titers of normal subjects, both in Japan and Taiwan, of NPC and BL patients, as illustrated in Fig. 1-A, dissociation in frequency distribution of healthy and abnormal subjects was found to be a maximum when the boundary of positive reaction was set at 1:640 dilution of the test sera (*3*). However, in the work of Dr. Henle's group, it was set at 1:160, as shown in Fig. 1-B. This may suggest that our conjugate and fluorescence microscope are more sensitive than theirs.

As shown in Fig. 2, a higher prevalence of persons with high HTV antibody titers was also found in healthy persons in Taiwan than in Japan (*1–3*). That is, the incidences reacting at a higher dilution than $\geq 1:640$ were 85.7% in BL (7 cases), 66.5% in Chinese NPC in Taiwan (173 cases) and 73.3% in Japanese NPC (15 cases). These values were extraordinarily higher than those in other neoplastic diseases (20%) or than those in normal subjects (ranging from 5.4 to 17.7%). On the other hand, a moderately high rate of positive incidence was observed in infectious mononucleosis (42.8%) and in malignant lymphoma (43.6%). In other diseases, such as measles, rubella, and syphilis, the incidences were even lower than those in normal subjects. As the morbidity of NPC in Taiwan has

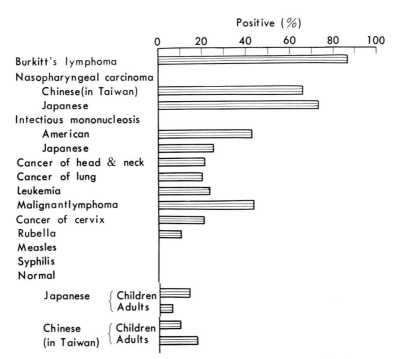

FIG. 2. Anti-HTV positive rate of sera from patients of Burkitt's lymphoma, nasopharyngeal carcinoma, other diseases and from normal subjects.

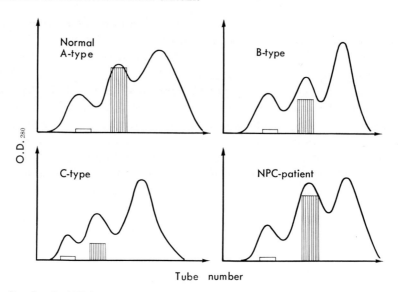

O.D. .280

Fig. 3. Anti-HTV reactivity in the fractions of the test sera separated by Sephadex G-200 gel filtration.   ▨, anti-IgG ;   ▢, anti-IgM.

been known to be nearly 100 times higher than that in Japan, the incidences of positive fluorescent antibody reaction among normal subjects in Taiwan and in Japan were compared.   The rate of positiveness in Chinese adults in Taiwan was 17.7%.   This is significantly higher than that of Japanese adults (5.4%).   On the other hand, there was essentially no difference between the incidences in the children of both countries.

An immunological characterization of the cell membrane was made.   Antibodies reacting with the membrane and other antigens in the cell were studied by fluorescent antibody techniques, immunoelectron microscopy, and immune adherence.   That is, antibodies reacting with an acetone-fixed smear of HTV carrying cells were found only in the IgG fraction of the sera of NPC and BL patients, and of normal subjects with high anti-HTV antibody titers, by means of the indirect fluorescent antibody method (1, 2).   The chromatography patterns of the results are shown in Fig. 3.   A serum sample with an anti-HTV titer of 1 : 2,560 is shown in (A), a serum with an anti-HTV titer of 1 : 160 in (B), and a serum with an anti-HTV titer of 1 : 40 in (C).   When the IgM fractions were tested after concentration to one-tenth of the original volume, no positive fluorescence was observed with acetone-fixed smears.

When the smears of the BL-cultured cell line (P3HR-1) with HTV were fixed by acetone and reacted with patients sera in the indirect fluorescent antibody technique, the specific fluorescence was observed on the surface of the BL cells in most of the cases, and only rarely observed in the cytoplasm.   However, when the acetone-fixed smears of P3HR-1 cells were directly reacted with fluorescein isothiocyanate-conjugated IgG fractions of BL, NPC sera, or healthy adult sera with a high anti-HTV antibody titer, three types of immunofluorescence were observed.   These were: specific fluorescence on the cell surface, diffuse or discrete specific fluorescence in the cytoplasm, and specific intranuclear fluorescence. One of these three types was observed separately, or two or three types were present in combined form. When the smear was stained with fluorescein isothiocyanate-conjugated IgG fractions of BL, NPC, or normal adult sera, no essential difference was observed. It was hard to measure the positive fluorescence quantitatively, but specific intracellar fluorescence was observed much more frequently with the direct fluorescent antibody technique, than with indirect fluorescent antibody technique. It has been suggested that, when compared with electronmicroscopic or immuno-electron microscopic observation, not all of these positive fluorescences correspond to virions of HTV (1). That is, as Dr. Suzuki *et al.* reported in this symposium, by immuno-electron microscopy, using the peroxidase-conjugated IgG fractions of BL, NPC, or normal adult sera with a high anti-HTV antibody titer, labeling was demonstrated not only in the complete virion in the cell but in the cytoplasm, in the nucleus, or on the membrane of HTV cells. These antigen-antibody relationships will be discussed by other participants of this symposium.

This, then, is the outline of the present status of the investigation of the Japan-China cooperative study group.

These studies have been supported by research grants from the Ministry of Public Health and Welfare, the Society for Promotion of Cancer Research, and the Princess Takamatsu Cancer Research Fund.

REFERENCES

1. Kawamura, A., Jr., Hamajima, K., Murata, M., Gotoh, A., Takada, M., Nishioka, K., Tachibana, T., Hirayama, T., Yoshida, T. O., Imai, K., Ito, Y., Yang, C.-S., Chu, C.-T., Wang, C.-H., Ho, S.-W., Tu, S.-M., Liu, C.-H., and Lin, T.-M. Studies on Nasopharyngeal Carcinoma and Burkitt Lymphoma by Immunofluorescence. Ann. N.Y. Acad. Sci., *177*: 250–267, 1971.
2. Kawamura, A. Jr., Hamajima, K., Gotoh, A., Murata, M., Takada, M., Sanpe, T., Takahashi, T., Yoshida, T. O., Ito, Y., Hirayama, T., Nishioka, K., Tachibana, T., Yang, C.-S., Wang, C.-H., Ho, S.-W., Chu, C.-T., Chen, H.-C., Hsu, M.-M., Linn, T.-C., Tu, S.-M., Lin, T.-M., and Liu, C.-H. Seroepidemiological Studies on Nasopharyngeal Carcinoma by Immunofluorescence. GANN Monograph, No. 10, 185–198, 1971.
3. Kawamura, A., Jr., Takada, M., Gotoh, A., Hamajima, K., Senpe, T., Murata, M., Ito, Y., Takahashi, T., Yoshida, T. O., Hirayama, T., Tu, S.-M., Liu, C.-H., Yang, C.-S., and Wang, C.-H. Seroepidemiological Studies on Nasopharyngeal Carcinoma by Fluorescent Antibody Techniques with Cultured Burkitt Lymphoma Cell. GANN, *61*: 55–71, 1970.

Discussion of Paper by Dr. Kawamura

Dr. Epstein: Really it is not right to say that Burkitt's lymphoma is a disease of Africans, that it only occurs in Africa, that it always affects the jaw. Far from that, it seems to affect everybody, anywhere, and if you happen to live in Africa, you may get it irrespective what ever your race is.

Dr. Ho: I would like to ask the last speaker about the peak age group of NPC. Is this or is this not just the peak of patients seen, because this should be quite different from the peak in the age specific morbidity curve as we see it in Hongkong and Singapore?

Dr. Lin: I think Dr. Kawamura presented data on the age specific morbidity rate.

Dr. Ho: The peak age groups is at 60 to 64? Does that apply to both male and female alike, or just both combined?

Dr. Lin: It's just combined; and I think we have separate male and female curves also, but, as I recall, the shape is about the same and there are no special differences.

Dr. Hirayama: I understand the meaning of Dr. Ho's question. We compared the age-specific morbidity rate of NPC for each sex between the data in Hongkong and the data in Taiwan. The pattern was found to be quite similar, and, as the feature common to both data, the peak age for males is somewhat younger than that for females.

Dr. Epstein: Have we any further questions? Well, then I think I will thank all speakers and contributors to the program this afternoon, and bring this session or a very successful first day to a close.

Listening here as session chairman to the interesting presentations we have heard today and to the stimulating and lively discussions which have followed each of them, I would like to record my pleasure at being here. I think we have all had a great privilege in being able to attend this meeting which is clearly serving such a useful and important role in the exchange of scientific ideas. Our subject matter is highly topical and I should like to thank the Princess Takamatsu Fund for Cancer

217

Research for having selected this topic and sponsored this meeting. We are all, I am sure, most grateful to the Fund and I should like to record my pleasure at the extremely successful way the Symposium is going.

RESEARCH ON NASOPHARYNGEAL CANCER: CLINICAL AND PATHOLOGICAL ASPECTS

Chairmen:

Werner Henle, J. H. C. Ho

Clinical Characteristics of Nasopharyngeal Carcinoma in Taiwan

Shih-Mien Tu

Department of Otolaryngology, National Taiwan University, Taipei, Taiwan, Republic of China

The term " nasopharyngeal carcinoma " usually calls our attention to two things. One is the Chinese and the other is lymphoepithelioma or undifferentiated carcinoma. Certainly, a number of reports have pointed to its high incidence among the Chinese and to a special relation between lymphoepitheliomas or transitional cell carcinomas, and nasopharyngeal carcinoma. In 1965, at the Eighth International Congress of Otorhinolaryngology, the writer presented an observation of 1,668 histologically verified nasopharyngeal carcinomas and discussed the peculiarity in incidence and pathology (4). During the following five-year period, from January 1965 to December 1969, more than 1,000 patients visited the National Taiwan University Hospital with symptoms and signs suggestive of nasopharyngeal cancer. The diagnosis was histologically confirmed chiefly by nasopharyngeal biopsy in 850 of these patients. There were 839 carcinomas and 11 sarcomas. This distribution amply demonstrated the tendency that sarcoma of the nasopharynx in the Chinese is far less common than in other populations. The present study is concerned with a review of the 839 cases of nasopharyngeal carcinoma.

Incidence

The yearly incidence of nasopharyngeal carcinoma is shown in Fig. 1. More than 150 cases visited us each year in a recent three year period; the average number of new patients was 168 per year. As compared with the data from the world literature, this is by far the highest incidence ever reported. For comparison, the data reported from each country was carefully reviewed and the average annual incidence was calculated. Although great care was taken to ensure that there was no case other than those with histologically proved carcinoma in this calculation, many authors appeared to collect the cases from two or more hospitals. In Japan, only three cases of nasopharyngeal carcinoma were seen per hospital per year.

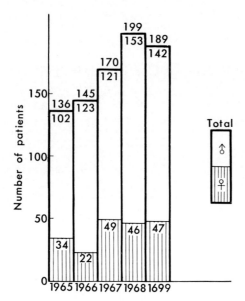

Fig. 1. Nasopharyngeal carcinoma: yearly incidence (1965–1969). Average yearly incidence, 167.8.

On the contrary, the incidence in Southern Asia, in such places as Hong Kong, Singapore, and Indonesia, appeared very high; the great majority of the victims were undoubtedly overseas Chinese. The figures available from the United States, 5.6 cases a year, also included some Chinese patients in the study. A relatively high incidence was reported from East Africa (23.4 in Kenya) (3), but in European

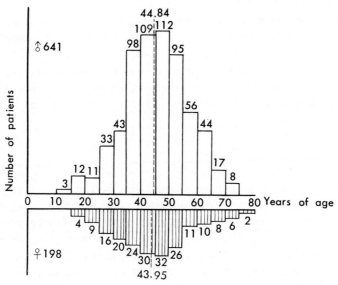

Fig. 2. Age distribution of nasopharyngeal carcinoma. Mean of age: mail 44.84, femail 43.95, all 44.63. The youngest age, 11 years; the oldest age, 76 years. ♂ : ♀=3. 24 : 1.

countries, as well as in other countries of Caucasian population, the average yearly incidence was less than 10 cases.

641 of our patients were male and 198 female, giving a ratio of 3.2 to 1. The male predominance is in accord with the figures which have appeared in many previous reports. The age of the patients ranged from 11 to 76 years and the average age was 44.6 years. The mean age of the women was a little less than that of the men (Fig. 2). There were 98 Chinese patients who came from 14 different provinces of mainland China after the war. The number of patients in this series varied greatly from province to province, but the greatest prevalence of the disease was found to be Southeast China. Kwangtung, Fukien and Chekiang were the order of frequency of occurrence.

Symptomatology

The signs and symptoms may be conveniently divided into six groups:
1. Cervical adenopathy
2. Pain in the head and neck
3. Bleeding from the nose and mouth
4. Nasal or nasopharyngeal symptoms
5. Aural symptoms
6. Neurological symptoms

In regard to initial symptoms and later developments of this series, 820 cases with detailed histories and complete records of observation were reviewed and analyzed (Table 1). Cervical metastasis was the first symptom in the majority of cases, 37.6%, and even one of the most common signs in the later course, 64.8%. The presence of a painless mass situated under the mastoid tip and the jaw angle and movable on palpation deep to the sternocleidomastoid muscle was usually an alerting and earliest symptom in the initial stage of the tumor. The second most frequent symptom was bleeding, occurring in 29.8% and 65.2%, respectively, in each stage. The patient was usually frightened by blood-tinged sputum in the morning and came to the doctor. Repeated bloody rhinorrhea or mild epistaxis followed soon.

Among 820 patients, 241 cases noticed the signs due to tubal obstruction as an

TABLE 1.   Frequency of Symptoms in 820 Cases of Nasopharyngeal Carcinoma

Symptoms	Initial		Later	
	No.	%	No.	%
1. Cervical adenopathy	308	37.6	531	64.75
2. Pain in the head and neck	129	15.7	400	48.8
3. Bleeding from the nose or mouth	244	29.8	535	65.2
4. Nasal or nasopharyngeal symptoms	190	23.2	422	51.4
5. Aural symptoms	213	25.97	560	68.3
6. Neurological symptoms	38	4.6	192	23.4
7. Miscellaneous	9	1.97	78	9.51

initial symptom. It ranked next to the above-mentioned symptoms, but ear symptoms might persist throughout the treatment and even lasted for a long time after the irradiation. Impaired hearing, tinnitus and a sensation of stuffiness of the ear were the most frequent complaints in the later stage of our patients (68.3%). Nasal obstruction, purulent nasal discharge, and nasal twang could be a first symptom of this disease. However, it was sometimes difficult to differentiate these from those symptoms due to purulent sinus infection. Headache often occurred unilaterally as a type of hemicrania. It was sometimes so severe as to prevent the patient from working.

The neurological symptoms present one of the most interesting aspects of nasopharyngeal carcinoma. The nerve is usually involved at the later stage by intracranial extension of the growth or backward invasion along the skull base. Consequently, only 38 cases (4.6%) of our 839 patients showed neurological symptoms at an initial stage. However, 192 cases (23.4%) were later proved to have palsies or paralyses of their cranial nerves. Because of their anatomical position, the fifth, and twelfth nerves were the ones most frequently involved and were followed by the nerves of the jugular foramen group and orbital cavity group (Table 2).

Owing to the variety of early symptoms, to the relative lack of initial symptoms related to the primary lesion, and to the inaccessibility of the nasopharynx, early diagnosis of nasopharyngeal carcinoma is usually difficult. In this study, there was an average delay of 8.2 months from the onset of symptoms to the institution of the correct diagnosis. Although more than 75% of the patients got an accurate diagnosis within one year after the onset of initial symptoms, there was still a long delay in diagnosis, more than two years in 41 cases (5%) (Table 3).

TABLE 2. Frequency of the Involvement of the Different Cranial Nerves

Authors	Cases involved/ Total	I	II	III	IV	V	VI	VII	VIII	IX	X	XI	XII	S
Mekie et al. (1954)	54/120	3	11	16	8	16	31	12	5	10	7	6	19	—
Scanlon et al. (1958)	37/88	—	1	5	4	10	29	6	0	10	8	3	9	—
Lederman (1961)	58/218	1	9	20	17	35	31	7	2	13	20	17	13	—
Bloom (1963)	26/57	2	4	11	6	19	14	7	6	14	5	4	8	8
Clifford et al. (1964)	31/85	—	8	10	9	13	17	8	7	8	6	7	13	
Total	206/568	6	33	62	44	93	122	40	20	55	46	37	62	8
Tu (1965)	373/915		38	80	91	190	227	39	8	109	89	60	167	30
Tu (1970)	192/820	1	10	32	28	145	129	14	1	45	52	20	67	8

TABLE 3. Time Elapsed from Initial Symptom to Accurate Diagnosis

Duration	No. of cases	Percentage (%)
Up to 3 months	216	25.74
3 months — 6 months	210	25.03
6 months — 1 year	215	25.62
1 year — 2 years	120	14.30
Over 2 years	41	4.88
Unknown	37	4.43

Pathology

The nasopharynx has been called the great " blind spot " in the diagnosis, since the nasopharynx is not entirely accessible for examination, since the primary lesion is often small or indefinite, since there is sometimes an island or mass of normal lymphatic tissue resembling a new growth, and since certain individual characteristics of the patient, such as a hypersensitive gag reflex, short velopharynegeal distance, elongated uvula, or trismus, may prevent a detailed examination. Eventually, many controversial opinions may exist among pathologists and clinicians, concerning the shape and location of the new growth. In 1947, Ackerman and del Regato (*1*) divided the tumors of the nasopharynx into three types: ulcerated, lobular, and exophytic. Since then, many reports have used this system to describe the gross appearance of nasopharyngeal carcinoma, though some used the terms infiltrative or polylobulated instead of lobulated.

Over the years, tracing the successive daily mirror findings of every patient, we have found this description unsatisfactory and sometimes incorrect. Furthermore, we have added a routine radiographic study of the nasopharynx with an opaque contrast media for the diagnosis of every case. To our surprise, the majority of the patients have shown a smooth or prominent swelling on the posterior wall of the nasopharynx. The change usually spreads to a wide extent on the posterior wall and sometimes infiltrates submucously to the roof and/or lateral wall. Without doubt, these changes can be easily overlooked by routine mirror examination, though the radiogram is not a good diagnostic aid for demonstrating the change of the posterior nostril and anterior wall of the nasopharynx. With the aid of Storz's electric laryngo-pharyngoscope, nasopharyngoscopic photography became another helpful weapon for this study in 1963. Since then, we have tried to take more than ten pictures in different directions for every case of nasopharyngeal carcinoma. Analyzing the findings obtained through these three methods, we have come to the conclusion that the primary growth of the nasopharynx can be grouped into three types: exophytic, infiltrative, and granular, and that the ulcerative lesion, which was considered by many authors as the common type in these tumors, should be disregarded. In this study we also found ulcerative changes in a few cases. But all of them were secondary ulcerations and infections found at the superficial layer of fungating or infiltrative swellings or were deep necrotic ulcerations seen after excessive irradiation.

In 206 cases of this series, the gross appearance and site of the primary growth could be classified rather accurately using the above-mentioned procedure. In the case of mixed figures, the most typical and predominant change was selected as the type of the tumor. Exophytic lesions were most commonly seen in our study, in 111 out of 206 cases. The submucous infiltration type came next, with 87 cases, and the granular type included 8.

As shown in Table 4, the exophytic change was most frequently seen in the roof of nasopharynx. The posterior wall appeared to be an unfavorable location for this type, but 85 out of 87 cases with submucous infiltration occupied the posterior wall. Granular change was commonly in evidence at the roof and anterior wall.

TABLE 4.   Relation of Site of Growth to Gross Appearance

Shape \ Site	Roof	Posterior wall	Lateral wall	Anterior wall	Total
Exophytic	79	16	37	39	111
Infiltrative	26	85	22	7	87
Granular	7	1	2	4	8
Total	112	102	61	50	206

TABLE 5.   Histological Classification of Nasopharyngeal Carcinoma (by H.C. Chen)

	Type
A) Adenocarcinoma	1
B) Anaplastic Carcinoma	
a) Carcinoma simplex	2
b) Majority of cells containing secretory granules	3
c) Mixed type	4
d) Majority of cells containing tonofibrils	5
C) Classical Epidermoid Carcinoma	6

However, it was sometimes noticed on the posterior well and roof at the limited area of the surface of other two types.

The histophathological classification of nasopharyngeal carcinoma is still confusing and perplexing.   In an attempt to abandon the term " lymphoepithelioma," our pathologist, Dr. Yeh, studied 1,000 consecutive biopsy specimens of these tumors in 1962 and set up a new histopathological classification.   However, it was complicated and impractical for clinical use (5).   Recently, based on electron microscopic studies of normal nasopharyngeal tissues and of biopsy specimens obtained from a certain number of patients with nasopharyngeal carcinoma, Dr. Chen reevaluated the light-microscopic structure of these tumors, and another classification was proposed (2).   Table 5 shows his new typing.

In this series, 133 specimens were available for re-evaluation and classification by Dr. Chen, and they were grouped histologically according to his method.   No adenocarcinoma was seen in this group (Type 1).   The majority of cases, 109 of 133, fell into the category of anaplastic carcinoma (Type 2–5).   The remainder, 24, were classsical epidermoid carcinomas (Type 6).   The relationship between the site of the growths, the gross appearance, and the histological classification was analyzed and is shown in Tables 6 and 7.   From this analysis, we could not come to any general conclusion.   Anaplastic carcinoma of the nasopharynx seems to prefer the exophytic

TABLE 6.   Comparison of Histology with Gross Appearance of Nasopharyngeal Carcinoma

Shape \ Type	1	2	3	4	5	6	Total
Exophytic	—	6	35	10	12	10	73
Infiltrative	—	4	24	4	11	14	57
Granular	—	1	1	—	1	—	3
Total	0	11	60	14	24	24	133

TABLE 7.   Relation of Site of Growth to Histological Classification

Type \ Site	1	2	3	4	5	6
Roof	—	6	30	9	13	12
Posterior wall	—	6	31	7	16	16
Lateral wall	—	1	15	8	9	4
Anterior wall	—	3	18	4	4	1

shape and may arise from any place in the nasopharynx, while epidermoid carcinoma seems to prefer the infiltrative or lobulated type as to gross appearance, and the roof and posterior wall as to the location in the nasopharynx.

SUMMARY

During the five-year period, 1965 to 1969 inclusive, 839 patients with nasopharyngeal carcinoma visited the National Taiwan University Hospital. There were 641 males and 198 females, giving a ratio of 3.2 to 1. The age of the patients ranged from 11 to 76 years; the average age was 44.6 years. 98 of 839 patients were mainland Chinese, and the greatest prevalence was found in Southeast China. The average yearly incidence was 168. This was the highest incidence ever reported.

The signs and symptoms in the initial and later stages were analyzed and divided into 6 groups. Cervical metastases and bleeding from the nose and mouth were the most commonly encountered initial symptoms. In the later stages, ear symptoms and bleeding were complained of most frequently. The neurological symptoms presented one of the most interesting aspects and usually developed in the later stages. Because of the anatomical position, the fifth, sixth, and twelfth nerves were most often involved. There was an average delay of 8.2 months from onset of symptoms to diagnosis.

With the aid of three diagnostic methods, i.e., successive daily mirror examinations, contrast radiography of the nasopharynx, and nasopharyngoscopic photography, the gross appearance and site of the primary growth was classified rather accurately in 206 cases.

The Exophytic type was most frequently seen, in 111 out of 206 cases, and was commonly located in the roof of the nasopharynx. Infiltrative change came next, with 87 cases, 85 of which demonstrated the change on the posterior wall. The granular type was rather rare and it seemed to prefer the roof and anterior wall. Dr. Chen's histological classification was briefly introduced, and the relation between the shape and site of the tumor was studied, but we could not arrive at a general conclusion.

REFERENCES

1.   Ackerman, L. V., and del Regato, J. A.   Cancer: Diagnosis, Treatment and Prognosis.   3rd Ed., C. V. Mosby Company, St. Louis, 1962.

2. Chen, H.-C., Yeh, S., and Sugano, H.   Histogenesis of Anaplastic Epidermoid Carcinoma and Stromal Reaction in the Nasopharynx.   GANN Monograph, *10*: 215–233, 1971.
3. Clifford, P.   Malignant Diseases of the Nasopharynx and Paranasal Sinuses in Kenya. UICC Monograph Series, *1*: 82–94, 1967.
4. Tu, S.-M.   Nasopharyngeal Carcinoma in Taiwan, Proceed. Eighth Intern.   Cong. Series, *113*: 184–185, Oct. 1965.
5. Yeh, S.   A Histological Classification of Carcinomas of the Nasopharynx with a Critical Review as to the Existence of Lymphoepithelioma.   Cancer, *15*: 895–920, Sept.–Oct. 1962.

Carcinoma of the Nasopharynx in Japan

Haruo Sugano, Shuji Sawaki, Goi Sakamoto, and Takeshi Hirayama

Department of Pathology, Cancer Institute, Tokyo, Japan [H. S., G. S.]; Department of Otolaryngology, Yokohama City University Medical School, Yokohama, Japan [S. S.]; Epidemiology Division, National Cancer Center Research Institute, Tokyo, Japan [T. H.]

It is well known that carcinoma of the nasopharynx (NPC) is very common in the Chinese, especially in southern China (*5, 9, 17*). In Japan, however, NPC is not common and only a few people have been interested in the pathology, diagnosis, and treatment of this lesion (*1, 6–8*). In 1961, Dr. Yeh gave a magnificent paper on the histological classification of NPC in Taiwan at the Meeting of the Japanese Pathological Society in Tokyo (*17*). We were deeply impressed with this interesting form of cancer.

At that time, a peculiar fatal necrotic lesion of the nasopharynx, called progressive gangrenous rhinitis, had attracted interest in this country (*11*). Although extensive microbiological examinations of this lesion were carried out, no clear results had been obtained. The studies concluded that this lesion should be understood as a clinical syndrome; lymphoma for the most part, sometimes carcinoma, and chronic inflammation, including Wegener's disease of the nasopharynx, revealed such a progressive necrotic lesion clinically (*12*). Through these studies, our knowledge of nasopharyngeal tumors gradually accumulated; evidence that NPC is closely associated with the EB virus (*13, 14*) has recently aroused much interest in NPC (*3*).

In this paper, the pathology, incidence, and some problems of NPC in Japan will be described and discussed. The study described in this paper is based on an analysis of 1,129 cases of NPC in the following four groups:

Group 1: 75 cases of biopsy materials from the Cancer Institue during the 20 years from 1947 to 1967, and selected from 117 cases of epipharyngeal tumor among 1172 cases of malignant tumors of the upper respiratory tract.

Group 2: 99 cases of autopsy records obtained from all the medical schools and major hospitals in Japan for 11 years from 1950 to 1966, and selected from 113 cases of nasopharyngeal tumors.

Group 3:   227 cases found from replies to questionnaires sent out by the out-patient clinics of the oto-rhinolaryngology departments of all the medical schools and major hospitals in Japan for 1969 and 1970, and selected from 347 cases of malignant nasopharyngeal tumors.

Group 4:   678 cases from national death records for the 17 years from 1948 to 1965. All the cases in each group, except the 678 cases in Group 4, were confirmed by histopathology.

Histology

Nasopharyngeal tumor in Japan is characterized by two prominent features when viewed histologically: predominance of squamous cell carcinoma, especially of undifferentiated squamous cell carcinoma, and a relatively high incidence of lymphoma. As Table 1 shows, squamous cell carcinoma was the most frequent, and accounted for 60–80% of all cases. Undifferentiated squamous cell carcinoma occurred in about one-half of all malignant nasopharyngeal tumors in all the groups. One-third of this undifferentiated carcinoma was transitional cell carcinoma and lymphoepithelioma, and the remaining two-thirds was spindle and polygonal-shaped carcinoma which are similar to carcinoma of the uterine cervix. Lymphoma was found in 12–30%, among which reticulum cell sarcoma occurred with twice the frequency of lymphosarcoma. Plasmocytoma was very rare, while Hodgkin's disease was not observed.

TABLE 1.   Histology of Nasopharyngeal Tumors

Source No. of cases	Group 1 117	Group 2 113	Group 3 347
Squamous cell *ca.*			
„ diff.	17.1(%)	38.0(%)	30.6(%)
„ undiff.	47.1	43.4	46.7
Other carcinoma	3.4	5.3	3.7
Lymphoma	30.1	12.4	18.2
Other sarcoma	2.3	0.9	1.4

TABLE 2.   Malignant Tumors of the Nasopharynx (%)

Reporters	(No. of cases)	Sq. cell *ca.*	Anapl. *ca.*	Other *ca.*	Malig. lymph.	Others
Vaeth, Cal.[a]	(82)	17.1	70.8	2.4	4.9	4.8
Wang, Mass.[b]	(115)	22.5	61.4	7.0	3.5	5.6
Shedd, Conn.[c]	(213)	51.4	12.2	14.5	5.6	13.6
Lederman, Lond.[d]	(327)	21.5	45.5		20.5	12.5
Yeh, Taiwan[e]	(1,437)	17.5	68.7	12.6	1.1	0.1
JAPAN						
Hatori[f]	(262)	37.1	15.6	7.7	32.0	7.6
Ootuka[g]	(90)	21.1	40.0	3.4	22.2	13.3
Group 1	(117)	17.1	47.1	3.4	30.1	2.3
Group 2	(113)	38.0	43.4	5.3	12.4	0.9
Group 3	(347)	30.0	46.7	3.7	18.2	1.4

[a],[b],[c],[d,e],[f] and [g] correspound to reference *1, 4, 8, 10,* and *15–17* respectively.

TABLE 3. Histological Type of Squamous Cell Carcinomas of the Upper Respiratory Tract in Group 1

	Nasal cavity	Naso-pharynx	Meso-pharynx	Tonsil	Hypo-pharynx	Maxilla	Total
No. of cases	58	75[a]	6	84	173	497	893
Well differentiated (%)	54	27	50	70	82	74	70
Poorly differentiated (%)	46	73	50	30	18	26	30

[a] Including four Chinese cases.

Table 2 shows a histological classification of nasopharyngeal tumors in various countries. In general, anaplastic squamous cell carcinoma is predominant in all the countries. On the other hand, the frequency of lymphoma in countries other than Japan is very low, only several per cent, except in Dr. Lederman's report from London. In contrast, lymphoma is rather common in Japan.

Among malignant tumors of the upper respiratory tract, as Table 3 shows, squamous cell carcinoma is most common in the maxilla and not so frequent in the nasopharynx. The high incidence of well-differentiated carcinoma of the maxilla in Japan is considered to be related to chronic inflammation of the accessory sinuses and squamous metaplasia of the lining epithelium, which are common in this country. On the other hand, anaplastic or poorly differentiated squamous cell carcinoma is predominant only in the nasopharynx. It is interesting that the histology of carcinoma of the nasopharynx is similar to that of the uterine cervix. Histogenesis of both carcinomas is also similar because they develop in the multi-layered columnar epithelium, often associated with squamous metaplasia. There have also been reports of the association of nasopharyngeal carcinoma with EB virus, and of cervical carcinoma with Herpes simplex type-2. A comparative study of these two cancers would be of interest and should be of value.

Sex ratio

NPC was dominant in the male. The sex ratio varied with groups and was 1.9: 1, 3.0: 1, 1.6: 1, and 1.7: 1 in Groups 1, 2, 3, and 4, respectively. On the average, it was twice as high in the male as in the female.

Age incidence

NPC is rarely found in childhood, but was common in the 30 to 60 year age group; the peak age group in both sexes was in the 50's in every group. The peak age of lymphoma was also in the 50's. Figure 1 indicates the age distribution of 279 cases of carcinoma, including 12 cases of adenocarcinoma and 63 cases of lymphoma in Group 3. The curve shows a plateau for carcinoma, while lymphoma forms a sharp peak. Figure 2 shows the age-specific death rate of NPC per 100,000 population of Group 4 in Japan and in Taiwan. In both sexes of the two countries, the mortality rate sharply increases with age. It decreases after the 60's in the male, and it always increases with age in the female. As for the difference in the incidence according to sex, the peak age group of the male and female in Group 1 was in the 50's and 30's; respectively; for Japan, 1965, the mortality rate showed a

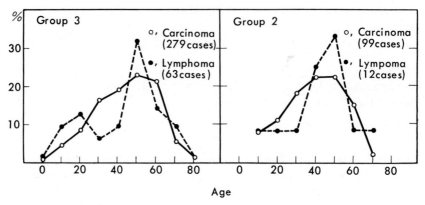

FIG. 1.   Age incidence of nasopharyngeal tumors.

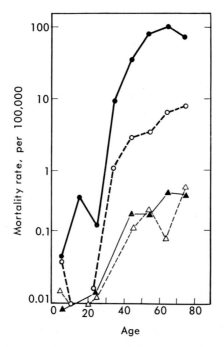

FIG. 2.   Age specific death rate of carcinoma of the nasopharynx.   ●, Taiwan, male ; ○, Taiwan, female ; ▲, Japan, male ; △, Japan, female.

peak in the 60's and 50's, respectively, for males and females.   Therefore, the peak age group in the female seems to be one decade younger than that in the male.

Incidence

Concerning the frequency of NPC in Japan, the rate of NPC found by autopsy was 0.146% of all tumor cases in Group 2.   Data from out-patient clinics in Group 3 revealed that 138 new cases of NPC were found in one year.   The mortality rate of NPC in 1965 was 0.054 per 100,000 population in the male and 0.044 in the female.

In the peak age group, it was 0.212 per 100,000 population of the males in the 60's and 0.132 of the females in the 50's.

Therefore, it can be concluded that the incidence of NPC in Japan is very low, but has shown a tendency to increase in recent years.

Geographic distribution

Geographic distribution of the patients with NPC in Group 3 is shown in

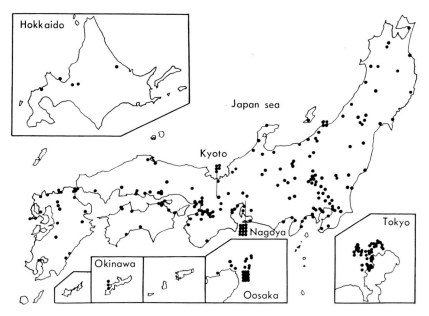

FIG. 3.   A geographic distribution of patients with NPC in Japan (Group 3).

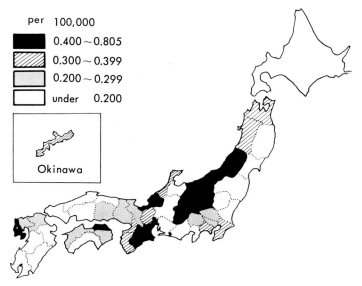

FIG. 4.   Morbidity rate of carcinoma of the nasopharynx (1969, 1970).

Fig. 3. Many patients were found in large cities, such as Tokyo, Nagoya, Osaka, and the northern part of Kyushu. It is interesting that it seems to be frequent in the areas along some large rivers, such as the Tone-Arakawa, Shinano, and Mogami rivers, and also around the Inland Sea; this finding may suggest a water-borne nature for NPC, or may only reveal the density of population in Japan. Therefore, the morbidity rate of NPC per 100,000 population was calculated by districts. This process revealed a significant geographical distribution showing a relatively high morbidity rate in the northern districts facing the Japan Sea and the districts in the central part of Japan. The Morbidity rate in Okinawa is not so high. The number of cases of NPC taken up in this study was limited and a larger number of cases should be accumulated.

Racial incidence

With regard to the racial incidence of NPC, 7 out of 277 cases of NPC in Group 3 were Chinese while none of the 63 cases of lymphoma was Chinese. The population of Chinese in Japan is 44,000 (*2*). Therefore, the incidence of NPC is almost 60 times higher in the Chinese than in the Japanese. This finding was also supported by the fact that 4 out of the 75 cases with NPC were Chinese in Group 1, as shown in Table 3. On the other hand, 3 out of 277 cases of NPC in Group 3 were Koreans. The population of Korean in Japan is 608,000 (*2*). Thus, there is no significant difference in the incidence between the Korean and the Japanese.

As Fig. 2 indicates, the incidence of NPC is roughly 100 times higher in the Chinese in Taiwan than in the Japanese. This shows that, although the incidence of NPC in overseas Chinese is still high, it is still lower than that for natives of Taiwan and the southern part of China. It is interesting that the incidence of NPC in Okinawa, which is geographically close to Taiwan and had been closely related to the mainland China in its history, is the same as that in the main islands of Japan.

SUMMARY

Carcinoma of the nasopharynx in Japan was studied in 1,129 cases obtained from biopsy, autopsy, questionnaires, and national death records. Among the malignant tumors of the nasopharynx, squamous cell carcinoma, especially anaplastic carcinoma, was predominant, and malignant lymphoma, especially reticulum cell sarcoma, showed a much higher relative frequency than in other countries. The sex ratio was 2.0 and the peak age group was in the 50's in both sexes. The incidence of carcinoma of the nasopharynx in Japan is very low, but its mortality rate has been gradually increasing, the rate in 1965 being 0.054 per 100,000 population in the male and 0.044 in the female. The autopsy rate of carcinoma of the nasopharynx among all tumors was 0.146%. Furthermore, 138 new cases visited outpatient clinics in one year. A geographical distribution of the patients showed that they were frequent in large cities, as well as in the areas along some rivers, and a relatively high morbidity rate was found in some particular districts in Japan. The incidence in Okinawa was not so high. Incidence of nasopharyngeal cancer in the Chinese in Japan is about 60 times higher than that in the Japanese, whereas its incidence in the Korean is almost the same as that in the Japanese.

REFERENCES

1. Hatori, H.   Statistics of Malignant Tumors of the Epipharynx.   Jibi-Rinsho, *59*: 581–584, 1966 (in Japanese).
2. Hirayama, T., Fukazawa, T., and Kimura, M.   Population Analysis of Foreigners in Japan.   Kōsei-no-Shihyo (Guide to Welfare), *12*: 8–14, 1965 (in Japanese).
3. Hirayama, T.   "Epidemiological Approach in the Research on Nasopharyngeal Carcinoma," 1969 (personal communication ; in Japanese).
4. Lederman, M.   Cancer of the Pharynx ; A Study Based on 2,417 Cases with Special Reference to Radiation Treatment.   J. Laryng. & Otol., *81*: 151–172, 1967.
5. Muir, C. S., and Shanmugaratnam, K., Eds.   Cancer of the Nasopharynx.   UICC Monograph Series, Vol. 1, Munksgaad, Copenhagen, 1967.
6. Miyaji, T. Carcinoma of the Nasopharynx and Related Organs in Japan Based on Mortality, Morbidity and Autopsy Studies.   Cancer of the Nasopharynx.   UICC Monograph Series, Vol. 1.   Eds. Muir and Shanmugaratnam, Munksgaad, Copenhagen, 29–32, 1967.
7. Ootuka, H.   On the So-called Lymphoepithelioma of the Nasopharynx.   Saishin-Igaku, *19*: 1708–1719, 1964 (in Japanese).
8. Ootuka, H.   Clinicopathological Study of Pharyngeal Cancer.   Gan-no-Rynsho (Cancer Clinics), *14*: 633–640, 1968 (in Japanese).
9. Shanmugaratnam, K.   Cancer of the Nasopharynx.   Proc. 9th Intl. Cancer Congress, UICC Monograph Series, Vol. 10, Springer-Verlag, Berlin-Heidelberg-New York, 1967, pp. 110–116.
10. Shedd, D. P., Essen, C. F., and Eisenberg, H.   Cancer of the Nasopharynx in Connecticut ; 1935 through 1959.   Cancer, *20*: 508–511, 1967.
11. Sugano, H., Enomoto, M., and Watanabe, T.   Four Autopsy Cases of Diffusely Metastasizing " Progressive Gangrenous Rhinitis "—Reticulum Cell Sarcoma of the Nose.   Acta Pathol. Japon., *7*, Suppl.: 817–834, 1957.
12. Sugano, H.   Burkitt Tumor and Allied Disorders in Japan.   GANN Monograph, *7*: 35–47, Maruzen Co., Tokyo, 1969.
13. Sugano, H., Takata, M., Chen, H.-C., and Tu, S.-M.   Presence of Herpes-type Virus in the Culture Cell Line from a Nasopharyngeal Carcinoma in Taiwan.   Proc. Japan Acad., *46*: 453–457, 1970.
14. de-Thé, G., Ambrosioni, J. C., Ho, H.-C., and Kwan, H.-C.   Lymphoblastoid Transformation and Presence of Herpes-type Viral Particles in a Chinese Nasopharyngeal Tumor Cultured *in vitro*.   Nature, *221*: 770–771, 1969.
15. Vaeth, J. M.   Nasopharyngeal Malignant Tumors : 82 Consecutive Patients Treated in Period of 22 Years.   Radiology, *74*: 364–372, 1960.
16. Wang, C. C., Little, J. B., and Schulz, M. D.   Cancer of the Nasopharynx: Its Clinical and Therapeutic Considerations.   Cancer, *15*: 921–926, 1962.
17. Yeh, S.   A Histological Classification of Carcinomas of the Nasopharynx with a Critical Review as to the Existence of Lymphoepitheliomas.   Cancer, *15*: 895–920, 1962.

Anaplastic Carcinoma of the Nasopharynx

Hai-chin CHEN, Shu YEH, Shih-mien TU, Mow-ming HSU, Tsong-chou LYNN, and Haruo SUGANO

Department of Pathology, College of Medicine, National Taiwan University, Taipei, Taiwan, Republic of China [H. C., S. Y.] ; Department of Otolaryngology, College of Medicine, National Taiwan University, Taipei, Taiwan, Republic of China [S. T., M. H., T. L.] ; Department of Pathology, Cancer Institute, Tokyo, Japan [H. S.]

For years, the question has occurred of why the majority of the nasopharyngeal carcinomas in Chinese are anaplastic carcinomas, and the proportion of adenocarcinoma is extremely rare (*53*). To discuss histogenesis of the various types of anaplastic nasopharyngeal carcinoma, it is necessary to understand the normal histology of the nasopharyngeal mucosa. In previous investigations (*26, 46,*), ultrastructural observations of nasopharyngeal carcinomas have shown a variety of cytoplasmic organelles in the neoplastic cells.

Concerning the etiology of nasopharyngeal carcinoma, no significant information has been elucidated. Although many factors may be implicated, it is of interest to observe that patients with nasopharyngeal carcinoma demonstrate high titers of antibody in sera against the EB virus (*55*). In order to know more about this problem, an electron microscopic study was attempted on cancer cells and tissue culture cells. The results of the tissue culture have been reported in a separate paper (*45*).

This paper is primarily concerned with the histogenesis of component cancer cells at an ultrastructural level vis-'a-vis their appearance as revealed by conventional light microscopy. With regard to the development of antibody producing cells in patients with nasopharyngeal carcinoma, attention was particularly paid to the behavior of lymphoid tissue in the stroma, and its response to the infiltration of cancer cells.

MATERIALS AND METHODS

During an 85 day period of cooperative study by Chinese and Japanese specialists in otolaryngology, pathology, virology, immunology, microbiology, hematology, and epidemiology, carried out at the National Taiwan University Hospital, Taipei, Taiwan, in the spring and summer of 1969, 49 patients with nasopharyngeal malig-

237

nancy were seen in the Out-Patient Department of Otolaryngology of the National Taiwan University Hospital. Three of these 49 patients were cases of malignant lymphoma. Of the remaining 46 patients with nasopharyngeal carcinoma, 3 exhibited well-differentiated epidermoid carcinoma. In addition, there were 3 patients who had already received radiotherapy, 1,000 r to 6,000 r divided doses, at other hospitals when first examined. These 9 cases were excluded from this study.

Biopsies, histologically proved to be anaplastic nasopharyngeal carcinoma prior to irradiation, consisted of 28 males and 12 females, varying in ages from 12 to 65 years. As controls, biopsies from 10 patients, from 14 to 65 years of age with diseases other than nasopharyngeal carcinoma were taken, and proved to be of normal mucosa. All the biopsies were processed separately for light and electron microscopic studies, immunofluorescent reactions, and tissue cultures.

Light microscopy was performed on paraffin sections, stained with hematoxylin and eosin, mucicarmine, reticulum, Masson's trichrome and Schiff's stains, as indicated.

For electron microscopy, specimens were immersed in cold 3% glutaraldehyde, buffered in phosphate or cacodylate buffer for 2 hr, washed in buffer solution overnight, postfixed in 1% osmium tetroxide, dehydrated through graded concentrations of ethanol, bathed in propylene oxide, and embedded in Epon-Araldite. Sections were cut with a Porter-Blum microtome, doubly stained with uranyl acetate

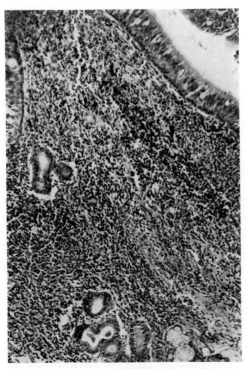

Fig. 1. A low power light photomicrograph shows normal nasopharyngeal mucosa covered by pseudostratified ciliated columnar epithelium overlying well-developed lymphoid tissue which contains sero-mucinous glands. × 80.

and lead hydroxide, and examined with a Hitachi U-11 electron microscope, operated at 75 kv.

OBSERVATIONS

Normal nasopharyngeal mucosa

Pseudostratified columnar ciliated epithelium—The findings presented here were based upon the biopsy specimens of nasopharyngeal mucosa from 10 noncancerous patients. In only 2 specimens was the nasopharynx covered exclusively by pseudostratified columnar ciliated epithelium overlying well-developed lymphoid tissue which contained scattered sero-mucinous glands (Fig. 1).

The cilia were uniformly and abundantly distributed over the surface of the columnar ciliated epithelium. Cross sections of the cilia showed the characteristic

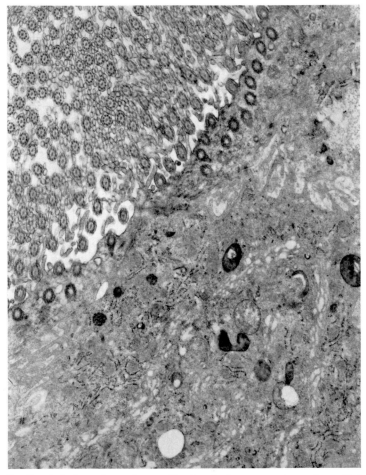

Fig. 2. Apical portions of two ciliated cells from normal pseudostratified ciliated columnar epithelium. The cell at the center contains abundant endoplasmic reticulum and secretory granules varying in size and shape. × 14,000.

"nine plus two complex" of microtubules with basal bodies at their rootlets. Mitochondria were found most abundantly in the apical cytoplasm. Endoplasmic reticulum, both rough and smooth-surfaced, was present, aggregated in small clusters. Golgi complexes were prominent, consisting of characteristic stacks of flattened cisternae and vacuoles. Secretory granules, limited by unit membranes, were frequently observed scattered in the cytoplasm, but varying in number and size (Fig. 2). Annulate lamellae (*14*) had formed occasionally in the supranuclear region, but their origin from nuclear envelopes could not be clearly demonstrated (*2*). The amount of annulate lamellae seen in any one cell varied from a single cisterna to one or several stacks, each consisting of 5 to 10 layers.

The small basophilic cells abutting on the basement membranes were rich in free ribosomes (Fig. 3). Mitochondria and rough endoplasmic reticulum were moderate in number and the Golgi complex was small. A few small secretory granules were occasionally recognizable, indicative of a progenitor of the ciliated epithelial cells. These cells were apparently different from the basal cells in the stratified squamous epithelium, because of the less marked cytoplasmic projections without intracytoplasmic tonofilaments.

In the nasopharyngeal mucosa there were present collections of mixed mucous and serous secretory glands below the level of the tunica propria (Fig. 1) and, occasionally, between the muscle bundles, although their proportion and distribution varied from case to case. Where the lymphoid tissue was well developed, the acinar

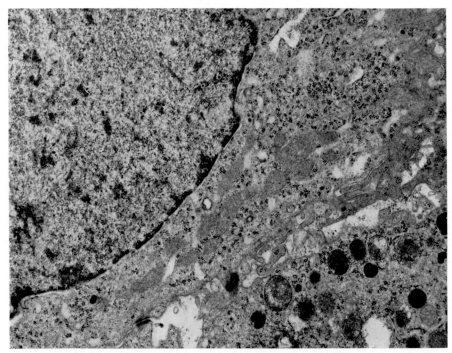

Fig. 3. A small basophilic cell rich in free ribosomes and a part of ciliated epithelial cell with many secretory granules (right lower corner) are shown. × 15,000.

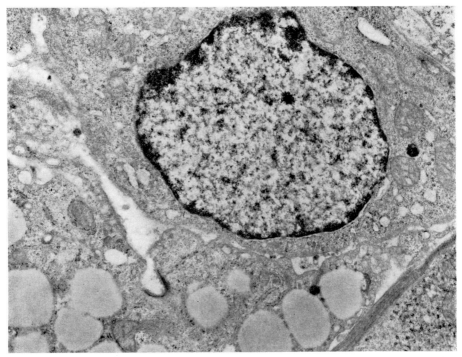

Fig. 4. A small basophilic cell with well-developed rough endoplasmic reticulum and a part of glandular epithelial cell containing many secretory granules are shown.   × 13,000.

cells were typical serous glands as a rule.   Most of the secretory granules that accumulated, especially in the apical cytoplasm of the serous secretory cells, appeared in electron micrographs as large, spherical granules, although their density and size varied considerably.

Goblet cells showed an increase in number with the progression of fibrosis and a decrease in lymphoid tissue in the tunica propria.   The cytoplasm was distended with mucous globules in an ordinary fashion.   Both kinds of secretory cells were characterized by a prominent Golgi complex and a well-developed rough endoplasmic reticulum.   Basophilic cells, which were closely apposed to the basement membrane of the acini and ductules, were easily discernible by the details of their fine structure, similar to those seen in the pseudostratified columnar ciliated epithelium, with or without granules in the cytoplasm (Fig. 4).

Stratified squamous epithelium—Yeh (*53*) has explained that focal or diffuse replacement of the pseudostratified columnar ciliated epithelium by squamous epithelium increases with age.   It has been stated by Ali (*1*) that 60% of the total epithelial surface of the nasopharynx is lined by stratified squamous epithelium under normal conditions.   Concerning the mechanism of squamous metaplasia in the mucosal epithelium and glandular epithelium, an electron microscopic study has been made of 13 satisfactory biopsy specimens: 11 from cancer cases and 2 from noncancer patients in an age group of from 21 to 46 years.

The ultrastructural appearance of a transitional area between the columnar

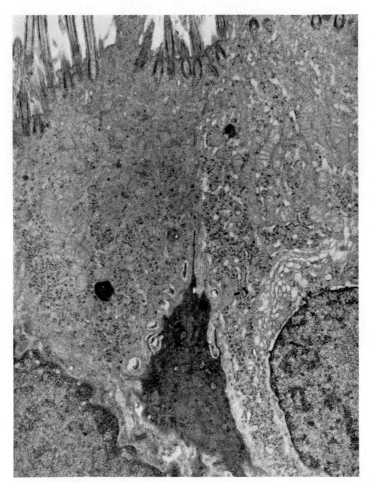

Fig. 5.   A basal cell with high density appears lying freely between two ciliated columnar epithelial cells.   × 11,000.

ciliated and squamous epithelia is illustrated in Figs. 5–7.   The intercellular spaces were moderately dilated, and basal cells appeared lying free among the columnar ciliated epithelial cells at all levels (Fig. 5).   With the proliferation of basal cells, the ciliated epithelial cells were shrunken and detached from the lining.   The basal cells were really active and moved upwards from the basal layer through the intercellular spaces to the superficial layer, finally overlapping and impinging upon the columnar epithelial cells (Fig. 7).

The migrating and proliferating basal cells had a fine structure very similar to that of the basal cells in human skin, except for occasional secretory granules in their cytoplasm.   Thus there were many half-desmosomes (43), or basal attachment plates, on the cell membrane facing the basement membrane.   The cytoplasm, with many slender cytoplasmic processes, was characterized by its extremely high density, owing to the abundance of the ribosomes.   Mitochondria were moderate in number, and rough endoplasmic reticulum was not conspicuous.   Tonofilaments were

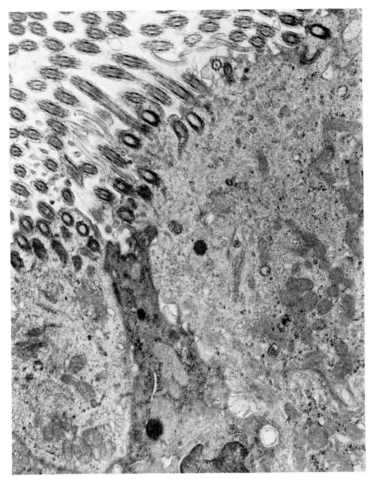

FIG. 6. A basal cell migrating in the superficial layer of pseudostratified ciliated columnar epithelium. × 13,000.

fine and delicate, often not recognizable, particularly in the case of noncornified squamous epithelium. The shape of these cells varied greatly in different areas, even becoming amoeboid in the intercellular spaces.

The basal layer showed melanin pigment deposition in 2 of the 13 cases examined. Langerhans cells with specific rods (*29, 56, 57*) and melanocytes, identified by the presence of melanosomes and premelanosomes (*49*) in the cytoplasm, were occasionally found in the basal layer. The pigment was chiefly confined to the basal layer, but was occasionally scattered in the intercellular spaces of the superficial cornified layers (*33*).

The transitional cells (*30*) in transitional areas were larger and less dense than the basal cells. Their cytoplasm was rather abundant, showing slender cytoplasmic processes extending into intercellular spaces. The fine structure of the desmosomes (*10, 12*) (Fig. 8) was not specific. The nucleus was spherical or ovoid in shape, with diffusely distributed chromatin and a small nucleolus. The cytoplasm was

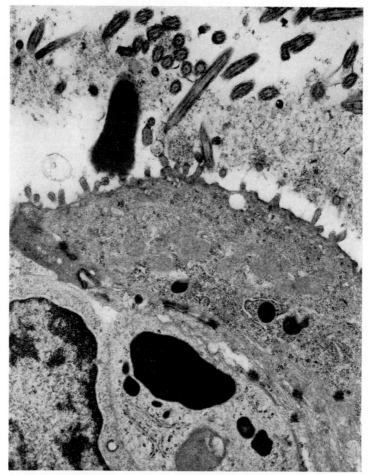

FIG. 7. Three transitional cells with secretory granules are shown. The superficial one seems to be converted from basal cell.   × 14,000.

slightly vesicular due to mild dilatation of the cisternae of the rough endoplasmic reticulum. Apparently different from the prickle cells with thick bundles of tonofibrils (Fig. 9) in the stratum spinosum of squamous epithelium, the tonofilaments in the transitional cells were delicate.   Mitochondria were not so conspicuous and a Golgi complex was occasionally recognized.   The free ribosomes were abundant and melanin and/or secretory granules were occasionally encountered.

In the case of cornified squamous epithelium, the cells of the stratum granulosum, usually two or three cells thick, was characterized by the presence of large, irregularly-shaped granules of keratohyalin in close contact with both tonofibrils and free ribosomes. Of particular interest is that mucous globules were scattered occasionally in this area, giving rise to a positive result with Schiff's and mucicarmine stain.   The presence of secretory granules in the basal cells and transitional cells, we presumed, indicated that a series of squamous epithelial cells are derived from

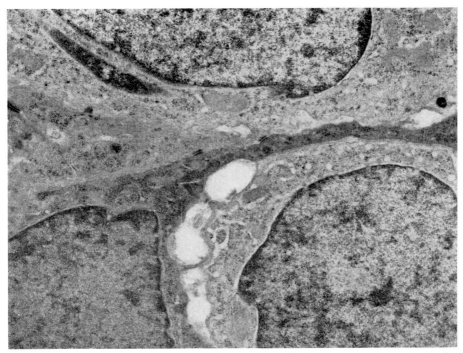

FIG. 8.   Two transitional cells separated by the cytoplasmic processes of two basal cells. × 13,000.

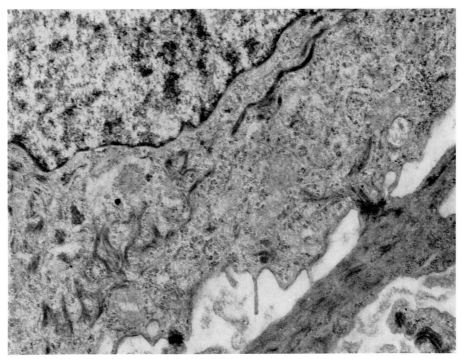

FIG. 9.   A prickle cell with bundles of tonofibrils in a stratified squamous epithelium. × 16,000.

the small basophilic cells which are thought to be the progenitors of secretory cells in the seromucinous glands.

The cellular component of anaplastic carcinoma

Histologically, a diagnosis of anaplastic carcinoma was made on biopsy specimens obtained from 40 patients, including one case of carcinoma simplex. According to the criteria as set forth by Yeh (*53*), all of these cases could be divided into 5 subgroups: combined cell carcinoma (13 cases), spindle cell carcinoma (13 cases), transitional cell carcinoma (12 cases), lymphoepithelioma (1 case) and carcinoma simplex (1 case).

Since there was a considerable overlap among these subtypes and since individual neoplasms showed mixed cellular constituents (*41*), the usual light microscopic classification at the tissue level could not always be correlated to cell typing as achieved with the aid of an electron microscope. A cytogenetic classification has been made in this study by taking cognizance of the fact that tonofibrils are present in the squamous epithelium and secretory granules in the ciliated or glandular epithelium from which the individual component cancer cells seem to have arisen. As a result of electron microscopic examination, the following groups of cancer cells are proposed.

Group A: Cancer cells with secretory potential

1)   Polyhedral basophilic cancer cells—The investigators were impressed by the fact that these cells possessed a fine structure simulating that of the small basophilic

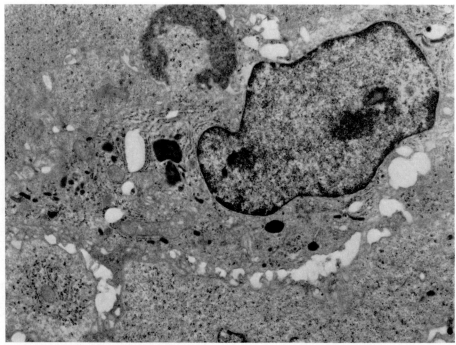

FIG. 10.   A polyhedral basophilic cancer cell is characterized by a prominent cytoplasmic vacuolar system and secretory granules.   × 11,000.

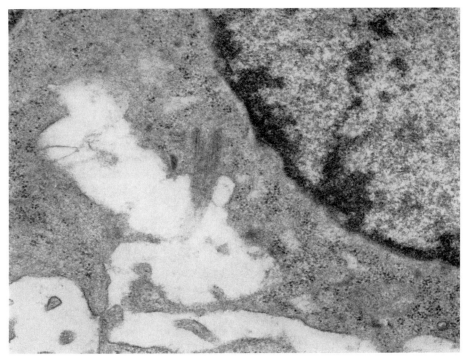

Fig. 11. Two abortive cilia in the cytoplasm of a polyhedral basophilic cancer cell.
× 31,000.

cells in the ciliated or glandular epithelium.   Their cellular density was comparatively high owing to the abundance of free ribosomes, occasionally interspersed with
polyribosomal aggregates, in the cytoplasm.   The nucleus, rather large in comparison to the size of its cell body, was mostly ovoid or spherical in shape, and was
characterized by a fine dispersion of chromatin with or without a small nucleolus.
The Golgi complex was prominent, often with vesicles or secretory granules in the
vicinity (Fig. 10).   Rough endoplasmic reticulum was randomly distributed and
mitochondria were occasionally recognized, apparently indicative of potential
ciliogenesis 25 in these cells (Fig. 11).

Indeed, this type of cell was the main component of the cancer nests in carcinoma
simplex.   However, it is also true that similar cells, varying in number, were
often recognized, intermingling within other types of cancer cells.   On careful scru-
tiny of the sections under the electron microscope, 13 cases of combined cell carcinoma and 8 cases of transitional cell carcinoma had this kind of cell situated
somewhere in the cancer nests.

2) *Large clear cancer cells*—These cells were actually variants of the polyhedral
basophilic cancer cells: the only difference was the large vesicular nucleus containing one or two prominent nucleoli (Fig. 12).   Secretory granules were present, but
tonofibrils were absent.   In contrast with distinct nuclear membranes, the cell
boundaries were often obscured as viewed under the light microscope.

Large clear cancer cells were often coexistent with large vesicular (transitional

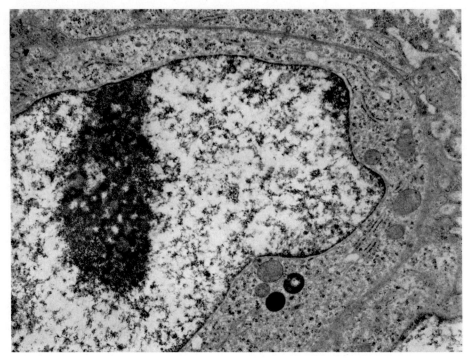

FIG. 12.   Two secretory granules in a large clear cancer cell with a vesicular nucleus containing a prominent nucleolus.   × 14,000.

cell: Group B, 3) and/or polyhedral basophilic cancer cells (Group A, 1) in varying proportions; in the 6 cases of transitional cell carcinoma, 3 cases of combined cell carcinoma, and one case of lymphoepitholioma, these cells were seen admixed with other types of cancer cells.

Group B :   Cancer cells with tonofibrils
    1)   Atypical basal cells—The ultrastructural features of these cells were almost the same as those of the basal cells in the squamous epithelium.   The cells in the cancer nests differed from the normal basal cells in three principal ways: First, the nucleus was indented (Fig. 13). Second, no half-desmosome or basement membrane at the junctional region with the stroma was present.   Third, mitotic activity was revealed.

    Generally speaking, atypical basal cells were commonly seenin the peripheral portion of the cancer nests of classical epidermoid carcinoma; next to these were atypical prickle and cornified cells.   In other words, the cells in the central areas of cancer nests of classical epidermoid carcinoma were more polyhedral, or flattened with keratohyalin granules.   In this series of cases, however, no atypical prickle or cornified cells were demonstrable, although atypical basal cells were observed in areas of cancer cell aggregations in 6 cases of combined cell carcinoma, 4 cases of transitional cell carcinoma, and 2 cases of spindle cell carcinoma.

    2)   Spindle cancer cells—Spindle cell carcinoma was characterized by sheets or

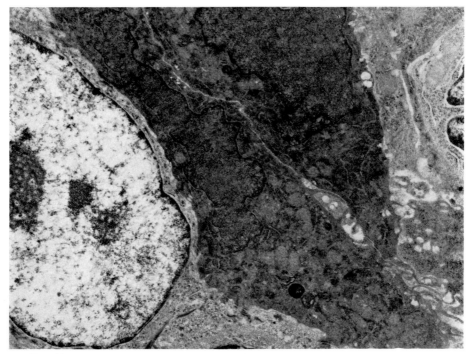

FIG. 13.   Two atypical basal cells, of which one contains secretory granules, are present in the peripheral portion of a cancer nest.   × 10,000.

strands of interlacing bundles of spindle-shaped cells which varied in size.   These tumor cells were elongated and their nucleus was fusiform, usually with finely granular chromatin and a small spherical or irregularly-shaped nucleolus (Fig. 14). The cytoplasm contained a moderate number of mitochondria, rough endoplasmic reticulum, and free ribosomes.   The tonofibrils were rather coarse, forming bundles running in the same direction, parallel to the plasmalemma.   Mitosis and multinucleated giant cells were not infrequently encountered.

These cells were, undoubtedly, the chief cellular component of the socalled " spindle cell carcinoma."   Attention should be called, however, to the fact that these cells were seen also amidst cellular populations of the other types of anaplastic nasopharyngeal carcinoma.   Therefore, some spindle-shaped cancer cells were found to be present in the 11 cases of combined cell carcinoma and the 4 cases of transitional cell carcinoma examined.

3)   *Vesicular cancer cells*—These tumor cells were relatively large and showed a vesicular nuclear structure.   The large nuclei were usually round or oval, rather poor in chromatin but containing 1 or 2 large nucleoli, and often with a network of nucleolonema (Fig. 15).   The cytoplasmic matrix was low in density and rich in small vesicles.   Mitochondria were grouped in perinuclear areas and the cisternae of the rough endoplasmic reticulum were slightly dilated.   Fine tonofilaments and coarse tonofibrils with bundle formation were abundant.   Although the Golgi complex was not prominent, some cells apparently contained small secretory granules.

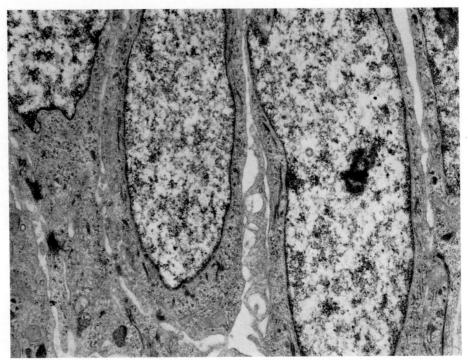

FIG. 14. Four spindle cancer cells with elongated nuclei are shown in this picture. × 14,000.

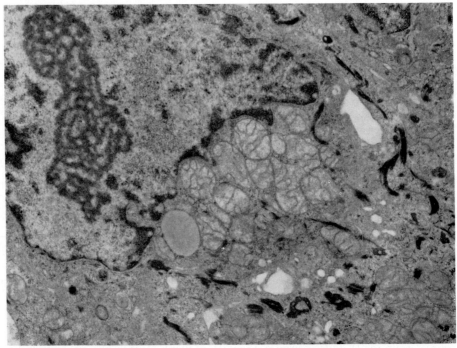

FIG. 15. A large nucleolus with a network of nucleolonema in the nucleus of a vesicular cancer cell.   × 13,000.

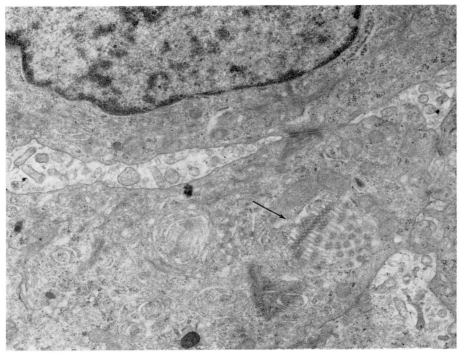

Fig. 16. An annulate lamella (arrow) is present in a vesicular cancer cell. Tonofibrils and secretory granules are coexistent in the cytoplasm. × 17,000.

Moreover, occasional annulate lamellae were present in the cytoplasm (Fig. 16). Considering the coexistence of tonofibrils, secretory granules, and annulate lamellae, these vesicular cancer cells are probably potentially bivalent and able to differentiate into cells of both squamous and columnar natures.

Microscopically, the tumor cells, with large pale-staining vesicular nuclei and poorly delimited cytoplasm, were closely packed and often arranged in solid groups (Fig. 17) or in anastomosing columns. Mitotic figures were common, and bizarre multinucleated giant cells were formed in places. These cells, apparently, were consistent with the component cells of transitional cell carcinoma including lymphoepithelioma, as described by Capell (4, 5). Like the large population of spindle-shaped cancer cells in various types of anaplastic nasopharyngeal carcinoma, the vesicular cancer cells were also widely distributed as a part of the component cells in the combined cell carcinoma (12 cases), spindle cell carcinoma (8 cases), and carcinoma simplex (1 case).

Stroma of anaplastic carcinoma

Generally speaking, anaplastic nasopharyngeal carcinoma, usually infiltrating the pre-existing well-developed lymphoid tissue in an early stage, consisted of two parts, the ill-defined cancer nests and the poorly-developed fibrous stroma. However, in the later stages, the amount of fibrous stroma varied considerably. Based on an analysis of the quantity of the fibrous stromal tissue, three basic types of stroma were proposed for classification.

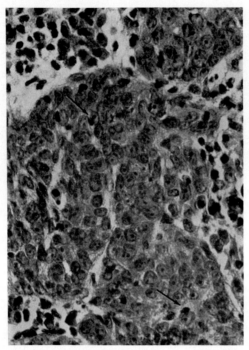

FIG. 17. Transitional cell carcinoma with comparatively distinct alveolar structure. In the loosely-textured connective tissue stroma there is lymphocytic infiltration, including a number of plasma cells. A few distorted lymphoid cells (arrows) are discernible scattered in the cancer nests.   × 300.

Type I stroma—Regardless of what cellular type the tumors (3 transitional cell carcinomas, 2 combined cell carcinomas, 2 spindle cell carcinomas, and 1 lymphoepithelioma, totaling 8 cases) might be, their stroma was made up of lymphoid cells, including a few plasma cells. Except for a little delicate connective tissue accompanying blood vessels, there was no discernible fibrous stroma at all. The ultrastructure of the lymphoid cells corresponded to mature lymphocytes, small or medium in size.

The cancer nests were ill-defined and small, often forming anastomosing trabeculae. In extreme cases, as in lymphoepithelima of Schmincke's type (*40*), the cancer cells were separated from each other, giving rise to a loosely packed sarcomatous appearance (Fig. 18), correlating with a marked decrease in the number of desmosomes seen under the electron microscope.

Type II stroma—The stroma was composed of loosely-textured connective tissue, relatively small in amount. The cancer cells were aggregated in strands or masses with a rather distinct alveolar structure, though no basement membrane was formed. As compared with Type I stroma, the number of lymphoid cells was very much reduced and plasma cell infiltration became conspicuous. A few lymphoid cells were scattered in the cancer nests (Fig. 17), but most of them were degenerated and distorted, occasionally being engulfed by tumor cells (Fig. 19).

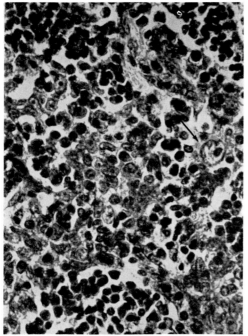

FIG. 18. Lymphoepithelioma of Schmincke type. Note the isolated transitional cells scattered in lymphoid tissue. A large clear cancer cell with a vesicular nucleus containing a prominent nucleolus is present (arrow). × 300.

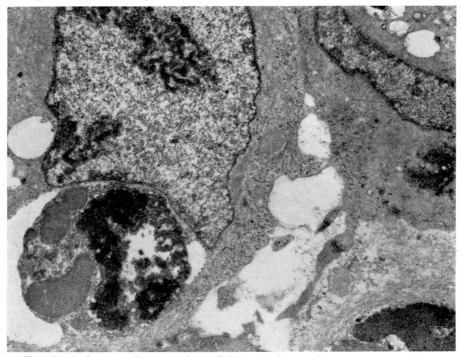

FIG. 19. A degenerated mononuclear cell is engulfed by a phagosome in a spindle cancer cell. × 11,000.

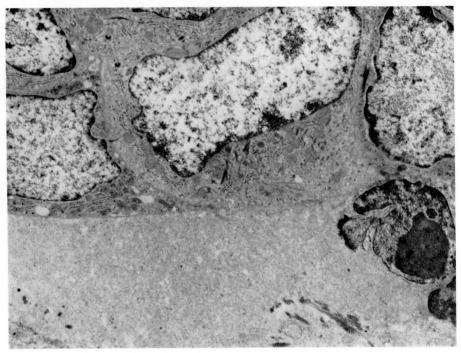

FIG. 20.   A degenerated lymphoid cell in the fibrous stroma. $\times$ 8,000.

It is of interest to note that most of the 22 patients (10 combined cell carcinomas, 6 spindle cell carcinomas, 6 transitional cell carcinomas) in this category possessed high titers of antibody in their sera against the EB virus.

Type III stroma—Most of the cases (5 spindle cell carcinomas, 1 transitional cell carcinoma, 1 combined cell carcinoma, and 1 carcinoma simplex) showed compact sheets or strands composed of various types of cancer cells.   The stroma was always distinct and densely fibrous, though varying in amount.   Lymphoid cells were very few and most of them were degenerated (Fig. 20).

Virus-like particles in cancer cells

1)   Intranuclear virus-like particles—A few intranuclear crystalline arrays (*28*) of virus-like particles (Fig. 21) were demonstrated in the large clear cancer cells (Group A, 2) and in the vesicular cancer cells (Group B, 3) from 3 patients who possessed high anti EB titers (Table 1).   They were usually interspersed among skeins of chromatin granules.   The particles occurred in two forms.   The first was found in the large clear cells (Group A, 2) measuring about 600–1,100 Å in diameter, often appearing hexagonal in profile (Fig. 22).

The second, measuring 700–800 Å in size, were found incidentally in a vesicular cancer cell (Group B, 3).   Their architecture was very similar to that of the larger particles described above (Fig. 23).   Empty particles were not encountered.

2)   Intracytoplasmic virus-like particles—A few single-coated, virus-like particles (Fig. 24) were encountered in the large clear or in the vesicular cancer cells from 2

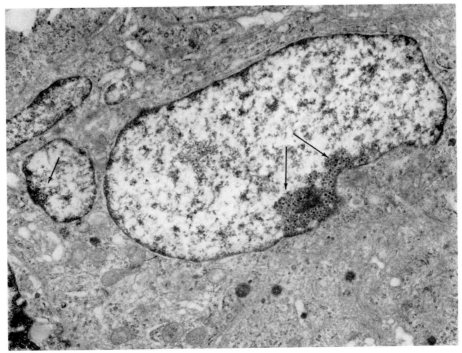

Fig. 21. Two intranuclear crystalline arrays of virus-like particles (arrows) in the vesicular nuclei. × 13,000.

TABLE 1. Cancer Cells with Virus-like Particles

Case No.	Patient Age	Patient Sex	Anti EB titers (u)	Virus-like particles Nuclear	Virus-like particles Intra-cytoplasmic	Type of cancer cell	Type of stroma	Undulating tubules
5	58	M	640	(+) L	(+)	A, 2	II	(+)
12	37	M	2,560	(卌) L	(−)	A, 2	II	(+)
13	38	M	610	(卅) S	(+)	B, 3	II	(−)
21	49	F	640	(−)	(−)	B, 3	II	(卅)

L, large intranuclear virus-like particles;   S, small intranuclear virus-like particles.

patients.   They were fewer in number but larger in size, with a diameter between, 1,400 and 1,900 Å, surrounded by a distinct envelope.   In most cases, a dense round or elongated core, measuring about 650 to 1,200 Å across, was prominent. These particles were invariably intracytoplasmic.

3)   *Undulating tubules*—These unusual inclusions, designated as " undulating tubules " (*21*) and related to the endoplastic reticulum, could be divided into three subtypes: (1) There were seen one or two large, electron-opaque bodies, like a virus nest (*17*), in the cytoplasm of the large clear cells, simultaneously with intranuclear and intracytoplasmic virus-like particles as described above.   These bodies showed a distinct architecture with crystalline arrays containing many electron-dense

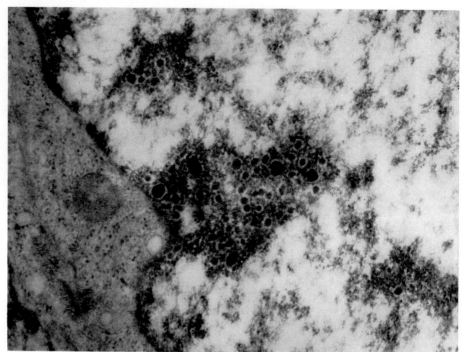

FIG. 22. Large virus-like particles without envelopes are grouping at the margins of a vesicular nucleus. × 37,000.

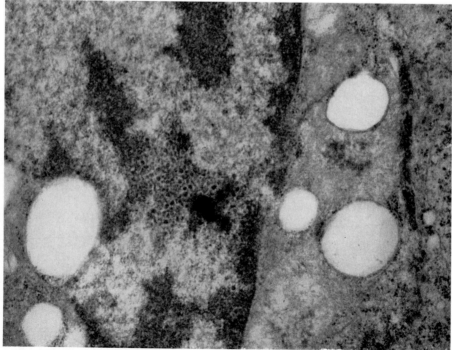

FIG. 23. Small virus-like particles scattered in the chromatin clumps of a vesicular nucleus. × 29,000.

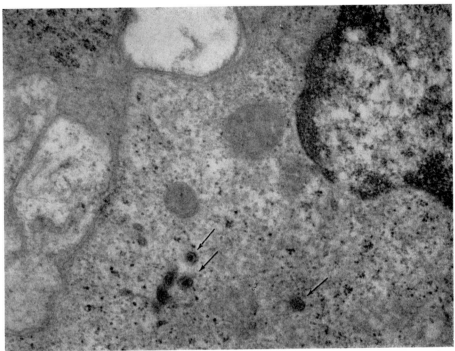

FIG. 24. Three single-coated virus-like particles (arrows) in the cytoplasm of a large clear cancer cell. × 36,000.

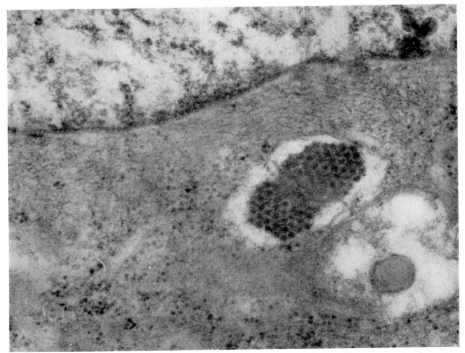

FIG. 25. Undulating tubules with a distinct architecture of crystalline arrays in the cytoplasm of a large clear cancer cell. × 63,000.

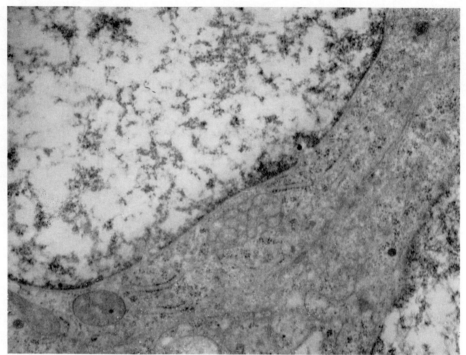

FIG. 26.   Lace-like undulating tubules in the cytoplasm of a large clear cancer cell.
× 24,000.

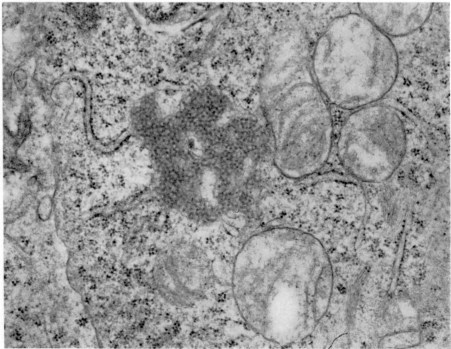

FIG. 27.   Vesicular undulating tubules connected with rough endoplasmic reticulum in
the cytoplasm of a vesicular cancer cell.   × 36,000.

hexagonal granules.   The granules were of similar size, about 500 Å in diameter, and were disposed with the dominant morphologic characteristics arranged in palisaded fashion, or as a mesh-work (Fig. 25).   (2) The tubules, which were discovered in the large clear cells with intranuclear virus-like particles, appeared as a lace-like network structure (Fig. 26).   (3) The third one, consisting of aggregates of numerous vesicles with or without an electron-opaque core (Fig. 27), was found in the vesicular cancer cells (Group B, 3) without virus-like particles in the nuclei and cytoplasm.   The above mentioned inclusions were seen in three cases.

In addition to these intracytoplasmic inclusions, annulate lamellae (*23*) were sometimes observed in some of the vesicular cancer cells, as described above.

DISCUSSION

Modulation of normal nasopharyngeal epithelial cells

In tracing the origin of various types of cancer cells in anaplastic carcinoma of the nasopharynx, it is essential to understand the cytogenetic interrelationships between normal epithelial cells, especially the nature of the transitional cells and the mechanism of squamous metaplasia.

Based on the ultrastructural analysis of the squamous, columnar ciliated and glandular epithelia in the nasopharynx, it has been established that there are two salient components of the cytoplasm that determine the mode of cytodifferentiation in the epithelial cells.   One is the prevalence of tonofibrils or tonofilaments in the squamous epithelium, and the other is the prominence of secretory granules and rough endoplasmic reticulum in the ciliated and glandular epithelium.   Both components appear to compete with each other in their evolution in the cytoplasm of transitional cells, which lie between ciliated and squamous epithelia.

The nature of the small basophilic cells resting on the basement membrane has not been well understood.   Their fine structure was apparently different from that of myoepithelial cells (*38*) and basal cells, since they have secretory granules and rather well-developed rough endoplasmic reticulum instead of myofilaments (*8*) and a

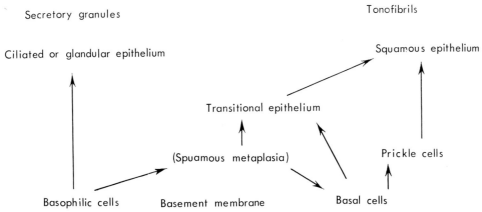

Fig. 28.   Modulation of normal nasopharyngeal epithelial cells.

tonofilaments, implying that they have the potential to develop into ciliated or glandular epithelium (see Fig. 28).

The presence of cytoplasmic tonofilaments in the basal cells should be regarded as prima facie evidence that they have a tendency towards cornification as a progenitor of other keratinocytes including prickle cells (see Fig. 28). As evidence of the activity of the basal cells, they are found migrating in the transitional areas, compressing and replacing the columnar ciliated epithelial cells. While controversy continues regarding the histogenesis of transitional cells and the interrelationships among the basal, small basophilic, and transitional cells, a schema of the possible directions of the histogenetic progression of the normal nasopharyngeal epithelia has been outlined in Fig. 28, for explaining the cytogenesis of individual anaplastic cancer cells.

Cytogenesis of anaplastic cancer cells

With the knowledge of two different biological behaviors shown by the normal epithelial cells in the nasopharynx, it is feasible to discuss the histogenesis of individual types of cancer cells.

The polyhedral basophilic cancer cells (Group A, 1) seem to be derived from the small basophilic cells on the pase of ciliated columnar epithelium and glandular epithelium. Provided there is a dominant cytoplasmic vacuolar system (6) including the Golgi complex and the endoplasmic reticulum, it does not matter whether the cells contain secretory granules or not. These cells are the chief component of a case of carcinoma simplex which did not show a positive mucin reaction. The exact origin of the large clear cells (Group A, 2) is still lacking concrete proof. If must be admitted, however, that most of the cells contain rather prominent secretory granules. This, probably, indicates that they originate from the secretory cells above the small basophilic cells.

The atypical basal cells (Group B, 1) are transformed from the basal cells of squamous epithelium, often showing a pavement-like arrangement along the margins of cancer nests. The spindle-shaped cancer cells (Group B, 2), which Krompecher (24) called basal cells, seem to be more differentiated than the atypical basal cells. The dominant feature of tumor cells is the accumulation of tonofibrils, which would lead, in a case of highly differentiated epidermoid carcinoma, to keratinization. This was not included in this study; however, it must be admitted that there exist transitions between the large spindle-shaped cancer cells and vesicular cancer cells.

The morphologic characteristics of vesicular cancer cells (Group B, 3) are almost the same as those of the transitional cells that lie in the transitional areas between the squamous and pseudostratified ciliated columnar epithelia, except for the presence of one or two prominent nucleoli in the large vesicular nucleus. The cell body is large and shows a light appearance. There are abundant tonofibrils and prominentsecretory granules. Hence, it is appropriate to call them " intermediate cells."

Histogenesis of anaplastic carcinomas

The component cells of anaplastic carcinoma are not as simple as is generally believed. Usually, they consist of collections of mixed cancer cells, in addition to

TABLE 2.   Distribution of Various Types of Cancer Cells in Anaplastic Carcinoma of the Nasopharynx

Cancer type	No. cases	A, 2	A, 1	B, 3	B, 2	B, 1
Spindle cell carcinoma	13			8	13*	2
Combined cell carcinoma	13	3	13*	12*	11*	6
Transitional cell carcinoma	13[a]	7	8	13*	4	4
Carcinoma simplex	1		1	1		

* Main component cancer cells.
[a] Including a case of lymphoepithelioma.

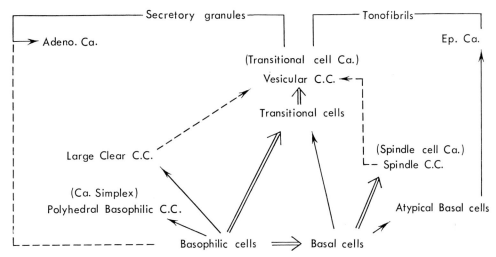

Fig. 29.   Histogenesis of anaplastic carcinoma in nasopharynx.   Arrows indicate the incidence: ⇒, extremely high ;   ⟶, high ;   ----→, low ;   - - - - questionable.   Ca., Carcinoma ;   C.C., Cancer cells.

the chief component cell.   The distribution of the aforementioned cancer cell types
in different types of anaplastic carcinoma is shown in Table 2.

From Table 2 the following conclusions can be drawn.

1) Spindle cell carcinoma is most probably epidermoid or squamous in origin.
The authors do not support the opinion of Frank et al. (13) that some spindle cells
might originate from the ciliated columnar epithelium.

2) Polyhedral basophilic cells (A, 1) and vesicular cells (B, 3) seem to have an
intimate interrelationship in their cytogenesis.   Both of them were often coexistent
in combined cell and/or transitional cell carcinomas and probably in carcinoma
simplex as well.   Therefore, it is suggested that transitional cells probably are derived
from small basophilic cells directly (Figs. 28, 29).

3) Considering the fact that transitional cell carcinoma contains a number of cells
which are derived from the ciliated columnar or glandular epithelial cells, it is reasonable to conclude that this tumor probably develops from the deep crypts in connection with the openings of the excretory ducts of the glands, in which squamous
metaplasia often occurs.

4) The origin of combined cell carcinoma may be multiple, probably arising either from the basal cells of the squamous epithelium or from the small basophilic cells in the pseudostratified ciliated columnar epithelium.

Indeed, the concept of the transitional cell is confusing. There is no unanimity of interpretation as to the cytogenesis of transitional cells among authors. Quick and Cutler (*36*) were the first to employ the term " transitional cell carcinoma " in nasopharyngeal carcinoma. They stated that the cells were small and uniform in size, with relatively large hyperchromatic nuclei, apparently different from the vesicular cancer cells (Group B, 3) in our category. From Ewing's illustration (*9*), the component cells of his transitional cell carcinoma are more spindle-shaped and hyperchromatic, probably indicative of the spindle cancer cells (Group B, 2) in our classification. The cancer cells described by Cappell (*4, 5*) are pale-staining epithelial cells of a syncytial type with round or ovoid vesicular nuclei, containing nucleoli, quite similar to the vesicular cancer cells (Group B, 3) or the large clear cells (Group A, 2) designated in this study. The authors would particularly like to emphasize that the term " transitional cells " should be confined to those cells characterized by a bivalent biological behavior, *i. e.*, that of evolving a cytoplasmic vacuolar system (*6*) and/or forming tonofibrils.

The reason why the majority of the nasopharyngeal neoplasms are anaplastic carcinomas and the proportion of adenocarcinoma is so extremely rare, may be a simple one, because the small basophilic cells at the base of pseudostratified ciliated columnar and glandular epithelia are easily transformed into transitional cells, from which most of the anaplastic carcinoma may arise (Fig. 29).

Stroma of anaplastic carcinoma

One of the objectives of this study was to elucidate the stromal reaction in nasopharyngeal cancers. The investigators do not wish to accept the theory that lymphoid cells in the cancer tissue represent the dominant stromal reaction, because these cells are nothing more than the pre-existing lymphoid tissue which will eventually be replaced by cancer and reactive stromal tissue. For this reason, it seems inadvisable to recognize the existence of lymphoepithelioma, (*7, 15, 18, 34, 41, 42, 47, 48, 51, 53*), although there are rhinologists, radiologists, and pathologists who have advocated it as a distinct tumor entity (*4, 5, 11, 13, 16, 27, 39, 44, 50*).

As can be seen from Table 3, no significant relationship between tumor type, clinical course, and amount of fibrous stromal tissue can be demonstrated, except in the cases of spindle cell carcinoma and carcinoma simplex, which tend to have a distinct fibrous stroma. Considering the fact that the fibrous stroma in the classical epidermoid carcinoma is constituted by rather compact cancer nests, often large in amount, both the composition of cancer nests and arrangement of cancer cells, compact or loose, would seem to influence the development of stroma.

Do local lymphoid tissue and stromal changes have any relationship with the formation of anti-EB virus antibody in the patients? This poses a very interesting problem from the viewpoint of tumor immunity. According to the anti-EB virus titers, the 38 patients examined by the technique of membrane immunofluorescent reactions (*19, 22, 54*) are divided into 5 classes: 40 U, 160 U, 640 U, 2,560 U, and

TABLE 3.   Three Types of Stroma in Anaplastic Carcinoma of the Nasopharynx

Type of cancer \ Type of stroma (amount)	I (small)		II (moderate)		III (large)		Total	
Spindle cell carcinoma	2	1–M 1–L	6	1–E 2–M 3–L	5	1–E 2–M 2–L	13	2–E 5–M 6–L
Combined cell carcinoma	2	1–E 1–M	10	5–E 1–M 4–L		1–L	13	6–E 2–M 5–L
Transitional cell carcinoma	4	1–M[a] 3–L	6	3–E 3–L	3	1–E 1–M 1–L	13	4–E 2–M 7–L
Carcinoma simplex						1–M		1–M
Total	8	1–E 3–E 4–L	22	9–E 3–M 10–L	10	2–E 4–M 4–L	40	12–E 10–M 18–L

E, early stage ;   M, moderately advanced stage ;   L, late stage.
[a] A case of lymphoepithelioma.

TABLE 4.   Anti-EB Virus Titers of Patients, Classified by Stromal Types

Type of stroma (amount) \ Anti-EB titers (u.)	40	160	640	2,560	> 2,560	Total (no. cases)
Type 1 (small)	1	1	6			8
Type 2 (moderate)		1	8	10	3	22
Type 3 (large)	1	3	4			8
Total (no. cases)	2	5	18	10	3	38[a]

[a] Two cases of transitional cell carcinoma are excluded because of inadequate serum.

>2,560 U.   It seems clear that the sera of patients in the category of Type II stroma possess significantly higher anti-EB virus titers than those in the other two groups (Table 4).

Under the light and electron microscopes, at least two cytologically different cells seem to be temporally related to the formation of antibody.   With a decrease in the number of lymphoid cells, plasma cells appear to increase and migrate at the margins of cancer nests, most significant in the cases of Type II stroma.   Although transformation of the small lymphoid cells into the mature plasma cells (*31, 32, 35, 37*) could not be demonstrated by the electron microscope, it is interesting that degenerated lymphoid cells are always found to be present either in the stroma or in the cancer nests.   It is unknown whether or not this phenomenon is related to the elevation of the anti EB virus titers in the sera of nasopharyngeal cancer patients. It is also difficult to answer the question of why the number of lymphoid cells in the cancer tissue decreases in cases with higher anti EB virus titers.

Virus-like particles in anaplastic carcinoma

EB virus, which was first recognized in the EB-1 cell line derived from Burkitt's lymphoma, is a member of the herpes virus group (*20*). The EB virus particles in the P3HR-1 lymphoma cell line (*52*) can occur in two forms: naked particles and less numerous, larger enveloped particles. The intranuclear and intracytoplasmic virus-like particles which have been detected by electron microscopy in a small proportion of cancer cells from 3 nasopharyngeal cancer patients are morphologically similar to one of the members of the herpes virus group.

Another unusual structure, although only very rarely encountered in the cancer cells, was the undulating tubules or crystalloid bodies in the form of a lace-like network or in the form of a mesh-work. Recently, these inclusions have been observed in human lymphoma cell lines by Bedoya *et al.* (*3*) and in the two " transformed " human embryonic cell lines, THE-2 and THE-3 cells harboring herpes-type virus particles (*21*). The biological significance of these inclusions is still undetermined.

There is no further indication yet that the intranuclear or intracytoplasmic virus-like particles observed in this study are EB virus. Even if these particles prove to be one of the oncogenic viruses, the problem of whether or not they are etiologically related to nasopharyngeal carcinoma will still remain open.

SUMMARY

Biopsy specimens from 40 Chinese patients with anaplastic nasopharyngeal carcinoma and normal nasopharyngeal mucosa from 10 noncancerous patients were studied with light and electron microscopes. Cytologically, the normal epithelial cells of the nasopharynx have two salient cytoplasmic components: tonofibrils, prevalent in the squamous epithelium, and secretory granules, prominent in the pseudostratified ciliated columnar epithelium. Cytogenetically, polyhedral basophilic cancer cells and large clear cancer cells, usually possessing a well-developed cytoplasmic vacuolar system, seem to be derived from the columnar epithelium. Atypical basal cells and spindle-shaped cancer cells are most likely squamous in origin. Transitional cells are potentially bivalent, characterized by the coexistence or admixture of tonofibrils and secretory granules in their cytoplasm. The pre-existing lymphoid tissue can be, and often is, replaced by cancer tissue with variably developed fibrous stroma. Herpes virus-like particles were observed in the cancer cells from 3 patients who possessed high titers of antibody in their sera against the EB virus.

This work was carried out under the project of the Committee of China-Japan Cooperative Study on Nasopharyngeal Carcinoma and was supported in part by grants from the National Council on Science Development, Republic of China ; the China Medical Board of New York, Inc. ; and the American Bureau for Medical Aid to China, Inc. The authors and indebted to Dr. Akiyoshi Kawamura, Jr. (Department of Immunology, Institute of Medical Science, University of Tokyo, Tokyo, Japan), Dr. Takato Yoshida (Laboratory of Viral Oncology, Aichi Cancer Center Research Institute, Nagoya, Japan) and Dr. Czau-Siung Yang (Department of Bacteriology, National Taiwan University, College of Medicine, Taipei, Taiwan) for their skillful technical assistance in the immunological studies. The advice of Dr. Yohei Ito (Laboratory of Viral Oncology, Aichi Cancer Center

Research Institute, Nagoya, Japan), Dr. Kusuya Nishioka (Virus Division, National Cancer Center Research Institute, Tokyo, Japan) and Dr. Takeshi Hirayama (Epidemiology Division, National Cancer Center Research Institute, Tokyo, Japan) is also gratefully acknowledged.

REFERENCES

1. Ali, M. Y.   Distribution and Character of the Squamous Epithelium in the Human Nasopharynx.   *In* Cancer of the Nasopharynx, C. S. Muir and K. Shanmugaratnam, eds. pp. 147–152,Copenhagen, Munksgaard, 1967.

2. Bal, A. R., Jubinville, F., Cousineau, G. H., and Inoué, S.   Origin and Fate of Annulate Lamellae in Arbacia Punctulata Eggs.   J. Ultrastruct. Res., *5*: 15–28, 1968.

3. Bedoya, V., Rabson, A. B., and Grimley, P. M.   Growth *in vitro* of Herpes Simplex Virus in Human Lymphoma Cell Lines.   J. Natl. Cancer Inst., *41*: 635–652, 1968.

4. Cappell, D. F.   On Lympho-epithelioma of Nasopharynx and Tonsils, J. Path. Bact., *39*: 49–64, 1934.

5. Capell, D. F.   Pathology of Nasopharyngeal Tumors. J. Laryng. Otol., *35*: 558–580, 1938.

6. DeRobertis, E. D. P., Nowinski, W. W., and Saez, F. A.   Cell Biology 4th ed. Chapt. 10.   The Cytoplasmic Vacuolar System an Microsomes. pp. 142–165, Philadelphia, W. B. Saunders Co., 1965.

7. Djojoparanoto, M., and Marchetta, F. G.   Nasopharyngeal Malignant Tumors in Surabaja and Vicinity (Indonesia) ; preliminary report.   AMA Arch. Otolaryng., *69*: 155–159, 1959.

8. Ellis, R. A.   Fine Structure of the Myoepithelium of the Eccrine Sweat Glands of Man.   J. Cell Biol., *27*: 551–563, 1965.

9. Ewing, J. Neoplastic Disease ; A Treatise on Tumor. 4th ed. pp. 784–785, 918–922, Philadelphia, Pa. W. B. Saunders Company, 1940.

10. Farquhar, M. G., and Palade, G. E.   Cell Junctions in Amphibian Skin.   J. Cell Biol., *26*: 263–291, 1965.

11. Fitzhugh, W. M., Jr.   Lymphoepithelioma (Schmincke tumor).   Arch. Otolaryng., *28*: 376–387, 1938.

12. Flax, M. H., and Caulfield, J. B.   Cellular and Vascular Components of Allergic Contract Dermatitis.   Amer. J. Path., *43*: 1031–1053, 1963.

13. Frank, I., Lev, M., and Blahd, M.   Transitional Cell Carcinoma of Upper Respiratory Tract.   Ann. Otol. Rhin. and Laryng., *50*: 393–420, 1941.

14. Frasca, J. M., Auerbach, O., Parks, V. R., and Stoeckenius, W.   Electron Microscopic Observations of Bronchial Epithelium.   I. Annulate Lamellae Exp. Molec. Path., *6*: 261–273, 1967.

15. Fursternberg, A. C.   Malignant Neoplasms of Nasopharynx.   Surg. and Gyne. and Obst., *66*: 400–404, 1938.

16. Geist, R. M., Jr., and Portmann, U. V.   Primary Malignant Tumors of Nasopharynx.   Amer. J. Roentgenol., *68*: 266–271, 1952.

17. Hassan, S. A., Rabin, E. R., and Melnick, J. L.   Reovirus Myocarditis in Mice : An Electron Microscopic Immunofluorescent, and Virus Assay Study.   Exp. Molec. Path., *4*: 66–80, 1965.

18. Hauser, I. J., and Brownell, D. H.   Malignant Neoplasms of Nasopharynx. pp. 49–54, Scotland, Oliver and Boyd., 1940.

19. Henle, G., and Henle, W. Immunofluorescence in Cells Derived from Burkitt's Lymphoma. J. Bact., *91*: 1248–1256, 1966.

20. Hinuma, Y. Biology of a Herpes-type Virus Associated with Burkitt Lymphoma Cell Lines. GANN Monograph, *7*: 66–76, 1969.

21. Kimura, I., and Ito, Y. Ultrastructural Studies on the Transformed Human Embryonic Cell Line, THE-2 and THE-3. GANN Monograph, *7*: 115–153, 1969.

22. Klein, G., Clifford, P., Klein, E., and Stjernwärd, J. Search for Tumor-specific Immune Reactions in Burkitt Lymphoma Patients by the Membrane Immunofluorescence Reaction. Proc. Natl. Acad. Sci. US, *55*: 1628–1639, 1966.

23. Koestner, A., Kasza, L., and Kindig, O. Electron Microscopy of Tissue Cultures Infected with Porcine Polioencephalomyelitis Virus. Amer. J. Path., *48*: 129–147, 1966.

24. Krompecher, E. Zür Vergleichenden Histologie der Basaliome. Z. Krebsforsch., *19*: 1–29, 1923.

25. Lin, H.-S., and Chen, I.-L. Development of the Ciliary Complex and Microtubules in the Cells of Rat Subcommissural Organ. Z. Zellforsch., *96*: 186–205, 1969.

26. Lin, H.-S., Lin, C.-S., Yeh, S., and Tu, S.-M. Fine Structure of Nasopharyngeal Carcinoma with Special Reference to the Anaplastic Type. Cancer, *23*: 390–405, 1969.

27. Martin, H. E., and Blady, J. V. Cancer of Nasopharynx. Arch. Otolaryng., *32*: 692–727, 1940.

28. McGavran, M. H., and Smith, M. G. Ultrastructural, Cytochemical and Microchemical Observations on Cytomegalovirus (Salivary Gland Virus) Infection of Human Cells in Tissue Culture. Exp. Molec. Path., *4*: 1–10, 1965.

29. Mishima, Y. Melanosomes in Phagocytic Vacuoles in Langerhans Cells. J. Cell Biol., *30*: 417–423, 1966.

30. Monis, B., and Zambrano, D. Ultrastructure of Transitional Epithelium of Man. Z. Zellforsch., *87*: 101–117, 1968.

31. Moore, R. D., Mumaw, V. R., and Schoenberg, M. D. Changes in Antibody Producing Cells in the Spleen during the Primary Response. Expt. Molec. Path., *4*: 370–390, 1965.

32. Movat, H. Z., and Fernando, N. V. P. The Fine Structure of the Lymphoid Tissue during Antibody Formation. Exp. Molec. Path., *4*: 155–188, 1965.

33. Motoltsy, A. G., and Parakkal, P. F. Membrane-coating Granules of Keratinizing Epithelia. J. Cell Biol., *24*: 297–307, 1965.

34. New, G. B., and Stevenson, W. End Results of Treatment of Malignant Lesions of Nasopharynx. Arch. Otolaryng., *38*: 205–209, 1943.

35. Nossal, G. J. V., Mitchell, J., and McDonald, W. Autoradiographic Studies on the Immune Response. 4. Single Cell Studies on the Primary Response. Australian J. Exp. Biol. Med. Sci., *41* (suppl): 423–435, 1963.

36. Quick, Q., and Cutler, M. Transitional Cell Epidermoid Carcinoma ; Radiosensitive Type of Intra-oral Tumor. Surg. Gyne. and Obst., *45*: 320–331, 1927.

37. Ringertz, N., and Adamson, G. A. The Lymphnode Response to Various Antigens. Acta Path. Scand., Suppl., *86*: 1–69, 1950.

38. Rowlatt, C., and Franks, L. M. Myoepithelium in Mouse Prostate. Nature (London), *202*: 707–708, 1964.

39. Schinz, H. R., and Zuppinger, A. Züricher Erfahrungen der Radiotherapie bei Bösartigen Epipharynx Tumoren. Hals- Hasen- u Ohrenh., *41*: 173–177, 1936.

40. Schmincke, A. Über Lymphoepitheliale Geschwülste. Beitr. Path. Anat., *68*: 161–170, 1921.

41. Shanmugaratnam, K., and Muir, C. S. Nasopharyngeal Carcinoma, Origin and Structure. *In* Cancer of the Nasopharynx, C. S. Muir and K. Shanmugaratnam, eds. pp. 153–162, Copenhagen, Munksgaard, 1967.

42. Simnons, M. W., and Ariel, I. M. Carcinoma of Nasopharynx ; Report of 150 Cases. Surg. Gyne. and Obst., *88* : 763–775, 1949.

43. Snell, R. An Electron Microscopic Study of the Human Epidermal Keratinocyte. Z. Zellforsch, *79* : 492–506, 1967.

44. Stout, A. P. Pathological Diagnosis of Nasopharyngeal Tumors. Laryngoscope, *51* : 446–450, 1941.

45. Sugano, H., Takada, M., Chen, H.-C., and Tu. S.-M. Presence of Herpes-type Virus in the Culture Cell Line from a Nasopharyngeal Carcinoma in Taiwan. Proc. Japan Acad., *46* : 453–457, 1970.

46. Svoboda, D., Kirchner, F., and Shanmugartnam, K. Ultrastructure of Nasopharyngeal Carcinomas in American and Chinese Patients—An Application of Electron Microscopy to Geographic Pathology. Exp. Molec. Patho., *4* : 189–204, 1965.

47. Teoh, T. B. Epidermoid Carcinoma of Nasopharynx among Chinese ; Study of 31 Necropsies. J. Path. and Bact., *73* : 451–465, 1957.

48. Tobek, A. Die Histologische Rückbildung der Lymphoepitheliome nach Röntgenbestrahlung (ein Beitrag zur Frag, ob die Sonderstellung der Lymphoepitheliome berechtigt ist). Z. Hals- Nasen- u Ohrenh., *30* : 182–196, 1931.

49. Toshima, S., Moore, G. E., and Sandberg, A. A. Ultrastructure of Human Melanoma in Cell Culture. Electron Microscopic Studies. Cancer, *21* : 202–216, 1968.

50. Vaeth, J. M. Nasopharyngeal Malignant Tumors ; 82 Consective Patients Treated in Period of 22 Years. Radiology, *74* : 364–372, 1960.

51. Willis, R. A. Pathology of Tumors, 3rd ed. pp. 300–302, Butterworth and Co. Ltd., London, 1960.

52. Yamaguchi, J. Electron Microscopic Studies on Herpes-type Virus in a Burkett Lymphoma Cell Line. GANN Monograph, *7* : 77–94, 1969.

53. Yeh, S. A Histological Classification of Carcinomas of the Nasopharynx with a Critical Review as to the Existence of Lymphoepithelioma. Cancer, *15* : 895–920, 1962.

54. Yoshida, T. O., and Ito, Y. Immunofluorescent Study on Early Virus-cell Interaction in Shope Papilloma *in vitro* System. Proc. Soc. Exp. Biol. Med., *128* : 587–591, 1968.

55. Yoshida, T. O., Liu, C.-H., Yang, C.-S., and Ito, Y. Membrane Immunofluorescence Reactions of Burkitt Lymphoma (P_3HR-1) Exposed to Sera of Tumor Patients and Healthy Normal Subjects : with Particular Reference to the Action of Sera of Nasopharyngeal Cancer Patients. GANN Monograph, *7* : 211–214, 1969.

56. Younes, M. S., Robertson, E. M., and Bencosme, S. A. Electron Microscope Observations on Langerhans Cells in the Cervix. Amer. J. Obst. and Gyne., *102* : 397–403, 1968.

57. Zelickson, A. S. The Langerhans Cell. J. Invest. Derm., *44* : 201–212, 1965.

Discussion of Papers by Drs. Tu, Sugano, and Chen

Dr. Ho: Dr. Tu, you have shown some extremely good pictures of the nasopharynx. How long does it take you to take one of your photographs?

Dr. Tu: Usually it takes 30 min at least. In some cases, the photography is
very difficult and it may take me half a day to take one picture.

Dr. de Thé: First of all, I wish to congratulate Dr. Chen on the enormous
material which he has presented. I think he has probably carried out the best
and most extensive electron microscopic study of nasopharyngeal carcinoma. I
wish to make a few comments. When studying the pathology of tumors by light
and electron microscopy you have to consider three points: one is the problem of
the target cell. What we call the target cell is the origin of the tumor; I think it
is extremely important indeed to understand the pathology of the tumor and define
the role of viral infection in these types of target cells in the development of the
tumor.

The second point is the differentiation of the tumor; you have described in
very elaborate tables the differentiation of tumors. Here I wish to make a few
comments. I was a pathologist early in my career and I might say that we
frequently spent many weeks, sometimes six months discussing problems concerning
the differentiation of some tumors.

When I entered the field of experimental oncology, I realized that the differentiation of a tumor had most probably nothing to do with the etiology of the
tumor. It may be important from the clinical point of view. I think differentiation
is under the control of the effectors of differentiation which are present in every
tumor tissue irrespective of whether a chemical or viral agent was the oncological
agent, as long as it will allow the cell to be receptive to the effectors of differentiation.

The third point I wish to comment on is the intranuclear structure you described.
I am sure you have noticed that the size is quite unlike that of a virus, and this is
certainly a criterion that an electron microscopist should take into account in order
to determine whether the particles under observation are virus-like or not. We
have recently discussed the virus-like particles revealed by EM in human tumors.
I think there are two different types of particles to consider. In one case what
you see is obviously a known virus corresponding to a known morphologic group
such as the Herpes group. In such a case there is absolutely no doubt and any
electron microscopist can identify it. The second type are the structures, which

look like virus particles and are found in human tumors.   In such cases I may say we have to be extremely cautious because there are many structural cellular particles which look like virus particles but we have absolutely no basis on which to say that they are virus particles.

DR. SOUTHAM: I wonder whether perhaps Dr. Tu or Dr. Chen could tell us a little more about the clinical course of the disease, whether it is characterized by local infiltrative growth only, by regional spread, or by distant metastasis.   My concern is what the cause of death is in these patients.   This is not purely a clinical question, because I am wondering whether this might have any possible relationship to host responses.   So, two specific questions: In your separation of exophytic and in-filtrative growths, is there any difference in the long-term pathogenesis of the disease, survival time, and manner of killing?   Then, considering what we have heard yesterday and today with respect to both BL and NPC, we see similar types of virus particles and similar antigenic responses, but we also see that they have, more or less, entirely different age distributions.   The prime age group for BL essentially ceases to exist before that for NPC starts.   From the standpoint of his-topathology, we might be dealing with variants of a common disease.

DR. CHEN: Dr. de Thé, I appreciate your comments.   I am a pathologist and, to be more precise, a morphologist rather than an etiologist.   Therefore, the question of what is the origin of a tumor is very important to me, especially in relation to tissue culture.   When we get many lymphoid cells but no epithelial cells growing, we pathologists must make the last judgment about what we have grown in our cultures;   we must determine what they are.   Therefore, I think histogenesis is very important.

At to the question about the factors deciding clinical prognosis, I should like to point out the reason why prognosis, such as radio-sensitivity, is so variable.   To me they are influenced by the proportions of adenomatous type and epithelial type cells, and as indicated by the secretory granules and tonofibrils present, respectively, under the electron microscope.   They are frequently coexisting in the same tumors. Therefore, from a simple histological diagnosis, it might be difficult to predict that anaplastic carcinomas would be uniformly radiosensitive and always of good prognosis.   We are now trying to review our materials and look for relationships between EM pathological pictures and clinical responses;   we will be reporting the results shortly.

DR. TU: About the clinical course of disease, many reports have said that lym-phoepitheliomas or anaplastic epidermoid cancer are radiosensitive and the prognosis is relatively favorable, but, actually, the prognosis is sometimes very poor and the tumor is not radiosensitive.   Some cases of NPC die of malignant cachexia or of massive bleeding from ruptured internal arteries of the nasopharynx, nasal cavity, or oral cavity.   Distant metastases are also very common.

DR. HO: May I supplement Dr. Tu's answers.   As for the clinical course of nasopharyngeal carcinoma, there are 3 types. The first is the mainly invasive type which occurs in about 8% of all cases. In this, the primary tumor remains mainly invasive, showing no sign of spread to regional lymph nodes, but in a minority of cases—in 4 out of 48 cases which we have studied recently, blood-borne metastases occurred later. In 2 they were found in the spine and in another 2, in the liver. In all 4 of them it was thought that the spread occurred when the tumor had invaded the venous sinuses at the base of the skull, as evidenced by the erosion seen in the bones adjacent to the sinuses, which normally communicate with the internal jugular veins and perivertebral venous plexus.

In the second type, the course is characterized mainly by lymphatic and blood-borne metastases with minimal or no infiltration of the adjacent structures. I have seen over five thousand cases of NPC, but have not yet encountered a single case with metastases occurring in the brain, although the brain is susceptible to local infiltration by the upward extension of the primary tumor through the base of the skull or to infiltration by adjacent meningeal metastases.

The third type has a mixed course: both local infiltration and metastases occurring in the same case, either one occurring before the other, or both occurring about the same time.

I have not found the histopathology of the biopsy specimens as revealed by light microscopy or the gross appearance of the primary tumor to be a useful guide to the clinical course or to radiosensitivity. The large crateriform primary tumors are, however, usually more radio-resistant.

DR. EPSTEIN: About undulated tubules, these are a specialized area of membrane bounded endoplasmic reticulum. These are not virus-like particles at all.

DR. AOKI: About virus-like particles, I think we should be careful. Have you examined for PPLO reaction?

DR. CHEN: In biopsies this is very difficult.

DR. NAKAHARA: No matter what kind of material you start with, cultivation appears to end in getting lymphoblastoid cells. I would like to ask whether you can recognize those lymphoblastoid cells in the original pathological material.

DR. CHEN: In non-cancerous cases, the lymphoid cells are occasionally recognizable, intermingled in the well-developed lymphoid tissue with enlarged germinal centers. As a rule, they show poor uptake of Janus Green B, and are apparently different from the reticulum cells. However, it is almost impossible to identify the existence of lymphoid cells in the stroma of cancer tissue.

DR. EPSTEIN: The difficulty lies in words only. The word lymphoblastoid is used because one does not want to say that they are lymphoblasts.

RESEARCH ON NASOPHARYNGEAL CANCER : ITS RELATION TO EBV

Chairmen :

J. H. C. Ho, Werner Henle

Genetic and Environmental Factors in Nasopharyngeal Carcinoma

J. H. C. Ho

Medical and Health Department, Institute of Radiology, Queen Elizabeth Hospital, Kowloon, Hong Kong

The majority of malignant neoplasms arising primarily in the nasopharynx of people of different races is carcinoma. In Europe and America where the incidence of nasopharyngeal cancer is low, the ratio of carcinoma to sarcoma is about 3: 1 in Europe (*28*), and in America it is between 8 and 9: 1 (*16, 43*). In Australia, Scott and Atkinson (*36*) found essentially no difference in the histopathological distribution of nasopharyngeal cancers in Caucasian and Chinese patients. Over 90% of the Australian patients had carcinoma. In Kenya, Africa, carcinoma is also the predominant tumor (*5*). In China and South East Asia, where the incidence is unusually high, about 99% of the malignant tumors are carcinomas. They are usually of the squamous type with varying degrees of differentiation. The undifferentiated type often shows, on electron microscopy, evidences indicative of its squamous origin (*41*). Although Friedmann (*17*) encountered occasionally similar evidences—desmosomes and cytoplasmic filamentous inclusions—in malignant lymphoma and chordoma, the mere facts that most nasopharyngeal carcinomas contain more than one histological variant in the same tumor, and that typical squamous features are not uncommonly found in sections among predominantly undifferentiated carcinoma cells support the belief, which is now widely held, that these undifferentiated carcinomas, including the so-called lymphoepitheliomas, are, histogenetically, variants of squamous carcinomas.

TABLE 1. Histological Types of Nasopharyngeal Cancers Diagnosed at Queen Mary Hospital, 1959–1963

	No. of cases	%
Carcinomas (squamous, undifferentiated and anaplastic)	1,571	98
Malignant melanoma	2	
Reticulum cell sarcoma	1	
Not histologically confirmed	32	2
Total	1,606	100

It is in nasopharyngeal carcinoma that a racial predilection has been found, and it is this tumor, and not the others arising in the nasopharynx, that this paper is concerned with.

Histogenesis

Liang *et al.* (*30*) thought, " Squamous metaplasia would be a prerequisite for

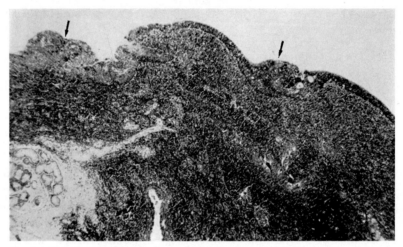

Fig. 1.   Before radiotherapy.   Two foci of carcinoma *in-situ* are indicated by arrows. Surface epithelium of ciliated respiratory type.

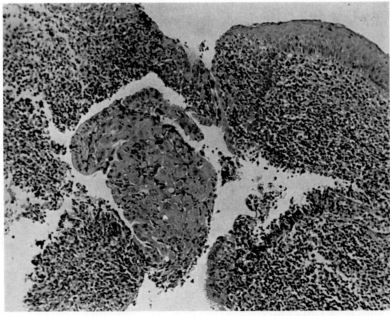

Fig. 2.   After radiotherapy.   Clump of degenerated carcinoma cells in center.   Surface lining of squamous type.

the formation of different types of nasopharyngeal carcinoma." This hypothesis is based on their finding that among 54 cases of malignancy (including precancerous change, carcinoma *in situ* and early invasive carcinoma) arising from the nasopharyngeal mucosa, 27, or 50%, arose from the squamous epithelium of the mucosa, and that at the most frequent site of carcinomatous origin, *i.e.*, the superior two-thirds of the nasopharynx, the mucosa was normally lined with cylindrical cell epithelium.

Shanmugaratnam and Muir (*37*), on the other hand, found that all forms of nasopharyngeal carcinoma, both the classical squamous cell carcinomas and the undifferentiated carcinomas, might arise from squamous, transitional, or respiratory epithelia lining the surface and crypts of the nasopharynx. Our experience in Hong Kong is in agreement with that of Shanmugaratnam and Muir. Figure 1 illustrates two foci of carcinoma *in situ* situated in the midst of ciliated respiratory epithelium in one single microscopic field. The patient was asymptomatic but had a family history of NPC. The discovery was accidental. A third focus, consisting of a clump of degenerated carcinoma cells, was discovered in a biopsy specimen obtained after a radical course of radiotherapy. This specimen was taken from the dorsal wall of the pharyngeal recess on the opposite side (Fig. 2). It is worth noting that after radiotherapy the mucosa was of the squamous type.

Genetic Factors

The role of heredity in human cancers is little known. It is doubtful that laboratory results obtained from inbred animals can be extrapolated to human beings with highly mixed genetic composition and environmental conditions. In the study of the genesis of nasopharyngeal carcinoma we are handicapped by the fact that only primates have an organ which resembles the human nasopharynx. Readily available laboratory animals, such as the rodents, do not. Consequently, we have to rely largely on human epidemiological studies.

Early cases

It is important to ascertain whether NPC was prevalent many centuries ago in certain parts of the world and in China, where the disease is now prevalent, because it will shed light on the relative importance of the genetic and environmental factors. It may well be that the prevalence in China now is a product of the Chinese environment over the last century.

Since the cancer is such a common disease in China (so much so that in the Chinese province of Kwangtung it has long been known as " Kwangtung tumor ") one would expect references to it in old Chinese medical writings. In the book " Etiology and Symptomatology of Diseases " by Chou Uen-Fung a royal physician of the *Sui* dynasty (AD 589–617), there was only a description of the various types of superficial tumorous swellings. Only in '*shu-lu*' or rat tumour was there a mention that these tumors appeared in the neck, but it was stated that the root was in the lungs. No mention had been made of the other clinical features of nasopharyngeal carcinoma. In a paper by Jung and Yu (*25*), which has often been cited, their only conclusion on this point was, " It has proved to be impossible for students of ancient

Chinese writings to determine whether all, some, or none of the cases of '*lo li* ' (glandular enlargement of the neck) were carcinoma metastases rather than tuberculosis, *etc.*''

We are, therefore, still left in doubt about whether the disease was also prevalent in China in the distant past.

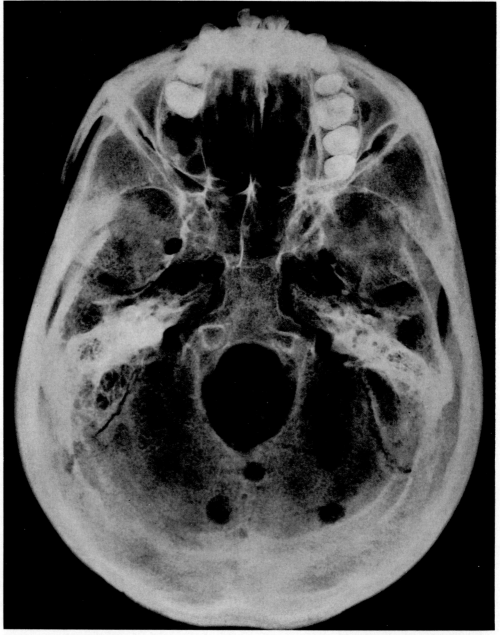

Fig. 3.   Supero-inferior axial projection of base of skull No. 236.   Destruction of posterior part of floor of left antrum indicated by black arrow.   Note rounded areas of bone destruction in occipital bone.

According to Clifford (7), the oldest pathological specimens of nasopharyngeal carcinoma at present known were derived from inhabitants of North East Africa and the Middle East from the period 3,500–3,000 B.C. Wells (45) states, " Only three or four cases of indubitable carcinoma have been recognized among the tens of thousands of ancient Egyptian mummies and skeletons which have been examined. Hardly a score of such cancers have been identified from all the cemeteries of the pre-Renaissance world." He thought that several of this very small number appeared to be of nasopharyngeal origin. Through the courtesy of Dr. J. C. Trevor, director of the Duckworth Laboratory, and the kind assistance of Prof. J. Mitchell and Mr. J. A. Fairfax Fozzard of the University of Cambridge, the author has had the opportunity to examine the radiographs of probably the most important specimen, skull No. 236, kept in the Duckworth Laboratory. The author is of the opinion that the destruction of the posterior part of the left maxillary alveolus and the floor of the antrum and the adjacent part of the hard palate and pterygoid laminae with antemortem loss of the second and third molars shown in Fig. 3 from the paper by Wells (44) is much more likely to be due to carcinoma or myeloma of the alveolus or of the antral floor than to nasopharyngeal carcinoma, because the bony destruction is found mainly in the parts in front of the nasopharynx, whereas those bones which overlie the nasopharynx, and are most commonly involved in nasopharyngeal carcinoma, remained intact. As for the multiple circular holes in the cranial vault without evidence of sclerotic reaction around them, they are more typical of myelomatous deposits than of metastases from nasopharyngeal carcinoma. A "strongly probable " one from Tepe Hissar, Iran, c. 3,000 B.C., according to Wells (45), was actually described by Krogman (26) as a condition which might be primarily due to sinus infection brought about by dental disease. The sites of bony destruction described are typical of those found in antral disease and certainly not in nasopharyngeal carcinoma.

Racial susceptibility

No race is known to be immune to the disease. A high incidence is found among all people of Mongoloid stock with the exception of the Japanese (32) and probably the Koreans (7); the incidence is low in other races. Although the frequency is highest among people of Chinese descent, both in and outside China, in China itself there is a drop in frequency from south to north, according to the relative frequency rates expressed as percentages of all malignant tumors diagnosed by biopsies reported by the major hospitals and medical schools for certain cities and provinces. For instance, Hsieh *et al.* (23) considered nasopharyngeal carcinoma to rank first in frequency in the two southern provinces of Kwangtung and Kwangsi with relative frequency rates of 30.87% (collected papers of Chung Shan Medical College, (23) and 19.24% (23) respectively. While in Taiwan (47), Fukien and Hunan to the north (23) the corresponding rates are respectively 13.32%, 10.3%, and 9.74%.

Table 2 gives a list of the relative frequency rates expressed as percentages of all malignant tumors diagnosed by biopsies reported by Hu and Yang (24) for cities and provinces in the Chinese mainland and by Yeh (48) for Taiwan. The rates show a fall from south to north.

TABLE 2.   Relative Frequency of Nasopharyngeal Carcinoma in Chinese Mainland and Taiwan Estimated in % of All Malignant Tumors Diagnosed by Biopsy

Place	Per cent of all cancers by biopsy	
	Male	Female
South		
Canton (Kwangtung province)	56.9% of 3,010	17.4% of 4,026
Kwangsi province	31.1 of 672	10.0 of 748
Central		
Fukien province	16.2 of 1,010	4.7 of 1,068
Taiwan	23.2 of 5,436	5.2 of 8,636
Shanghai (Kiangsi province)	7.3[a) of 8,332	—
Sian (Shensi province)	6.7 of 879	—
North		
Tsinan (Shangtung province)	5.1 of 2,738	—
Tientsin (Hopei province)	7.9 of 1,562	—
Peking	4.0 of 5,137	—

[a) Would be 6.28% instead if the 1,189 cases seen at the 2nd Medical College, Shanghai, were included. This college has no radiotherapy facilities and hence no NPC cases were likely to be referred to it.

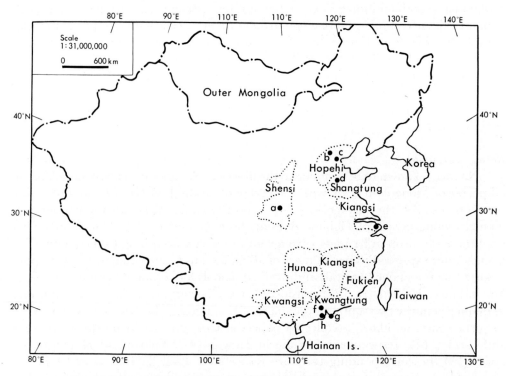

FIG. 4.   Map of China.   a, Sian;   b, Peking;   c, Tientsin;   d, Tsinan;   e, Shanghai; f, Canton;   g, HongKong;   h, Macao.

The difference in frequency could be due to a difference in geographic locality of domicile or to a difference in ethnic origin.   It is, therefore, important to determine whether there is a difference in the frequency of the cancer among Chinese originating from different parts of China living in the same locality.   An analysis according to place of origin was made by Ho (*21*) of 345 Chinese patients who were domiciled in Hong Kong for at least six months before registration at the Radiotherapy Department of the Queen Mary Hospital in 1961, the year when a census of the population was taken.   It was found that Chinese originating from the province of Kwangtung had an incidence rate, standardized to the Hong Kong 1961 census population, over $3\frac{1}{2}$ times higher than that among people from the central coastal provinces of China, and that within the group originating from Kwangtung, those from Hong Kong, Macao and adjacent places, and the Sze Yap area have incidence rates almost double those from Chiu Chau (known as Teochew in Singapore).   These findings are in general agreement with those reported by Mekie and Lawley (*31*) for Chinese patients in Singapore.   They found that the people from Teochew and Fukien (Hokkien) have lower frequencies than the Cantonese, Khek, and the people from Hainan Island.   The latter three groups were from Kwangtung.

Effect of migration

   To investigate the relative importance of the genetic and environmental factors it is essential to study the effect of migration on the incidence rates among people of high risk such as the Chinese.   There is no doubt that the incidence among migrant Chinese populations domiciled in places, such as Hawaii, California, and Australia, far away from their homeland and subjected to an environment more likely to differ significantly from that of their place of origin, remains excessively high, but it is not certain that the locally born Chinese population in these places has a significantly reduced incidence.   In Australia, Scott and Atkinson (*36*) found little difference in the risk of suffering from the disease whether a person of Chinese descent is born in, or outside of, Australia.   On the other hand, Worth and Valentine (*46*) reported incidence rates for the population over the age of 14 years of Chinese descent to be 35.1 per 100,000 for males born in China and Hong Kong, and 10.2 for those born in Australia.   In the case of female patients, they are respectively 29.0 and 11.1. The corresponding crude rates are respectively 31.6 and 7.1 for males and 19.2. and 7.8 for females.   Their report was based on an analysis of 15 Chinese cases during a 10 year period, 1953 to 1963.   Of the 11 male cases born in China, it was only possible to ascertain that 5 had been in Australia more than 5 years when diagnosed; one had been in Australia only 1 month, and the duration of residence was unknown for the other 5.   However, they pointed out that if only the first 5 cases were included in the non-Australian-born group and the others excluded, this would give an over 14 age-adjusted rate of 16.0 which is only about 57% higher than the corresponding rate among the Australian-born Chinese.   In a place like Sydney, where all the case data were obtained, there is a definite likelihood of Chinese from S.E. Asia having traveled there specifically for treatment during the period of this study.   If these had been included in the non-Australian-born group this would have artificially inflated the rate for this group.   There is normally a vast difference between the incidence rates among

Chinese below the age of 25 and those in the 5th and 6th decades of life. In the case of Chinese males in Hong Kong, the rates during the 5 year (1965–1969) period for the 15–19 and 20–24 age groups are respectively, 1.6 and 4.1; whereas, in the 45–49 and 50–54 age groups, they are both 70.9. A significant difference in the age distribution of the two groups of population would have resulted in a several-fold difference in their incidence rates. An indication that the rates given by Worth and Valentine (46) might not be truly representative is to be found in their observed sex-incidence ratio. There is only a slight difference between the male and female rates, whereas the male: female ratio among Chinese patients reported anywhere else in the world is 2.4: 1 or higher, and this also applies to the Chinese cases in the series analysed by Scott and Atkinson (36) which gave a ratio of 4.4: 1.

In Hawaii, Quisenberry and Reimann-Jasinski (35) in an analysis of 14 cases of Chinese descent, 9 born on the U.S. mainland and Hawaii and 5 born elsewhere, reported to the Hawaii Tumor Registry during 1960–1962, found the rates for the latter to be 6 times higher than the former. In addition to the small number being analyzed, the annual rate of 54.2 per 100,000 for all age groups and both sexes combined for Chinese other than those born in the U.S.A. and Hawaii, which is about $3\frac{1}{2}$ times higher than the corresponding rate in Hong Kong of 14.89 for the period (1965–1969), makes one wonder whether this group might have included Chinese who were not domiciled in Hawaii but went there specifically for treatment. An alternative explanation is that Chinese, by migrating to Hawaii, had become more susceptible to the disease, whereas the locally born Chinese were no more susceptible than the Chinese in Hong Kong or South East Asia a most unlikely state of affairs.

In the State of California, U.S.A., Zippin et al. (49) investigated the place of birth of 31 Chinese male cases reported to the California Tumor Registry during 1942–1957, i.e., over a 16 year period, and found the ratio of observed-to-expected (O/E) number of cases by age group to be more than 8 times higher in Chinese under age 55 born outside the United States as compared with those born inside. No difference was found between the two groups over 55.

Unfortunately, the results were based on an analysis of a small series of cases spread over a long period. The interpretation must, therefore, be accepted with reservation. According to the authors themselves, a difference in coverage might exist between U.S. and non-U.S.-born Chinese, but they did not mention whether the non-U.S.-born group might have included patients who went to California from the Far East specifically for treatment. If only a few such cases were included, the difference would be considerably less. Two assumptions were made in the calculation of the O/E ratio. One was that the age-specific incidence rates for cancer of the nasopharynx for males in New York applies equally well to the Chinese population in California. This is not valid because the age-specific incidence rate for Chinese males reaches a peak at 50–54 in Hong Kong, whereas that for Caucasion males reached a peak 1–2 decades later. Furthermore, in Chinese, cancer is almost synonymous with carcinoma in the nasopharynx, whereas in Caucasians, it may include 5–30% of tumors other than carcinomas. The second assumption is that the age-distribution of the U.S.-born and foreign-born Chinese populations in California, according to the 1950 United States census, constitute the mean age-distribution for the two groups during 1943–1957. This is not necessarily valid. Furthermore, there might be a difference in the ethnic composition of the two groups which also could have accounted for the difference in incidence rates.

Buell (3), on the other hand, studied the California mortality records of deaths from cancer of the nasopharynx among 67 men and 13 women of Chinese descent during the 14 years from 1949 through 1962. The number of cases analyzed is again small and spread over a long period. He found that the risk of nasopharyngeal cancer in the locally born Chinese is considerably higher than in the white population, but lower than that in the immigrant Chinese. The factor of increase is about 20-fold for both men and women of Chinese descent born in the United States, and 30- to 40-fold for the men and women born in China. Buell further states that the Chinese immigrants to California have carried with them as much, if not more, risk of cancer of the nasopharynx as have the immigrants to Singapore.

While a lower incidence among the U.S.-born Chinese would support an environmental hypothesis, both Zippin et al. (49) and Buell (3) were of the opinion that it did not rule out a genetic etiology. It could be the result of a genetic-environmental interaction or a selection against a genotype as a cause of the reduction in the filial generation. Buell feels that there is no doubt that the immigrant generation had a lower fertility than their fathers, for, even as late as 1950, the ratio of single adult men to single women was 2 to 1 and several decades earlier the ratio was several times higher. He finds evidence that marriage was often postponed as revealed by the disparity in the parental age on some birth certificates of Chinese, with a paternal age of 40 or 50 and a maternal age of 20 or 30 being not infrequent. Also according to Buell, about 28% of the nasopharyngeal cancer cases were reported to have died unmarried, and some married men were separated from their wives for long intervals, partly due to the Extension Acts of 1882 and 1924 (28).

In conclusion, it could be said that we are still left in doubt as to whether distant migration has altered the risk of Chinese born in their country of adoption, but the risk of those born in their place of origin appears to be unaffected. Further studies are called for.

Incidence in people of part-Chinese ancestry

Ho (22) reported a crude average annual incidence rate estimated to be between 20.0 and 26.7 per 100,000 during 1959–1963 among Hong Kong " Macaonese " as a whole. " Macaonese " was a term used by the Macao Government until a few years ago to describe " local " Portuguese as distinct from " continental " Portuguese. Macao has been colonized by Portugal for over 4 centuries, and the " Macaonese " are largely products of intermarriage between the two races, but all of them are Catholics by religion. Many of them have migrated to Hong Kong. In fact, the large majority of the people of Portuguese nationality in Hong Kong are " Macaonese ". According to a communication dated 15th August, 1966, from the Commissioner of Registration of the Hong Kong Government, the number of persons resident in Hong Kong of Portuguese nationality who had registered with

TABLE 3.   Incidence of Nasopharyngeal Carcinoma in Macaonese in Hong Kong, 1959–1963

No. of cases	Estimated population	Cases/million/year
4	3,000–4,000	200–267

his department for Hong Kong Identity Cards consisted of 833 males and 735 females over the age of 6; those between 6 and 17 years of age numbered 117 males and 121 females.   Those below the age of 6 were not registered and it was not possible to ascertain the number of those who had adopted British nationality, and had not registered as Portuguese.   Those registered as Portuguese included, on the other hand, a small proportion of " continental " Portuguese.   With the help of some of the leaders of their community it has been estimated that the total Portuguese population in Hong Kong was somewhere between 3,000 and 4,000 at the time of the study. Even taking the lower estimate of 20.0 per 100,000, the crude incidence rate is unusually high; it is higher than the highest among the crude rates for the various ethnic groups of Chinese in Hong Kong, e.g., 13.2 for the people originating from the Sze Yap area (21).   There was probably an underestimation of the " Macaonese " population, accounting for its unusually high incidence, but there could be no doubt that it was much higher than that for the other non-Chinese ethnic groups in Hong Kong, because among the 53,230 persons classified as non-Chinese in the 1961 census there were 5 cases of nasopharyngeal carcinoma diagnosed during the 5 year period 1959–1963; 4 of them were " Macaonese," one was a Malay.   There was not a single case among the Caucasians which consisted largely of members of the expatriate British Armed Forces and Civil Service and their families and staffs of foreign business firms and consulates, numbering about 10 times the estimated population of " Macaonese."

In Thailand, Garnjana-Goochorn and Chantarakul (18) conducted a prospective survey of 1,000 consecutive cancer patients in the Tumor Clinic of the Siriraj Hospital in Dhonburi with the intention of determining relative frequencies of nasopharyngeal cancer among the three racial groups—Chinese, Chinese of part-Thai ancestry, and Thais.   Out of the 1,000 cases, there were 170 Chinese, 195 Chinese of mixed descent, 628 Thais, and 7 of other nationalities.   Nasopharyngeal cancer was found in 27 Chinese (15.9%), 20 Chinese of mixed descent (10.3%), and 29 Thais (4.6%).   From this study they estimated the ratio of relative frequencies in the three groups to be, respectively, 3.4: 2.2: 1.0; they believed that this estimation was as near the correct proportion as they could get in Thailand.   They further reported that nasopharyngeal cancer constituted 3.5% of all malignant neoplasms diagnosed at Siriraj Hospital during a 6 year period (1957–1962).

The Thais are a Mongoloid people and mostly Buddhists; the Portuguese are Caucasian and Catholics.   Yet in both, the products of intermarriage with Chinese appear to inherit at least a part of the high risk of their Chinese ancestors.

Familial aggregations

China has been ravaged by wars, rebellions, and revolutions over the last several decades, and over half of the present population of Hong Kong consists of either

TABLE 4.   Frequency of Family History of NPC in Patients with NPC and in Those with Other Cancers (OC) Diagnosed at M. & H.D. Institute of Radiology, Hong Kong (1969).

Cancer	Families with history	Families with no history	Total
NPC	12[a]	385	397[b]
OC	2	687	689[c]
Total	14	1072	1086

$\chi^2 = 14.77785$ $(P < 0.001)$ $t = 3.864234$ $(P = 0.00011)$

[a]   3 of the 12 families were " boat " people.

[b]   72 cases excluded because a family history was unobtainable, unreliable, or not obtained.

[c]   515 cases excluded, 230 for the above reasons and 285 because the cancers were sex-determined, *e.g.*, gynaecological, penile, *etc*.

refugees or descendants of refugees from China.   As a result, many of the patients in Hong Kong have either prematurely lost some or all of their close relatives through unnatural causes or lack of medical care, or have lost contact with them altogether. In some patients, the causes of death of their relatives were not ascertainable because of inadequate diagnosis, while in a few others they knew nothing about the condition of their blood-linked relatives because they were adopted by other families when they were very young.   The source of the present study consists mainly of medical records which are, as a rule, inadequate for genetic studies, because clinicians are usually more concerned with medical diagnosis and treatment than with obtaining a detailed family history of disease.   The medical staff had, however, been requested particularly to ask for family histories of nasopharyngeal carcinoma (NPC) in both groups of patients.   Positive questions were asked in order to counterbalance the memory bias of patients who tended to remember relatives suffering from a disease similar to their own better than ones suffering from other diseases.   In doubtful cases the patients were called back for further questioning by the author himself. Table 4 gives the incidence of a family history of NPC in families of patients with NPC and of those with other cancers (OC) diagnosed at the Medical and Health Department Institute of Radiology, Hong Kong, in 1969.   It shows a much greater risk (P <0.001) for NPC among blood-linked close relatives of patients with NPC than those of patients with other cancers.   It is interesting to note that a quarter of the families with aggregations of NPC cases were from the " boat " population which has always married within its own group until recently; the whole marine population constitutes only 2.76% of the total population, according to the Report of the By-Census 1966 of the Government of Hong Kong.

Table 5 shows the direction of the aggregation in the 12 families with a positive history.   If we accept the two cases with typical clinical histories (the mother and the father of families No. 2 and 8 respectively) as genuine NPC cases, then the incidence of aggregations in this series is as great in the vertical as in the horizontal direction. The actual relative incidence is likely to be even greater in the former, since in any family there is, invariably, a greater population at risk in the horizontal link than in the vertical; it is far more likely for a patient to know of or remember diseases suffered by relatives belonging to the same generation than those belonging to earlier generations, especially when facilities for medical diagnosis were poor in the early

TABLE 5. Familial Aggregations of NP Carcinoma in Patients Seen in 1969

Families	Vertical	Horizontal	Remarks
1)	daughter (II/2M+4F) & father	1 female paternal 1st cousin	
2)	son (V/2M+3F) & mother[a]		
3)		2 sisters (I & II/6M+3F)	"Boat" people
4)	son (IV/4M+5F) & mother		
5)		2 paternal 1st cousins: male (III/3M+2F) & M(2M)	
6)	son (V/4M+3F) & father		
7)		male (V/3M+2F) & bro. (II)	
8)	daughter (IV/1M+5F) & father[a]	& bro. (I)	
9)	son (only child) & father		
10)		male (only child) & his half bro. by same father, but latter's half bro. by same mother well.	"Boat" people
11)	mother (II/1M+3F) & daughter		
12)		bro. (?/4M+1F) & 1 bro.	"Boat" people
	Total = 7	Total = 7	

[a] Diagnosis based on typical history only. (II/2M+4F) means propositus is the 2nd child (II) of a family of 2 sons and 4 daughters.

days. Although age allows the older generations a longer duration at risk, it is unlikely that it would be an important bias factor favouring vertical aggregation, because the risk of getting NPC in Chinese declines after the 5th decade life. Actually, the incidence in the 4th decade is already greater than that in the 7th decade.

It would appear from the familial studies in Hong Kong, including the pedigree of one family with three successive generations affected (Fig. 5), that, if there were a vertical transmission in NPC risk, it does not appear to be sex-linked. The apparently random aggregation is indicative of a multi-factorial etiology; if genes are involved, they are likely to be polygenic.

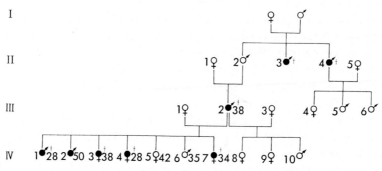

FIG. 5. Pedigree of a family with three successive generations affected by NPC. Numerals on right indicate age at diagnosis except where only age at death ascertainable. †, dead ; ●, nasopharyngeal carcinoma.

ABO blood group distribution

If a genetic etiology is suspected, then every effort should be exerted to study the genetic profiles of people with high and low risks, and of patients and normal controls. So far, only the ABO blood group distributions have been investigated. Clifford (8), in comparing the ABO blood group distribution in 233 Kenyan patients with nasopharyngeal carcinoma and in controls, found a significance level of 3% in the comparison A/O, and thinks that this is highly suggestive that in Kenya group-A persons are " protected " or at less risk of nasopharyngeal carcinoma, while persons with other blood-groups are consequently at greater risk.

In Hong Kong a study of the ABO blood-group distribution in 1,000 Chinese patients with nasopharyngeal carcinoma failed to reveal any significant difference in the distribution in this group when compared with normal controls in the A/O

TABLE 6. ABO Blood Group Distribution in Patients with Nasopharyngeal Carcinoma and Controls

Population (all Chinese)	0	A	B	AB	Total
NPC patients: males	291	197	205	57	750
NPC patients: famales	99	69	69	13	250
Total	390	266	274	70	1,000
Percentage (%)	39	26.6	27.4	7	100
Controls (19)	258	181	180	51	670
Controls (42)	5,747	3,650	3,515	856	13,768
Total	6,005	3,831	3,695	907	14,438
Percentage (%)	41.6	26.5	25.6	6.3	100

For A/O comparison: $t = 0.82093$ ($P = 0,41$), for B/O comparison: $t = 1.62801$ ($P = 0.104$).

TABLE 7. ABO Blood Group Distributions in Chinese Outside Hong Kong (After Mourant et al., 33) and in Chinese in Hong Kong

Place	Authors		Size	Percentage			
				O	A	B	AB
China							
Yangtse River	Yang, F.M.	1925	1,096	42.9	29.5	19.7	7.9
Hunan	,,	1928	93	43.01	31.18	19.35	6.45
Hupeh	,,	1928	197	42.13	32.49	17.26	8.12
Kiangsu	,,	1928	228	52.63	21.05	15.79	10.53
Kwangtung	,,	1928	196	40.82	32.65	18.37	8.16
Canton	Dormanns	1929	992	45.87	22.78	25.20	6.15
,,	Alley & Boyd	1943	101	45.54	29.70	18.81	5.94
Peking	Liu & Wang	1920	1,000	30.70	25.10	34.20	10.00
,,	Hung & Steffan	1928	427	65.34	4.68	19.67	10.30
Hong Kong	Grimmo & Lee	1961	670	38.51	27.02	26.86	7.61
,,	Tong & Pang	1963	13,768	41.74	26.51	25.53	6.22
Singapore	Allen & Scott	1947	624	43.11	24.04	27.72	5.13
Sumatra							
(East coast)	Bias & Verhoef	1924	592	40.20	25.00	27.33	7.26
New York City	Levine & Wong	1943	150	30.00	34.00	25.33	10.67

or B/O comparison (Table 6).   Shanmugaratnam (*39*) also failed to find any signifi-cant difference in this regard between NPC cases and controls in Singapore.

Table 7 shows the distribution of ABO blood-groups amongst Chinese in and outside Hong Kong.   A similar blood-group distribution in that the percentages of the A and B groups are about the same, was found in Hong Kong, Singapore, and Canton (*13*), all of which have an extremely high incidence of the carcinoma.   In the Yangtse River region, Hunan, Hupeh, and Kiangsu, all of which are in central China where the incidence of the cancer is lower (*24*), there is a definite excess of the A group over that of the B, whereas in Peking in northern China, where the relative frequency of the cancer, expressed as a percentage of all cancers, is the lowest (4.0%) according to Hu and Yang (*24*), there is a definite excess of the B group over that of the A.   It would appear, therefore, that if certain genetic factors were associated with a greater susceptibility in Chinese they are unlikely to be the ones linked with certain ABO blood-group gene frequencies.

Environmental Factors

Many environmental factors have been suspected but none has been proved to have a causal relationship with NPC.   First, Dobson (*12*) postulated that the cancer was caused by the smoke from burning grass, wood, tobacco, candles, incense (joss sticks), kerosene lamps, and lamps burning peanut oil in poorly ventilated houses in China.   Then Clifford and Beecher (*4*) suspected that the inhalation of smoke from the burning wood of exotic trees (eucalyptus and wattle) and indigenous acacias in ill-ventilated huts for several hours a day over a period of years might have some bearing on the distribution and incidence of the disease in Kenya, especially since significant quantities of carcinogenic substances such as benzopyrene, bezanthracene, *etc.*, have been found in the soot taken from the roof of the huts of 46 patients with nasopharyngeal cancer on analysis by Hoffman and Wynder (*4*) at the Sloane-Kettering Institute, New York.   On the other hand, Booth *et al.* (*2*) found a similar living condition among the one million and more people living in the Highlands of Australian New Guinea, but NPC is a rarity among them.   It might be argued that the smoke in the two cases contains different substances, but then the crude annual incidence rates of NPC for most Kenyan tribes are below 0.5 per 100,000, and even among the Nandi tribe, which has the highest, the rate was only 0.94 (*6*), only slightly higher than that for Swedes who live in well-ventilated houses.   Further-more, Ho (*21*) found the incidence rates for the marine population in general, and the ' boat ' people in particular, who live and spend most of their lives in sampans and junks and cook their food in the open air, to be significantly higher than that for the land-dwellers in Hong Kong.   It would appear, therefore, unlikely that domestic smoke plays a significant role in the genesis of NPC, and certainly it cannot account for the high incidence in Hong Kong Chinese.

Opium has also been suspected since it was first introduced into China in the early part of the nineteenth century through Kwangtung.   In a retrospective survey of 685 patients diagnosed as having NPC during the 2 year period, 1962 to 1963, at the M. and H.D. Institute of Radiology, Hong Kong, only 4 patients admitted having smoked opium. There may have been some under-recording, but it is unlikely to be more than slight. In Singapore, Shanmugaratnam and Higginson (*38*) found no significant difference between the NPC patients and control cases in their use of opium. In fact, in their survey they also found no significant difference between the two groups in their use of Chinese medicine, dietary and other habits, *e.g.*, the use of alcohol, cigarettes, pipe tobacco, cigars, snuff, Chinese anti-mosquito coils, and incense.

Occupation and economic status

Neither in Hong Kong nor in Singapore (*38*) did the cancer occur more frequently in any particular occupational group, and in Hong Kong the high incidence appears to occur in Chinese of all economic levels.

Oriental incense

Incense in the form of joss sticks (thin bamboo strips coated with a dried paste of sawdust from oriental sandal-wood) are burnt not only in Buddhist or Taoist temples in China but also on a small scale for ancestral and other forms of worship in many Chinese homes in Hong Kong. Sturton *et al.* (*40*) with the help of C. Zippin found a difference (significant at the 5% level) between incense burning and non-incense burning for males under the age of 50 and for males as a whole but not for males over 50 when a group of 29 male NPC patients was compared with a group of 38 male patients with other cancers. There was, however, no significant difference in the female patients of the two groups. On the other hand, there were evidences which did not support such incense smoke as being an important etiological factor: (a) Similar, though not necessarily the same, sort of incense burning is common in temples and some homes in other countries such as Japan and Ceylon where the incidence of NPC is very low, and in Burma where the incidence is relatively low (*27*). (b) The incidence in Macaonese, traditionally Catholics who do not burn joss sticks in their homes or go to Buddhist or Taoist temples for worship, was high; that in Malays, traditionally Muslims, was relatively high. (c) NPC is not at all common among Buddhist monks or nuns or among Taoist temple workers—there were only 1 Buddhist nun and 1 Taoist temple keeper among some 3,500 NPC patients seen at the M. and H.D. Institute of Radiology, Hong Kong, during 1956–1966. (d) The incidence of NPC is higher in the marine population and the 'boat people' engaged in fishing as a livelihood than in the land population in Hong Kong (*20*), and yet it is the latter which is more exposed to incense smoke. (e) Females are more exposed to incense and kitchen smoke than males and, the cancer has a male preponderant incidence.

Chronic infection of the upper respiratory passage and vasomotor rhinitis

Although nasal sinus infection is a common complication of NPC, only a minority of the patients in Hong Kong gave a past history of chronic upper respiratory infection or of vasomotor rhinitis. These diseases may be common in Chinese but they are certainly uncommon as antecedent conditions in NPC.

Nutritional state

Contrary to the findings of Clifford (*5*) among Kenyans, a good nutritional state without clinical evidence of vitamin A or B group deficiency was the rule rather than the exception among Hong Kong patients.

Virus

It is now established that there is among NPC patients an unusual frequency of high titer of antibodies to Epstein-Barr virus (EBV) (*10, 11, 19, 34*), but we are still ignorant of the nature of this relationship. This subject will be covered by other contributors to this symposium.

Pattern of age distribution

Figure 6 shows the male age-specific incidence patterns of nasopharyngeal carcinoma in Sweden, Singapore, and Hong Kong for comparison. The patterns in Singapore and Hong Kong are alike in that the incidence rate is low before the age of 25 years, after which there is a steep rise to a peak at 50–54. This is followed by a fall which is only slightly less steep. In Swedish males the steep rise begins two decades later and the peak is reached at 70–74 which is also two decades later than the peak in Singapore and Hong Kong cases.

It would seem from Fig. 6 that NPC in males have two different age distribution patterns. In Sweden, a low incidence area, it behaves like most other epithelial cancers in that there is an uninterrupted, fairly regular increase in incidence from childhood to beyond 70 (*9*). In high incidence areas, such as Hong Kong and Singapore, the pattern shows instead a rapid progressive increase in incidence in early adult life to a plateau-like peak at 45–54, the climacteric period, thereafter the incidence progressively decreases. The latter pattern strongly suggests that the cancer in high incidence areas was not due to continued exposure to an external carcinogen throughout life and that hormonal factors might have an influence on the incidence.

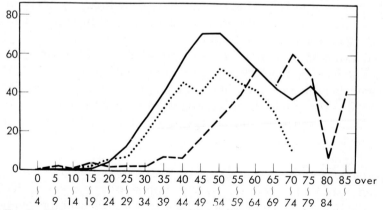

Fig. 6. Male age-specific incidence rates of nasopharyngeal carcinoma in Hong Kong, Sweden, and Singapore. ——, per 100,000, Hong Kong, 2019 cases (1965–1969) ; – – – –, per 2 million, Sweden (only transitional cell, squamous and undifferentiated carcinoma included), 202 cases (1959–1965) ; ······, per 100,000, Singapore, 839 cases (1950–1961).

DISCUSSION

That NPC occurs with unusually high frequency also in Chinese outside China is beyond doubt, but it is not clear whether distant migration has altered the frequency in Chinese born in their place of adoption.   Results of previous studies are far from conclusive.

People who have part-Chinese ancestry seem to share some of the high risk of their Chinese ancestors.   Family members of NPC patients have been found to have a higher risk of getting NPC than those of patients with other cancers, and vertical familial aggregation of the cancer is at least as frequent as horizontal.   These facts are suggestive, but not necessarily the result, of gene action.   They may be the result of social customs, dietary habits, family recipes for treating minor ailments, *etc.*, passed down to subsequent generations and shared by members of the same generation.   We should, therefore, look for external factors likely to affect all ethnic groups of high risk.   That such factors are also common among people of low risk does not necessarily exclude the possibility of their interacting with other factors, especially genetic, to play a causative role in the development of the cancer, but their absence or rarity among them would add weight to the circumstantial evidence in their favor.   Mosquito repellant coils have, until very recently, been frequently used by all people of high risk for many decades, but incense or joss sticks are still commonly burnt in their environment.   They should still remain on the suspected list of external etiological agents despite the fact that we now have only evidence which indicate their lack of importance.

We must not only look for substances which are normally inhaled, because it has been shown that chemical compounds of the nitrosamine group act systemically and are organ-specific (*14*).   They further showed that a single dose of such a carcinogen can initiate a train of events which will culminate in cancer development after a latent period without a further dose (*15*).   Bonser (*1*) suggests that nitrosamine is not itself carcinogenic but has to be converted enzymatically to an active carcinogenic metabolite.   The enzymes capable of effecting such a conversion are different for different nitrosamines, so that the location of specific enzymes determines the site of the cancer.

Nitrosamines are formed when nitrites and/or nitrates are used as food additives or preservatives.   Cantonese salt fish is a common and favourite item of food among most Chinese in and outside China, and also among most Macaonese and Malaysians.   Further epidemiological and laboratory investigation of this item as a possible etiological factor is called for.

CONCLUSION

The etiology of NPC is not known.   All we can say at this stage of our knowledge is that it is most likely to be multifactorial, and that if a genetic factor is involved it is certain to be polygenic.   There is an old saying: "A pinch of salt is worth a pound of precept."   What is needed now is more data and not immediate conclusions.

SUMMARY

It is squamous carcinoma which is the predominant malignant neoplasm of the nasopharynx of people of all races.   Squamous metaplasia does not appear to be an essential intermediate stage in its development.   It is this neoplasm, and not others, which has a predilection for persons of Chinese descent and also an association with a herpes-type virus infection.

A high incidence of the disease is found among all people of Mongoloid stock with the exception of the Japanese and probably the Koreans.   The frequency of the disease is not uniform in different parts of China.   People of mixed Chinese descent appear to have inherited at least part of the high risk of their Chinese ancestors.   Religious practice does not seem to influence the risk.

Close blood-linked relatives of NPC patients appear to have a higher risk of getting NPC than those of patients with other cancers.   In one study it was shown that vertical aggregation of NPC is at least as common as horizontal.   In one family in another study, three successive generations were affected.   The aggregations were quite random and did not appear to be sex-linked, suggesting a multifactorial and polygenic etiology.   There is no significant difference between the ABO blood group distribution in NPC patients and that in apparently normal controls of similar ethnic composition in Hong Kong.   Many environmental factors have been suspected but none has been proved to have a causal relationship with NPC.   In addition to EB virus or a herpes-type virus very similar to it in antigenic pattern, there were three other external factors likely to affect all ethnic groups of people of high risk, *e.g.*, Chinese incense or joss sticks, mosquito repellant coils and salted fish, deserve further investigation despite the fact that we have at present only evidence indicating the lack of importance of any one of these three.   The pattern of age distribution of NPC in people of high risk, *e.g.*, Hong Kong and Singapore Chinese males, differs significantly from that in Swedish males of low risk.   The former shows a rapid progressive increase in incidence in early adult life, followed by a progressive decrease after 50–54.   This pattern strongly suggests that the cancer was not due continued exposure to an external carcinogen throughout life and that hormonal factors might have an influence on the incidence.   The Swedish pattern behaves, on the other hand, like those seen in other epithelial cancers in that there is an uninterrupted, fairly regular increase in incidence from childhood to beyond 70.

The author is grateful to Dr. the Hon. Gerald Choa, Director of the Medical and Health Services of Hong Kong, for his permission to publish this paper, to the medical staff of his Institute for their special attention in obtaining the family histories of the cases, Mr. C. M. Lam for statistical assistance, Mr. R. Abessor for preparing Figs. 4 to 7, Mrs. P. Liu for careful secretarial assistance, Messrs. K. Fung and H. K. Tam for data collection, Messrs. K. W. Leung and A. Lam for photographic assistance and Mr. H. C. Kwan for Figs. 1 and 2.

The author is also indebted to the Swedish Cancer Registry and Prof. Nils Ringertz, Scientific Surveyor of the Registry, for their generous cooperation in supplying Swedish data, to Prof. J. Mitchell, F. R. S., and Mr. J. A. Fairfax Fozzard of Cambridge University for supplying the radiographs of skull No. 236 kept at Duckworth Laboratory, Cambridge, and to Mr. J. C. Trevor, Director of the Laboratory, for the facilities afforded, to Prof. R. Doll of Oxford University and Dr. T. Hirayama for helpful advice, to Prof. K. Shanmugaratnam and Dr. Myo Tint for supplying Singapore and Burmese data, respectively, and finally to Dr. L. Atkinson for helpful information regarding conditions in Australian New Guinea.

REFERENCES

1. Bonser, G. M. Factors Concerned in the Location of Human and Experimental Tumours. Brit. Med. J., *2*: 655–660, 1967.
2. Booth, K., Cooke, R., Scott, G., and Atkinson, L. Carcinoma of the Nasopharynx and Oesophagus in Australian New Guinea 1958 to 1965. *In* P. Clifford, C. A. Linsell, and G. L. Timms (ed.), Cancer in Africa, 319–322, E. Afr. Med. J.: East African Publishing House, Nairobi, 1968.
3. Buell, P. Nasopharynx Cancer in Chinese of California. Brit. J. Cancer, *19*: 459–470, 1965.
4. Clifford, P., and Beecher, J. L. Nasopharyngeal Cancer in Kenya. Clinical and Environmental Aspects. Brit. J. Cancer, *18*: 25–43, 1964.
5. Clifford, P. Carcinoma of the Nasopharynx in Kenya. E. Afr. Med. J., *42*: 373–396, 1965.
6. Clifford, P. Malignant Disease of the Nasopharynx and Paranasal Sinuses in Kenya. *In* C. S. Muir and K. Shanmugaratnam (ed.), Cancer of the Nasopharynx. UICC Monograph Series, 1: 82–94, Munksgaard, Copenhagen, 1967.
7. Clifford, P. A Review on the Epidemiology of Nasopharyngeal Carcinoma. Int. J. Cancer, *5*: 287–309, 1970.
8. Clifford, P. Blood-groups and Nasopharyngeal Carcinoma. Lancet, *2*: 48–49, 1970.
9. Cook, P. J., Doll, R., and Fellingham, S. A. A Mathematical Model for The Age Distribution of Cancer in Man. Int. J. Cancer, *4*: 93–112, 1969.
10. de Schryver, A., Freiberg, S., Jr., Klein, G., Henle, W., Henle, G., de-The, G., Clifford, P., and Ho, H. C. Epstein-Barr Virus-associated Antibody Patterns in Carcinoma of the Post-nasal Space. Clin. Exp. Immunol., *5*: 443–459, 1969.
11. de-The, G., Ho, H. C., Kwan, H. C., Desgranges, C., and Favre, M. C. Nasopharyngeal Carcinoma (NPC). I. Types of Cultures Derived From Tumour Biopsies and Non-Tumorous Tissues of Chinese Patients with Special Reference to Lymphoblastoid Transformation. Int. J. Cancer, *6*: 189–206, 1970.
12. Dobson, W. C. Cervical Lymphosarcoma. (Letter to the Editor). Chin. Med. J., *38*: 786, 1924.
13. Dormanns, E. A. *In* A. E. Mourant, A. C. Kopec, and K. Domaniewska-Sobczak (ed.), ABO Blood Groups, p. 146, Blackwell, Oxford, 1958.
14. Druckrey, H., Ivankovic, S., Mennel, H. D., and Preussmann, R. Selektive Erzeugung Von Carcinomen der Nasenhohle bei Ratten durch N,N'-Nitrosopiperazin, Nitrosopiperidin, Nitrosomorpholin, Methyl-allyl, Dimethyl-und-Methyl-vinyl-Nitrosamin. Z. Krebsforsch, *66*: 138–150, 1964.
15. Druckrey, H., Steinhoff, D., Preussmann, R., and Ivankovic, S. Erzeugung von Krebs durch eine einmalige Dosis von Methylnitroso-Harnstoff und verschiedenen Dialkylnitrosaminen an Ratten. Z. Krebsforsch, *66*: 1–10, 1964.

16. Fletcher, G. H., and Million, R. R. Malignant Tumors of the Nasopharynx. Am. J. Roentgonol. & Rad. Therapy, *93*, No. 1 : 44–55, 1965.

17. Friedmann, I. Nasopharyngeal Carcinoma. *In* A. A. Shivas (ed.), Racial and Geographic Factors in Tumour Incidence. Pfizer Medical Monographs, *2* : 189–206, University of Edinburgh, 1967.

18. Garnjana-Goochorn, S., and Chantarakul, N. Nasopharyngeal Cancer at Siriraj Hospital, Dhonburi, Thailand, *In* C. S. Muir and K. Shanmugaratnam (ed.), Cancer of the Nasopharynx. UICC Monograph Series, *1* : 33–37, Munksgaard, Copenhagen, 1967.

19. Grimmo, A. E. P., and Lee, S. K. A Survey of the Blood Groups in Hong Kong Chinese of Cantonese Origin. Oceania, *31* : 222–226, 1961.

20. Henle, W., Henle, G., Ho, H. C., Burtin, P., Cachin, Y., Clifford, P., de Schryver, A., de-The, G., Diehl, V., and Klein, G. Antibodies to Epstein-Barr Virus in Nasopharyngeal Carcinoma, Other Head and Neck Neoplasms, and Control Groups. J. Nat. Cancer Inst., *44* : 225–231, 1970.

21. Ho, H. C. Nasopharyngeal Carcinoma in Hong Kong. *In* C. S. Muir and K. Shanmugaratnam (ed.), Cancer of the Nasopharynx. UICC Monograph Series, *1* : 58–63, Munksgaard, Copenhagen, 1967.

22. Ho, H. C. Cancer of the Nasopharynx. *In* R. J. C. Harris (ed.), Panel II, Ninth International Cancer Congress. UICC Monograph Series, *10* : 110–116, Springer-Verlag, Berlin, Heidelberg, New York, 1967.

23. Hsieh, C. K., Li, C. C., Min, H. C., Chang, F. L., and Li, P. K. Clinical Analysis of 1,000 Cases of Nasopharyngeal Carcinoma. Chin. Med. J., *84* : 767–780, 1965.

24. Hu, C. H., and Yang, C. A. Decade of Progress in Morphologic Pathology. Chin. Med. J., *79* : 409–422, 1959.

25. Jung, P. F., and Yu, C. Nasopharyngeal Cancer in China. Postgrad. Med., *33* : A77–A82, 1963.

26. Krogman, W. M. The Skeletal and Dental Pathology of an Early Iranian Site. Bull. Hist. Med., *8* : 28–48, 1940.

27. Myo Tint. Personal communication, 1970.

28. Lederman, M. Cancer of the Nasopharynx. Thomas, Springfield, 1961.

29. Lee, R. H. The Chinese in the United States of America, Hong Kong University, 1960.

30. Liang, P. C. Studies on Nasopharyngeal Carcinoma in the Chinese. Statistical and Laboratory Investigations. Chin. Med. J., *83* : 373–390, 1964.

31. Mekie, D. E. C., and Lawley, M. Nasopharyngeal Carcinoma. I. Clinical Analysis of 120 Cases. Arch. Surg., *69* : 841–848, 1954.

32. Miyaji, T. Carcinoma of the Nasopharynx and Related Organs in Japan based on Mortality, Morbidity, and Autopsy studies. *In* C. S. Muir and K. Shanmugaratnam (ed.), Cancer of the Nasopharynx. UICC Monograph Series, *1* : 29–32, Munksgaard, Copenhagen, 1967.

33. Mourant, A. E., Kopec, A. C., and Domaniewska-Sobczak, K. ABO Blood Groups, 146–152, Blackwell, Oxford, 1958.

34. Old, L. J., Boyse, E. A., Oettgen, F. H., de Harven, E., Geering, G., Williamson, B., and Clifford, P. Precipitating Antibodies in Human Serum to an Antigen present in Cultured Burkitt's Lymphoma Cells. Proc. Nat. Acad. Sci. (Wash.), *56* : 1699–1704, 1966.

35. Quisenberry, W. B., and Reimann-Jasinski, D. Ethnic Differences in Nasopharyngeal Cancer in Hawaii. *In* C. S. Muir and K. Shanmugaratnam (ed.), Cancer of

Association between a Herpes-type Virus and Nasopharyngeal Carcinoma—Present Status of Studies

Guy de-Thé, J.H.C. Ho, Timothy Greenland, Anton Geser, and Nubia Munoz

International Agency for Research on Cancer (Unit of Biological Carcinogenesis), Lyon, France [G. T., T. G., A. G., N. M.]; Medical and Health Department Institute of Radiology, Queen Elizabeth Hospital, Kowloon, Hong Kong [J. H.]

The previous presentations have clearly demonstrated the unique position of nasopharyngeal carcinoma (NPC) among the human tumors. Dr. Ho (*4*) presented the epidemiology of NPC, giving evidence that one ethnic group (namely the southern Chinese) is particularly susceptible to this tumor. He also presented evidence of family clustering: in 1969, nearly 2.5% of the cases in Hong Kong occurred in families already having a case of NPC. This situation greatly stimulated our interest because it is reminiscent of the situation in mice where there are dramatic differences in the incidence of leukemia and lymphoma for different inbred strains. This was shown by Lilly *et al.* (*6*) to reflect a genetically determined susceptibility to tumor induction by oncogenic viruses.

Dr. Chen (*1*) has presented the histopathology of this tumor, stressing the importance of the infiltration of the tumor by lympho-plasmocytic elements, with great variations from one tumor to another and even within one tumor. This infiltration has been described by some pathologists as nontumoros, although this has not been formally proved yet. Other interesting histopathological properties of this tumor are the great variations in the state of differentiation from one tumor to another, and its apparent multifocal origin, as multiple carcinoma *in situ* can be found in systematic biopsies made on patients with early clinical signs of NPC.

Evidence of an Association between a Herpes-type Virus and Nasopharyngeal Carcinoma

In the past two years, evidence has accumulated regarding the association between a herpes-type virus (HTV), sharing structural antigens with the EBV, and nasopharyngeal carcinoma (NPC). Although these results have recently been

We would like to dedicate this paper to the memory of Dr. Nicole Granboulan, Maitre de Recherches at the CNRS, " Institut de Recherches Scientifiques sur le Cancer ", Villejuif, France, who was a personal friend of one of us (G. T.), and whose early and tragic death afflicted so many friends of hers.

TABLE 1. Types of Cultures Obtained from NPC Biopsies from Hong Kong between January 1969 and August 1970

Diganosis[a]	Successful cultures	Epithelioid growth	Early lymphocytic production	Fibroblastic growth	Permanent lymphoblastoid cultures
NPC	85	22	60	66	28
OT	7	3	2	6	1
NT	15	9	10	15	5
NNP	9	3	4	9	2

[a] NPC, nasopharyngeal carcinoma; OT, ENT tumors other than NPC; NT, diseased tonsils from Chinese children; NNP, 'apparently' normal nasopharyngenal mucosa of patients with either sub-clinical signs of NPC or family history of NPC.

published (16), it might be useful to review them rapidly and to discuss their respective values.

Tissue culture studies

The results obtained in tissue culture of NPC biopsies are shown in Table 1, which is a resumé of our findings of the past 18 months (15, 16).

a) Epithelial growth—such growth (Fig. 1) was obtained in 26% of the biopsies and was always of short duration (4 to 12 weeks) and of limited extent (a few mm around the explants). It was interesting to note that NPC biopsies obtained from Africa (Nairobi and Kampala) never gave rise to epithelial cultures, whereas the epithelial growths obtained in Singapore by Ian Jack (5) were much larger than those obtained in Lyon. This would suggest that the epithelial tumorous cells are quite fragile and do not survive well when kept in unnatural conditions. It should now be the primary aim of the laboratories concerned to attempt to establish long-term culture of epithelial cells.

b) Early lymphocytic production (ELP)—such production started from the first day of culture and clearly represented the division and survival of the lymphoid elements present in the tumor. As already mentioned (16), these early lymphoid cells disappeared gradually from the cultures within 2 to 3 weeks and never showed any sign of infection by HTV, either by electron microscopy or by immunofluorescence.

c) Fibroblastoid cultures—such growth was observed in 78% of the cultures and appeared either as a primary culture or as a secondary growth to the epithelial sheets. Besides their abnormal growth pattern (criss-cross orientation with various degrees of loss of contact inhibition), these fibroblastic cells showed rounded nuclei with indentations, giving them an abnormal appearance. Although we have no direct evidence, the possibility that epithelial cells could convert to fibroblastic

→ FIG. 1. Epithelial growth on the 9th day of culture of a NPC biopsy. Note that some of the cells are taking on a fibroblastoid appearance, whereas others are still clearly epithelial. × 400.

FIG. 2. Aspect of a long term lymphoblastoid culture showing the tendency of the round free-floating cells to grow in clumps, attach, and divide onto the fibroblastoid elements attached to the surface of the bottle. × 140.

FIG. 3. Aspect of the lymphoblastoid free-floating cells after Giemsa staining. × 1,700.

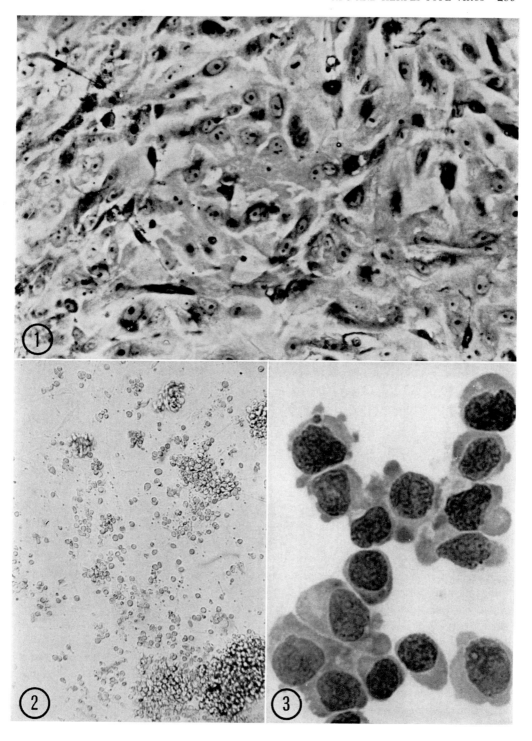

phenotypes should not be ruled out. Up to now, no sign of HTV infection has been found in these cells.

d) Lymphoblastoid transformation and establishment of permanent lines—such lines were derived from approximately 33% of the NPC cultures at periods varying from 40 to 120 days from the start of the culture. Their appearance (Figs. 2 and 3) and growth properties have been described (*16*) and we wish today to stress once more that in some of these lines lymphoblastoid cells showed reattachment to the glass, taking on a fibroblastoid appearance. We do not know the origin of the lympho-blastoid cells emerging from fibroblastoid cultures. Emperipolesis of lymphoid cells in fibroblasts has been occasionally observed but we wish to emphasize that morphological, phenotypic variation does indeed exist in some systems (*10*). We should not rule out the possibility that round free-floating lymphoblastoid cells might be derived from fibroblastic cells.

e) Cultures from control specimens—growths similar to those observed with NPC were obtained from other ENT tumors, tonsilitis surgical specimens, and biopsies from apparently normal nasopharyngeal mucosa (see Table 1). The fact that spontaneous lymphoblastoid transformation and establishment of permanent cultures were observed in these nontumorous specimens suggests that the development of permanent lymphoblastoid lines is not specific for tumorous tissues but merely re-flects the presence in the original material of a factor responsible for this transforma-tion. It has already been proposed (*16*) that this factor is a herpes-type virus with ' transforming properties.' In order to be considered as having oncogenic poten-tialities, such a virus does not have to be present only in tumorous tissue, as it is well established that animal oncogenic viruses can replicate in nontumorous cells.

Electron microscopy

The results of the studies with electron microscopy on NPC-derived cultures will be published elsewhere in detail. In the NPC biopsies three types of cells can be encountered: epithelial tumorous cells showing great variation in their state of differentiation—lymphoplasmatic elements, sometimes closely associated with the tumor cells—and fibroblastic elements showing abnormal nuclei.

The epithelioid sheets obtained *in vitro* clearly exhibit ultrastructural features of epithelial cells (Fig. 4), as keratin fibrils and junctional complexes including des-mosomes can be observed. No structures suggestive of a viral infection have been observed in these epithelial cells. The ultrastructural study of the ' early lymphoid cells ' showed a heterogeneous population of small lymphocytes, reticular cells, *etc*; no virus particles were found in these cultures. In contrast, as already published (*14, 16*), herpes-type capsids, nucleocapsids, and virions were observed in lympho-blastoid cell lines (Figs. 5, 6, and 7). The release of the virus particles occurred in two different ways: either by complete disruption of the cells and of the nuclei con-taining many capsids and nuclecapsids (Fig. 6), or by budding through the nuclear envelope and migration of the particles through cytoplasmic channels which the virus seemed to induce along its path. Dr. Roizman (*11*) has discussed the syn-thesis of membrane-associated glycoproteins induced by infection with herpes simplex virus (HSV). The apparent *de novo* synthesis of cytoplasmic channels by the HTV

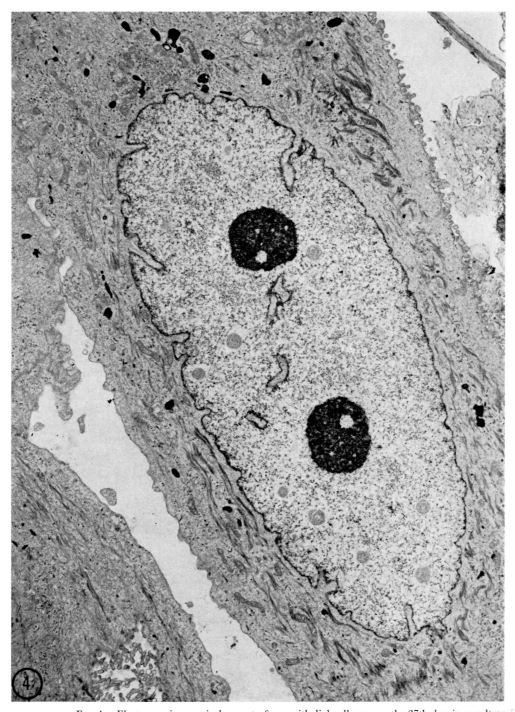

FIG. 4. Electron microscopical aspect of an epithelial cell seen on the 27th day in a culture originated from an NPC biopsy. Note the presence of round fibrillar bodies in the nucleus, and of intra-cytoplasmic tonofibrils. × 6,600.

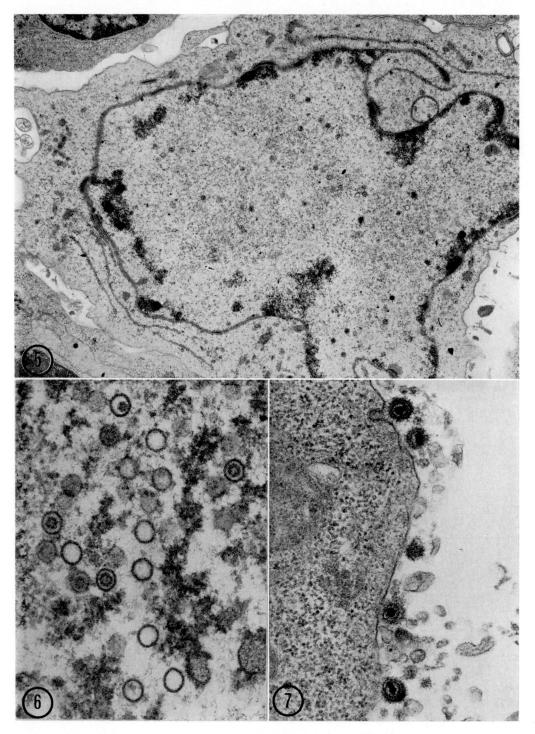

associated with NPC might represent an ultrastructural aspect of biochemical events similar to those induced by HSV. The negative staining of semi-purified HTV reveals viral structures apparently not different from those of HSV or EBV.

Serological and other immunological studies

Old *et al.* found in 1966 (*9*) that sera from NPC patients contained precipitating antibodies similar to those present in the sera of Burkitt's lymphoma (BL) patients. Henle, using sera from NPC patients from whom we obtained our cultures, showed that these sera had high antibody titers against EB-type structural antigens (*3*). De Schryver *et al.* (*12, 13*), at the Karolinska Institutet, found that NPC sera had high antibody activity against membrane-associated antigens when BL-derived or NPC-derived cultures were used as antigens.

Dr. G. Henle (*2*) has presented her fascinating results concerning early antigens induced by superinfection of an infected but nonproductive BL-derived cell line (Raji) and showed that antibodies against this type of antigen are present mostly in cancer patients (BL and NPC).

The results mentioned above establish that an association does exist between a herpes-type virus and NPC. Indeed these serological properties are not restricted to Chinese NPC patients, as they were also observed in NPC patients from Africa, Europe, and North and South America. Thus, the association seems to be specific for the disease itself. As will be discussed in the next section, we have initiated a large sero-epidemiological study in Southeast Asia aimed at establishing the prevalence and incidence of infection by this type of virus in populations at high and low risk of NPC. The immunofluorescence (IF) test of Henle will be used to evaluate the level of antibodies to antiviral capsid antigen(s) in the collected sera with a view to comparing the antibody levels in the various survey populations.

As these tests are to be carried out in different and distant laboratories (Hong Kong, Singapore, and Lyon), the statistical analysis of the results will not be an easy task, and it would be greatly eased if subjective evaluation of the observations could be avoided. With such a purpose in mind, we developed a test in which automatic counting of radioactive iodine uptake replaces the subjective search for fluorescent cells. In this test, a radio-iodine ' paired labeled mixture ' of rabbit anti-human gamma globulin antiserum and rabbit normal gamma globulin labeled with different isotopes of iodine replaces the goat anti-human gamma globulin antisera used in the indirect immunofluorescence test of Henle. Although details of the technique are still to be published (Greenland *et al.*, in preparation), in brief, the ratio of the uptake of the two isotopes represents the attachment of the gamma globulin from the patients' sera on to the fixed cells.

← Fig. 5. Typical cell in an NPC-derived long term lymphoblastoid line, showing the characteristic nuclear lesions : margination of the chromatin, multilayered reduplication of the nuclear membrane, and presence of herpes-type nucleocapsids.   × 12,800.

Fig. 6. High magnification of disintegrating nucleus showing the ultrastructure of empty capsids and nucleocapsids.   × 51,300.

Fig. 7. Extracellular virions showing the characteristic herpes-type ultrastructure.   × 39,000.

If the log of this ratio is plotted against the dilution of patients' sera, there is sometimes a high level plateau representing saturation of the cells by the sera: then there is always a region of linear descent which represents the dose responsive uptake of diminishing amounts of antibody in the serum dilutions, followed by a low-level plateau representing a background of nonspecific uptake of nonantibody gamma globulin from the patients' sera and/or production of gamma globulin by the antigenic cells. A cut-off point is chosen at a level higher than that at which the majority of sera begin to show their low-level plateau, and the titer of each serum is expressed as the last doubling dilution before its graph cuts this level. The result thus determined correspond well with the indirect immunofluorescence titers determined for the same sera by Dr. Henle.

Both the inherent linearity of the results for each serum within an experiment and studies on repeated dosage of the same sera suggest a satisfactory reproduceability. We are now starting to apply this technique to a small-scale seroepidemiological study to test its practicability and its suitability for statistical analysis.

Analysis of the histopathological features of the tumor biopsies with tissue culture and serological results

We carried out this analysis in order to see to what extent the lymphoblastoid transformation obtained *in vitro* with the NPC biopsies and the high antibody activities of the NPC sera were related to the degree of lymphoplasmocytic infiltration of the corresponding tumors. Details of this analysis will be published elsewhere (Munoz *et al.*, in preparation) but we can say that no correlation seems to exist between these different parameters, which would indicate that the sole presence of lymphoid elements mixed with epithelial tumor cells in NPC is not responsible for the immunological reactivity against HTV. It was interesting to note in this analysis that the degree of differentiation of the epithelial tumor cell seemed to influence the chance of lymphoblastoid transformation.

Nature of the Association between HTV and NPC

Two hypotheses can be put forward concerning the nature of the association between HTV and NPC:

HTV might be a passenger virus which grows in lymphoid elements present in the tumor. The lymphoid cells could be stimulated by the presence of epithelial tumors cells and could subsequently produce HTV, which would play no role in the development of this tumor. This hypothesis cannot be ruled out as there are examples of passenger viruses in animal tumors. Furthermore, it has been established that this type of virus may lie dormant in the lymphnodes of normal individuals (7). However, as a rule, such passenger viruses should not be present in all tumor-bearing individuals, as the population from which the tumor-bearing individuals derive does not seem to be infected at a 100% level. Similarly, if the virus were merely a passenger, other epithelial tumors of the ENT area with a similar lymphoid infiltration should have a serological pattern similar to that of NPC. This does not seem to be the case, as Klein *et al.* (mentioned by de Schryver *et al. 12*) have shown that sera obtained from Indian donors with tumors arising from the tonsils and the back of the tongue, where lymphoid tissue is also abundant, have a low reactivity as compared with NPC or BL sera.   Not supporting this hypothesis either is the fact that NPC cases all over the world, in South East Asia, Africa, North and South America, and Europe, have the same serological pattern.

HTV may be causally related to NPC either in a direct way as the prime on-cogenic agent, or in an indirect way, as a necessary co-factor helping another car-cinogen.   The establishment of the nature of such a relationship is certainly not an easy task: we cannot, in man, conduct experiments like those which are carried out in animal species to prove that a virus is oncogenic.   Therefore, we have, for studies in man, to develop a new tool, a new approach, a new way of thinking.   It appeared to us that the integration of field population studies with advanced labora-tory investigations might represent such an approach and that the international position of IARC might facilitate such an approach.

If direct proof of the causative relationship between a virus and a tumor cannot be obtained through experiments in man, we might avail ourselves of the experiments that Nature is carrying out for us, by analyzing the sequential events which occur between the time of infection by a given virus in man and the eventual development of the tumor.   Three phases could be described in studying such natural events:

Phase 1, which is now historical for NPC and BL, represents the establishment of the fact that an association does indeed exist between a given virus and a given tumor.

In Phase 2, the natural history of the virus in man should be elucidated by conducting epidemiological studies, in populations with both high and low risk of tumor.   This phase should yield information about the age at which virus infection takes place, the stability of immunity over a period of time and the probability of reinfection at various ages, and should show whether the risk of virus infection is correlated with the risk of tumor development from population to population.   When valid estimates of the various relevant parameters have been obtained during Phase 2, it will be possible to construct realistic models reflecting the virus epidemiology in the various study populations and to consider whether meaningful hypotheses re-garding the etiological role of the virus can be formulated and tested.

Phase 3 will consist of observing the sequence of events (virus infection, im-munological changes, tumor development) in large-scale prospective studies in human populations.   This will allow for an analysis of the time relationship bet-ween virus infection and tumor development and thus show whether the sequence of events is of such a nature that the hypothesis of causation can be maintained.

In the case of NPC, studies representing Phase 2 are now in progress in Hong Kong, Singapore, and Lyon, aimed at studying the dynamics of HTV infection under different conditions.   The study in Singapore is of particular interest since it covers the Chinese population which has a high incidence of NPC, as well as the Indo-Pakistanis, in which NPC is rare.   The situation regarding NPC etiology is somewhat more complicated than that of BL, since NPC occurs at a later age and thus may have a long latent period, whereas the latent period in BL must be re-latively short since this tumor occurs in children.   It is therefore essential to include persons of all ages in the NPC-oriented studies.   The on going surveys in Hong Kong and Singapore will be made large enough to yield fairly accurate estimates of the various epidemiological parameters required for the construction of epidemiological models.   Whether Phase 3 will be attempted or not, in connection with NPC, will depend upon what is found in the ongoing studies of the natural history of HTV infection.   If, for instance, a small group of males should be found to remain free of HTV antibodies up to the age of NPC manifestation, it might be postulated that they are those at risk of developing the tumor and a study aimed at testing such a hypothesis might be manageable.

In the case of BL, Phase 2 has already been carried out in Uganda, where the epidemiology of EBV-infection was investigated in the West Nile district in an 18-month follow up study, directed by Dr. G.W. Kafuko of the East African Virus Research Institute, Entebbe.   Although this study was too small to give precise estimates of the age-specific rate of infection, it showed that the virus antibody levels are sufficiently stable over time to permit a meaningful classification of the study population according to their immunological status.   A follow up study thus seems feasible and plans are now in preparation for a study representing Phase 3 in the West Nile district.   It is proposed to collect serum from approximately 30,000 children under 6 years of age and to follow these children for a period of five years, during which time it is expected that approximately 35 cases of BL will develop.   The sera from the affected children will then be examined in order to determine their EBV antibody levels prior to tumor development.

The hypothesis that virus infection is a prerequisite for the development of BL, or that the tumor only develops in children who have had a high virus antibody level for a prolonged period can then be tested by observing in which immunological subgroups the BL cases actually occur.   If the cases should happen to be randomly distributed between the various serological groups, it would obviously be difficult to maintain the concept that the virus plays an etiological role, unless one postulates more complex hypotheses, such as those involving long and varying latent periods between virus infection and tumor manifestation; such complex hypotheses would, however, appear untestable in epidemiological studies of a manageable size.

One of the major problems in such field sero-epidemiological studies is to ensure that we are measuring the right and relevant antibody.   Actually, in the IF test, we are detecting antibodies against viral capsid antigens but we do not know to what extent these antibodies are protecting against new viral infection, even if they are meaningful in the development of the disease.   It is possible that, as described by G. Henle (2), antibodies directed against early antigens are more relevant in this connection.

In order to make a more thorough analysis of the antigens present in the long-term cultures derived from NPC or BL, we carried out experiments using radioactive iodine labeled antibodies (Greenland et al., in preparation).   A panel of, for example, 6 sera was divided into 2 aliquots from each serum, one being labeled with ^{125}I and the other with ^{131}I.   All possible mixtures were then made up by combining these aliquots (36 mixtures).   Specimens from a panel of 12 coded cell lines derived from NPC or from BL were treated with every one of the paired mixtures and then the relative uptake of each serum in the mixtures was calculated for each cell line.

As there was no competition between the sera—there being an excess of antigen—it was possible to class the sera according to their strength on a given line. The place of a given serum in the order of strength for a given cell line should be independent of the serum with which it is paired, and of the isotope used to label it. This was in fact the case.

The order of the sera should be the same with all cell lines if there were no antigenic difference between them, but would change if lines were antigenically different. The latter situation was observed. By computer analysis, as well as by estimating the weight of the gamma globulin taken up from each serum by each cell line, it was possible to estimate the number of antigenic differences necessary to fit the results. Thus, it appears that at least 4 and possibly 6 different antigens were present in these lines. One antigen, designated 'A', was certainly related to capsid antigen(s), as it was regularly present in all IF positive lines and absent in IF negative lines. Another antigen, designated ' C ', was present in all tested NPC-derived lines from Hong Kong or from Africa, and absent in all BL and IM derived lines tested. As this experiment represented a very large amount of work, only 7 lines from NPC, 4 lines from BL, and 1 line from IM have been tested so far by these sera.

The difference observed between NPC- and BL-derived cell lines might represent either a difference in the origin of the cells, or a different virally induced antigen. In the latter case, this could be an indication of a strain difference between the virus associated with NPC and the EBV associated with BL.

These results should be considered together with those presented by Dr. Nishioka (8), in which he found that NPC- and BL-derived cell lines behaved differently in immuneadherence tests. The differences found by Dr. Nishioka may also point to a difference in cellular origin or a difference induced by differing viral strains. Future studies will, we hope, clarify the situation, as it is of prime importance to establish whether one single virus, namely the Epstein-Barr virus, is responsible for different human tumors or if there is a family of closely related viruses, each strain or member having different biological activities, including tumor-inducing capacities.

The work described has involved most of the members of the Unit of Biological Carcinogenesis, International Agency for Research on Cancer, and Mr. H. C. Kwan, M. & H. D. Institute of Radiology, Kowloon, Hong Kong, to whom the authors' grateful thanks are due.

This research was supported by Contract NIH-70–2026 within the Special Virus-Cancer Program, National Cancer Institute, National Institutes of Health, U.S.A.

REFERENCES

1. Chen, H.-C. *et al*. Anaplastic Carcinoma of the Nasopharynx. Proceedings of the 1st International Symposium of The Princess Takamatsu Cancer Research Fund, pp. 237, University of Tokyo Press, Tokyo, 1971.
2. Henle, G. Antibodies to EBV-induced Early Antigens in Infectious Mononucleosis, Burkitt's Lymphoma and Nasopharyngeal Carcinoma. Proceedings of the 1st International Symposium of The Princess Takamatsu Cancer Research Fund. pp. 343,

University of Tokyo Press, Tokyo, 1971.

3. Henle, W., Henle, G., Ho, H.-C., Burtin, P., Cachin, Y., Clifford, P., de Schryver, A., de-Thé, G., Diehl, V., and Klein, G.   Antibodies to Epstein-Barr Virus in Nasopharyngeal Carcinoma, Other Head and Neck Neoplasms, and Control Groups.   J. Nat. Cancer Inst., *44*: 225–231, 1970.

4. Ho, J. H. C.   Genetic and Environmental Factors in Nasopharyngeal Carcinoma. Proceedings of the 1st International Symposium of The Princess Takamatsu Cancer Research Fund, pp. 275, University of Tokyo Press, Tokyo, 1971.

5. Jack, I.   Personal communication.

6. Lilly, F.   The Histocompatibility-2 Locus and Susceptibility to Tumor Induction. Nat. Cancer Inst. Monograph, *22*: 631–642, 1966.

7. Nilsson, K., Pontén, J., and Philipson, L.   Development of Immunocytes and Immunoglobulin Production in Long-term Cultures from Normal and Malignant Human Lymph Nodes.   Int. J. Cancer, *3*: 183–190, 1968.

8. Nishioka, K. *et al.*   Immunological Studies on the Cell Membrane Receptors of Cultured Cells Derived from Nasopharyngeal Cancer, Burkitt's Lymphoma, and Infectious Mononucleosis.   Proceedings of the 1st International Symposium of The Princess Takamatsu Cancer Research Fund, pp. 401, University of Tokyo Press, Tokyo, 1971.

9. Old, L. J., Boyse, E. A., Oettgen, H. F., de Harven, E., Geering, G., Williamson, B., and Clifford, P.   Precipitating Antibody in Human Serum to an Antigen Present in Cultured Burkitt's Lymphoma Cells.   Proc. Nat. Acad. Sci. U.S.A., *56*: 1699–1704, 1966.

10. Paraf, A., Moyne, M. A., Duplan, J. F., Scherrer, R., Stanislawski, M., Bettane, M., Lelievre, L., Rouze, P., and Dubert, J. M.   Differentiation of Mouse Plasmocytomas *in vitro*: Two Phenotypically Stabilized Variants of the Same Cell. Proc. Nat. Acad. Sci. U.S.A., *67*: 983–990, 1970.

11. Roizman, B.   Biochemical Features of Herpesvirus-infected Cells.   Proceedings of the 1st International Symposium of The Princess Takamatsu Cancer Research Fund, pp. 103, University of Tokyo Press, Tokyo, 1971.

12. de-Schryver, A., Friberg, S., Jr., Klein, G., Henle, W., Henle, G., de-Thé, G., Clifford, P., and Ho, H.-C. Epstein-Barr Virus-associated Antibody Patterns in Carcinoma of the Post-nasal Space.   Clin. exp. Immunol., *5*: 443–459 ,1969.

13. de Schryver, A., Klein, G., and de-Thé, G.   Surface Antigens on Lymphoblastoid Cells Derived from Nasopharyngeal Carcinoma.   Clin. exp. Immunol., *7*: 161–171, 1970.

14. de-Thé, G., Ambrosioni, J. C., Ho, H.-C., and Kwan, H.-C.   Lymphoblastoid Transformation and Presence of Herpes-type Viral Particles in a Chinese Nasopharyngeal Tumor Cultured *in vitro*.   Nature, *221*: 770–771, 1969.

15. de-Thé, G.   Establishment of Long-term Lymphoblastoid Cultures from Nasopharyngeal Carcinoma (NPC).   GANN, *10*: 145–148, 1971.

16. de-Thé, G., Ho, H.-C., Kwan, H.-C., Desgranges, C., and Favre, M. C.   Nasopharyngeal Carcinoma (NPC).   I. Types of Cultures Derived from Tumor Biopsies and Non-tumorous Tissues of Chinese Patients with Special Reference to Lymphoblastoid Transformation.   Int. J. Cancer, *6*: 189–206, 1970.

Antibodies of Herpes-type Virus in Nasopharyngeal Carcinoma and Control Groups in Taiwan

Tong-Ming Lin, Czau-Siung Yang, Shen-Wu Ho, Jwo-Farn Chiou, Chiu-Hwa Wang, Shih-Mien Tu, Kung-Pei Chen, Yohei Ito, Akiyoshi Kawamura, Jr., and Takeshi Hirayama

College of Medicine, National Taiwan University, Taipei, Taiwan, Republic of China [T-M. L., C-S. Y., S-W. H., J-F. C., C-H. W., S-M. T., K-P. C.]; Aichi Cancer Center Research Institute, Nagoya, Japan [Y. I.]; Institute of Medical Science, University of Tokyo, Japan [A. K.]; Epidemiology Division, National Cancer Center Research Institute, Tokyo, Japan [T. H.]

The etiology of nasopharyngeal carcinoma (NPC) still await clarification. So far, the influence of genetic factors as well as environmental factors on the disease is far from being conclusively understood. Recently, however, it has been found that the herpes-type virus (HTV) antibody titer of NPC patients is significantly higher than that of normal healthy controls in Africa, Hong Kong, Japan, and Taiwan (*2, 4*).

The present paper reports the results of a comparative study of anti-HTV antibody titers in NPC patients as well as three control groups in Taiwan.

MATERIALS AND METHODS

Sera were collected by the heparinized capillary tube method from patients with NPC, neighborhood controls matched by age and sex, patient families, and neighborhood control families. Alltogether 117 cases of NPC, 306 neighborhood controls, 303 patient families, and 538 neighborhood control families were available for the study. Of the 117 cases of NPC (91 males and 26 famales) 106 cases (91%) were proved histologically, while 11 cases (9%) were diagnosed clinically only.

The indirect immunofluorescent antibody method established by Henle and Henle (*3*) was employed with slight modification. The target cells used for the experiment were from the P3HR-1 (*5*) cell line derived from Burkitt's lymphoma and supplied by Dr. Y. Hinuma.

RESULTS

Percentage distribution of anti-HTV antibody titers

Figure 1 shows the percentage distribution of anti-HTV antibody titers at each level for the NPC patients and the three control groups. A definite dissociation was

309

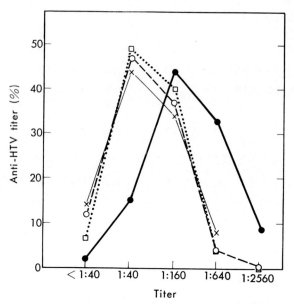

Fig. 1.   Percentage distribution of anti-HTV antibody titer (age adjusted).   ●, NPC patients ; ○, control ; □, NPC families ; ×, control families.

noted among the curves of the NPC patients and the three control groups.   No definite differences were observed among the three control groups.   From the figure it is apparent that the limiting value of anti-HTV antibody titer for sensitivity is at 1: 160 and for specificity is at 1: 640.   Accordingly, these with anti-HTV antibody titers of more than 1: 640 were considered " sero-positive."

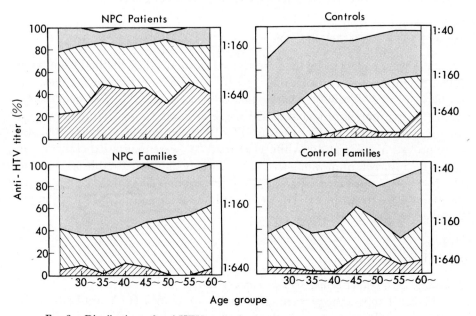

Fig. 2.   Distributions of anti-HTV antibody titer by age groups.

TABLE 1. Percentage Distribution of the Anti-HTV Antibody Titers and Their Geometric Means by Sex in NPC Patients and Three Control Groups

Group	Titer	Anti-HTV titer (%)					Geom. mean
		< 1 : 40	1 : 40	1 : 160	1 : 640	1 : 2,560	
NPC patients	M	2	12	44	34	8	1 : 253
	F	0	23	42	27	8	1 : 210
	T	1	15	44	32	8	1 : 242
Neighborhood controls	M	11	45	38	5	1	1 : 67
	F	14	51	29	6	0	1 : 58
	T	12	47	36	5	0	1 : 65
NPC patient families	M	10	49	38	2	1	1 : 64
	F	8	47	38	7	0	1 : 74
	T	9	48	38	5	0	1 : 69
Neighborhood control families	M	18	51	26	5	0	1 : 51
	F	13	41	38	8	0	1 : 70
	T	16	45	33	6	0	1 : 61

The percentage distributions of anti-HTV antibody titer by age are illustrated in Fig. 2. A slight increase of the titer with age was noted. The percentage of " sero-positive " titers was significantly higher in the NPC patients than the other groups of controls. Table 1 shows the distribution by sex. It can be seen that 40% of the NPC patients show positive reactions, while only 5%, 5%, and 6%, respectively, for the neighborhood controls, patient families, and neighborhood control families show positive reactions. Though statistically not significant, there was a difference in the " sero-positive " cases for the NPC patients by sex, namely 42% for males and 35% for females, but no sex difference was noted in the control groups or else the percentage of " sero-positive " cases was a little higher in females.

Geometric mean titers

Geometric mean titers of anti-HTV antibody are also shown in Table 1. For the NPC patients the value of the titer is 1:242, while only 1:65, 1:69, and 1:61, respectively, were recorded for the neighborhood controls, patient families, and neighborhood control families. About a 1.2 times higher value of antibody titer was noted for males than females in the NPC patients, namely 1:253 for males and 1:210 for females, but nearly no differences were observed in the three control groups by sex.

Statistical analysis of the distribution of anti-HTV antibody titer

Ridit analyses (*1*) were performed for the NPC patients and the three control groups (Fig. 3). The neighborhood controls at all ages were taken as identified distribution. The results indicated that the sera of NPC patients exhibited a higher ridit scale in each age group. No large differences were observed among the three control groups.

The summary χ^2 test of Mantel and Haenzel (*8*), and Mantel (*7*) was used for the calculation of the distribution of anti-HTV antibody titers of the NPC patients

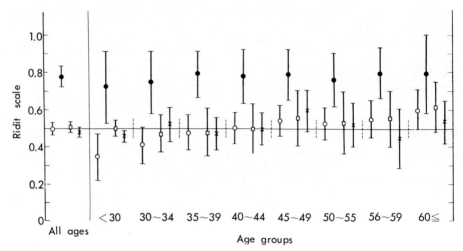

FIG. 3. Ridit analysis of anti-HTV antibodies in nasopharyngeal carcinoma and controls. ●, NPC patients; ○, controls; □, NPC families; ×, control families; |———|, 95% confidence interval.

and neighborhood controls, the NPC patients and patient families, and the NPC patients and neighborhood control families. The values were 92.0, 81.5 and 90.5 respectively ($P<0.001$).

Association of relative risk of nasopharyngeal cancer with anti-HTV antibody titer

The relative risks of NPC at various anti-HTV antibody levels are illustrated in Table 2. The data indicated that there was a close association of risk of NPC with increasing anti-HTV antibody titers, namely, those with antibody titers of 1:640 and 1:2,560 have more than 30 times and 200 times, respectively, the NPC risk of those with antibody titers of less than 1:40.

TABLE 2. Observed and Expected Number of NPC Cases and the Association of Relative Risk with Anti-HTV Antibody Level

Group Titer	Observ. NPC[a] No	Exp. N[b] controls		Exp. NPC families		Exp. N.C.[c] families	
		No.	R.R.[d]	No.	R.R.	No.	R.R.
< 1: 40	2	13.5	1.0	8.5	1.0	16.1	1.0
1: 40	17	54.7	2.1	57.3	1.3	51.7	2.6
1: 160	51	43.8	7.9	46.5	4.7	39.8	10.3
1: 640	38	4.8	53.4	4.8	34.4	9.4	32.5
1: 2,560	9	0.3	202.5	0.1	382.5	0	—

Expected values were estimated from the distribution of controls specific for age.
[a] NPC, nasopharyngeal carcinoma.
[b] N, neighborhood.
[c] NC, neighborhood control.
[d] R.R., relative risk.

Household aggregation of " sero-positive " cases

Household aggregation of "sero-positive" anti-HTV antibody titer was analyz-

TABLE 3.   Analyses of Household Aggregation of "Sero-positive" Cases

Group / No. of sero-positive cases	P.[a] families Obs.	P.[a] families Exp.	C.[b] families Obs.	C.[b] families Exp.	Total Obs.	Total Exp.
0	67	69.1	265	263.1	332	328.9
1	39	34.4	34	38.0	73	78.0
2	6	8.1	5	2.8	11	9.2
3	0	1.3	0	0.1	0	0.8
4	1 (7)	0.1 (9.5)	0 (5)	0 (2.9)	1 (12)	0 (10.0)
5	0	0	0	0	0	0
6	0	0	0	0	0	0
Total	113	113	304	304	417	416.9
Statist.	$\chi^2 = 1.33$ df $= 1$		$\chi^2 = 1.36$ df $= 1$		$\chi^2 = 0.75$ df $= 1$	
Analysis	$0.3 > P > 0.1$		$0.3 > P > 0.1$		$P > 0.3$	

[a] P, patient.
[b] C, Control.

ed by the binomial distribution method (6).   Table 3 shows the results.   The results indicated that there was no evidence to suggest any household aggregation of "sero-positive" anti-HTV antibody.

DISCUSSION

The present data confirmed earlier reports on the unusually high frequency of high anti-HTV antibody titer among patients with NPC.   In this survey the economic status of the NPC patients and control groups was partially matched, as our neighborhood controls were obtained from neighbors living near the patients and matched by age and sex.   Percentage distribution of "sero-positive" cases, geometric means, ridit analyses, summary χ^2 tests, and relative risks of different antibody titer level to NPC, all indicate that there is a strong association of "sero-positive" anti-HTV antibody titer with NPC.   Though these results can not exclude the possibility of a passenger role of HTV in NPC, they may suggest a causal relationship between HTV and NPC.   A possibly genetically determined predisposition to develop NPC among Chinese may be associated with factors which permit HTV to have either a direct function in the transformation of target cells or a priming role for the subsequent action of carcinogenic or co-carcinogenic agents.

Although there are significant differences in the anti-HTV antibody titers among the NPC patients and the three control groups, it is worth pointing out that in spite of differences in the age, there is little difference in the distribution of antibody titers and geometric mean titers among the three control groups.   Moreover, there were no definite differences in the distribution of antibody titers and geometric mean titers by sex among the three control groups.   This means there was no significant difference in the infection rate to HTV virus between the sexes.   However, our results indicated that, though statistically not significant, there was a male excess of "sero-positive" cases and geometric means in the NPC patients, the percentage of " sero-positive " cases was 42% for males and 35% for females, and the geometric mean titer was 1:253 for males and 1:210 for females.   Whether these results have special meanings or are due to other variables, such as the small number of the female patients or the stage of the disease, must await further study.   At all events, this point should be clarified before a hypothesis of HTV etiology to NPC can be established.   Furthermore, there were no indications of household aggregation of " sero-positive " cases in either the patient families or the neighborhood control families. This means that the infection of HTV may be a sporadic one in nature.

At any rate, the use of cell lines derived from NPC instead of those lines derived from Burkitt's lymphoma, and a prospective study of the natural history of HTV infection and the patterns of HTV related serological reactions in a population of high risk, such as that in Taiwan, may help us to clarify the relationship between the virus and NPC.

SUMMARY

Sera collected from patients of nasopharyngeal carcinoma (NPC) in the northern and southern parts of Taiwan were titrated for antibodies to the herpes type virus (HTV) in a Burkitt's lymphoma cell line (P3HR-1) by the indirect immunofluorescent antibody technique.   The results were compared with those of neighborhood controls matched by age and sex, patient families and neighborhood control families.   Dissociations in the frequency distribution of NPC and healthy control groups were found to become maximum when the limiting value was set at 1:640 There were no significant differences in the frequency distribution among the three control groups.   Of 117 NPC patients, 40% had " sero-positive " titers ($\geqq$ 1:640), while the same appeared only in 5%, 5%, and 6% for neighborhood controls, patient families, and control families, respectively.   Though statistically not significant, there was a difference in the percentages of " sero-positive " cases for the NPC patients by sex, namely 42% for males and 35% for females, but either no sex difference was noted in the three control groups or else the percentage was slightly higher in females.   The geometric mean titers were 1:242, 1:69, 1:65, and 1:61, respectively, for the NPC patients, neighborhood controls, patient families, and neighborhood control families.   There were differences in the geometric means by sex in the patients, namely 1:253 and 1:210, respectively, for males and females, while no differences by sex were noted in the three control groups.   Ridit analysis and the summary χ^2 test showed definite differences between the NPC patients and the three control groups.   The relative risks indicated that persons with antibody titers of 1:2,560 had more than 200 times the NPC risk of those with antibody titers of less than 1:40.   There were no indications of household aggregation of high anti-HTV titers ($\geqq$ 1:640) in the patients and control families.   The significance and implications of these findings are discussed.

This study was partly supported by grants from the Ministry of Health and Welfare and the Society for the Promotion of Cancer Research, Japan, and partly by the National Science Council, Republic of China.   We are grateful to the doctors and staffs of the pathological units, hospitals, and clinics in the study area for permission to interview their patients.   The technical assistance of Mrs. S. Y., Chen, C. Z. Sung, T. S. Tsai, and Miss M. N. Cheng was greatly appreciated.

REFERENCES

1. Bross, I. D. J.   How to Use Ridit Analysis.   Biometrics, *14* : 18–38, 1958.
2. Kawamura, A., Jr., Takada, M., Gotoh, A., Hamajima, K., Sanpe, T., Murata, M., Ito, Y., Takahashi, T., Yoshida, T., Hirayama, T., Tu. S.-M., Liu, C.-H., Yang C.-S., and Wang, C.-H.   Seroepidemiological Studies on Nasopharyngeal Carcinoma by Fluorescent Antibody Techniques with Cultured Burkitt Lymphoma Cell.   GANN, *61* : 55–71, 1970.
3. Henle, G., Henle, W., and Diehl, V.   Relation of Burkitt's Tumor-associated Herpes-type Virus to Infectious Mononucleosis.   Proc. Nat. Acad. Sci., U.S., *59* : 94–101, 1968.
4. Henle, W., Henle, G., Ho, H.-C., Burtin, P., Cachin, Y., Clifford, P., De Schryver, A., De-Thé, G., Diehl, V., and Klein, G.   Antibodies to Epstein-Barr Virus in Nasopharyngeal Carcinoma, Other Head and Neck Neoplasms, and Control Groups.   J. Nat. Cancer Inst., *44* : (*1*) : 225–231 1970.
5. Hinuma, Y., and Grace, J. T., Jr.   Cloning of Immunoglobulin-producing Human Leukemic and Lymphoma Cells in Long-term Culture. Proc.   Soc. Expl. Biol. Med., *124* : 107–111, 1967.
6. Hirayama, T.   Ekigaku ni okeru Tokey teki Hoho, *In* Ekigaku to Sono O-you, *2* : 96–100 ; Tokyo, Nanzando, 1963 (in Japanese).
7. Mantel, N.   Chi-square Test with One Degree of Freedom ; Extension of the Mantel-Haenzel Procedure.   J. Amer. Stat. Assoc., *58* : 690–700, 1963.
8. Mantel, N., and Haenzel, W.   Statistical Aspects of the Analysis of Data from Retrospective Studies of Disease.   J. Nat. Cancer Inst., *22* : 719–748, 1958.

The Natural History of HTV Infection
and Its Clinical, Immunological, and Oncological Manifestations

Takeshi HIRAYAMA, Kusuya NISHIOKA, Akiyoshi KAWAMURA, and Tong-Ming LIN

Epidemiology Division, National Cancer Center Research Institute, Japan [T. H.], Virology Division, National Cancer Center Research Institute, Japan [K. N.], Department of Immunology, Institute of Medical Science, University of Tokyo, Japan [A. K.], Department of Public Health, College of Medicine, National Taiwan University, Taiwan [T.-M. L.]

This paper was written in order to clarify our present position in the flow of herpes-type virus (HTV) tumor research programs and to emphasize the necessity of conducting a seroepidemiological population prospective study on the natural history of HTV-infection and the immunological response flow reflected in its clinical manifestations, such as infectious mononucleosis and Izumi fever, and in its oncological manifestations, such as Burkitt's lymphoma, childhood leukemia, and nasopharyngeal cancer.

Anti-HTV Titers in Selected Neoplasms

The recognition of the close association of HTV-infection and selected neoplasms such as Burkitt's lymphoma (BL), childhood leukemia, and nasopharyngeal cancer (NPC) has really opened a new page in the history of the epidemiological study of these neoplasms (4, 6, 7, 11–14, 16–18, 20–22). With regard to BL, the association with a high anti-HTV antibody titer has clearly been shown by the data of Henle and his co-workers (4, 14). With regard to childhood leukemia, a significantly higher anti-HTV titer was observed by fluorescent antibody techniques for the study group as compared to normal controls in Japan (8, 10). Out of 6 confirmed cases of acute childhood leukemia and 504 cases of normal controls tested, all under age 15, an anti-HTV of 1: 640 was found in 3 and 10, 1: 160 in 1 and 107, 1: 40 in 2 and 223 and 1: 40 in 0 and 158. The chi-square value for linear regression was calculated as 13,828 with 1 degree of freedom. As this is significant at less than the 0.001 level, such a striking deviation in the anti-HTV titer in the leukemia group is extremely unlikely to be the product of random occurrence.

In the case of NPC, as shown by Shanmugaratam and Higginson, none of the environmental and host factors studied were noted to be significantly related to NPC (19). The higher incidence rate among Chinese, especially those of southern origin,

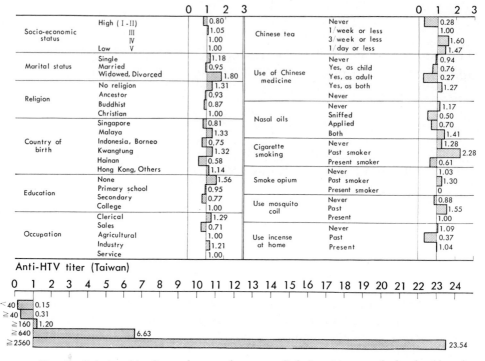

FIG. 1. Relative risk of nasopharyngeal cancer. Relative risk was calculated taking the mean morbidity rate as the unit risk. Materials: Singapore study. upper figures, calculated on (19); lower figures, calculated from Table 1.

was the only known epidemiological characteristic of the disease. Under such circumstances, it has been confirmed during the past few years that NPC patients carry unusually high titers of anti-HTV antibody (6, 12, 13, 18, 20, 21) and the relative risk of NPC varied far more strikingly by anti-HTV titers than by any factors so far studied (Fig. 1).

Serological case control studies conducted recently in various areas and for various ethnic groups on sera from patients of NPC and hospital and field controls by us and by other researchers consistently showed a higher anti-HTV titer in the former as shown in Tables 1, and 2, Figs. 2, 3, 4, and 5. Table 1, Fig. 2, and Fig. 3 indicate the frequency distribution of the NPC patient group and control group according to their anti-HTV antibody titers. The geometric mean, mean ridit and its 95% confidence interval are also shown. It is very clear from these that the average anti-HTV titer of NPC patients is significantly higher than that for controls in any ethnic group and in any geographical area where the study was performed. Table 2 shows the result of the Chi-square test for linear regression. From this table one can safely state that the frequency of NPC goes up with the increase in anti-HTV antibody titers. Figure 4 shows anti-HTV titers of NPC patients and controls by sex and Fig. 5 illustrates these by age groups. Consistency of association is apparent in both figures.

TABLE 1. Anti-HTV Titers of NPC Patients and Controls

Country			Titers						Geom mean	Mean ridit	95% Confidence interval
			$<1:40$	$1:40$	$1:160$	$1:640$	$1:2,560$	Total			
Japan		C	34	119	92	13	1	259	1: 63	0.500	0.536–0.464
		S	0	1	3	5	6	15	1: 701	0.901	1.000–0.752
Taiwan	(1) {	C	15	112	147	54	5	333	1: 115	0.500	0.532–0.468
		S	0	8	50	75	40	173	1: 519	0.805	0.849–0.761
	(2) {	C	36	143	111	15	1	306	1: 64	0.500	0.533–0.467
		S	2	17	51	38	9	117	1: 241	0.779	0.832–0.725
Hong Kong[a]		C	63	64	12	2	0	141	1: 24	0.500	0.549–0.451
		S	3	22	64	71	5	165	1: 249	0.917	0.962–0.872
Singapore[b]		C	7	18	7	4	1	37	1: 59	0.500	0.595–0.405
		S	0	5	11	12	5	33	1: 326	0.806	0.906–0.705
East Africa[a]		C	63	91	19	1	0	174	1: 28	0.500	0.544–0.456
		S	2	8	23	36	1	70	1: 267	0.912	0.981–0.843
France[b]		S	207	87	40	1	0	335	1: 19	0.500	0.532–0.468
		S	1	2	2	1	0	6	1: 79	0.780	1.000–0.544

Taiwan (1): hospital study; Taiwan (2): systematic field study; S: study group (Nasopharyngeal cancer); C: control;   [a] Henle et at. (6).   [b] Sohier et al. shown in (1).

TABLE 2. Anti-HTV Titers of NPC Patients and Controls

	Source of variation	
	Due to linear regression	Departure from regression line
Degree of freedom	1	4
Japan	$\chi^2 = 54.59$	$\chi^2 = 57.76$
	$p < 0.01$	$p < 0.01$
Taiwan (1) {	$\chi^2 = 141.13$	$\chi^2 = 6.59$
	$p < 0.01$	$p > 0.05$
(2) {	$\chi^2 = 93.66$	$\chi^2 = 11.04$
	$p < 0.01$	$p > 0.01$
Hong Kong	$\chi^2 = 166.06$	$\chi^2 = 14.02$
	$p < 0.01$	$p \doteqdot 0.01$
Singapore	$\chi^2 = 20.16$	$\chi^2 = 1.58$
	$p < 0.01$	$p > 0.05$
East Africa	$\chi^2 = 125.68$	$\chi^2 = 17.70$
	$p < 0.01$	$p < 0.01$
France	$\chi^2 = 10.94$	$\chi^2 = 20.28$
	$p < 0.01$	$p < 0.01$

Taiwan (1), hospital study;   Taiwan (2), systematic field study.

In summary, so far as the association is concerned, we can say that conclusive evidence is already available for BL and NPC, and also for selected types of childhood leukemia.   Whether such association does or does not indicate a causative relationship is a matter for further study.   There is no question that a serological follow-up study of a high risk group is essential to answer the question.   To prepare

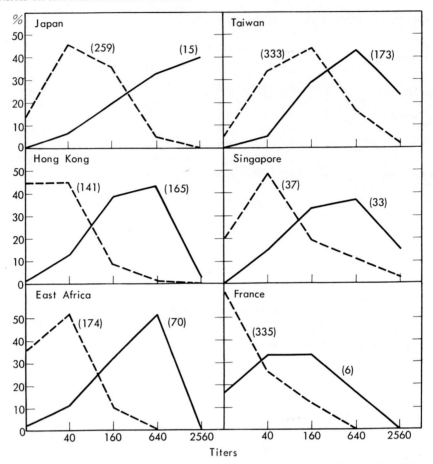

FIG. 2. Percentage distribution according to anti-HTV titers in patients with NPC and controls. ······, controls; ———, NPC. Number in parentheses shows total cases.

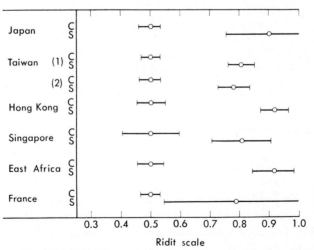

FIG. 3. Anti-HTV titers of NPC patients and controls. Taiwan (1), hospital study; Taiwan (2), systematic field study. S, study group (nasopharyngeal cancer); C, control.

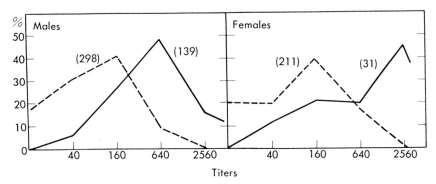

FIG. 4. Percentage distribution according to anti-HTV titers in patients with NPC and controls in Taiwan. ······, controls ; ———, NPC. Number of parentheses shows total cases.

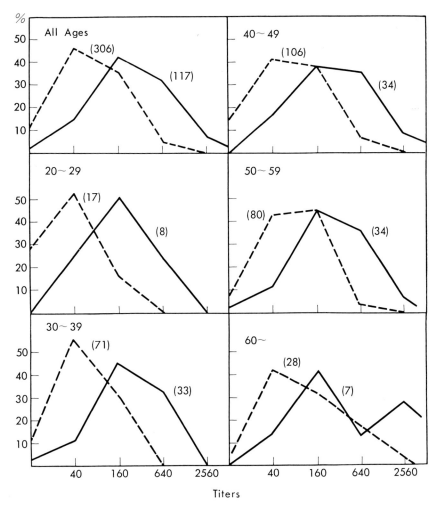

FIG. 5. Percentage distribution according to anti-HTV titers in patients with NPC and controls in Taiwan. ······, controls ; ———, NPC. Number of parentheses shows total cases.

a blue print for future population prospective studies, speculation as to the ultimate results expected to be obtained from such a long range project was felt to be necessary at the present moment.

The Natural History of HTV-Infection with Special Reference to an Izumi Fever Outbreak

Supposing the project is started by bleeding a large population what kind of epidemiological patterns might we get as to the spread of HTV-infection? What sort of clinical manifestations will occur immediately following infection? That the virus is causatively related to Infectious Mononucleosis has already been shown by laboratory studies and epidemiological survey (2, 3, 5, 15). A partial answer to these questions was also obtained by analyzing the recent Izumi fever outbreak in early 1970 on an island near Nagoya.

Izumi fever is a scarlatina-like disease first described by Izumi and his colleagues in 1929 (23). Atypical lymphocytes usually increase in the peripheral blood. It occurs endemically or in the form of an outbreak mostly in rural populations in Japan. Evidence that it is water-borne was obtained frequently by epidemiological studies.

In January 1970, an outbreak of febrile disease occurred on Toshi Island, which is situated in the middle part of Japan, surrounded by Ise Bay and the Pacific Ocean. The first survey was carried out by us in January and revealed that the clinical features of the disease were typical of Izumi fever. Out of 20 cases of Izumi fever, 1 case was under age 5, 12 cases were 5–9 years, and 7 cases were 10–14 years; there were none in older age groups. The number of patients by date of onset was

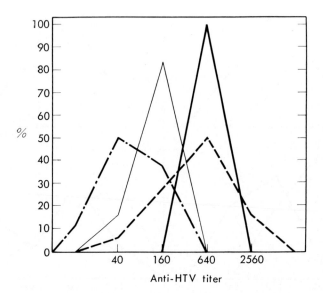

FIG. 6. Distribution of anti-HTV titers for Izumi fever patients and controls on Toshi Island, Mie Prefecture, Japan. Paired sera for Izumi fever patient (1970). –·–·–, non-patient school children ; ———, acute ; ▬▬▬, convalescent ; ······, total Izumi fever patients convalenscent sera.

as follows: January 14–15, 3 cases; January 16–17, 6 cases; January 18–19, 4 cases; January 20–21, 2 cases; January 22–23, 2 cases; and after February 2, 3 cases; the total was 20 cases.

The causative role of HTV-infection was clearly shown by the sharp titer rise in paired sera taken at acute and convalescent stages as shown in Fig. 6. Sera taken on January 22 from 6 cases of Izumi fever and stored by freezing were compared with paired sera taken on May 17 from the same patients. The early sera

TABLE 3. Anti-HTV Titer by Age Groups in Toshi Island, Mie Prefecture, Japan (1970)

Age Groups	Number of persons	< 1 : 40	1 : 40	1 : 160	1 : 640	1 : 2,560	?
Male							
0– 4	15	6	3	2			4
5– 9	101	32	48	17	4		
10–14	116	40	43	33			
15–19	15	5	4	5	1		
20–24	16	7	1	7	1		
25–29	14	8	5		1		
30–34	24	11	5	8			
35–39	23	10	4	7	1		1
40–44	44	19	14	8	3		
45–49	24	9	7	5	2	1	
50–54	11	5	2	3		1	
55–59	11	4	4	3			
60–64	10	4	3	3			
65–69	14	5	4	3	2		
70–74	7	2	5				
75–79	7	4	1	1			1
80–84	3	1	1		1		
85–							
Total	455	172	154	105	16	2	6
Female							
0– 4	15	10	4				1
5– 9	83	29	36	17			1
10–14	95	21	49	24	1		
15–19	10	2	5	2	1		
20–24	15	6	4	4		1	
25–29	21	11	5	5			
30–34	18	10	5	2			1
35–39	27	8	10	6	2	1	
40–44	43	26	6	7	3		1
45–49	20	9	7	4			
50–54	33	20	6	4	3		
55–59	30	13	2	9	6		
60–64	21	11	8	1	1		
65–69	29	14	7	6	2		
70–74	15	8	2	4	1		
75–79	6	4	1	1			
80–84	3	1		1	1		
85–89	2				2		
Total	486	203	157	97	23	2	4

were actually of about 2 weeks after the infection; the next serum samples were taken 4 months later.   Cases showing an anti-HTV titer of 1: 40, 1: 160 and 1: 640 were 1, 5, 0 in the former and 0, 0, 6 in the latter.   As shown in Fig. 6, the antibody titer was noted to have increased significantly ($p=0.001$ by Fisher's direct propability method).   In total, the sera of 18 patients of Izumi fever taken at the convalescent stage, and the sera of 419 non-patient children under age 15 in the same island were compared.   Cases showing an anti-HTV titer of $<1: 40$, 1: 40, 1: 160, and 1: 640 were 0, 1, 5, 9, and 3 for Izumi fever patients and 136, 192, 86, 5, and 0 for the controls.   The chi-square value for linear regression was calculated as 85,327 with 1 degree of freedom which is significant at less than the 0.001 level.

A community-wide seroepidemiological study was conducted for 449 male and 482 female inhabitants on this island in June 1970 (Table 3).   Cases showing an anti-HTV titer of less than 1: 40, 1: 40, 1: 160, 1: 640, and 1: 2,560 were 172, 154, 105, 16, and 2 in males and 203, 157, 97, 23, and 2 in females.   While there was no significant difference in the rate of infection between males and females the result clearly showed that the epidemic attacked age groups under 24 more frequently than older age groups.   319 out of 475 (67.2%) showed anti-HTV titer 1: 40 or higher in age groups under 24 while it was only 237 out of 456 (52.0%) in older age groups. $\chi^2=41.7$ $p<0.001$ (Fig. 7).   The result also strongly suggested the existence of subclinical infection in the case of an Izumi fever outbreak.   Neither the disease nor the infection showed familial aggregation, indicating that the epidemic was spread by a common vehicle (Fig. 8).   On the other hand, district aggregation was noted to exist to a certain extent.   The time of exposure was estimated as January 10, 1970, by analyzing the epidemic curve (Figs. 9, and 10) under the

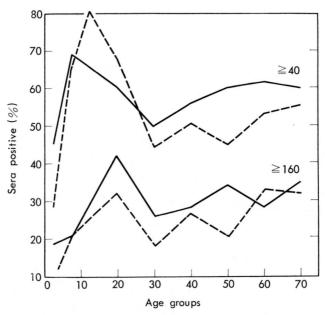

Fig. 7.   Anti-HTV titer by age groups on Toshi Island, Mie Prefecture, Japan (1970).
——, male ; ⋯⋯, female.

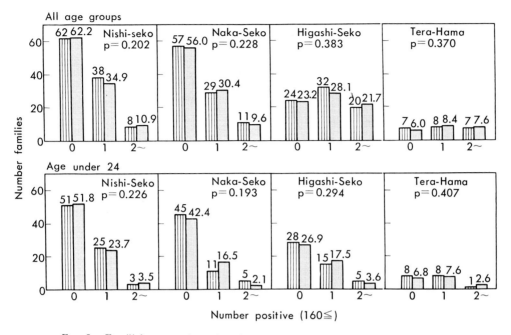

FIG. 8. Familial aggregation of anti-HTV antibody positive reactors, Toshi Island, Mie Prefecture, Japan (1970). Expected value was calculated from binomial distribution. ▥, actual; ▱, expected.

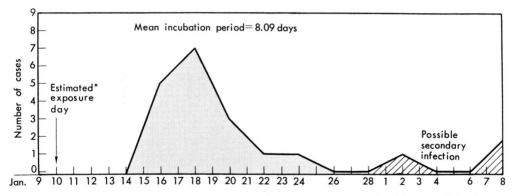

FIG. 9. Number of new cases of Izumi fever by date of onset Toshi Island, Mie Prefecture, Japan (1970). Other evidence of Jan. 10 exposure. (1) One confirmed case visited this island only Jan. 10 and 11. (2) One confirmed case came back to the island on Jan. 7. * Assuming the distribution of incubation period fits to log-normal distribution.

hypothesis that the distribution of the incubation period fits to log-normal distribution. This estimation is compatible with the fact that a typical Izumi fever case visited this island only on January 10, and 11. There was also another typical case which returned to this island on January 7. Most of the previous Izumi fever outbreaks were found to have been caused by drinking contaminated water. Apparently this was also the case in this episode. All the Izumi fever patients drank water from the same water supply of this island which was quite unsanitary. Due

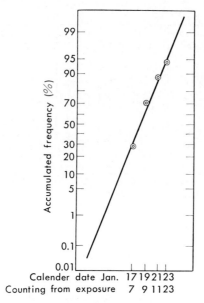

FIG. 10. Accumulated frequency distribution of Izumi Fever, Toshi Island, Mie Prefecture showing linear arrangement on probability paper (1970). Number of days from estimated exposure is taken in log scale.

to the water shortage, the daytime water supply was almost cut off entirely around January 10. To make matters worse, the untreated water running along the rice paddies was added to the water supply. In addition to this, the characteristic epidemic curve, geographical distribution, and the lack of familial aggregation all point to the possibility that the disease is water-borne. In short, as a lesson from this epidemic, the possibility of spread by water should be seriously considered as the mode of infection of HTV along with extrafamilial close contact. About the latter mode of infection it may not be necessary to mention Dr. Henle's beautiful study of the seroepidemiology of infectious mononucleosis in Yale University students (3, 15).

Low Herd Immunity as an Important Component of the Epidemic Constitution

Coming back to the anti-HTV titer curve by age groups on Toshi Island shown in Fig. 7, if one extrapolates the curve for adults back wards to younger age groups, one can get an estimated curve for children before the onset of the Izumi fever outbreak. From this estimate one can understand the reason why such an epidemic took place on this island. The density of susceptibles prior to the outbreak must have been quite high as about 60–70% of the children had probably been without anti-HTV antibody. Such a high density of susceptibles plus the sudden exposure to environmental pollution must have been the reason for the outbreak of Izumi fever on this island.

In relation to this experience, the authors wish to point out the importance of the study of herd immunity with regard to the HTV antibody level as one of the possible factors in the clustering of related malignancies such as Burkitt's lymphoma, and nasopharyngeal carcinoma.   In a recent clustering episode of childhood leukemia in Yugawara in 1968–69 (*8, 9, 10*), in which 5 cases of leukemia occurred out of 970 children of 2–6 years of age during a period of two years, the anti-HTV antibody level was noted to be far higher among leukemia cases as compared to controls. Only 4 out of 31 healthy children tested (12.9%) showed titers higher than 1:160 compared to 75% of the leukemia cases (2 out of 3 tested).   Those found negative were 14 out of 31 or 45.2% compared to 0% in leukemia cases.   Thus healthy children in the district showed extraordinarily low titers when tested in October of 1968, but a considerable rise in the titers was noted in August of 1969.   Thus the high density of susceptibles at the time of the outbreak should be counted as an important factor in this leukemia clustering together with a high dose exposure to HTV.   Similar considerations might be fruitful for a study of the reasons for time-space clustering of Burkitt's lymphoma and also for higher incidence of NPC in low titer families.

Cancer Risk by anti-HTV Titers and by Various Risk Factors—A Blue Print for Future Population Prospective Studies

Next, let us speculate as to the magnitude of the risk of developing neoplasms after infection for each population subgroups classified by anti-HTV titer, taking nasopharyngeal cancer as the example.   As a method for such speculation, first the relative risk was calculated, according to the selected risk factors based on the available results of serological case control studies in many countries, taking the

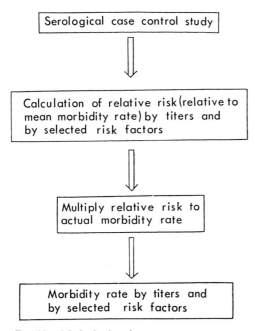

Fɪɢ. 11.   Method of study.

mean morbidity rate as the unit risk.   As the second step, the relative risk was
applied to the actual morbidity rate obtained by a special survey or cancer registry
(Fig. 11).

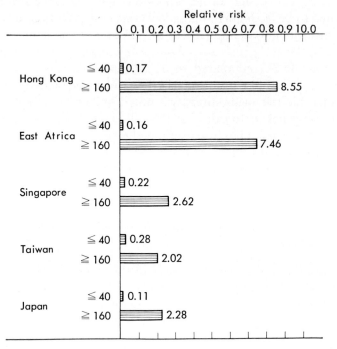

Fig. 12.   Relative risk of nasopharyngeal cancer by anti-HTV antibody titer.   Relative risk
was calculated taking the average incidence rate in each area as the unit risk.

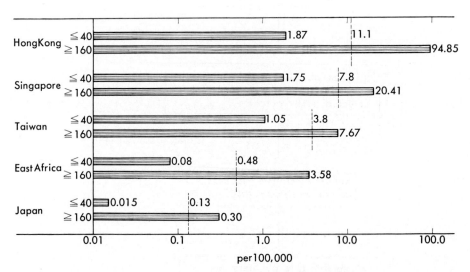

Fig. 13.   Absolute risk of nasopharyngeal cancer by anti-HTV titer.   Absolute risk was obtained by applying the relative risk for each group to the actual mean morbidity rate in each
area.

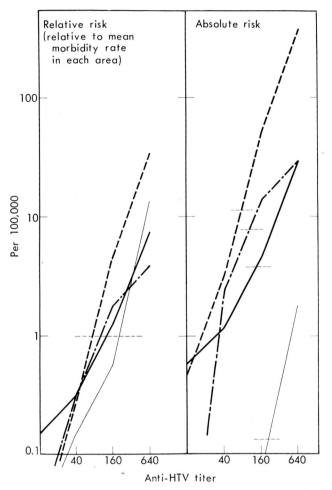

FIG. 14.   Risk for nasopharyngeal cancer by anti-HTV antibody titer.   ----, Hong Kong ;
——, Japan ;   ——, Taiwan ;   –·–·–, Singapore ;   ······ mean morbidity rate.

A higher risk in Chinese in Hong Kong as compared to Chinese in Taiwan and Singapore (Figs. 12, 13, and 14, and Table 4) was observed even in the same category of anti-HTV titer groups.   A higher risk for males compared to females was observed mainly in the high titer group (Fig. 15).   These results indicate the need for searching out the co-factors closely related to race and sex in addition to the factor of HTV infection.   The absolute risk for positive reactors was noted to increase in older age groups more than in younger age groups (Fig. 16).   Since there is a tendency for the titer to be lower in younger NPC patients compared to older NPC patients (Table 5), the backward extrapolation of the curve of the age specific negative rate obtained in a recent field seroepidemiological study in Taiwan was attempted (Fig. 17a, b).

The result showed that most of the NPC patients had probably already reached to high anti-HTV titers by the end of the teen age period.   The oncogenic process appeared to start its operation from this age period.   Whether or not such specula-

TABLE 4.   Risk for Nasopharyngeal Cancer by Anti-HTV Antibody Titer

		Relative[a] risk	Absolute risk	Mean morbidity rate per 100,000
Japan	< 40	0.00	0.00	0.13
	40	0.15	0.02	
	160	0.56	0.07	
	640–	13.57	1.76	
Taiwan	< 40	0.15	0.55	3.8
	40	0.31	1.18	
	160	1.20	4.56	
	640–	7.68	29.19	
Hong Kong	< 40	0.04	0.45	11.10
	40	0.29	3.26	
	160	4.56	50.39	
	640–	32.47	360.45	
Singapore	< 40	0.00	0.00	7.80
	40	0.31	2.43	
	160	1.76	13.74	
	640–	3.81	29.73	
East Africa	< 40	0.08	0.04	0.48
	40	0.22	0.10	
	160	3.01	1.44	
	640–	91.97	44.15	

[a] Relative to mean morbidity rate, obtained by serological case-control study.

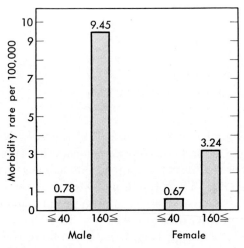

FIG. 15.   Nsopharyngeal cancer morbidity rate by anti-HTV antibody titer in Taiwan.

tion is correct, *e.g.*, the tumor formation is really a late effect of HTV-infection during late childhood or adolescence, and the risk of NPC is really higher for the risk group mentioned above should all be confirmed by a population prospective study in the nearest possible future.   Hopefully the expected pattern described here could serve as a guideline in planning such a large-scale population study.

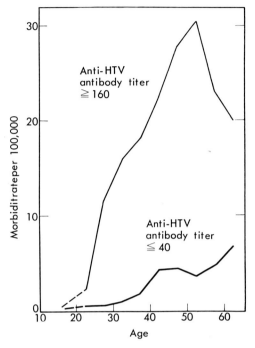

Fig. 16. Nasopharyngeal cancer morbidity rate by age groups. Sources of calculation: (1) Morbidity survey in Taiwan (1966–68). (2) Relative risk by anti-HTV antibody titers for each age group are based on seroepidemiological survey results.

TABLE 5. anti-HTV-antibody Titers of NPC Patients and Controls In a Blind Study in Taiwan

	Anti-HTV Titer	Age Group			Total	
		-34	35–59	60–		
NPC Patients	1 : 2,560	0	7	2	9	$\chi^2 = 21.16$
(Index cases)	1 : 640	5	32	1	38	$n = 6$
	160	12	36	3	51	$p \doteqdot 0.001$
	≦ 1 : 40	4	14	1	19	
Total		21	89	7	117	
%	1 : 2,560	0	7.87	28.57	χ^2 due to linear regression	
					5.60	$p < 0.05$
Controls	2,560	0	0	1	1	$\chi^2 = 32.11$
	640	0	10	5	15	$n = 6$
	160	12	90	9	111	$p < 0.001$
	≦ 40	44	122	13	179	
Total		56	222	28	306	
%	640 & up	0	4.50	21.43	χ^2 due to linear regression	
					13.80	$p < 0.001$

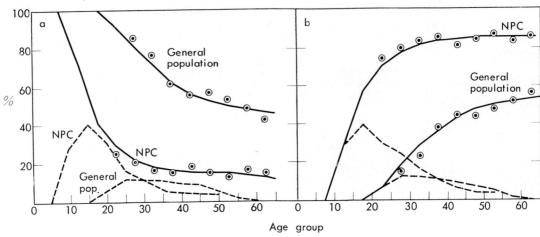

FIG. 17. a: Anti-HTV antibody percent negative (1 : 40 or lower). b: Extrapolation of anti-HTV antibody positive rate (1 : 160 and higher) in nasopharyngeal cancer group and control group. - - -, positive conversion rate.

HTV-tumor Research Programs—Where Do We Stand Now?

Finally we should like to ask ourselves that where do we stand now in HTV research programmes. Table 6 is the recommended HTV-tumor study project; the present position in this research flow is indicated in the table. So for (1), the association between HTV and the selected tumors in question has been well demon-

TABLE 6.   HTV-tumor Study Project

	Phase I Association study	Phase II Causation study	Phase III Control study
Laboratory study	① demonstration of association (T.C ; E.M ; IM) ② identification of virus	① titration of virus ② study of oncogenic properties of virus ③ detection of antigens in infected cell	❶ selection of safe and potent mutants ❷ separation of antigens for sub-viral vaccine ❸ experimental model study
Field study	③ seroepid. study for hospital population ④ descriptive epidemiology ⑤ analytic epidemiology	④ field seroepid. study for natural history of virus infection (including mode of spread) ⑤ field seroepid. study for relative risk by titers and by selected risk factors ❻ study of clinical, immunological, and oncological response flow after infection ❼ study of co-factors (high risk group)	❹ Population prospective study a) to evaluate immunization programme b) to confirm causation

○ : result already available ;   ● : remained to be studied.

strated by tissue culture study, electron microscopic study, and immunological studies; (2) HTV particles of typical morphology have been identified in cultured material derived from biopsy (*20, 21*); (3) a seroepidemiological study of a hospital population has already been completed; and (4) descriptive and (5) analytic epidemiology of these neoplasms have also been well explored and documented. Therefore, we are definitely not in Phase I (Association Study Phase) and must be in Phase II which is the Causation Study Phase. In Phase II (1) titration of virus has already become possible and (2) much progress has been made in the study of the oncogenic potential of virus, including a DNA-DNA hybridization experiment (*24*). (3) Detection of various key antigens in infected cells, including one apparently not associated with the virus, has become possible. (4) A field sero-epidemiological study of the natural history of virus infection, including the mode of spread, has already been in progress as was partly introduced in this paper. (5) A field sero-epidemiological study for relative risk by titers and by selected risk factors has also been carried out as described in this paper. (6) A Study of the clinical, immunological, and oncological response flow after infection and (7) a study of co-factors and high risk groups have definitely not been finished and will be subjects for immediate future study. The time to move in to Phase III, which is the Control Study, is around the corner. In Phase III, aims must be focused on the exploration of the launching of vaccination programs by (1) selection of safe and potent mutants and by (2) separation of antigens for sub-viral vaccine. In connection with this, (3) experimental model studies have already been done as is shown in Table 7. In Table 7 experimental models for protection against Marek disease are summarized. Marek disease was shown to be completely protected against by the use of selected vaccines. Such models should also be cultivated for other animal tumors and be fully utilized in the planning of human tumor control pro-

TABLE 7. Experimental Model for Protection against HTV Oncogenesis

Author	Disease	Vaccine	Result	Tested	Marek after challenge[a]	Antibody response	Virus isol
(1) Churchill et al. (1969)	Marek	MDHV attenuated by continuous passage	vaccinated	74	7	V-virus+ C-virus+	+ +
			unvaccinated	110	77	C-virus+	+
(2) Kottaridis et al. (1969)	Marek	MDHV in chick embryo fibroblast	vaccinated	223	39	—	—
			unvaccinated	211	107		
(3) Okazaki et al. (1970)	Marek	Turkey herpes V	vaccinated	31	0	V-virus+ C-virus−	+
			unvaccinated	36	24	C-virus+	+

(1) Nature, *221*, 744–747, 1969. (2) Nature, *221*, 1258–59, 1969. (3) Avian Disease, *14*(2): 413–429, 1970.
V-virus, Vaccine virus; C-virus, Challenge virus.
[a] Challenged either by inoculation or by contact.

grams. Finally, it is the view of the authors that (4) a population prospective study should carefully be planned and implemented (a) to evaluate immunization programs and at the same time (b) to confirm causation.

In short we are definitely at the later stage of Phase II or at the beginning of Phase III as shown in Table 6. What is urgently needed now is the development of tools applicable for field epidemiological study: reliable and pracical markers of both productive and non-productive infection of HTV, markers for the operation of co-factors, and specific markers indicating cell transformation toward malignancy. Without such key markers or tools of immunology it appears un likely that an efficient, profitable sero-epidemiological population prospective study could be planned and implemented.

The result of such an epidemiological study aimed at the confirmation of the the viral oncogenesis of NPC as well as the evaluation of selected immunization programs is expected to furnish us with a solid basis for moving into the next potential project, which is the eradication program for these malignancies.

REFERENCES

1. Annual Report, International Agency for Research on Cancer. World Health Organization, pp. 39–40, 1969.
2. Diehl, V., Henle, G., Henle, W., and Kohn, G. Demonstration of a Herpes Group Virus in Cultures of Peripheral Leukocytes from Patients with Infectious Mononucleosis. J. Virol., *2*: 663–669, 1968.
3. Evans, A. S., Niederman, J. C., and McCollum, R. W. Sero-epidemiologic Studies of Infectious Mononucleosis with EB Virus. New Eng. J. Med., *279*: 1121–1127, 1968.
4. Henle, G., Henle, W., Clifford, P., Diehl, V., Kafuko, G. W., Kirya, G., Klein, G., Morrow, R. H., Munube, G. M. R., Pike, P., Tukei, P. M., and Ziegler, J. L. Antibodies to Epstein-Barr Virus in Burkitt's Lymphoma and Control Group. J. Nat. Cancer Inst., *43* (5): 1147–1157, 1969.
5. Henle, G., Henle, W., and Diel, V. Relation of Burkitt's Tumour-associated Herpestype Virus to Infectious Mononucleosis. Proc. Nat. Acad. Sci., *59*: 94–101, 1968.
6. Henle, W., Henle, G., Ho, N.-C., Burtin, P., Cachin, Y., Clifford, P., de Schryver, A., de-Thé, G., Diel, V., and Klein, G. Antibodies to Epstein-Barr Virus in Nasopharyngeal Carcinoma, Other Head and Neck Neoplasms. J. Nat. Cancer Inst., *44* (1): 225–231, 1970.
7. Hinuma, Y. Biology of Herpes-type Virus Associated with Burkitt Lymphoma Cell Lines. GANN Monograph, *7*: 65–76, 1969.
8. Hirayama, T. An Epidemiological Study of Leukemia in Japan, with Special Reference to the Problem of Time-space Clustering. GANN Monograph, *7*: 1–19, 1969.
9. Hirayama, T. Epidemiological Study of Leukemia in Japan with Special Reference to the Problem of Time-space Clustering. Acta Haemat., *31* (5): 737–747, 1968 (In Japanese).
10. Hirayama, T., Hitosugi, M., Kadohira, Y., Moriya, Y., Kawamura, M., Sanpe, T. Hanawa, Y., Ise, Y., Kasuga, S., Narita, I., and Ishida, M. A Clustering Episode of Childhood Acute Leukemia in Yugawara, Kanagawa Prefecture, Japan. Igaku

no Ayumi, *70* (7) : 303–305, 1969 (in Japanese).

11. Ito, Y., Kurita, I., and Osato, T. Herpes-type Virus Particles and Chromosome Markers in Two Human Cell Lines Derived from Embryonic Cultures Exposed to Human Leukemic Culture Fluid *in vitro*. GANN, *60* (3) : 247–251, 1969.

12. Ito, Y., Takahashi, T., Tu, S.-M., and Kawamura, A., Jr. High Anti-EB Virus Titer Sera of Patients with Nasopharyngeal Carcinoma ; A Small Scaled Sero-epidemiological Study. GANN, *60* : 335, 1969.

13. Kawamura, A., Jr., Takada, M., Gotoh, A., Hamajima, K., Sanpe, T., Murata, M., Ito, Y., Takahashi, T., Yoshida, O., Hirayama, T., Tu, S.-M., Liu, C.-H., Yang, C.-S., and Wang, C.-H. Sero-epidemiological Studies on Nasopharyngeal Carcinoma by Fluorescent Antibody Techniques with Cultured Burkitt Lymphoma Cells. GANN, *61* : 55, 1970.

14. Klein, G., Pearson, G., Henle, G., Henle, W., Goldstein, G., and Clifford, P. Relation between Epstein-Barr Viral and Cell Membrane Immunofluorescence in Burkitt Tumour Cells. J. Exp. Med., *129* (4) : 697–705, 1969 ; *129* (4) : 707–718, 1969.

15. Niederman, J. C., McCollum, R. W., Henle, G., and Henle, W. Infectious Mononucleosis, Clinical Manifestations in Relation to EB Virus Antibodies. J. Am. Med. Ass., *203* : 205–209, 1968.

16. Osato, T. Herpes-type Infection in Human Embryo Cells *in vitro* : Entry, Replication and Chromosomal Aberrations. GANN Monograph, *7* : 173–182, 1969.

17. Osato, T., and Ito, Y. Transformation *in vitro* of Human Embryo Tissues by Human Leukemic Culture Fluid. GANN Monograph, *7* : 95–103, 1969.

18. de Schryver, A., Frieberg, S., Jr., Klein, G., Henle, W., Henle, G., de Thé, G., Clifford, P., and Ho, H.-C. Epstein-Barr Virus-associated Antibody Pattern in Carcinoma of the Post-nasal Space. Clin. Exp. Immunol., *5* (5) : 443–459, 1969.

19. Shanmugaratnam, K., and Higginson, J. Aetiology of Nasopharyngeal Carcinoma : Report on a Retrospective Survey in Singapore. " Cancer of the Nasopharynx " UICC Monograph, Series Vol. 1, pp. 130–137, Munksgaard, Copenhagen, 1967.

20. Sugano, H., Takada, M., Chen, H.-C., and Tu, S.-M. Presence of Herpes-type Virus in the Culture Cell Line from a Nasopharyngeal Carcinoma in Taiwan. Proc. Japan Acad., *46* : 453–457, 1970.

21. de Thé, G., Ambrosioni, J. C., Ho., H-C., and Kwan, H.-C. Presence of Herpes-type Virions in Chinese Nasopharyngeal Tumour Cultured *in vitro*. Proc. Amer. Ass. Cancer Res., *10* : 19, 1969.

22. de Thé, G., Ho, H.-C., Desgranges, C., and Favre, M. C. Nasopharyngeal Carcinoma (NPC) 1. Types of Cultures Derived from Tumour Biopsies and Non-tumourous Tissues of Chinese Patients with Special Reference to Lymphoblastoid Transformation. Int. J. Cancer, *6* : 189–206, 1970.

23. Wilson, G. S., and Miles, A. A. Topley and Wilson's Principle of Bacteriology and Immunity, II. 5th Ed., p. 2217, London, 1964.

24. zur Hausen, H., and Schulte-Holthausen. Presence of EB Virus Nucleic Acid Homology in a " Virus-free " Line of Burkitt Tumour Cells. Nature (London), *227* (5255) : 245–248, 1970.

Discussion of Papers by Drs. Ho, de Thé, Lin, and Hirayama

DR. NISHIOKA: I would like to add some comments on Izumi fever, which Dr. Hirayama has discussed.

A scarlatine-like disease was described by Izumi and his colleagues in 1929. It occurs endemically in the rural population of Japan and also in the form of outbreaks common among school children or young people living in barracks or dormitories. Clinically, there are two forms, one is severe with a diphasic febrile curve and a shorter course. Gastrointestinal disturbances are observed. No serological findings indicating streptococcal or other bacterial or viral infections have as yet been reported; the Paul-Bunnell test is negative.

An increase of atypical lymphocytes in the peripheral blood has been reported in this disease. A similar hematological pattern was induced in mice experimentally injected with patients' materials and with the spleen of rats and field mice collected in the endemic area of the disease. Evidence of a water-borne spread was obtained frequently by epidemiological studies but conclusive evidence of the nature of the causative agent of the disease has not yet been found.

Based on the blood picture characterized by the appearance of atypical lymphocytes in the patients' blood as seen in patients with infectious mononucleosis and infectious hepatitis and on comparative epidemiological and clinical studies, I am of the opinion that Izumi fever and these two diseases belong to the same group of diseases which have been called " lymphotropic viral diseases " by Kissel and Arnould in 1952. At that time, they postulated that rubella and acute infectious lymphocytosis might also belong to the same category of viral diseases, but, at present, it has been clearly demonstrated that these two disease entities have no association with EBV-infection etiologically.

In an outbreak of Izumi fever on Toshi Island, anti-EBV titers in convalescent patients' sera were as high as in sera of NPC, BL, and IM patients and significantly higher than in healthy controls. Increases of antibody titer, observed in paired sera, indicated that a causative association exists between this virus and Izumi fever.

DR. YAN: In connection with anti-HTV titer in Taiwan, I would like to report on some anti-HTV titers in Chinese monkeys. The frequency and height of HTV titers in 273 adult Taiwan monkeys was found to be lower than in Taiwanese human sera titer, showing that monkeys can be used as experimental animals.

Maternal anti-HTV antibodies in new-born Taiwan monkeys, separated from their mothers immediately after birth and fed artificially, was tested. Blood specimens were taken at 5 week intervals and tested for anti-HTV titers. HTV or HTV-carrying cells were given subcutaneously to one-day old Taiwan monkeys and at the same time Immuran was given orally (3–5 mg per kg body wt. per day for 35 days) and blood specimens were tested at 1–3 week intervals; serum was tested at 5 week intervals for anti-HTV titers. These tests are in progress.

DR. FUJII: Dr. Ho, you showed no correlation between ABO blood group distribution and the incidence of NPC. What do you think of the HLA system?

DR. HO: That is an important system to be examined next.

DR. W. HENLE: Dr. Hirayama, you mentioned that the relative risk of NPC goes up as the anti-EBV titer goes up. This is actually putting the cart before the horse, because in stage I, according to Dr. Ho's classification, the antibody titers are usually low and they go up stepwise as the disease develops ultimately to stage V. The question is, what is the risk before getting the disease and what is the titer then?

DR. HIRAYAMA: I think I should make it clear that the present exercise in showing this type of relative risk is working on the hypothesis that the virus concerned is not a passenger and that the propagation of the virus takes place before the occurrence of the disease. Of course, another hypothesis is also possible. For the present I just want to know what kind of results we will get by utilizing the available data. If we bear in mind that we are dealing with one particular hypothesis I think this kind of maneuver is permissible.

I think I should like to make one comment on the familial aggregation of NPC patients. When we study the familial aggregation of gastric cancer patients, we get aggregations in many instances of 2 cases in one family, and sometimes 3 or even 4–5 cases; this is due to random distribution and such distribution tends to level off. But in addition to that kind of distribution we may run across some families which show a very, very high concentration of patients, sometimes more than 10 or even 16 cases in the same family, like Napoleon's family. The pedigree in which Dr. Ho found 9 cases in one family with 6 out of 7 children from 1 mother affected could be one such case of extreme aggregation.

DR. HO: It is very important to study twins. Unfortunately, in my series we have only one pair of probable dizygotic twins. Both developed the disease. One was my patient and the other was not.

DR. YOSHIDA: Dr. de Thé, I am very interested in your technique for detecting new antigens. How did you obtain floating cells from tissue cultures? Did you try to test also the presence of membrane-specific antigens simultaneously with your technique?

DR. DE THÉ: As I said, no attempt has been made to investigate this in the living cell because of technical difficulties. This finding does not mean that the antigen is necessarily located in or on the cell because technical difficulty prevented a conclusion from being drawn at present. Also it does not mean that the antigen located at the cell membrane does not interfere with our newly discovered antigen.

DR. YOSHIDA: Could your new antigen be located in the nucleus?

DR. DE THÉ: We have absolutely no idea.

DR. YAN: Dr. de-Thé, I would like to know whether the cells derived from your NPC cultures and used in the antigen analysis were cloned. In short, did you do cell cloning in your antigenic analysis?

DR. DE THÉ: No. We have only just started cell cloning.

DR. HO: Nasopharyngoscopic photography produces excellent visual records of nasopharyngeal tumors, but it suffers from the disadvantage that it is very time-consuming. For this reason it is unlikely to be adopted as a routine procedure, especially in a busy department.

It is interesting to note from the report by Sugano *et al.* that Chinese in Japan have a risk almost 60 times that of Japanese. If all 7 Chinese cases were local residents and did not include among them patients who went to Tokyo for treatment, then an explanation should be sought for the extremely low risk in Japanese when practically all other people of Mongoloid stock, *e.g.*, Chinese and Malays, have a high risk, and a close association between Japanese and Chinese has been in existence for the past many centuries. The finding that NPC patients in Japan have a significantly higher anti-EBV titer than control groups in Japan, like in the case of NPC patients elsewhere, is in support of a widely held belief that the close association between HTV-infection and NPC is world-wide and not confined to any particular racial groups or environmental conditions.

Dr. Chen suspects that prognosis and radiosensitivity of the tumor might be influenced by the relative proportions of the adenomatous and squamous elements, *i.e.*, secretory granules and tonofibrils, respectively, present in the tumor cells. The result of the review which is now being carried out by him and his colleagues of the material in Taiwan is awaited with interest. There is, however, disagreement that the particles observed by electron microscopy in the cells derived from NPC biopsies from 4 Taiwan patients with high anti-EBV titers are viral particles.

It is quite likely that the " lymphoblastoid " cells derived from NPC cultures are lymphoblasts, but, as Prof. Epstein has rightly pointed out, the word, "lymphoblastoid " is used to describe those cells which closely resemble lymphoblasts because one does not want to say that they are lymphoblasts. It is the correct attitude to take before we are absolutely sure that they are.

It is of importance to note, as Dr. de Thé has pointed out, that the specific association between HTV and NPC lies only in the serological response of NPC patients' sera which regularly show antibodies against EB viral capsid- and membrane-associated antigens, usually in high titer.   Immunofluorescence tests have shown that this virus shares with the virus associated with BL the same viral capsid antigens, but the HTV particles observed in long-term NPC cultures have also been observed from control cultures from adenolymphoma and tonsillitis.   Consequently, it would appear that it is not the apparently ubiquitous virus infection *per se* but rather a certain as yet unknown factor or factors which determine the type of response in the patient to the HTV infection that matter.   More data are required.   Dr. de Thé and his colleagues have carried out a comparative analysis of antigens using pair-labeled mixtures of NPC sera and have shown that lymphoblastoid cells derived from NPC shared an antigen, regularly absent in BL-derived cultures.   It is, however, not possible to tell whether this antigen is cell-specific or virus-specific. The tumor cells in NPC are of epidermoid origin, whereas those of BL are of lymphoid origin.   So far, in NPC only HTV particles and HTV-associated antigens have been demonstrated in the lymphoblastoid cells derived from NPC cultures, as in the case of BL, and not in the epithelial cells.   From the histo-pathogenetic point of view, there is no likelihood that NPC and BL are variants of the same disease.

Tong *et al.* found no indication that there was any household aggregation of high anti-EBV titers in families of patients and controls.   This is not unexpected, since the titer, which rises with advancing stages of the disease, according to Ho's stage classification, is usually low at first.

The report by Hirayama *et al.*, which was later amplified by Dr. Nishioka during the discussion, that Izumi fever, a scarlatine-like disease, is due to HTV-infection is based on data obtained from a sero-epidemiological study of an outbreak of the fever in early 1970 on Toshi Island and also on the appearance of atypical lymphocytes in patients' peripheral blood.   It would seem that we have now one other benign disease which gives rise to antibodies against EBV in convalescent patients' sera in titers as high as those in NPC, BL, and infectious mononucleosis.

In the search for genetic factors, wider studies on the genetic profile of people with high and low risks of NPC and of NPC families and patients and of controls are called for.   My findings of a significantly higher aggregation of cases in families of NPC patients than in families of patients with other cancers, and also of a higher risk in people of mixed Chinese ancestry, *e.g.*, Macaonese, than in people of Caucasian stock domiciled in Hong Kong are in support of a genetic hypothesis, but these findings do not exclude a non-genetic or a genetic-environmental interpretation. The evidence so far obtained does not allow the conclusion to be drawn that HTV-infection is essential for the malignant transformation of the epithelial cells in the nasopharynx, although it is quite possible that HTV-infection plays a role in the genesis of NPC together with other factors.

EBV INTRACELLULAR ANTIGENS

Chairmen:

George Klein, Takeshi Hirayama

Antibodies to EBV-induced Early Antigens in Infectious Mononucleosis, Burkitt's Lymphoma and Nasopharyngeal Carcinoma

Gertrude HENLE

The Children's Hospital of Philadelphia and The School of Medicine, University of Pennsylvania, Philadelphia, Pennsylvania, U.S.A.

It has been shown recently that lymphoblastoid cells of lines free of EBV antigen-producing cells, but not necessarily devoid of EB viral genomes, can be infected with virus derived from EBV carrier cultures. It was noted, however, that the infectious process is aborted at an early stage in most, if not all of the invaded cells (7); *i.e.*, EBV-induced early antigens (EA) are synthesized but not viral capsid antigens (VCA). Differentiation between these two groups of antigens, both detectable in indirect immunofluorescence tests with acetone-fixed cell smears, has become possible by the use of selected human sera. Sera from many patients with infectious mononucleosis (IM), Burkitt's lymphoma (BL), and nasopharyngeal carcinoma (NPC), but rarely from other donors, have antibodies to EA and to VCA in that they elicit brilliant immunofluorescence in abortively infected cells (EA), as well as in virus-producing cells of EBV carrier cultures, such as the EB3 line (VCA and EA). In contrast, pooled human γ-globulin preparations or sera from certain healthy donors have antibodies to VCA but not to EA, since they fail to react with abortively infected cells but give strong fluorescence with virus containing cells of carrier cultures. The "donor reagents" were proven to possess antibodies to viral capsid antigens by electron microscopically demonstrable antibody coating and agglutination of nonenveloped viral nucleocapsids (6, 14).

The synthesis of EA may be followed in a small proportion of the invaded cells by production of VCA, depending on the cell line used for infection as well as on the dose of virus inoculated. When both types of antigen are produced, as in Raji cells exposed to a large dose of EBV, the appearance of EA-containing cells precedes that of VCA-containing cells by about 4 hr; the maximal number of EA-positive cells reached in 24 hr exceeds that of VCA-positive cells by a factor of at least 10. With a small inoculum of EBV, aimed to yield from 5–15% EA-synthesizing cells, VCA fails to become detectable or appears at most in a negligible number of cells.

Abortively infected Raji cells have been used for detection and titration of

343

antibodies to EA in parallel with virus-producing cells of EB3 carrier cultures for measuring anti-VCA.   It appears that anti-EA reflects to some extent current EBV-associated disease processes and their severity.   The present status of these studies will be summarized below.

Anti-EA Responses in Heterophil Antibody-positive Infectious Mononucleosis

It has been shown previously (*5, 15*) and confirmed by others, that sera obtained well in advance of the onset of IM are free of anti-VCA, whereas in the acute phase of illness all patients have anti-VCA in titers of at least 1:40 and as high as 1:1,280. These antibodies persist after recovery at readily detectable levels for years, if not for life.   Anti-EA also was found to be absent in all preillness sera (*9*).   It appears in the acute stage in no more than about 70% of the patients however, and then with some delay and at relatively low titers as compared to anti-VCA.   Furthermore, in contrast to anti-VCA, the anti-EA response is transitory in that these antibodies, as a rule, disappear within a few months.   The delay in anti-EA development, as well as its early disappearance, are useful in the sero-diagnosis of IM, in that 4-fold or greater increments or declines in titer, indicative of a current EBV-infection, are observed with greater frequency than corresponding changes in anti-VCA titers. Furthermore, the mere presence of anti-EA in titers of ≧1:20 denotes, with few exceptions, a concurrent or very recent EBV-infection.   Such a finding may be especially helpful in the diagnosis of EBV mononucleosis in patients without heterophil antibody responses, as seen frequently in children.   It should be noted that heterophil antibody-negative IM may often be due to another virus of the herpes group, cytomegalovirus (*12*), and at times to other, as yet unidentified, infectious agents (*1, 13*).

There is evidence that anti-EA responses in IM depend to some extent upon the severity of the illness (*9*).   Patients were subdivided according to their peak anti-VCA and anti-EA responses which were then compared with respect to the duration of illness, frequency of splenomegaly, need for steroid therapy, and frequency of various hematological features.   On the basis of these comparisons, patients with anti-VCA titers of ≧1:160 and anti-EA titers ≧1:80, taken as one extreme, tended to have more severe illnesses than patients with anti-VCA titers of 1:40–1:80 and no detectable anti-EA, taken as the other extreme.

Antibodies to EA in Burkitt's Lymphoma

All African patients with this disease thus far examined were found to possess antibodies to VCA, mostly at titers ≧1:160, with a geometric mean of 1:320 (*2, 4*). In contrast, anti-VCA was non-detectable in an appreciable number of African control children and, in those who had these antibodies, the titers were generally low, with a geometric mean of <1:40.   Recent tests for anti-EA were positive in about 80% of 124 BL patients at titers which were usually lower than the anti-VCA titers but on occasion matched them (*3*).   The anti-EA titers were found to persist, with few exceptions, for as long as the patients survived.   Among control children, anti-EA was rarely found and, if detected, the titers did not exceed 1:20 as a rule, even in the few instances in which very high anti-VCA titers were measured.

In order to clarify the question of why some BL patients had anti-EA and others not, the available data were assorted according to the following criteria: (a) data obtained at the time of admission; (b) data collected shortly before death; and (c) data derived from patients who had survived for at least 2 years and some for as long as 6 years after first admission. The anti-VCA and anti-EA titers were then correlated with the future fate and the past clinical histories of the patients, depending upon the group under study. The following results have emerged from these comparisons.

(a) *Sera obtained at the time of admission*—Among patients admitted without anti-EA were some who were moribund or died within a few weeks; that is, they arrived too late for successful chemotherapy. Those admitted in a less advanced stage of the disease were found to have a better chance of survival for at least one year than patients admitted with high anti-EA titers. The mortality within one year among patients with high anti-EA levels was nearly twice that of patients admitted without anti-EA.

(b) *Sera collected shortly before death*—The majority of dying patients had high anti-EA titers. Sera had also been collected from most of these patients at the time of admission which, with few exceptions, also contained high anti-EA titers. A few patients, however, had no anti-EA at admission but subsequently developed high titers. Among the patients who died without detectable anti-EA were some who had been admitted in a moribund state as already discussed. Several others in this category succumbed to invasion of the central nervous system, drug toxicity, or intercurrent infections, while the presenting tumor was in marked or complete regression. In a few patients admitted with high anti-EA levels, a decline in anti-EA titer was noted before death.

(c) *Sera collected from patients who survived for at least two years*—Among these patients were some who to date have survived for as long as 9 years. More than half of these had no or only low levels of anti-EA in spite of often very high anti-VCA titers. Yet, an appreciable proportion of these patients had high anti-EA titers. A review of the records revealed that tumor recurrences were substantially more frequent among patients with high anti-EA titers (60%) than among patients with no or low levels of anti-EA (18%).

The low or negative anti-EA reactions in this group of patients could not be ascribed, as a rule, to a loss of these antibodies during the years intervening since first admission. Sera were available from some of these patients which had been collected at admission. These, with few exceptions, also had low or non-detectable levels of anti-EA. A few, however, had been admitted with antibodies to EA which subsequently declined in titer or were lost.

From these various observations it appears that antibodies to EA reflect to a considerable extent the prognosis of the patient with respect to recurrences of the tumor after successful initial chemotherapy. Patients who maintain high anti-EA levels or develop them in the course of time are prone to have one or more recurrences, some as late as 5 years after the initial remission and at times with fatal consequences. In contrast, patients who have low or non-detectable levels of anti-EA or who show declines in titer in the course of time, tend to have relatively few, generally early recurrences which usually respond again well to chemotherapy.

The apparent prognostic implications of antibodies to EA cannot be explained at present.   The anti-EA levels appear to be unrelated to the stage of the disease at admission, to the localization of the tumor, or to the total tumor burden.   Some of the patients admitted in a moribund state had widely disseminated large tumor masses, yet revealed no anti-EA.   Other patients admitted in Stage I had high anti-EA titers.   Furthermore, patients who had been free of detectable tumors for years, maintained constant high anti-EA titers.   The persistent EBV-infection undoubtedly is not restricted to the tumor but involves presumably also the lymphoreticular system, as postulated for healthy carriers of the virus.   While high levels of persistent EBV infection might conceivably affect, in time, the immunological resistance of patients, there is no clear-cut evidence at present that humoral or cellular immune responses are significantly impaired in BL patients.   It is unlikely that anti-EA plays the role of an enhancing antibody since it appears to be directed solely against intracellular antigens.   It is possible, however, that anti-EA serves indirectly as an indicator of the presence of other antibodies for which no tests are available at present, among them, plssibly, tumor enchancing antibodies.   If this were true and involved an EBV-induced antibody, the virus could no longer be considered a mere passenger in the tumor, since it would be diffcult to explain why an antibody induced by a passenger virus should reflect the prognosis of the patient.

Antibodies to EA in Nasopharyngeal Carcinoma

NPC is the third disease which is regularly associated with antibodies to EBV-related antigens.   Anti-VCA titers are generally high with a geometric mean of 1:340 (5, 8).   In contrast, patients with carcinomas of similar histology elsewhere in the head and neck region do not show such an association and the incidence of high anti-VCA titers and the geometric mean levels are similar to those seen in appropriate controls.   As in BL, some NPC patients do not have antibodies to EA, but in the 75% who do, the titers of anti-EA are often very high.   In contrast to BL, the frequency of high anti-VCA and anti-EA titers in NPC as well as the geometric mean levels seem to be related to the stage of the disease.   The antibody levels are lowest in Stage I and increase stepwise as the disease progresses ultimately to Stage V.   It thus appears that in NPC the antibody titers might reflect the total tumor burden, but before accepting this interpretation it will be necessary to correlate the serological data with various clinical features such as the results of therapy and their resistance, similar to the studies carried out in Burkitt's lymphoma.

Antibodies to EA in Other Malignant or Non-malignant Diseases

High anti-VCA titers have been observed also in certain other diseases at a greater frequency than expected in controls, but at a lesser frequency than noted in IM, BL, or NPC.   This has been evident especially in Hodgkin's disease (HD) (11), chronic lymphocytic leukemia (CLL), and sarcoidosis (10).   In HD, high titers were regularly seen in the sarcomatous (lymphocyte depletion) form of the illness, whereas in the paragranuloma type the antibody pattern resembled that found in controls. In the granuloma type of illness, intermediary results were obtained. Anti-EA was found in many of the patients with high anti-VCA titers, but the anti-EA levels were usually relatively low.

In CLL nearly 40% of the patients had high anti-VCA titers accompanied usually by some anti-EA reactivity but often at low levels. No relation between high titers and clinical features has become evident (unpublished).

Of the sarcoidosis patients, examined in collaboration with Drs. Wahren and Espmark (16), about 30% had anti-VCA titers of 1:160 or higher, but few of these showed anti-EA and, if found, the titers did not exceed 1:20. It should be noted that in this disease the levels of antibodies to herpes simplex and cytomegaloviruses are also somewhat higher than in appropriate controls.

SUMMARY

These studies have revealed different patterns of anti-VCA and anti-EA reactivities in the various diseases discussed. Infectious mononucleosis clearly represents a primary EBV infection. Sera obtained prior to illness are devoid of antibodies to EBV-related antigens. Anti-VCA develops regularly in the acute phase of illness and anti-EA in about 70% of the patients. Anti-VCA persists thereafter at readily detectable levels, but anti-EA, with few exceptions, disappears again within a few months. In control groups of young adults or children, one may find on occasion high anti-VCA titers accompanied by low levels of anti-EA which presumably denote recent silent or non-recognized primary EBV-infection. Yet, in rare instances, anti-EA may persist at low levels for years, perhaps depending upon the extent of the persistent viral carrier stage, which, as a rule, follows primary infections.

Whether or not Burkitt's lymphoma arises as a consequence of a recent primary EBV-infection is unknown at present. Once the tumor has developed, generally high anti-VCA titers are found which tend to persist at nearly constant levels as long as the patient survives. Anti-EA is found in about 80% of these patients and high levels of these antibodies consitute an apparently unfavorable prognostic sign. High titers of both antibodies seem to be unrelated to the stage of the disease, the site of the tumor, or the total tumor burden. These data together with other observations discussed elsewhere in this symposium suggest, but by no means prove, an etiologic role of EBV in BL. None of the available data rigidly exclude, however, the alternate possibility that EBV is merely a passenger in this tumor. If EBV should ultimately be found to be causally related to BL, it would most likely exert its oncogenic activity only in combination with other, as yet unknown, factors.

As to nasopharyngeal carcinoma, it seems less likely than in BL that this malignancy arises in consequence of a recent preceding primary EBV infection. Patients developing NPC fall into an older age range than BL patients and the vast majority of primary EBV infections occurs early in life. All NPC patients have antibodies to VCA, usually at high titers but only 70% reveal, in addition, anti-EA. The height of titers and the geometric means in this malignancy increase with the advance of the disease from Stage I to Stage V, which reflects to a considerable extent the increase in total tumor burden. While these observations would be compatible with a passenger role for the virus in this malignancy, a correlation of the serological data with clinical features has yet to be attempted and an explanation has to be sought for the lack of a similar association of EBV with carcinoma of comparable histology elsewhere in the head and neck.

Finally, increased frequencies of high anti-VCA titers, rarely accompanied by high anti-EA levels, have been observed in some other malignant or non-malignant diseases; that is, Hodgkin's disease, chronic lymphocytic leukemia, and sarcoidosis.

It would be difficult, and indeed not necessary, to provide a unifying explanation for the multitude of apparently " EBV-associated diseases." What might be a causal relation of EBV in some diseases, possibly influenced by the type of target cell involved, might be a passenger role in other diseases or a nonspecific stimulation of immune responses in yet others. Certainly much remains to be done before clarification of these problems can be attained.

The work reported was supported by research grant CA 04568 and Contract PH-43-66-477 within the Special Virus Leukemia Program, National Cancer Institute, U.S. Public Health Service ; and by the U.S. Army Medical Research and Development Command, Department of the Army, Contract DA-49-193-MD-2474 under the sponsorship of the Commission on Viral Infections, Armed Forces Epidemiological Board.

REFERENCES

1. Evans, A. S., Niederman, J. C., and McCollum, R. W. Seroepidemiologic Studies of Infectious Mononucleosis. New England J. Med., *279*: 1121–1127, 1968.
2. Henle, G. and Henle, W. Immunofluorescence in Cells Derived from Burkitt's Lymphoma. J. Bact., *91*: 1248–1256, 1966.
3. Henle, G., Henle, W., Klein, G., Gunvén, P., Clifford, P., Morrow, R. H., and Ziegler, T. L. Antibodies to EBV-induced Early Antigens in Burkitt's Lymphoma. J. Natl. Cancer Inst., *46*: 861–871, 1971.
4. Henle, G., Henle, W., Clifford, P., Diehl, V., Kafuko, G., Kirya, B., Klein, G., Morrow, R., Munube, G. M. R., Rike, P., Tukei, P. M., and Ziegler, J. L. Antibodies to Epstein-Barr Virus in Burkitt's Lymphoma and Control Groups. J. Natl. Cancer Inst., *43*: 1147–1157, 1969.
5. Henle, G., Henle, W., and Diehl, V. Relation of Burkitt's Tumor-associated Herpes type Virus to Infectious Mononucleosis. Proc. Nat'l. Acad. Sci., *59*: 94–101, 1968.
6. Henle, W., Hummeler, K., and Henle, G. Antibody Coating and Agglutination of Virus Particles Separated from the EB3 Line of Burkitt Lymphoma Cells. J. Bact., *92*: 269–271, 1966.
7. Henle, W., Henle, G., Zajac, B., Pearson, G., Waubke, R., an Scriba, M. Differential Reactivity of Human Serums with Early Antigens Induced by Epstein-Barr Virus. Science, *169*: 188–190, 1970.
8. Henle, W., Henle, G., Ho, H.-C., Burtin, P., Cachin, Y., Clifford, P., de Schryver, A., de-Thé, G., Diehl, V., and Klein, G. Antiboieds to Epstein-Barr Virus in Nasopharyngeal Carcinoma, Other Head and Neck Neoplasms, and Control Groups. J. Nat'l. Cancer Inst., *44*: 225–231, 1970.

9. Henle, W., Henle, G., Niederman, J. C., Klemola, E., and Haltia, K. Antibodies to Epstein-Barr Virus-induced Early Antigens in Infectious Mononucleosis. J. Inf. Dis., *124*: 58–67, 1971.

10. Hirshaut, Y., Glade, P., Viera, L. O. B. D., Ainbender, E., Dvorak, B., and Siltzbach, L. E. Sarcoidosis, Another Disease Associated with Serologic Evidence for Herpes-like Virus Infection. New England J. Med., *283*: 502–505, 1970.

11. Johanson, B., Klein, G., Henle, W., and Henle, G. Epstein-Barr Virus (EBV)-associated Antibody Patterns in Malignant Lymphoma and Leukemia. I. Hodgkin's Disease. Int. J. Cancer, *6*: 450–462, 1970.

12. Klemola, E., and Kääriäinen, L. Cytomegalovirus as a Possible Cause of a Disease Resembling Infectious Mononucleosis. Brit. J. Med., *2*: 1099–1102, 1965.

13. Klemola, E., von Essen, R., Henle, G., and Henle, W. Infectious-mononucleosis-like Disease with Negative Heterophil Agglutination Test. Clinical Features in Relation to Epstein-Barr Virus and Cytomegalovirus Antibodies. J. Inf. Dis., *121*: 608, 614, 1970.

14. Mayyasi, S. A., Schidlovsky, G., Bulfone, L. M., and Buscheck, F. I. The Coating Reaction of the Herpes-type Virus Isolated from Malignant Tissues with an Antibody Present in Sera. Cancer Res., *27*: 2020–2024, 1967.

15. Niederman, J. C., McCollum, R. W., Henle, G., and Henle, W. Infectious Mononucleosis. Clinical Manifestations in Relation to EB Virus Antibodies. J. Amer. Med. Assoc., *203*: 205–209, 1968.

16. Wahren, B., Carlens, E., Espmark, A., Lundbeck, H., Löfgren, S., Madar, E., Henle, G., and Henle, W. Antibodies to Various Herpes-group Viruses in Sera from Sarcoidosis Patients. Submitted for publication.

A New Antigen Induced by the Epstein-Barr Virus and Its Reactivity with Sera from Patients with Malignant Tumors

Yorio Hinuma,* Takeshi Sairenji,* Tsuyoshi Sekizawa, and Shiroh Ida

Department of Microbiology, Tohoku University School of Dentistry, Sendai, Japan

Gerber, *et al.* (*2*) reported that a human hematopoietic cell line, NC-37 could be infected with Epstein-Barr virus (EBV) produced from a Burkitt lymphoma cell line, P3HR-1. During the course of our confirmation of their findings, a new antigen in the infected cells was found. This antigen was formed by EBV infection but was distinct from the EB virion antigen. Antibody against the new antigen was detected in sera from patients with certain types of malignant disease.

In this paper, we present experiments on the formation of the new antigen in EBV-infected NC-37 cells and the results of examination of human sera for their reactivity with the new antigen. A part of these studies has previously been reported elsewhere (*8*).

MATERIALS AND METHODS

Cells—The NC-37 cell line (*1*) was used. The cells were confirmed to be negative for EB virion antigen and for immunoglobulins (γ, μ and α chains) by means of immunofluorescence (*6*). The cells were also negative for membrane immunofluorescence with the serum from a healthy adult, VO-7 (*10*). The cells were maintained in stationary suspension cultures in Eagle's MEM plus 20% fetal bovine serum.

Virus—Culture fluids of P3HR-1 cells (*6*) were used for the EBV preparations, since it has been known that relatively large amounts of the enveloped EBV particles are produced into the culture fluids (*9*). Procedures for the concentration of virus have been described in a previous paper (*5*). In some experiments, the EBV preparations were passed through a Millipore membrane (0.8 μ) and then used for the infection.

---

* Present address: Department of Microbiology, Kumamoto University Medical School, Kumamoto, Japan

Immunofluorescences

The indirect immunofluorescent method was employed (*6*). For the detection of EB virion antigen in the experimentally infected cells, a reference serum, VO-7, was used as stated above. For detection of the new antigen, three reagent serums, No. 2 from an African patient with Burkitt's lymphoma, NPC-114 from a Chinese patient with nasopharyngeal carcinoma and P-62 from a Japanese patient with an unclassified malignant lymphatic disease were used. Antibody against the virion antigen was titrated by using an acetone-fixed smear of P3HR-1 cells as described previously (*6*). Antibody against the new antigen was examined by using acetone-fixed smears of NC-37 cells infected with EBV which were prepared as described in the text.

RESULTS

Formation of a new antigen in NC-37 cells inoculated with EBV

About 6×10^5 NC-37 cells per ml in a fresh growth medium were mixed with an equal volume of the culture fluid of P3HR-1 cells; then one portion of the EBV-inoculated cells was incubated at 33°C and the other at 37°C. During the incubations, cells were sampled at intervals and examined for immunofluorescence with two reagent serum, VO-7 in 1:10 dilution and No. 2 in 1:20 dilution. Results of a typical experiment are summarized in Figs. 1, 2, and 3. The incubated cells grew more rapidly at 37°C than at 33°C, as seen in Fig. 1. Percentages of fluorescent cells reacted with No. 2 serum were much higher than those with VO-7 serum both at 37°C and 33°C, as shown in Fig. 2. For instance, in the culture at 33°C 6 days after infection, about 8% of the cells were positive with No. 2 serum but only about 0.5% were positive with VO-7 serum. Since both reagent serums contained about an equally high titer (1:160 and 1:320) of antibody against EB virion an-

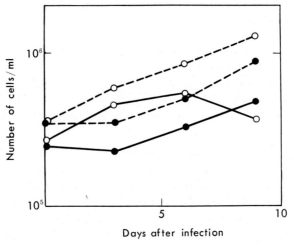

FIG. 1. Growth curves of NC-37 cells inoculated with EBV at 37°C and 33°C. O⋯⋯O, 37°C total cells ; ●⋯⋯●, 33°C total cells ; O——O, 37°C viable cells ; ●——●, 33°C viable cells.

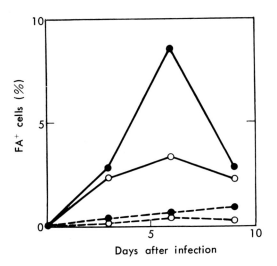

FIG. 2. Differential reactivity of 2 human sera, VO-7 and No. 2, with NC-37 cells infected with EBV in the experiments shown in Fig. 1. FA$^+$ cells indicates number of positive fluorescent cells. ●——●, 33°C No. 2 ; ○——○, 37°C No. 2 ; ●······●, 33°C VO-7 ; ○······○, 37°C VO-7.

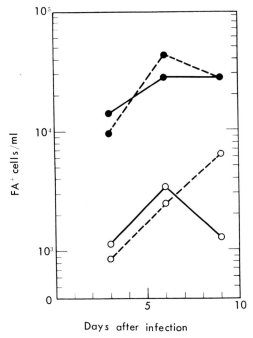

FIG. 3. Growth curves of the new antigen-bearing cells in the experiments shown in Fig. 1. FA$^+$ cells indicates number of positive fluorescent cells. ●······●, 33°C No. 2 ; ●——●, 37°C No. 2 ; ○······○, 33°C VO-7 ; ○——○, 37°C VO-7.

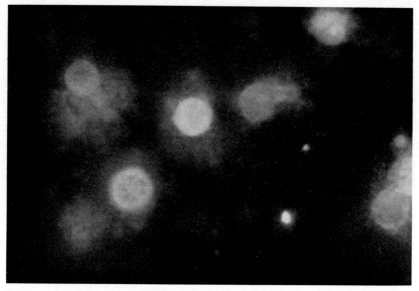

Fig. 4. Immunofluorescent staining with P-62 serum of NC-37 cells infected with EBV. Note cytoplasmic and nuclear brilliance.

tigen, the antigen stainable with No. 2 serum should be distinct from the virion antigen. As shown in Fig. 3, the number of new antigen-bearing cells did not increase after the time when the maximum percentage of such fluorescent cells was observed, even though the total number of cells was still increasing.

The new antigen of infected cells was distributed not only in the cytoplasm but also in the nucleus, as illustrated in Fig. 4.

Infectivity of EBV preparations from P3HR-1 cell cultures

Nineteen different culture fluids from the P3HR-1 cell line were examined for their infectivity to NC-37 cells. Procedures for infection were similar to those described above. The virus-inoculated cells were incubated at 33°C for 5 days and then cell smears were made. After the immunofluorescent staining with P-62 serum, the percentages of fluorescent cells were counted. As a control, VO-7 serum for staining of the virion antigen was also used. As shown in Table 1, the infectivity greatly varied with each preparation. Of all the preparations, those

TABLE 1. Infectivity of EBV Preparations from P3HR-1 Cell Cultures

P3HR-1 cell culture fluid No.	Concentration	Storage before infection	Percent[a] of fluorescent cells
1	1	fresh	8.5
2	1	fresh	2.4
3	1/500	fresh	12
4–19	1	−20°C for 6 to 12 months	0.2–1.2

[a] Maximum percent of positive cells after immunofluorescence with P-62 serum.

freshly harvested generally gave high titers of infectivity, whereas the long-stored (at $-20°C$) one did not. In the case of the concentrate of fresh preparation (No. 3), it showed the highest titer of infectivity. It was roughly calculated that more than 10^5 infectious units/ml of EBV were contained in the No. 1 culture fluid.

Detection of antibody against the new antigen in various human sera

It has been shown in a previous paper (7) that antibody against the virion antigen could be detected in more than 90% of healthy persons over 3 years old in

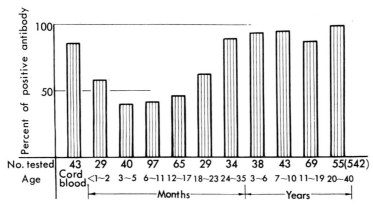

FIG. 5. Age specific incidence of healthy persons with antibody against the EB virion antigen in Japan.

TABLE 2. Incidence of Antibody against The EBV-induced New Antigen in Various Human Sera

Diagnosis	No. of patients tested	No. of positive anti-new antigen
Healthy donors :		
with anti-virion	15	0
without anti-virion	8	0
total	23	0
Infectious mononucleosis like disease and other unidentified non-malignant lymphoid diseases	14	0
Malignant lymphoma :		
reticulum cell sarcoma	7	3
lymphosarcoma	6	0
Hodgkin's disease	7	4
unclassif. malignant lymphoma	5	2
total	25	9
Burkitt's lymphoma	4	2
Nasopharyngeal carcinoma	13	11
Leukemia :		
acute lymphatic leukemia	9	4
acute myelogeneous leukemia	4	0
chronic lymphatic leukemia	3	2
chronic myelogeneous leukemia	3	2
total	19	8
Histiocytosis X	1	1

Japan. This was confirmed by further studies, as shown in Fig. 5. Preliminary study indicated that sera from some patients with malignant tumors but not those from healthy adult donors showed a reactivity with the new antigen. This prompted us to screen a number of sera from healthy persons and from various patients for antibody against the new antigen. As the antigen preparation, EBV infected NC-37 cells smears were made. The smears showed about 5% fluorescent cell with P-62 serum (1:10), but scarcely any (less than 0.1%) cells were stained with VO-7 serum. All sera were tested in 1:10 dilution. The results of the screening of 99 sera are shown in Table 2. None of the sera from 23 healthy donors, including 15 adults with a high titer of anti-EB virion antigen and 8 infants lacking anti-virion antigen, which were selected from the samples shown in Fig. 5, showed anti-new antigen. All of the 14 patients with non-malignant lymphatic involvement, some of whom were suffering from an infectious mononucleosis like disease, showed negative anti-new antigen. In contrast, a high incidence of anti-new antigen was found in the sera from patients with malignant lymphoid diseases; anti-new antigen was detected in 3 out of the 7 patients with reticulum cell sarcoma, 2 out of 5 with unclassified malignant lymphoma, and 4 out of 7 with Hodgkin's disease, none was positive in the 6 patients with lymphosarcoma. The anti-new antigen was also positive in 2 out of 4 patients with Burkitt's lymphoma and 11 out of 13 with nasopharyngeal carcinoma. Among 19 patients with various types of leukemia, 8 showed positive anti-new antigen. The antibody was not detected in the sera from the 4 patients with acute myelogeneous leukemia. It should be stressed that a high incidence of positive anti-new antigen was observed not only in patients with nasopharyngeal carcinoma or Burkitt's lymphoma but also in other malignant diseases, such as reticulum cell sarcoma, Hodgkin's disease, unclassified malignant lymphoma, and various types of leukemia.

Difference between the anti-new antigen and the anti-virion antigen in human sera

The titer of anti-virion antigen in the sera with positive anti-new antigen was determined by using P3HR-1 cell preparations. As shown in Table 3, 6 out of the 14 sera tested showed a nigher titer of the antibody than the normal range (1:160

TABLE 3. Titer of Anti-virion Antigen in Sera of Patients with Positive Anti-new Antigen

Titer of anti-virion antigen	No. of sera
1,280	1
640	2
320	3
160	3
80	2
40	2
20	0
10	0
Total	14

TABLE 4.   Relation between The Titers of Anti-virion Antigen and Anti-new Antigen

Serum No.	Titer of antibody against	
	Virion antigen	New antigen
A–352	<10	<10
VO–7	160	<10
P–62	1,280	40
A–240	320	160
NPC–114	640	640

or less), but the other did not.   No serum free from anti-virion antigen was observed among them.   The titers of both anti-new antigen and anti-virion antigen in 5 selected human sera were determined.   The results are shown in Table 4.   There were no constant parallel relationships between the titers of the two antibodies.

DISCUSSION

It seems to be clear in the present paper that the new antigen which appeared in EBV-infected NC-37 cells was a non-virion antigen, induced by EBV.   All of the tested serum specimens from healthy persons, even though they possessed high titers of antibody against the virion antigen, did not react with the new antigen.   However, a considerable number of sera in patients with certain malignant diseases did react with the new antigen, as well as with the virion antigen.   In the same cultures, the virion antigens could be detected in a small fraction of the infected cells.   This suggests a heterogeneous infection in the cells infected with EBV; a majority of the infected cells only form the new non-virion antigen and another minor fraction of the cells in the same culture synthesize the virion antigen or both the virion and new antigens.   The former type of infection may be called "abortive infection." However, with respect to the latter type of infection, it is not definite yet whether it is a process of producing infectious virus, even though virion antigen is produced, as revealed by immunofluorescence.   Reasons for the occurrence of such heterogenous infection in the single NC-37 cell cultures inoculated with EBV are unknown. However, there may be at least two possibilities, the heterogenous population of the infectious virus, and the heterogeneity of the susceptive cells.   It should be noticed that the actual number of the new antigen-bearing cells did not increase after the time when the total number of cells still continued to increase (Fig. 3), suggesting that most new antigen-bearing cells could not multiply.   This may suggest that the cessation of cell growth was caused by a direct or indirect inhibition of the synthesis of cellular macromolecules in the host cells by the new antigen induced by EBV.   However, the present experiments do not completely exclude the possible continuous growth of a small portion of the new antigen-bearing cells in the cultures.

Henle et al. (4) reported that "early antigens" appeared in Raji or 64–10 cells infected with EBV, which were produced from P3HR-1 cell cultures.   The early antigens seem to be analogous to the new antigen in the present paper.   Both the antigens are distinct from the virion antigen and are definitely induced by

EBV infection of human lymphoblastoid cells. The antibody against these antigens was found in sera from patients with Burkitt's lymphoma and nasopharyngeal carcinoma but not in those from healthy donors. However, the identity of the new antigen and the early antigen should be clarified by further studies. There are several similarities between the new antigen and the T antigen induced by adenoviruses, polyoma virus or SV40. These were non-virion antigen, localization within cells, and detection of antibody to the antigen in tumor-bearing animals or humans (3). However, we do not yet have evidence of the formation of cells which are capable of continuous multiplication and which harbor the new antigen, but not the virion antigen, like the known DNA tumor virus-transformed cells.

The present paper indicated no incidence of antibody against the new antigen in sera from healthy donors and patients with non-malignant lymphatic involvement, although the number of sera tested was not very high. On the other hand, however, there was an approximately 50% incidence of the antibody in sera from patients with malignant lymphoma, including reticulum cell sarcoma, Hodgkin's disease, Burkitt's lymphoma, and unclassified malignant lymphoma. Also, about 50% of the sera from patients with various types of leukemia, except for acute myelogeneous leukemia, gave positive reactions with the new antigen. Patients with nasopharyngeal carcinoma showed the highest incidence (80%) of antibody. These results may suggest a new territory for the search for human tumors suspected to be caused by EBV. In other words, the present data lead to the prospect that EBV may play a possible etiologic role not only in certain localized tumors; Burkitt's lymphoma or nasopharyngeal carcinoma, but also in other more general malignancies including malignant lymphatic diseases and certain types of leukemia.

SUMMARY

A hematopoietic cell line, NC-37 infected with Epstein-Barr virus (EBV), which was produced in the culture fluid of a P3HR-1 Burkitt's lymphoma cell line, formed a new antigen distinct from the EB virion antigen. The new antigen was seen both in the nucleus and in the cytoplasm by immunofluorescence. Antibody against the new antigen was detected in sera from patients with nasopharyngeal carcinoma, Burkitt's lymphoma, reticulum cell sarcoma, Hodgkin's disease, unidentified malignant lymphatic tumors, and various types of leukemia, in incidences of about 50% or more. The antibody, however, was not found in sera from healthy persons or patients with non-malignant lymphatic involvements. The new antigen may be analogous to the EBV-induced early antigen in other hematopoietic cell lines which has been reported by Henle and co-workers.

Aided partly by the grants from the Ministry of Education and the Ministry of Health and Welfare of the Japanese Government.

REFERENCES

1. Chandra, S., Liszczak, T., and Monroe, J. H. Small Particulate Debris Adhering to Cell Surface in Human Leukocytes Cultures: Relationship with Presence of

Herpes-type Virus Particles. J. Natl. Cancer Inst., *44*: 497–505, 1970.

2. Garber, P., Whang-Peng, J., and Monroe, J. Transformation and Chromosome Changes Induced by Epstein-Barr Virus in Normal Human Leukocyte Cultures. Proc. Natl. Acad. Sci., *63*: 740-746, 1969.

3. Habel, K. Antigen of Virus-induced Tumors. Adv. Immunol., *10*: 229–250, 1969.

4. Henle, W., Henle, G., Zajac, B. A., Pearson, G., Waubke, R., and Scriba, M. Differential Reactivity of Human Serums with Early Antigens Induced by Epstein-Barr Virus. Science, *169*: 188–190, 1970.

5. Hinuma, Y., Konn, M., Yamaguchi, J., and Grace, Jr. J. T. Replication of Herpes-type Virus in a Burkitt Lymphoma Cell Line. J. Virol., *1*: 1203–1206, 1967.

6. Hinuma, Y., Konn, M., Yamaguchi, J., Wudarski, D. J., Blakeslee, Jr., J. R., and Grace, Jr., J. T. Immunofluorescence and Herpes-type Virus Particles in the P3HR-1 Burkitt Lymphoma Cell Line. J. Virol., *1*: 1045–1051, 1967.

7. Hinuma, Y., Ohta-Hatano, R., Suto, T., and Numazaki, Y. High Incidence of Japanese Infants with Antibody to a Herpes-type Virus Associated with Cultured Burkitt Lymphoma Cells. Japan. J. Microbiol., *13*: 309–311, 1969.

8. Hinuma, Y., Sairenji, T., and Ohta-Hatano, R. Detection of Antibody to a New Antigen Induced by Epstein-Barr Virus in Serums from Patients with Malignant Lymphoid Diseases. Proc. Japan Acad., *46*: 980–992, 1970.

9. Konn, M., Yamaguchi, J., Grace, Jr., J. T., and Hinuma, Y. Factors Influencing the Formation of Immunofluorescent Antigen in a Burkitt Lymphoma Cell Line. Japan. J. Microbiol., *13*: 215–217, 1969.

10. Takahashi, H., and Hinuma, Y. Nature of Antigens of Cultured Burkitt Lymphoma Cells, as Revealed by Membrane Immunofluorescence. GANN, *61*: 337–346, 1970.

Evidence for A Relation of The Epstein-Barr Virus to Burkitt's Lymphoma and Nasopharyngeal Carcinoma

Werner HENLE*

The Children's Hospital of Philadelphia and The School of Medicine, University of Pennsylvania, Philadelphia, Pennsylvania, U.S.A.

The facts that the Epstein-Barr virus (EBV) has a world-wide distribution and is the cause of infectious mononucleosis (*2, 11, 23*) do not negate the possibility that this virus may be involved also, on rare occasions, in the induction of malignancies, although most likely in conjunction with other factors. Most oncogenic animal viruses also seem to be widely disseminated among their host species, yet rarely cause tumors under natural conditions. EBV is not a highly cytocidal virus and readily establishes persistent, latent infections which constitutes one requirement for an oncogenic agent. Since EBV appears to be restricted for its replication to cells of the lymphoreticular system it would be expected, if oncogenic, to induce such malignancies as lymphomas. Indeed, EBV, as will be discussed below, has a growth stimulating effect on cells of the lymphocytic series. It thus may not be a mere coincidence that Burkitt type ovarian tumors were detected recently in an American patient 16 months after the onset of infectious mononucleosis (*1*). Induction of these tumors must no doubt have preceded their detection by many months.

Efforts to relate a suspected oncogenic virus, such as EBV, to human malignancies, such as Burkitt's lymphoma (BL) or nasopharyngeal carcinoma (NPC), depend to a large extent upon experiences gained in the study of animal tumor viruses. The extensive research activities in this area have provided various approaches to the search for human tumor viruses which can be listed as follows:

1. Detection of virus, or of virus-determined antigens, or of virus-related nucleic acids in human tumors;
2. Induction of tumors in non-human primates or other animals by inoculation of virus;
3. Transformation of normal cells by virus *in vitro*; and

---

* Career Award 5–K6–AI–22,683 from The National Institutes of Health, U.S. Public Health Service.

4. Demonstration of antibodies to virus related antigens at higher frequency and/or higher titers in patients with given malignancies than in healthy individuals or patients with other tumors.

In the following sections, the present status of the evidence linking EBV with BL and NPC will be summarized according to these four general approaches.

Search for Traces of EBV in BL and NPC

Herpes-type virus particles have rarely, if ever, been found in BL or NPC biopsies upon electron microscopic examination. The more sensitive EBV-specific immunofluorescence test (*8, 13*), with few exceptions, likewise has failed to detect EBV antigen-containing cells in acetone-fixed cell smears derived from BL biopsies (*22*). Only in 6% of nearly 80 biopsies were occasional cells observed (<1 in 100,000) which showed characteristic and specific staining for EB viral capsid antigens (VCA) and/or EBV-induced early antigens (EA). Yet, when BL biopsy cells are placed in culture, VCA and/or EA-containing cells appear regularly, often within 3–5 days of incubation, and at times involving up to 5% of the cell population (*22*). Lymphoblastoid cell lines derived from NPC biopsies likewise have shown the regular presence of EBV (*26*).

It was shown by Klein and his associates that a large proportion of cells in the majority of BL biopsies have cell membrane antigens, detectable by immunofluorescence tests with live cells, which are not present in other cells of these patients (*19*). These antigens are present also in cultured BL cells and were shown to be EBV-determined (*17, 18*). When BL biopsy cells apparently failed to reveal EBV-determined membrane antigens, they usually were found to be coated with immune gamma globulin G, that is, the patients's antibodies.

Recently, zur Hausen and Schulte-Holthausen (*6*) reported the hybridization of ^{3}H labeled EB viral DNA with cellular DNA derived from cultured BL cells, including cells of the Raji line, which up to then had been thought to be free of EBV on the basis of electron microscopic examination and immunofluorescence tests (*4*). The equivalent of about 6 viral genomes were calculated to be in each Raji cell on the average. That every cultured BL cell indeed may harbor the EB viral genome was demonstrated by Zajac and Kohn (*28*) who raised clones from singly picked EB2 cells in the presence of antibodies to EBV at an efficiency of well over 40%. In an extension of the observations of Hinuma and co-workers (*16*) with cloned sublines of the P3J line of BL cells, every clone was found to contain a small proportion of VCA-producing cells, in spite of the fact that the parent culture revealed less than 1% VCA-positive cells.

Most recently, zur Hausen and co-workers (*7*) extended the DNA-DNA hybridization experiments to BL and NPC biopsies as well as to various control materials. All of 13 BL and 10 NPC biopsies revealed the presence of EB viral DNA equivalent to 1–26 viral genomes per cell. No EB viral DNA was found in biopsies of 10 other tumors, including 4 lymphoma and 3 Hodgkin's disease biopsies, even though all these patients had antibodies to EBV-related antigens and thus presumably were carriers of the virus.   No hybridization was observed between EBV ^{3}H-DNA and DNA derived from a Marek's disease tumor or from cells infected with herpes simplex (HSV) or cytomegalo viruses.   Furthermore, HSV ^{3}H-DNA failed to anneal with DNA derived from BL or NPC biopsies.   Thus, the EBV-specificity of the hybridization experiments seems assured.

These various studies have clearly shown an intimate association of EBV with Burkitt's lymphoma and NPC.   It remains to be ascertained whether the association of the virus with NPC is restricted to the lymphocytic elements of these tumors or extends also to the anaplastic carcinoma cells.

Induction of Tumors by EBV in Nonhuman Primates or Other Animals

In spite of numerous efforts in many laboratories, inoculation of EBV-containing materials into non-human primates or other animals have failed to date to produce tumors.   The failures in nonhuman primates may be ascribed, at least in part, to the fact that many of these animals were shown to have antibodies reacting with EBV-related antigens (5) and thus had been infected previously with EBV or a closely related agent.   In spite of its lack of success thus far, this approach deserves further exploration in view of the fact that several other members of the herpes group of viruses by now have been proven to possess oncogenic potentials.

Transformation of Lymphocytes by EBV

There is mounting evidence that EBV has a growth-stimulating effect on cells of the lymphocytic series in vivo as well as in vitro.   Cultures initiated with peripheral leucocytes from patients in the acute stage of infectious mononucleosis (IM) were shown to develop regularly and rapidly into continuous lines of lymphoblastoid cells, all harboring EBV in a small proportion of the cells (2, 3).   Leukocytes from healthy donors or patients with diseases other than IM also developed at times into lymphoblastoid cell lines, but growth commenced in these cases only after many weeks of cultivation.   These cultures, too, harbored EBV, indicating that the virus often persists in the lymphoreticular system after the primary infectious process and indeed, the presence of the virus most likely was responsible for the establishment of these lines.   This interpretation is supported by the observation that leucocytes from antibody-negative donors (not previously exposed to EBV) rarely grew in culture.

The growth-stimulating effect of EBV on leucocytes of antibody negative donors has been examined experimentally with the use of 3 different procedures: (a) by co-cultivation of leucocytes with lethally X-irradiated blastoid cells from EBV-positive lines (3, 15); (b) cultivation of leucocytes in cell free media from EBV-positive blastoid cell lines (24);   and (c) exposure of leucocytes to EBV separated from EBV-carrier cultures (12, 27).   Each of these techniques has led to the establishment of lymphoblastoid cell lines with a variable degree of frequency.   The EBV-specificity was documented variously by the facts that lethally X-irradiated cells from EBV-negative lines had no growth stimulating effect; that growth was prevented when EBV had been removed by filtration, or inactivated by heat or ultraviolet light, or neutralized by antibodies to EBV. All lines established by these procedures revealed the presence of EBV-related antigens in small proportions of the cells; that is, viral capsid antigens, EBV-induced early antigens, and EBV-determined cell membrane antigens. Those lines appropriately examined also showed the C-group marker chromosome (15) previously observed in cultured BL cells (21). While these results fulfill severall of the criteria established for transformation of normal cells by oncogenic animal viruses, they are insufficient to indicate that the lymphoblastoid cell lines so obtained are of a truly malignant nature.

Antibodies to EBV-related Antigens in Burkitt's Lymphoma and Nasopharyngeal Carcinoma

All African patients with BL (8, 10) as well as all African or Hong Kong Chinese patients with NPC (11, 14) were shown to have antibodies to VCA, usually at high titers with geometric means between 1:320 and 1:350. Nearly all of these patients were found to possess, in addition, antibodies to EBV determined cell membrane antigens (19, 25) and over 75% to have antibodies also to EBV-induced early antigens (9, 13). These serological data were in striking contrast to results obtained with appropriate control groups or patients with other malignancies of the lymphoreticular system or carcinomas of the head and neck other than NPC. Among the controls or patients with malignancies other than BL or NPC, some were found who had no detectable antibodies to EBV-related antigens and the others showed, as a rule, only low titers. Yet, a few individuals in every one of these groups had relatively high antibody titers which might reflect recent primary or superinfections or high levels of latent, persistent EBV carrier states.

Recent observations, discussed elsewhere in this symposium, indicate that the levels of antibodies to EA reflect to a considerable extent the prognosis of BL patients with respect to the likelihood of recurrent tumors after chemotherapeutically induced remissions. The data revealed that patients with persistently high or rising anti-EA titers are more prone to show relapses, at times as late as 5 years after the initial treatment, than patients with no or low and declining levels of anti-EA (9).

These observations provide further impetus to horizontal studies on patients with BL or NPC from the time of admission through remissions and recurrences. Frequent determinations of antibodies to the viral capsid, early, and cell membrane antigen complexes as well as of precipitating antibodies might reveal changes in titers or patterns of these reactivities referable to preceding or subsequent clinical events and, in turn, provide further evidence of the role played by EBV in these malignancies. That this approach may yield significant information is suggested by the results obtained with the first BL patient so studied (20). During a period of tumor remission of more than 3 years the patient maintained high levels of antibodies to VCA, EA, and MA but the precipitation test was negative. Anti-MA then declined to insignificant levels a few months prior to the detection of a recurrent tumor to which the patient succumbed. Antibodies to MA reappeared, the anti-VCA and anti-EA titers increased to some extent, and precipitating antibodies now became detectable as the recurrent tumor grew in size. While the persistence of anti-EA was in line with its prognostic implications, the loss of anti-MA might have been responsible for the regrowth of the tumor from surviving malignant cells. Before this interpretation can be accepted many additional patients must be studied in this manner to determine whether the pattern observed in this patient is reproducible in other similar cases.

The data discussed have indicated a close association of EBV certainly with BL and, to a considerable extent, also with NPC. Whether this association reflects an etiologic role of EBV in these malignancies or whether the virus represents merely a passenger is still an unsettled question. While evidence in favor of the first alternative seems to be growing, none of the observations rigidly exclude the second possibility.

The author's work was supported by research grant CA-4568 and contract PH-43-66-477 within the Special Virus Leukemia Program, National Cancer Institute, National Institutes of Health, U. S. Public Health Service.

REFERENCES

1. Cohen, M. H., Hirshaut, Y., Stevens, D., Hull, E. W., and Carbone, P. P. Infectious Mononucleosis Followed by Burkitt's Tumor. Annals Int. Med., *73*: 591, 1970.

2. Diehl, V., Henle, G., Henle, W., and Kohn, G. Demonstration of a Herpes Group Virus in Cultures of Peripheral Leukocytes from Patients with Infectious Mononucleosis. J. Virol., *2*: 663, 1968.

3. Diehl, V., Henle, G., Henle, W., and Kohn, G. Effect of a Herpes Group Virus (EBV) on Growth of Peripheral Leukocyte Cultures. *In vitro*, *4*: 92, 1969.

4. Epstein, M. A., Achong, B. G., Barr, Y. M., Zajac, B., Henle, G., and Henle, W., Morphological and Virological Investigations on Cultured Burkitt Tumor Lymphoblasts (Strain Raji). J. Nat. Cancer Inst., *37*: 547, 1966.

5. Gerber, P., and Birch, S. M. Complement-fixing Antibodies in Sera of Human and Nonhuman Primates to Viral Antigens Derived from Burkitt's Lymphoma Cells. Proc. Nat. Acad. Sci., *58*: 478, 1967.

6. zur Hausen, H., and Schulte-Holthausen, H. Presence of EB Virus Nucleic Acid Homology in a " Virus-free " Line of Burkitt Tumour Cells. Nature, *227*: 245, 1970.

7. zur Hausen, H., Schulte-Holthausen, H., Klein, G., Henle, W., Henle, G., Clifford, P., and Santesson, L. EB-virus DNA in Biopsies of Burkitt Tumours and Anaplastic Carcinomas of the Nasopharynx. Nature, *228*: 1056–1057, 1970.

8. Henle, G., and Henle, W. Immunofluorescence in Cells Derived from Burkitt's Lymphoma. J. Bact., *91*: 1248, 1966.

9. Henle, G., Henle, W., Klein, G., Gunven, P., Clifford, P., Morrow, R. H., and Ziegler, J. L. Antibodies to Early EBV-induced Antigens in Burkitt's Lymphoma. J. Nat. Cancer Inst., *46*: 861–871, 1971.

10. Henle, G., Henle, W., Clifford, P., Diehl, V., Kafuko, G., Kirya, B.G., Klein, G., Morrow, R. H., Munube, G. M. R., Pike, P., Tukei, P. M., and Ziegler, J. L. Antibodies to Epstein-Barr Virus in Burkitt's Lymphoma and Control Groups. J. Nat. Cancer Inst., *43*: 1147, 1969.

11. Henle, G., Henle, W., and Diehl, V. Relation of Burkitt's Tumor-associated Herpes-type Virus to Infectious Mononucleosis. Procd. Nat. Acad. Sci., *59*: 94, 1968.

12.   Henle, W., and Henle, G.   Evidence for a Relation of Epstein-Barr Virus to Burkitt's Lymphoma and Nasopharyngeal Carcinoma.   IVth International Symposium on Comparative Leukemia Research, Cherry Hill, N. J. S. Karger AG Basel, 1969.

13.   Henle, W., Henle, G., Zajac, B., Pearson, G., Waubke, R., and Scriba, M.   Differential Reactivity of Human Serums with Early Antigens Induced by Epstein-Barr Virus.   Science, *169*: 188, 1970.

14.   Henle, W., Henle, G., Ho, H.-G., Burtin, P., Cachin, Y., Clifford, P., de Schryver, A., de Thé, G., Diehl, V., and Klein, G.   Antibodies to Epstein-Barr Virus in Nasopharyngeal Carcinoma, Other Head and Neck Neoplasms, and Control Groups. J. Nat. Cancer Inst., *44*: 225, 1970.

15.   Henle, W., Diehl, V., Kohn, G., zur Hausen, H., and Henle, G.   Herpes-type Virus and Chromosome Marker in Normal Leukocytes after Growth with Irradiated Burkitt Cells.   Science, *157*: 1064, 1967.

16.   Hinuma, Y., Konn, M., Yamaguchi, J., Wudarski, D. J., Blakeslee, J. R., Jr., and Grace, J. T., Jr.   Immunofluorescence and Herpes-type Virus Particles in the P3-HR-1 Burkitt Lymphoma Cell Line.   J. Virol., *1*: 1045, 1967.

17.   Klein, G., Pearson, G., Henle, G., Henle, W., Goldstein, G., and Clifford, P.   Relation between Epstein-Barr Viral and Cell Membrane Immunofluorescence in Burkitt Tumor Cells.   III. Comparison of Blocking of Direct Membrane Immunofluorescence and Anti-EBV Reactivities of Different Sera.   J. Exper. Med., *129*: 697, 1969.

18.   Klein, G., Pearson, G., Nadkarni, J. S., Nadkarni, J. J., Klein, E., Henle, G., Henle, W., and Clifford, P.   Relation between Epstein-Barr Viral and Cell Membrane Immunofluorescence of Burkitt Tumor Cells.   I. Dependence of Cell Membrane Immunofluorescence on Presence of EB Virus.   J. Exper. Med., *128*: 1011, 1968.

19.   Klein, G., Clifford, P., Klein, E., Smith, R. T., Minowada, J., Kourilsky, F. M., and Burchenal, J. H.   Membrane Immunofluorescence Reactions of Burkitt Lymphoma Cells from Biopsy Specimens and Tissue Cultures.   J. Nat. Cancer Inst., *39*: 1027, 1967.

20.   Klein, G., Clifford, P., Henle, G., Henle, W., Geering, G., and Old, L. J.   EBV-associated Serological Patterns in a Burkitt Lymphoma Patient during Regression and Recurrence.   Int. J. Cancer, *4*: 416, 1969.

21.   Kohn, G., Mellman, W. J., Moorhead, P. S., Loftus, J., and Henle, G.   Involvement of C Group Chromosomes in Five Burkitt Lymphoma Cell Lines.   J. Nat. Cancer Inst., *38*: 209, 1967.

22.   Nadkarni, J. S., Nadkarni, J. J., Klein, G., Henle, W., Henle, G., and Clifford, P.   EB Viral Antigens in Burkitt Tumor Biopsies and Early Cultures.   Int. J. Cancer, *6*: 10, 1970.

23.   Niederman, J. C., McCollum, R. W., Henle, G., and Henle, W.   Infectious Mononucleosis.   Clinical Manifestations in Relation to EB Virus Antibodies.   J.A.M.A., *203*: 205, 1968.

24.   Pope, J. H., Horne, M. K., and Scott, W.   Identification of the Filtrable Leukocyte-transforming Factor of QIMR–WIL Cells as Herpes-like Virus.   Int. J. Cancer, *4*: 255, 1969.

25.   de Schryver, A., Fribert, S. Jr., Klein, G., Henle, W., Henle, G., de-Thé, G., Clifford, P., and Ho, H.-C.   Epstein-Barr Virus-associated Antibody Patterns in Carcinoma of the Post-nasal Space.   Clin. Exper. Immun., *5*: 443, 1969.

26.   de-Thé, G., Ho, H.-C., Kwan, H.-C., Desgranges, D., and Favre, M. C.   Nasopharyngeal Carcinoma (NPC).   I. Types of Cultures Derived from Tumour Biopsies and

Nontumorous Tissues of Chinese Patients with Special Reference to Lymphoblastoid Transformation.   Int. J. Cancer, *6*: 189, 1970.

27. Gerber, P., Whang-Peng, J., and Monroe, J. H.   Transformation and Chromosome Changes Induced by Epstein-Barr Virus in Normal Human Leukocyte Cultures. Proc. Nat. Acad. Sci., *63*: 740, 1969.

28. Zajac, B. A., and Kohn, G. Epstein-Barr Virus Antigens, Marker Chromosome, and Interferon Production in Clones Derived from Cultured Burkitt Tumor Cells. J. Nat. Cancer Inst.   Cancer Inst., *45*: 399, 1970.

Discussion of Papers by Drs. G. Henle, Hinuma, and W. Henle

DR. NAKAHARA: Where do infectious mononucleosis cells come from? Are there any primary foci somewhere in the body? I think that just because mononucleosis is infectious, there is no reason why it must be excluded from the territory of cancer research. I am interested in increasing the territory of cancer research.

DR. G. HENLE: One problem here is that infectious mononucleosis is not often fatal and is a disease of children; this does not permit unnecessary procedures such as biopsies, lymph node punctures, *etc.*, without the parents' permission. By the time the parents' permission is obtained it would be too late. It is likely that information must be obtained on the question you have been asking. One might consider infectious mononucleosis as an abortive neoplastic disease; I would like to know what is going on there. Factors that limit cell proliferation in mononucleosis may be lacking in neoplastic disease and their identification would be important.

DR. G. KLEIN: As we shall hear later during the symposium, Dr. Nishioka and his group have evidence of a receptor on the surface of cells derived from infectious mononucleosis (IA receptor) that is similar to the lymphoblastoid lines derived from NPC and different from the lines derived from BL that have another (IgG) receptor.

DR. SOUTHAM: In the original definition, the term tumor-specific transplantation immunity has been used in relation to a compatible host, autochthonous or syngeneic. If we extend " compatibility " to other allogeneic xenogeneic hosts that do not have an intact rejection mechanism, we have a broader possibility. To immunologically depressed recipients, there may be a correlation between transplantability and the malignancy of the transplanted tissue. I refer to cortisone-treated animals and to the cheek pouch of the untreated hamster and also to my own work in patients with advanced cancer who are in an immunologically depressed state. More recently, we have used immunologically tolerant rats made tolerant by the intravenous injection of the cell line that is being studied with reference to transplantability. On the assumption that there was a correlation between malignancy and transplantability, we studied about 75 lymphoblastoid cell lines by intravenous inoculation of newborn rats and subcutaneous or intraperitoneal transplantation into tolerant rats. We obtained positive takes with many Burkitt cell lines and acute leukemia lines, with tumor growth and involvement of many organs, particularly when the cells were given intravenously.

Many lines from Burkitt's lymphoma and leukemia could not be transplanted; however, I do not think this is particularly bothersome because we cannot assume that all lines really represent the malignant cell. They may be derived from non-malignant cells, even though they carry virus or viral genome.

We tested approximately 20 cell lines established by Dr. George Moore and his group, derived from normal peripheral blood leucocytes. None of these grew. Some other lines of nonmalignant origin did grow in both kinds of recipients. One of them was a normal cell line established from the normal lymph node of a donor with pernicious anemia and no evidence of neoplastic disease. We also had growth from 3 of 4 cell lines derived from infectious mononucleosis.

Our initial interpretation was that the transplantability was not an acceptable criterion of malignancy. Perhaps this conclusion was hasty, since these cell lines were probably infected with EBV and carried the viral genome.

DR. EPSTEIN: I am very glad that this was brought up. About this technique, sometimes I have the feeling that a large number of cells are needed for growth to occur. Is there any evidence that what you see histologically in these animals is lymphoma or some other type of malignant disease?

DR. SOUTHAM: Cytologically, the cells are identical; they are readily recognized and increase in involved organs exactly as they grow in tissue culture. Chromosome analysis confirms that the transplanted cells grow. When transplanted subcutaneously, they remained localized, intact, and did not grow. Given intraperitoneally, there was local invasion throughout the abdominal cavity but no metastasis. We did obtain true metastasis with one cell line derived from cancer but not with Burkitt or leukemia lines. When the cells were injected intravenously, we got widespread growth involving the eye, brain, adrenals, lungs, and sometimes the kidney. Tissue distribution was different with different cells, but we cannot say whether this is an equivalent of metastasis or infiltration because the cells moved as the direct result of inoculation. In short, I don't think that we have any other parameter in transplantation experiments than the fact of growth and the cytological character of the cell that has grown.

DR. G. KLEIN: Dr. Southam, your work on the xenograft system was very interesting. I was convinced that you have demonstrated a maligant potential in the tumor-derived lines where you obtained positive takes. The lines derived from nontumor patients may often either represent dormant tumor cells or malignant transformation *in vitro* due either to EBV or other, unknown causes. Absence of proliferative growth is more difficult to interpret; however, it may be due to rejection or to the lack of malignant potential, at least in relation to the rat host. I think it would be necessary to scrutinize the negative lines very carefully for the presence of EBV and associated antigens. If negative lines are found, after the application of all methods, including CF tests and perhaps nucleic acid hybridization as well, one could try to infect such lines with EBV, and see whether this makes any difference. If no EBV antigen-free lines can be found, this would be interesting as well.

DR. YAN: I have two questions. First to either Dr. Hinuma or Dr. G. Henle. Do you have any idea of the type of immunoglobulin reacting with the EA of Henle or the new antigen of Hinuma?

DR. G. HENLE: It reacted with Hyland's anti-IgG.

DR. KLEIN: Is it mono-specific?

DR. G. HENLE: No.

DR. G. KLEIN: Does Dr. Hinuma have the same situation?

DR. HINUMA: Yes.

DR. YAN: Second, how do you standardize your target cell for detecting anti-EA antibody?

DR. G. HENLE: Given numbers of cells were infected with virus dilutions adjusted to induce EA antigen but no VCA. The cultured virus came from Pfizer's laboratory. We use a 1:50, a 1:100 or a 1:200 dilution of the virus, depending upon the batches. The virus was stored in a very large number of ampoules in a liquid nitrogen container because the virus is not stable at $-70°C$ and we had to have a very large number of ampoules which had been titrated first. We used the same ampoule to make 400 to 600 smears at any one time by one technician and we used the same batch of antigens.

DR. G. KLEIN: I would like to ask Dr. Hinuma to comment on his procedure; I would also like to ask the following question. You said your antigen might be identical with Henle's EA antigen but you were not quite sure. You showed a slightly different reactivity distribution in relation to the various patients' sera in comparison with Dr. Henle but these differences may not be significant and depend on the relatively small number of samples. Do you have any other reason to say whether yours and Henle's antigen are different or identical?

DR. HINUMA: I have no idea what to say about this because I have only data that the antigen is different from the virion antigen. That is all. I don't know whether our antigen is the same as Henle's EA or not. My feeling is that our antigen appears a little later, around five days.

DR. G. KLEIN: I think that the difference in the time of the appearance of the antigen may be entirely dependent on the dose of the virus. It seems to me that you are probably dealing with the same early antigen as Dr. Henle.

DR. DE THÉ: Dr. Henle, you said that it was not possible to obtain lympho-blastoid lines from sero-negative donors. I think that K. Nilsson obtained lym-phoblastoid lines from anti-VCA-negative individuals. Am I wrong?

DR. W. HENLE: This is true, but the patient from whom this cell line was obtained was 64 years old and may have been previously sero-positive. Also, very low antibody titers are not detectable at 1:10 dilutions of sera. Dr. Nilsson has now set up 27 human embryonic spleen and lymph node cultures. None of these cultures grew, whereas he had 100% success with lymph node cultures obtained from operations on adults. None of the embryo sera had anti-VCA antibody.

DR. DE THÉ: The is very important in any seroepidemiological study, because when VCA type antibody is negative, this would mean that the patient has no virus. On the other hand, if you can establish permanent lines from EBV negative patient, this does not hold.

DR. G. HENLE: I don't quite think so, because Dr. Nilsson explants lymph nodes from patients under surgery and this is a somewhat different situation. With other viruses, a few cells can contain virus with no/or only small quantities of meas-urable antibody.

DR. DE THÉ: The only criterion we now have to say that a child has not been infected by EB virus is the negativity of the available serological tests. If the serological tests do not reflect this, i.e., if negativity does not mean that the individual has not been infected, the whole seroepidemiological and prospective study can be questioned. Sero-conversion does not have to mean new infection in that case. It can be due to internal reinfection as in herpes simplex. For internal reasons, when a boostering occurs, the antibody titer might rise without external infection.

DR. G. KLEIN: The distribution of the anti-EBV(VCA) titers may give some information on this question. In Dr. Henle's test, the cut-off point is at a 1:10 serum dilution. If one looks at the distribution curve, the extreme left of the Gaussian curve is lacking, indicating that a <10 titer category contains both sera that are really positive and sera that may be truly negative. The prospective studies of Niederman and Evans are relevant in this respect, because they show that true negatives really exist. Whereas sero-positive students did not develop any cases of mononucleosis in the course of 2 years, 20% of the sero-negative (by the <10 criterion) students developed infectious mononucleosis. This must mean that at least 20% of the negative (<10) group must be truly negative. If all the Burkitt's lymphoma developed in the small negative group, this would be meaningful no matter how many false negatives were included in this group. Is there any other comment?

DR. HINUMA: I would like to ask a question of Dr. Henle. We don't have a high incidence of infectious mononucleosis in Japan but you have many cases in your country. Someone has called it the "kissing disease" indicating probably that the free virus may infect some particular type of cells of individuals whose EBV antibody titers are negative. Do you believe in horizontal transmission? Do you have any virologically suggestive data that free virus can be isolated by some susceptible cells?

DR. W. HENLE: As you pointed out, the genetic factor in relation to susceptibility is to be considered but you have antibody, haven't you? Don't be afraid of "kissing disease." We really do not know the transmission. Of course, originally, we did not have any techniques to transmit the virus of infectious mononucleosis. It is now time to try again since at least it is possible to transmit something to the proper cells such as Raji or other cells.

DR. EPSTEIN: One thing might be useful at this point. Surely, isn't the situation of human mononucleosis at the same stage as Marek's disease a few years ago?

At that time, it was quite clear that the disease was infectious because of the evidence of explosive outbreaks among chickens kept together in close quarters, but nobody at that time could find any site of infectious viruses. It only became apparent when the virus was produced in the cells lining the feather follicles and was shed into the atmosphere that the chickens were inhaling. In that way, we could be sure where the infectious virus was elaborating. I am quite sure that the situation in human infectious mononucleosis is the same. I am not suggesting the feather follicles but there must be some undetected site where the virus is elaborated in humans.

DR. G. HENLE: We have been trying to isolate EB virus from tonsils obtained from our otolaryngologists but there, millions of adenovirus particles are present and overgrow everything.

DR. NELSON: I wonder if one of the criteria Dr. Henle mentioned for cheering the virus-causes-tumor-idea could be extended to include criteria which are consistent with viral etiology in the demonstration of a common tumor-specific antigen within the tumor, regardless of whether we suspected a particular virus or not. I mention this because I want to refer to our work on nasopharyngeal cancer done in Singapore, looking at the tumor cells themselves, not the lymphoblastoid type derived from biopsy, but tumor cells in frozen section. We looked at patient's sera by indirect immunofluorescence to try to detect anti-tumor autoantibodies. In about half the patients, 28 sera we got at the initial bleeding at the time of biopsy, 4 had antibodies to tumor cell nucleus. Of those, one was anti-nuclear factor, generally not tumor-specific, and 9 had antibodies reacting with tumor cell membranes in the frozen section. When we tested these sera against sections from patients from whom the sera were not obtained, we found that the antigens were common to tumor cells. This actually means that carcinoma or epithelial cells have common tumor-specific antigens. In fact, it is not a completely tumor-specific antigen, and occasionally normal epithelial cells from normal biopsies reacted; the other thing we found was that 1 out of 10 normal blood donors also had antibodies to nucleus or cytoplasm. This is consistent with the general idea that the nasopharyngeal carcinoma itself is caused by, or associated with, the virus.

DR. G. KLEIN: I am not sure at present that such a thing as a completely tumor-specific antigen exists. Certainly, as far as the virus-associated antigens are concerned, and perhaps in some chemically-induced tumors as well, the tumor-associated antigen can be found in certain normal cells as well. This is the case for polyoma, SV40, the various murine leukemia agents, etc. In this respect, EBV antigens are no different from the classical tumor-associated antigens.

DR. YOSHIDA: I would like to ask if you hvae data on anti-EA antibody titers in other cancer patients?

DR. G. HENLE: We have tested chronic lymphocytic leukemia and Hodgkin's disease but we have not yet looked at other cancers.

DR. G. KLEIN: Could we ask Dr. Green about two points? What techniques would you advise using to detect EBV-specific messenger RNA in cells that carry the viral genome, have virus determined antigens, but make no virus? The second question is what approach you would suggest in studying the question of whether EBV-DNA is integrated with the host cell DNA.

DR. GREEN: First, you need to have standard early and late transformed mRNA able to be recognized in hybridization competition. And, perhaps you need lots of by bridization competition, otherwise in doing this with polyacril amidgel, you cannot recognize the specific messengers. We now characterize all the messengers produced in adenovirus-infected cells and we can identify the early transformed and late messengers.

Secondly is you have a more sensitive procedure if you use hybridization competition; where you are using unlabeled RNA in various biopsy materials you can't label the RNA there, so that you should use direct hybridization in this case. Using a known population of mRNA in that case and in the case of DNA, this might be very easily done by taking very small amounts of Burkitt's. EBV-DNA and making complementary copies; we did this with adenovirus. Under these conditions you can detect very, very small numbers of messenger molecules per cell, on the order of 10 to 100. Concerning the second question of integration, it is very easy. All you need there is, again, about a microgram of DNA of which you make complementary RNA copies. This is very, very radioactive and the complementary RNA will be detected in 0.01 μg of viral DNA and cell DNA population. There you can take cultures and immobilize on a filter and identify this RNA complementary to EBV-DNA; this has been done, first with SV40, then polyoma and adenovirus, the procedure, which has just been reported by Galbin and Martin, detects one SV40 genome in an SV40 transformed cell. This is reassociation kinetics combined by complementary RNA. You take the cell DNA from biopsy material and you reassociate it *in vitro* and, depending upon the number of copies of viral DNA you get associated at a certain time interval, you can detect this by using viral DNA or complementary RNA just to find out what frequency. I am not sure I have come across very clearly. It is complex and difficult to explain but it is easy to do.

DR. G. KLEIN: zur Hausen is presently making complementary RNA to EBV-DNA. So the reagent should be available. With regard to early " transformed " and late mRNA populations, the early product might be obtained from infected cells where DNA synthesis has been inhibited. The late could be obtained from permissive cultures and the " transformed " form Raji or from viable biopsy specimens.

DR. GREEN: The system is ready for molecular biology where we are now working. We don't have to say much about it. We are making complementary RNA and we are tying up with such an experiment. I think it is a good system and should yield further information.

EBV-INDUCED MEMBRANE ANTIGENS

Chairmen:

Takeshi Hirayama, George Klein

Membrane Antigen Changes in Burkitt Lymphoma Cells

George KLEIN

Department of Tumor Biology, Karolinska Institutet, Stockholm, Sweden

The studies of the author and his associates have been supported by the Swedish Cancer Society, by Grant CA-04747 and Contract No. NIH-69–2005 from the National Institutes of Health and a grant from the Damon Runyon Foundation.

Most of the work reported here has been carried out in collaboration with Drs. Peter Clifford, W. Henle, G. Henle, J. Yata, J. Stjernswärd, E. Klein, T. Tachibana, K. Nishioka, G. Goldstein, G. Pearson, L. Gergely, A. de Schryver, B. Johansson, P. Gunvén, and Nina and Jerzy Einhorn, as reported in the technical publications listed.

After it had become clear that all virus induced experimental tumors carry a common, group specific transplantation antigen, we asked the question whether it would be possible to obtain evidence, by testing the reactivity of live Burkitt's lymphoma (BL) cells, with patients' sera, and in comparison with appropriate controls, that would indicate the existence of characteristic cell membrane associated antigens, in analogy with the virally induced murine leukemias and, if so, whether this information could help to elucidate the etiology of the disease, as well as the possible role of host defense reactions that may influence its clinical course. To approach this problem, we chose the technique that was most sensitive in the experimental leukemia studies (*45, 59*), *viz.*, membrane immunofluorescence with viable target cells (*70*). The findings, summarized briefly in the following chapters, essentially confirmed the expectations, but they have also led to many unexpected observations and raised new dilemmas. Some of them may serve to exemplify the problems encountered during the transition from the experimental to the human situation.

Studies on BL Biopsy Cells

During the first phase of this work, fresh BL biopsy cells were exposed to the sera of BL patients and various other donors; we were looking for attached immunoglobulins by the indirect membrane fluorescence technique (*44, 53, 54*).   The sera of BL patients reacted more frequently than African control sera from donors with other neoplastic or non-neoplastic diseases.   The possibility that the reactivity of the BL sera was due to isoantibodies became unlikely when it was found that autochthonous serum-cell combinations gave positive reactions in five of six cases where this could be tested.   It turned out, furthermore, that the most regularly positive sera have been derived from patients whose tumors have gone to total regression after chemotherapy.   For this reason, the autochthonous target cell was frequently unavailable as far as the highly positive serum donors were concerned. To exclude isoantibodies, such sera were tested in parallel series against lymphoma cells and normal bone marrow cells derived from the same allogeneic BL donor. Lymphoma cells, but not bone marrow cells, reacted regularly in such tests, thus increasing the probability that the reactivity of the BL serum-cell combinations could not be simply due to the presence of isoantibodies.   This was further reinforced by the finding that lymphoid cells of normal donors and of donors with different types of leukemias and other lymphoreticular diseases also failed to react.

While this was encouraging, further studies on the specificity of the reaction were hampered by the great variability of the biopsy preparations.   One major source of the difficulty was the variable degree of the immunoglobulin coating on the surface of the biopsy cells.   This coating was detected by direct membrane immunofluorescence with conjugated anti-immunoglobulin reagents.   It could be of two basically different kinds: IgM and/or IgG, showing not only a difference in class specificity but also a difference in behavior in relation to the course of the disease (*46, 51*).   In the cases where the cell surface reacted with anti-IgM conjugates, reactivity was usually expressed in 100 percent or nearly 100 percent on the cells.   When such cells were converted into established lines *in vitro*, their " IgM-ring " was maintained during longterm propagation.   The membrane-IgM reactive lines did not secrete IgM into the medium (*17*).

The IgG coat behaved quite differently.   It was rarely present on untreated BL biopsy cells, but tended to appear if the tumor persisted in spite of treatment. It accumulated following a recurrence that was presumably due to the selection of a tetraploid, probably immunoresistant, BL cell variant (*10, 51*).   " Self-enhancement," *i.e.*, the accumulation of " blocking " antibodies that prevent the access of immune lymphoid cells (*30*) is an obvious possibility.

Whether these considerations are realistic or not, the changing pattern of IgG coating with time and its failure to persist on derived *in vitro* lines (*46, 71*), indicate that it is due to coating from the outside, unlike the membrane associated IgM, which appears to represent a special type of production from the inside.

The presence of preformed immunoglobulin on the cell surface may interfere with the indirect membrane immunofluorescence reaction and, when present in subliminal degree, it probaly explains some of the variability encountered when biopsy cells are used as targets.   In order to avoid this variability, we started looking for more standardized target cells and turned to established culture lines.

Experiments with Established Tissue Culture Lines

A number of BL-derived lymphoblastoid cell lines growing in stationary suspension cultures were tested against BL sera that reacted regularly with BL biopsy cells and were free of demonstrable isoantibodies (*52*). The pattern appeared strange but interesting. Four BL-derived lines gave positive membrane immunofluorescence reactions in the indirect test, after exposure to the reference serum " Mutua " (derived from a BL patient in long-term regression), whereas three BL-derived lines were negative. Eight control lines derived from various leukemias and, in one case, from a normal donor, were negative as well. At first, we could not understand this pattern. A clue was obtained, however, when these results were compared with the reactivity of the same cell lines in the Henle test (*31*) known to detect EB-viral (probably nucleocapsid) antigens. In carrier cultures, these antigens are present in a small frequency of the cells, as a rule. These cells show degenerative features and, when simultaneous immunofluoresence and electron microscopy is performed (*25, 32*) turn out to contain herpes-type Epstein-Barr (EB) virus (*13*) particles. The first comparison of the membrane and EBV test revealed (*60*) that the four membrane positive lines contained EBV antigens in more than 1% of the cells, whereas the membrane-negative lines were either EBV-negative or contained a very small frequency of positive cells (less than 1%).

This suggested that the membrane antigen detected by this reference serum may be determined by the genome of the EB virus. More conclusive evidence was obtained in a prospective study (*60*). Fourteen new lines were established from biopsies received from Nairobi, and the frequency of EBV positive and of membrane reactive cells was determined in parallel, on coded specimens, at two different laboratories. The same relationship was found as in the preliminary retrospective study: only the lines that carried a relatively high " EBV-load " showed a positive membrane antigen reactivity. In the reactive lines, the frequency of membrane positive cells was approximately ten times higher than the frequency of EBV-positive cells. The biopsies from which the lines were derived were membrane positive, but EBV-negative, as a rule. EBV reactivity appeared during the first week in culture. This suggests that the production of the viral nucleocapsid antigen is suppressed in the tumor cell *in vivo*. The suppressive factor could be antibody, but there are many other possibilities. Another curious observation was that repeated establishment of parallel lines from the same patient, derived from successive biopsies, led to lines with fairly similar EBV levels, whereas lines derived from different patients were quite different (*72*). This suggests that the viral " load " per cell, or the activatability of the virus, or both, are characteristic for the individual tumor. Since the membrane-associated IgM marker, mentioned above, and another study with G6PD-isozyme markers (*16*) strongly indicate that the BL process has a clonal origin, this may reflect the virus-cell relationship that characterizes a particular clone. This is also suggested by the closely similar levels of EBV-DNA hybridizable cellular DNA in repeated biopsies taken from multiple tumors from the same BL patient (*27*).

The postulate that the membrane antigen is determined by the EB virus was directly confirmed when it was found that it could be induced to appear in EBV negative lines by the admixture of heavily irradiated EBV carrying cells (*58*), or by infection with EBV concentrates (*19, 37*).   In the infected cells, membrane antigens appeared after 20–24 hr.   DNA-inhibitors, such as cytosine arabinoside (Ara C) or IUDR, did not prevent its appearance, whereas puromycin inhibited it completely.   It behaves, in other words, like an " early " product of the viral genome, not requiring viral DNA synthesis.   In this respect, it shows certain parallels with membrane and T antigens found in experimental oncogenic DNA virus systems (*11, 66, 86*).

Although the relationship between EBV and the membrane antigen was clarified by these studies, this applies only to the EBV-carrier cultures *in vitro* and it must be kept in mind that similar compelling evidence is lacking about the connection between the membrane antigens detected on the biopsy cells and thè virus, although there are strong indications that the biopsy cells probably express the same membrane antigen as the carrier cultures (*96*).

The antigenic components entering the EBV-determined membrane and the intracellular nucleocapsid complex differ with regard to immunological specificity. By absorbing sera that reacted with the membrane and the intracellular EBV complex as well, with large numbers of intact, viable membrane antigen-positive cells it was possible to remove the membrane reactive antibodies, with only a minor reduction in the anti-EBV titer (*82*).   Moreover, some sera could be found with antibodies against the membrane antigen, or the EBV antigen, but not both.   Although such " discordant " sera were in the minority, their existence is in line with the immunological distinctness of the two antigen types.

Further analysis of the two antigen systems revealed (*100*) that both the membrane and the intracellular antigens must be regarded as antigen complexes, with several distinct subcomponets.   Sera that contain antibodies against several subcomponents of the intracellular EBV complex also tend to carry, as a rule, several antibody components against various parts of the membrane antigen complex, but the relationship is not absolute and many combinations can be found.   Patients with large, persisting tumors frequently had a larger number of serum antibody components against both antigen complexes than sera from healthy, EBV positive individuals, or convalescent sera from donors after infectious mononucleosis, or sera from BL patients whose tumors have gone to long term regression following chemotherapy.

The nature of the membrane antigen, particularly its specification by the viral or the cellular genome remains to be clarified.   Recently, indirect evidence has accumulated suggesting that it may represent a viral envelope component.   The ability of different sera to neutralize an artificial EBV infection of EBV negative culture lines (such as Raji or 6410) was related to the titer of membrane reactive antibody, and not to the anti-EBV titer (*81*).   This was particularly apparent when a series of sera were tested that were discordant with regard to their anti-EBV and membrane reactivity.   In another series of tests, the sera of rabbits immunized with EBV concentrates were able to block the membrane antigen reaction specifically

(*3*). This indicated that the membrane antigen was present in the immunizing material, either as a constituent or as a contaminant of the viral particles.

It has been shown that herpes simplex virus (HSV) is capable of inducing new membrane antigens in the cells it infects (*89*). Viral mutants with different envelope characteristics induce different membrane changes, in a way that closely parallels their envelope properties (*88*). It has been concluded that the appearance of envelope material is responsible for the changes in the cell membrane. Presumably, the virus changes the cellular membrane in order to facilitate the process of its own envelopment. In view of the parallel between EBV neutralization and membrane reactive antibody levels, it is conceivable that the EBV associated membrane antigen represents viral envelope material as well. This is of interest, because, for HSV, a relationship has been demonstrated between the changed " social behavior " of infected cells and their membrane modifications after exposure to different mutants of HSV (*88*). The understanding of the role EBV induced membrane changes might play for cell behavior may elucidate the relationship between this agent and the neoplastic diseases with which it is most regularly associated.

Disease-related Serological Patterns

This can be discussed at two levels: a) the relationship between EBV-associated serological reactivity and the clinical and pathological diagnosis; and b) changes in EBV-related serological patterns during the clinical course of EBV-associated diseases.

a) The relationship between EBV-associated serological reactivity and the clinical and pathological diagnosis

Concerning a), it can be first stated that the serological anti-EBV reactivity, as determined by the Henle test (*31*) is extremely widespread in all human populations. If the level of significant reactivity is set at a 1:10 serum dilution, as is customary (*33*), the large majority of adult populations are EBV-positive. It may be questioned whether the 10–15% negatives (with titers $<$10) are real or spurious. Specific antibodies may occur at titers below 10 and may be missed, due to the various test artifacts that arise at high serum concentrations (*33*). On the other hand, whereas some of the $<$10 " negatives " may hide specific reactivity, at least some of them must be real negatives in the biological sense. A prospective study (*74*) has shown that EBV-positive young adults are protected from infectious mononucleosis, whereas a considerable proportion of the " EBV-negatives " (*i.e.* $<$10) developed the disease and became EBV-positive, in the course of a 2–4 years' observation period.

The causal relationship between EBV and at least one form of infectious mononucleosis (*34*) is most clearly established by this prospective study. If this is accepted, it immediately leads to the question of whether EBV plays any role in other diseases, particularly the neoplastic diseases with which it is most regularly associated.

The serological patterns that are now known can be evaluated in different ways. In the Henle type anti-EBV test, Burkitt's lymphoma (BL) and nasopharyngeal carcinoma (NPC) are distinguished by outstandingly high anti-EBV titers, so far unparallelled amongst other lymphoproliferative diseases and other carcinomas of the head and neck region (33, 38, 42, 91). The geometric mean anti-EBV titer of BL patients was eight times higher than in various control groups. There were no significant differences between control sera collected from areas with a high or a low incidence of Burkitt's lymphoma. With the exception of a few, moribund cases, low (<1:80) anti-EBV titers were very rare among BL patients and there are no histologically confirmed cases with negative (<1:10) titers. Occasionally, long term regression cases tended to show falling titers after some years, but this was by no means the rule. The serological behavior of BL and NPC is also exceptional in the precipitin test developed by Old, Oettgen et al. (77, 78), performed against a soluble antigen extracted from the EBV-carrying P3J line. NPC sera from African and American patients were positive in 85–87% and 59% of the African BL sera gave positive precipitin reactions. Other neoplasms, including lymphoproliferative diseases and carcinomas of different kinds gave a much lower incidence of positives, with the exceptions of chronic lymphatic leukemia and lymphosarcoma that came close to the reactivity of the BL sera. Two distinct precipitin lines (B and P) could be identified regularly but there was no obvious disease related difference between the two.

The antibodies against the EBV-associated membrane antigens can be most easily evaluated by the blocking of the direct membrane fluorescence reaction, obtained with specific reference conjugates (21, 55). When the Mutua conjugate was used, already referred to in a previous paragraph, Burkitt's lymphoma (22) and nasopharyngeal carcinoma sera (91) showed a high blocking activity, whereas the sera of normal African controls, Burkitt patients relatives, and African tonsillitis patients showed mostly negative reactions, even though occasional positives were encountered. Head and neck tumors, other than Burkitt's lymphoma and nasopharyngeal carcinoma, were also largely negative but occasional highly positive sera have been encountered in this material as well. The difference between the regularly high-reactive African or Chinese nasopharyngeal carcinomas and the predominantly low-reactive Indian hypopharyngeal and oropharyngeal carcinomas was particularly remarkable (91).

In a " tripartite " study, the anti-EBV (Henle)-test, the blocking of direct membrane fluorescence, and the precipitin reaction have been compared in 151 coded sera (56). There was a clear overrepresentation of BL and NPC sera within the " triple-high " reactivity group and they were virtually absent from the " triple-low " group. The opposite was true for the two main groups of control sera, derived from healthy relatives of BL patients and from donors with head and neck tumors other than BL and NPC.

One interesting question concerns the relationship between geographical localization and serological reactivity. Nasopharyngeal carcinomas are more easily to evaluated in this respect, since they represent a clear pathological entity and are not readily confused with other conditions. The EBV-associated serological reactivity of African, Swedish, French, Chinese, and American cases was uniformly high and appeared to be characteristic for the anaplastic or poorly differentiated type (38, 77, 91).

The evaluation of Burkitt's lymphoma outside Africa presents a more difficult problem, because the pathological picture alone does not permit a sharp distinction against other lymphomas. The combined clinical and pathological picture has readily recognizable features in the high endemic areas, but they are less characteristic in other regions and the classification becomes more arbitrary. If one nevertheless examines the data on the serological behavior of " Burkitt-like " lymphomas outside Africa, it appears that the results are partly in line with the African Burkitt lymphomas (2, 56), and partly differ from the African cases, i.e., have no distinctively high EBV-associated reactivity (defined as high anti-EBV titer and/or high membrane blocking index) and thus resemble ordinary lymphosarcomas rather than " true " Burkitt's. This picture cannot be interpreted meaningfully at present since serology cannot serve as the basis for classification if the problem is to decide whether non-African cases have an African-Burkitt-like serology or not; the argument becomes circular. Speculatively at least, one may nevertheless consider the possibility that the non-African Burkitt-like cases are heterogeneous. Some of them would be " true Burkitt's," i.e., have the same etiology as the African cases, whereas other would be different and comparable to " ordinary " lymphosarcomas. Whether this classification can be based on the EBV-associated serological patterns will, of course, depend on the question of whether the relationship of the EB virus to Burkitt's disease is of an essential or of an accidental nature.

b) Changes in EBV-related serological patterns during the clinical course of EBV-associated diseases

Another approach to the study of disease related EBV patterns is to follow the antibody titers against the various EBV-associated antigens horizontally, during the course of " EBV-associated " diseases, such as BL and NPC. For comparison, one may choose EBV-positive individuals with more or less related neoplastic diseases that are not regularly associated with high anti-EBV titers. Studies of this type are now becoming feasible; some preliminary information is already available. In BL, the indirect membrane test, performed with biopsy cell targets, has indicated at an early stage (53, 54) that the most highly reactive sera can be found in patients whose tumors have gone to long term regression. Later, when the more specific and sensitive blocking of direct membrane fluorescence replaced the indirect test as the main method for detecting antibodies against the EBV-associated membrane antigen complex in established culture lines, it turned out (22, 55, 56) that nearly all histologically confirmed African BL sera have a high blocking activity, i.e., show a complete or nearly complete cross reactivity with the reference conjugate. The few exceptions have come from moribund patients. This monotonously uniform blocking activity, obtained with the undiluted sera, hides large quantitative differences, however. When compared by serial titration against the same reference conjugate, the blocking titer of various BL patients sera (taking a blocking index of 0.5 as the endpoint) can vary between 1:1 and 1:600 (22). In the individual patient, the titers may change considerably in the course of the disease, but, as a rule, they remain within the same order of magnitude: most changes are restricted to relatively few dilution steps up or down and the patients can be therefore classified into groups of low, medium, and high reactivity.

Our preliminary findings indicate that the blocking titer differences between patients, as well as the horizontal changes, are influenced by a number of factors. In the course of rapid and extensive tumor growth, antibody levels probably fall, due to adsorption on tumor cell membranes. When the patient receives chemotherapy and the tumor regresses, there is often an increase in titer. At first sight, this may seem paradoxical, in view of the immunosuppressive effect of chemotherapy. It is known, however, that chemical immunosuppression inhibits new primary antibody responses against antigens administered after the drug, but is much less efficient against immune reactions established before treatment.

An increase in blocking antibody titers was particularly apparent in BL and NPC patients who received local radiotherapy (12), including cases where therapy did not lead to complete tumor regression. In view of the fact that X-irradiated tumor cells are relatively good immunogens in experimental systems (61) this is of considerable interest. It may also be relevant that in EBV-carrier cultures with a relatively low membrane antigen reactivity, X-rays can induce the appearance of the membrane antigen on a large fraction of the cells (104).

In BL patients with recurring tumors that continue to grow in spite of chemotherapy, blocking antibody levels that have fallen to low levels at or around the time of recurrence can rise again (e.g., 51). Subsequently, the lymphoma cells become coated with IgG, as a rule, if the tumor persists. It is conceivable that such cells represent immunoresistant variants, similar to what has been found in experimental systems (15). This is supported, indirectly at least, by the history of two patients whose tumors recurred after several years of total regression and contained a high frequency of near-tetraploid cells (10), in contrast to more than 20 other BL biopsies examined (63), with a shorter clinical history, that were all in the near-diploid range. Tetraploid cells can frequently outgrow host responses that efficiently reject diploid cells of the same lineage (24).

The immunoglobulin coat acquired by the tumors that persist in spite of therapy may be the equivalent of enhancing antibody or of blocking antibody in Hellström's sense (30). This is not necessarily an alternative to the possibility that membrane-reactive antibodies may have a growth inhibitory action but is rather, another facet of the same complex picture. An antibody that has cytotoxic or growth inhibitory properties against immunosensitive cells may exert an enhancing effect (i.e., protect the target cell against the cell-mediated immune response) when it interacts with an immunoresistant cell without killing it. In addition, different antibodies no doubt differ; some can be cytotoxic and others enhancing towards the same target cell. In the course of chemotherapy that falls short of a total tumor kill, and the subsequent regrowth of the residual tumor with more antigen release and antibody binding, the immunosensitivity of the tumor cell population and the killing vs. enhancing power of the antibody population must obviously change in a complex way. This would require a multicomponental experimental analysis that is not yet within reach.

In addition to the changes in membrane reactive antibody levels brought about by the tumor itself (i.e., changes due to absorption, antigen release, effect of tumor growth on the immune response, *etc.*), the antibody titer may change for other, tumor-unrelated reasons, and this may, in turn, influence tumor growth. This possibility has been brought into focus by the history of a BL patient (*51*) who was in total tumor regression for a period of four and a half years and subsequently developed widespread abdominal metastases. Her membrane reactive antibody level, determined by the blocking test, fell markedly more than 6 months prior to recurrence, at a time when there was no reason to suspect the presence of any metastases. When the abdominal recurrence became manifest half a year later, the membrane reactive antibody level was still low, and the tumor cells were not yet coated with IgG. In the course of the subsequent two months, the serum antibody level increased again and the lymphoma cells became IgG-coated. This secondary sequence of events decreases the probability that the fall of the antibody level that preceeded recurrence by 6 months was due to absorption on an as yet cryptic tumor, because, in that case, a period of slow tumor growth would have followed during the subsequent 6 months' period, and the secondary increase in antibody level, as well as the coating of the lymphoma cells with immunoglobulins would be expected to have occurred in the interim, appearing already at the time of clinical recurrence. Indirect as this reasoning is, it has nevertheless raised the question of whether a fall in antibody levels may be sometimes the cause, rather than merely the consequence, of tumor recurrence, and whether it could act by facilitating the outgrowth of " dormant " neoplastic cells.

There is some preliminary evidence indicating that the antibodies against the soluble EBV-associated antigens detected by immunoprecipitation show a different disease related pattern, appearing at the time of progressive tumor growth and frequently absent in patients whose tumors are in complete regression (*51, 56*). Although there are numerous exceptions to this, a relationship of this type appeared clearly when the horizontal history of the patient already mentioned above was followed during long term regression and subsequent recurrence (*51*). This may also explain why high anti-EBV titered NPC sera are more frequently precipitin positive than BL sera with comparably high titers: in NPC, the serum material is mainly derived from patients with residual or progressively growing tumors, while a collection of BL sera include progressor and regressor sera as well.

Recently, Henle *et al.* have described yet another EBV-associated antigen, designated as EA (early antigen) (*39*), detected in EBV-infected Raji or 6410-cells. The sera of some EBV-positive donors, but not of others, contained antibodies against it. EA precedes the classical Henle-type " EBV-antigen " during the infectious cycle; the latter has been renamed as " VCA " (viral capsid antigen). The appearance of EA is readily prevented by puromycin but not by DNA inhibitors (*19*). The behavior of EA is thus not unlike what has been mentioned above for MA, with one important exception: whereas MA is compatible with continued cell growth and DNA synthesis, EA inhibits host macromolecular synthesis, as shown by a combination of immunofluorescence and autoradiography (*20*) and thus probably signals the entry of the cell into the lytic cycle. In contrast to EA, VCA is dependent on DNA synthesis and therefore probably represents a " late " viral product.

The tumor-related presence of precipitating and of anti-EA antibodies (35) is reminiscent of some DNA-virus-induced experimental tumor systems, particularly the case of antibodies against " T-antigens." In polyoma-, SV40-, and ade-novirus induced tumors, it is the " tumored hamster ", *i.e.*, the host of non-virus producing, T-antigen positive tumors that tends to develop antibodies againts T-antigens. The antibody levels usually fall when the tumor is removed or rejected and eventually disappear. T-antigens are intracellular, like the soluble antigens in the present system. They are also " early " components of the viral cycle, independent of DNA synthesis (86) and they are regularly present in transformed cells. In the former respect, (independence of DNA synthesis) they are similar to, in the latter respect (compatibility with cell multiplication) they are different from, the EA antigens. As far as the T antigens are concerned, it is not known whether t hey are released from growing tumor cells by some kind of secretory process, or are only liberated from dead and dying cells. A release of the EA antigen may well be related to an abortive virus cycle, perhaps induced in tumor cells on their way to necrosis, *i.e.*, under circumstances where the virus cycle cannot proceed to completion. The frequent absence of anti-T and anti-EA antibodies after tumor removal is in sharp contrast to the membrane reactive antibodies, which tend to remain high, or even increase following rejection in experimental systems, and, as far as this has been studied, probably in the BL system as well. This may be related to the continued presence of " dormant " tumor cells with a preserved, virally determined, foreign membrance antigen, held in check, but not killed by the host immune mechanism.

Further clarification of the relationship between the dynamics of antibody formation against different EBV-determined antigens and the clinical course of the " high-EBV-associated diseases," such as BL and NPC, may be helpful in elucidating important virus-tumor-host relationships, particularly if compared to EBV-positive sera from patients with other tumors that are not characterized by a regularly high EBV-association.

Implications and Dilemmas

Four main dilemmas arise from this pattern of findings; they are interrelated but all have their specific aspects. They can be briefly stated as follows:

a) *The etiological dilemma*—Can the occurrence of distinctive, tumor associated antigens give any clues about the etiology of the disease?

b) *The problem of neoplastic behavior*—Are the changes in the composition of the cell membrane, or other cellular organelles, as reflected by the appearance of new antigenic specificities, fundamentally involved in the neoplastic behavior of the cell, or, in other words, does the unresponsiveness of the cell to growth control depend on the change in composition or structure that is revealed by the immunological tests?

c) *The therapeutic problem*—Can any of the immunological reactions now identified serve to measure the patient's reactivity to his own tumor, in connection with various therapeutic procedures, including attempts at immunotherapy; and

d) Are there any *preventive* approaches in sight?

Concerning the etiological dilemma, it is a useful point of departure that all virally induced experimental tumors share the same antigen, as long as they are induced by the same virus, at least as far as the transplantation-type, membrane associated antigens are concerned. The reverse, the assumption of a common viral etiology on the basis of common antigens found in tumors of unknown origin is not necessarily justified, however. It has been shown (*64, 79, 94, 99, 101*) that virally induced new antigens can be made to appear by superinfecting normal cells or tumors of unrelated etiology with oncogenic and even with some non-oncogenic viruses. The only difference between this secondary " antigenic conversion " and the primary event that occurs in direct relation to tumor induction, is the lesser stability of the former, particularly in immune hosts (*93*), as well as a more irregular association between antigen and tumor, depending on the accidental nature of superinfection.

As discussed above, high anti-EBV titers and high antibody levels against EBV-associated membrane antigens and soluble antigens are regularly associated with at least two neoplastic diseases: Burkitt's lymphoma and nasopharyngeal carcinoma. For nasopharyngeal carcinoma, it is clear that this serological pattern is independent of geographical or ethnic origin. A similar situation may exist for Burkitt's lymphoma, but the lack of reliable criteria by which the identity of the disease can be established outside the endemic areas and distinguished from ordinary lymphomas makes a similar evaluation of the non-African cases more difficult.

It is important to stress that the main difference between BL and NPC and other normal or neoplastic serum donor categories investigated is not EBV-positivity, nor the occurrence of high titered reactions in occasional donors, since such donors may be found in most other categories as well, but the *regular and consistent association of high titered reactions according to all three tests*. Looking at it from this angle, BL and NPC are unique. One may question, however, whether this angle can be justified or, more specifically, what it implies.

As a starting point, we may take the convincing demonstration that EBV is causally related to at least one form of infectious mononucleosis (*34, 74*). This form afflicts EBV-sero-negative adolescents, as a rule, it is frequently positive for heterophile antibodies and is regularly accompanied by sero-conversion to anti-EBV positivity. As indicated by a prospective study (*74*), anti-EBV individuals are apparently protected from the disease.

The serological screening of many different human populations also showed (*33, 37*) that there is another, " early " sero-conversion to anti-EBV positivity, culminating around 4 years of age, and particularly frequent in low socioeconomic groups. This early infection does not lead to infectious mononucleosis or any other disease entity so far recognized.

Hypothesis

Viewed against this background, the relationship of EBV infections to BL and NPC may be considered in terms of the following alternatives:

a) The virus that causes infectious mononucleosis is also responsible for these two tumors; if this is true, intrinsic or extrinsic co-factors have to be postulated to explain the malignant conversion (the " *co-factor hypothesis* ");

b) Different virus subtypes are responsible for the different clinical entities (the " *multiple virus hypothesis* "); or

c) The virus is a relatively harmless inhabitant of lymphoid tissues, although it may cause temporary proliferation (mononucleosis) under certain conditions. When lymphoid tissues proliferate for other reasons, *e.g.*, in malignancies due to other, unrelated causes, the virus travels along as a passenger, with increased antigen production and high-titered antibody formation as a result.   This " *passenger hypothesis* " is the logical analogue of the " antigenic conversion " of established tumors by etiologically unrelated viruses, discussed above.   In view of the high regularity of association, a requirement for a particular trophic relationship between EBV and the target (lymphoid) tissue may be added in the present case.

Passenger Virus Hypothesis

The *passenger hypothesis* cannot be excluded at present, but it appears less likely in view of the fact that lymphoproliferative diseases other than BL and anaplastic carcinomas other than NPC do not show a regular high-titered EBV-association. This statement includes malignancies occurring in the same or closely adjacent ana-tomical areas, such as reticulum cell sarcoma, lymphosarcoma, *etc.*, and carcinomas that arise in, or close to, the tissues of the Waldeyer ring, such as the hypopharynx, oropharynx, the tonsil, base of the tongue, soft palate, *etc*. Carcinoma of the maxilla is a possible exception, but larger groups remain to be investigated.   Hodgkin's disease represents a very interesting case in itself.   Recently it has been found that the sarcomatous form, *i.e.*, the lymphocyte poor type with the worst prognosis, shows a high anti-VCA and anti-MA reactivity, quite comparable to BL and NPC, whereas the lymphocyte rich and relatively more benign paragranulomatous form is low-reactive in both tests and thus resembles the control material (*42*).   The granulo-matous form was intermediate, both with regard to histological type and serologi-cal reactivity.   This means, as far as the serology is concerned, that it represents a mixture of high-and low-reactive cases.   Whereas it is thus possible that EBV plays some special role in the etiology of Hodgkin's sarcoma, the inverse correla-tion with lymphocytic predominance would not be in line with a simple passenger hypothesis.

None of this reasoning excludes the passenger hypothesis conclusively, of course, but quite a number of *ad hoc* assumptions have to be made to maintain it in face of this evidence.   One would have to postulate some specific trophic relationship bet-ween the virus and the kind of lymphocyte that gives rise to BL and is particularly abundant in NPC, that would not apply to the lymphoid cells that proliferate in the various other malignancies, used as controls.   No valid objection can be raised against such a hypothesis, but it appears rather far fetched in view of the fact that EBV-carrying blastoid cell lines can be regularly isolated from EBV positive indivi-duals, including donors with lymphoreticular malignancies of the " control " type, *i.e.*, diseases that do not show a consistently high EBV-positive serology. The sarcomatous form of Hodgkin's disease is also very hard to explain.

Co-factor Hypothesis

The possibility that EBV acts together with some *co-factor* in causing neoplastic disease or, to phrase the same thesis differently, it acts by increasing the likelihood of neoplastic transformation brought about by other factors, has been recently proposed by Burkitt (*6*) as far as the etiology of BL is concerned. In order to fit the geographic distribution of the disease with an ubiquitous virus, Burkitt proposed that an insect-transmitted co-factor is responsible for the malignant manifestation and specified it as chronic holoendemic malaria. This was based on the absence of BL from certain areas where malaria control has been enforced for some time and its presence in adjacent regions where malaria control was not regularly practiced.

It may be agreed that interactions between viruses and other agents, capable of stimulating the proliferation of a target tissue may lead to malignant transformation in experimental systems where neither the virus nor the other agent is oncogenic *per se* (*97*). Since chronic malaria exerts a strong proliferative stimulus on the RES, Burkitt's modified theory is reasonable, although it may be objected that the same picture would result from the transmission of *any* etiological factor or co-factor mediated by the appropriate insect, and this includes other viruses. Recently, some preliminary evidence has been obtained concerning the frequency of the sickling trait in BL patients (*43*), however, that indicates a possible role of malaria in the causation of the disease.

Multiple Virus Hypothesis

The third possibility, the multiple virus hypothesis, implies the existence of closely related but biologically different EBV-viruses with differences in their oncogenic power and their target tissue preference. In light of the information derived from experimental oncogenic viruses, this is a realistic alternative as well. As far as leukemia viruses of the RNA type are concerned, it will be recalled that, prior to the discovery of the interference test for avian leukosis virus classification (*90*), it was not possible to distinguish by morphological or immunological means between the viruses that were responsible for the different lympho- and myeloproliferative diseases or for fowl sarcoma. It is now known that the avian leukosis—sarcoma virus group has many closely related members; some induce solid tumors with highly distinctive properties, others are responsible for myeloid or erythromyeloid leukemia, or lymphomatosis, and still others cause no recognizable disease at all. A closely similar development can be noticed in the murine leukosis-sarcoma field. The Friend, Rauscher, Gress, Moloney, Kaplan, Rich, Graffi, Mazurenko, *etc.*, agents are similar antigenically and indistinguishable by ultrastructure, but they induce characteristic clinical and pathological disease entities, specific for the viral agent (*87*). In the DNA field, a possibly relevant example is the series of herpes simplex mutants, studied by Roizmann and his colleagues. Although this is not known to be an oncogenic system, it is important that different viral mutants induce different membrane changes in infected cells and, concomitantly, the cells are altered in their " social behavior " in ways that are characteristic for the virus mutant.   Although a lytic virus obviously cannot transform its targets, the cellular changes are nevertheless concerned with intercellular relationships.   Conceivably, other, non-lytic viruses of the same family might induce membrane changes compatible with cellular viability and reproductive integrity, and a social behavior changed in the direction of disobediance to growth regulation—or, in other words, neoplasia.   It may be recalled in this connection that the agents of at least two neoplastic diseases, Marek's neurolymphomatosis in the chicken (*8*) and Lucké's carcinoma in the frog (*67*) were recently identified as herpes type viruses.   A simian lymphoma is also probably due to a herpes-type virus (Herpes virus saimiri) (*40*).

The immunological tests so far performed on EBV-associated antigens, including those referred to in the previous sections, are not necessarily competent to reveal finer differences between closely related but biologically different agents with cross-re-active or overlapping antigenic components.   A preliminary study of the membrane antigens carried on EBV-positive lymphoblastoid cell lines derived from BL and NPC did not show any difference in the reactivity patterns (*92*), but this may simply re-flect the insufficient discriminating ability of the test.

Further studies are needed to distinguish between these possibilities.   In order to narrow down the passenger hypothesis, more extensive tests are desirable on tumor categories where occasional sera gave high EBV-associated reactivity, but only limited samples have been tested.   It is also desirable to conduct nucleic acid hybridization studies on the corresponding tumors.   More refined analytical methods are needed for the attempts to detect different virus variants.   The recent developments in the herpes simplex field suggest that biochemical studies on viral envelopes and altered cell membranes may be particularly rewarding.

Concerning the relationship between EBV and nasopharyngeal carcinoma, the same types of hypotheses can be discussed as for BL.   The multiple virus hypothesis would imply an NPC-specific EBV-variant.   The co-factor hypothesis would lead to a consideration of both genetic and environmental factors, in light of the information on the incidence of the disease in migrant high-risk populations (*69*). A prospective serological study of this question would be very difficult at the present time, since NPC, unlike BL, occurs over an extremely wide age-range.

The possible significance of the cell membrane changes, reflected by the ap-pearance of new antigens, for the understanding of neoplastic cell behavior cannot be assessed at present, but it may be pertinent to point out that cell membrane changes are among the most seriously considered parameters of neoplastic behavior at pre-sent.   They are almost invariably found when comparable normal and transformed cells are studied in parallel.   They may concern changes in behavior, such as contact inhibition (*1*), or altered expression of phytoagglutinin receptors (*4, 41*) that may reflect a change in the synthesis of certain glycolipids (*23*), and are perhaps linked to the appearance of new surface antigens (*68*).   Membrane antigen changes have been demonstrated in all experimental tumors that have been thoroughly studied (*11, 30, 47, 49, 76, 80, 93*), and although the details concerning antigenic strength and patterns of cross reactivity vary from system to system, they must reflect some remodeling of the membrane structure. Growth regulating mechanisms, including both the forces that act *via* long range, humoral arms and the short range, contactual signals as well, must transmit their message to the target cell *via* receptors on the outer membrane. Nonlytic virus-cell interactions may result in the incorporation of virally determined (or virally derepressed) components into the membrane that render the appropriate receptors insensitive to regulation and, if this is compatible with continued cell growth and division, it may trigger neoplastic development. Since infection with potentially oncogenic viruses and the concomitant surface antgenic changes are not limited to the oncogenic target tissue but can occur in other cells as well that remain normal (*i.e.*, subject o regulation), a tissue or cell type specificity must be added to explain transformation. Since different tissues must obey different types of growth regulation, this is not surprising. Also, virally determined antigens may be retained while *in vivo* tumorigenic properties decrease or are lost from cell hybrid lines (*50, 57, 102*) or from the " revertant " forms that may arise from transformed cultures *in vitro* (*62, 83, 85*). Further studies on such systems will be most interesting, not only for the understanding of neoplastic behavior and the possible role of membrane changes in it, but also for the understanding of normal growth responsiveness at the cell level.

Meanwhile, the question of whether EBV associated membrane antigens are essential for the neoplastic behavior of BL and NPC cells is not clear. As far as NPC is concerned, such membrane antigens have been demonstrated in derived lymphoblastoid cell lines (*92*) but it is not known whether they are present on the surface of the carcinoma cells. Established culture lines of BL cells carry EBV, as a rule, although at very different levels (*60, 72*). The membrane antigen can only be demonstrated in lines with a relatively high " EBV-load " (*60*) and is subject to environmental fluctuations (*103*). There is at least one BL line (Raji) which contains no EBV antigen demonstrable by immunofluorescence or virus particles (*14*) although it carries DNA that hybridizes specifically with EBV-DNA, as already mentioned (*26*). Since the Raji line can be superinfected with EB virus (*39*), the absence of virus production is presumably not due to repressors. If it carries genetic information derived from EBV, it is probably a defective viral genome, lacking the cistrons that specify the membrane, capsid, and early protein antigens. If there could be any assurance that the Raji line represents a neoplastic cell, this would imply that the membrane antigen is not required for neoplastic behavior. Since this question cannot be tested directly with a human cell, however, a conclusive answer is not available. Further studies on the presence of viral DNA and virus specific RNA in BL derived lines, in comparison with EBV carrying blastoid cell lines of other origin may prove very informative. In this connection, it is interesting that IM derived lines are reportedly more prone to lose their EBV than BL derived lines (*37*). Thus, whereas EBV is clearly helpful in inducing lymphoblastoid transformation and facilitates the establishment of stationary suspension cultures (*18, 36, 37, 84*), there is no doubt that blastoid cell lines *can* exist without a productive EBV cycle.

Therapeutic Problems

Turning now to the *therapeutic problems*, it seems clearly established that the host immune response plays an important part in Burkitt's lymphoma. This is indicated by the documented occurrence of spontaneous regression (*7*) by a substantial fraction of long term survivors, sometimes after only mild chemotherapy (*5, 9, 73*), by the reactivity of the autochthonous host against its own tumor cells, indicated by the presence of humoral antibodies reacting with the surface of viable cells (*53, 54*), by the positive C'1-a fixation test (*75*), and by the transformation of host lymphocytes when confronted with mitomycin treated autochthonous lymphoma cells in the mixed lymphocyte-target cell interaction test (*98*). In addition, the progressive accumulation of an IgG coating on the cell surface of tumors that persist in spite of therapy (*46, 51*) together with the tetraploid (immunoresistant?) constitution of tumors that have recurred after long-term regression (*10*) suggests that the dynamics of immunoselection may also apply to this human system as they do for experimental tumors (*24*). Immunoresistance may be as important as drug resistance, if not more so, in frustrating therapy.

The host response to an autochthonous tumor is no less complex than other immune responses against viable cells. Different effector components interact in such a way that rejection, or its opposite, enhancement, will dominate the eventual outcome. Humoral antibodies are cytotoxic in some situations, whereas in others they lack demonstrable growth inhibotory effects but nevertheless manage to attach and thereby prevent the access of host lymphoid cells (*48, 76*). Recent evidence indicates that such a " blocking antibody " may play an important role in counteracting the cell mediated host response in experimental (*28*) and human (*29*) tumors as well.

The main therapeutic dilemma is what the proper stimuli are, specific or non-specific, and how they are best administered to the immune system in order to achieve the objective, rejection, and avoid its opposite, enhancement. The rationale of introducing immune stimuli at a time when the tumor load confronting the host is minimal, *i.e.*, after regression has been induced by chemotherapy, is obvious (*65, 95*), but the optimal form of stimulus and the best mode and timing of its administration is not. No *a priori* guidance can be given from experimental studies, because the same mode of administration, dosage, vehicle, *etc.* of the same preparation may favor rejection in one system and enhancement in another, and the differences, depending on host species, tumor type, and individual characteristics of the tumor line, are immense. Ideally, it would be desirable to develop methods that allow the quantitative assessment of cell bound immunity and the synergistic or antagonistic action of humoral antibodies in relation to it, in each untreated patient and follow it subsequently during treatment. While this should be feasible, at least in principle, its practical application is still in the future. Meanwhile, an empirical approach, based on as much rational reasoning as the experimental models will allow, may yield important information, as the work of Mathé and his group clearly indicates (*65*).

Obviously, the prevention approach will have to await the further clarification of the relationship between serum conversion and tumor development, preferably from a prospective study. A discussion of this beyond the general statement that the ultimate goal an immunological approach must be prevention rather than therapy appears premature at the present time.

REFERENCES

1. Abercrombie, M. Contact Inhibition: The Phenomenon and Its Biological Implications. The Second Decennial Review Conference on Cell Tissue and Organ Culture, Bedford, Penna, p. 249, 1966.
2. Ahlström, C. G., Andersson, T., Klein, G., and Åkerman, M. Malignant Lymphoma of " Burkitt Type " in Sweden. Int., J. Cancer, 2: 583, 1967.
3. Bremberg, S., Klein, G., and Epstein, A. Direct Membrane Fluorescence Reaction of EBV-carrying Human Lymphoblastoid Cells: Blocking Tests with Xenogeneic Antisera. Int. J. Cancer, 4: 761, 1969.
4. Burger, M. M. Isolation of a Receptor Complex for a Tumor Specific Agglutinin from the Neoplastic Cell Surface. Nature, 219: 49, 1968.
5. Burkitt, D. Chemotherapy of Jaw Tumors. In Treatment of Burkitt's Tumor, UICC Monograph Series, ed. by J. H. Burchenal. Heidelberg: Springer Verlag, Vol. 8, p. 94, 1967.
6. Burkitt, D. Etiology of Burkitt's Lymphoma—An Alternative Hypothesis to a Vectored Virus. J. Nat. Cancer Inst., 42: 19, 1969.
7. Burkitt, D., and Kyalwazi, S. K. Spontaneous Remission of African Lymphoma. Brit. J. Cancer, 21: 14, 1967.
8. Churchill, A. E. Herpes-type Virus Isolated in Cell Culture from Tumors of Chickens with Marek's Disease. I. Studies in Cell Culture. J. Nat. Cancer Inst., 41: 939, 1968.
9. Clifford, P. Further Studies in the Treatment of Burkitt's Lymphoma. E. African Med. J., 43: 179, 1966.
10. Clifford, P., Gripenberg, N., Klein, E., Fenyö, E. M., and Manolov, G. Treatment of Burkitt's Lymphoma. Lancet II: 517, 1968.
11. Deichmann, G. I. Immunological Aspects of Carcinogenesis by Deoxyribonuleic Acid Tumor Viruses. Adv. Cancer Res., 12: 101, 1969.
12. Einhorn, N., Klein, G., aud Clifford, P. Increase in Antibody Titer against the EBV Associated Membrane Antigen Complex in Burkitt's Lymphoma and Nasopharyngeal Carcinoma after Local Irradiation. Cancer, 26: 1013, 1970.
13. Epstein, M. A., Achong, B. G., and Barr, Y. M. Virus Particles in Cultured Lymphoblasts from Burkitt's Lymphoma. Lancet, 1: 702, 1964.
14. Epstein, M. A., Achong, B. G., Barr, Y. M., Zajac, B., Henle, G., and Henle, W. Morphological and Virological Investigations on Cultured Burkitt Tumor Lymphoblasts (Strain Raji). J. Nat. Cancer Inst., 37: 547, 1966.
15. Fenyö, E. M., Klein, E., Klein, G., and Swiech, K. Selection of an Immunoresistant Moloney Lymphoma Subline with Decreased Concentration of Tumor Specific Surface Antigens. J. Nat. Cancer Inst., 40: 69, 1968.
16. Fialkow, P. J., Klein, G., Gartler, S. M., and Clifford, P. Clonal Origin for Individual Burkitt Tumors. Lancet, 2: 384, 1970.
17. van Furth, R., Gorter, H., Nandkarni, J. S., Nandkarni, J.J., Klein, E., and Clifford,

P.   Synthesis of Immunoglobulins by Biopsied Tissues and Cell Line from Burkitt's Lymphoma. Submitted for Publication.

18. Gerber, P., Whang-Peng, J., and Monroe, J. H.   Transformation and Chromosome Changes Induced by Epstein-Barr Virus in Normal Human Leukocyte Cultures. Proc. Nat. Acad. Sci., 63: 740, 1969.

19. Gergely, L., Klein, G., and Ernberg, I.   Appearance of EBV-associated Antigens in Infected Raji Cells.   Virology, 45: 10, 1971.

20. Gergely, L., Klein, G., and Ernberg, I.   Host Cell Macromolecular Synthesis in Cells Containing EBV-induced Early Antigens Studied by Combined Immunofluorescence and Radioautography. Virology, 45: 22, 1971.

21. Goldstein, G., Klein, G., Pearson, G., and Clifford, P.   Direct Membrane Immunofluorescence Reaction of Burkitt's Lymphoma Cells in Culture.   Cancer Res., 29: 749, 1969.

22. Gunven, P., Klein, G., Henle, G., Henle, W., and Clifford, P.   Antibodies to Epstein-Barr Virus (EBV) Associated Membrane (MA) and Viral Capsid (VCA) Antigens in African Burkitt Lymphoma Patients and Controls.   Nature, 228: 1053, 1970.

23. Hakamori, S. I., and Murakami, W. T.   Glycolipids of Hamster Fibroblasts and Derived Malignant-transformed Cell Lines.   Proc. Nat. Acad. Sci., 59: 254, 1967.

24. Hauschka, T. S., Kvedar, B. J., Grinnel, S. T., and Amos, D. B.   Immunoselection of Polyploids from Predominantly Diploid Cell Populations.   Ann. N.Y. Acad. Sci., 63: 683, 1956.

25. zur Hausen, H., Henle, W., Hummeler, K., Diehl, V., and Henle, G.   Comparative Study of Cultured Burkitt Tumor Cells by Immunofluorescence, Autoradiography and Electron Microscopy.   J. Virology, 1: 830, 1967.

26. zur Hausen, H., and Schulte-Holthausen, H.   Presence of EB Virus Nucleic Acid Homology in a " Virus-free " Line of Burkitt Tumor Cells.   Nature, 227: 245, 1970.

27. zur Hausen, H., Schulte-Holthausen, H., Klein, G., Henle, W., Henle, G., Clifford, P., and Santesson, L.   EB-virus DNA in Biopsies of Burkitt Tumors and Anaplastic Carcinomas of the Nasopharynx.   Nature, 228: 1056, 1970.

28. Hellström, I., and Hellström, K. E.   Colony Inhibition Studies on Blocking and Non-blocking Serum Effects on Cellular Immunity to Moloney Sarcomas.   Int. J. Cancer, 5: 195, 1970.

29. Hellström, I., Hellström, K. E., Evans, C. A., Heppner, G. H., Pierce, E. G., and Yang, J. P. S.   Serum-mediated Protection of Neoplastic Cells from Inhibition by Lymphocytes Immune to Their Tumor-specific Antigens.   Proc. Nat. Acad. Sci., 62: 362, 1969.

30. Hellström, K. E., and Hellström, I.   Cellular Immunity against Tumor Antigens. Adv. Cancer Res., 12: 167, 1969.

31. Henle, G., and Henle, W.   Immunofluorescence in Cells Derived from Burkitt's Lymphoma.   J. Bact., 91: 1248, 1966.

32. Henle, G., and Henle, W.   Immunofluorescence, Interference, and Complement Fixation Techniques in the Detection of Herpes-type Virus in Burkitt Tumor Cell Lines.   Cancer Res., 27: 2442, 1967.

33. Henle, G., Henle, W., Clifford, P., Diehl, V., Kafuko, G. W., Kirya, B. G., Klein, G., Morrow, R. H., Munube, G. M. R., Pike, P., Tukei, P. M., and Ziegler, J. L.   Antibodies to Epstein-Barr Virus in Burkitt's Lymphoma and Control Groups.   J. Nat. Cancer Inst., 43: 1147, 1969.

34. Henle, G., Henle, W., and Diehl, V. Relation of Burkitt's Tumor-associated Herpes-type Virus to Infectious Mononucleosis. Proc. Nat. Acad. Sci., *59*: 94, 1968.

35. Henle, G., Henle, W., Klein, G., Gunvén, P., Clifford, P., Morrow, R. H., and Ziegler, J. L. Antibodies to Early EBV-induced Antigens in Burkitt's Lymphoma. J. Nat. Cancer Inst. *46*: 861, 1971.

36. Henle, W., Diehl, V., Kohn, G., zur Hausen, H., and Henle, G. Herpes-type Virus and Chromosome Marker in Normal Leukocytes after Growth with Irradiated Burkitt Cells. Science, *157*: 1064, 1967.

37. Henle, W., and Henle, G. Evidence for a Relation of EBV to Burkitt's Lymphoma and Nasopharyngeal Carcinoma. Proc. of the Intern. Symposium of Comparative Leukemia Research, Cherry Hill, 1969, pp. 706–713. S. Karger, Basel, 1970.

38. Henle, W., Henle, G., Burtin, P., Cachin, Y., Clifford, P., de Schryver, A., de-Thé, G., Diehl, V., Ho, H.-C., and Klein, G. Antibodies to Epstein-Barr Virus in Naso-pharyngeal Carcinoma, Other Head and Neck Neoplasms, and Control Groups. J. Nat. Cancer Inst., *44*: 225, 1970.

39. Henle, W., Henle, G., Zajac, B. A., Pearson, G., Waubke, R., and Scriba, M. Dif-ferential Reactivity of Human Sera with EBV-induced " Early Antigens." Science, *169*: 188, 1970.

40. Hunt, R. D., Meléndez, L. V., King, N. W., Gilmore, C. E., Daniel, M. D., William-son, M. E., and Jones, T. C. Morphology of Disease with Features of Malignant Lymphoma in Marmosets and Owl Monkeys Inoculated with Herpesvirus Saimiri. J. Nat. Cancer Inst., *44*: 447, 1970.

41. Inbar, M., and Sachs, L. Structural Differences in Sites on the Surface Membrane of Normal and Transformed Cells. Nature, *223*: 710, 1969.

42. Johansson, B., Klein, G., Henle, G., and Henle, W. Epstein-Barr Virus (EBV)-associated Antibody Patterns in Malignant Lymphoma and Leukemia. I. Hodgkin's Disease. Int. J. Cancer, *6*: 450–462, 1970.

43. Kafuko, G. W., and Burkitt, D. Burkitt's Lymphoma and Malaria. Int. J. Cancer, *6*: 1, 1970.

44. Klein, E., Clifford, P., Klein, G., and Hamberger, C. A. Further Studies on the Membrane Immunofluorescence Reaction of Burkitt Lymphoma Cells. Intern. J. Cancer, *2*: 27, 1967.

45. Klein, E., and Klein, G. Antigenic Properties of Lymphomas Induced by the Mo-loney Agent. J. Nat. Cancer Inst., *32*: 547, 1964.

46. Klein, E., Klein, G., Nadkarni, J. J., Nadkarni, J. S., Wigzell, H., and Clifford, P. Surface IgM-kappa Specificity on a Burkitt Lymphoma Cell *in vivo* and in Derived Culture Lines. Cancer Res., *28*: 1300, 1968.

47. Klein, G. Tumor Antigens. Ann. Rev. Microbiol., *20*: 223, 1966.

48. Klein, G. Humoral and Cell-mediated Mechanisms for Host Defense in Tumor Immunity. Viruses Inducing Cancer, Implications for Therapy, ed. by W. J. Burdette, Univ. of Utah Press, Salt Lake City, *379*: 323, 1966.

49. Klein, G. Experimental Studies in Tumor Immunology. Fed. Proc., *28*: 1739, 1969.

50. Klein, G., Bregula, U., Wiener, F., and Harris, H. The Analysis of Malignancy by Cell Fusion. I. Hybrids between Tumour Cells and L Cell Derivatives. J. Cell Science, *8*: 659, 1971.

51. Klein, G., Clifford, P., Henle, G., Henle, W., Old, L. J., and Geering, L. EBV-associated Serological Patterns in a Burkitt Lymphoma Patient during Regression and Recurrence. Int. J. Cancer, *4*: 416, 1969.

52. Klein, G., Clifford, P., Klein, E., Smith, R. T., Minowada, J., Kourilsky, F. M., and Burchenal, J. H.   Membrane Immunofluorescence Reactions of Burkitt Lymphoma Cells from Biopsy Specimens and Tissue Cultures.   J. Nat. Cancer Inst., *39*: 1027, 1967.

53. Klein, G., Clifford, P., Klein, E., and Stjernswärd, J.   Search for Tumor Specific Immune Reactions in Burkitt Lymphoma Patients by the Membrane Immunofluorescence Reaction.   *In* Treatment of Burkitt's Tumor, UICC Monograph Series, ed. by J. H. Burchenal, Vol. 8, p. 209, Heidelberg: Springer Verlag, 1967.

54. Klein, G., Clifford, P., Klein, E., and Stjernswärd, J.   Search for Tumor Specifie Immune Reactions in Burkitt Lymphoma Patients by the Membrane Immunofluorescence Reaction.   Proc. Nat. Acad. Sci., *55*: 1628, 1966.

55. Klein, G., Pearson, G., Henle. G., Henle. W., Goldstein, G., and Clifford, P.   Relation between Epstein-Barr Viral and Cell Membrane Immunofluorescence in Burkitt Tumor Cells.   III. Comparison of Blocking of Direct Membrane Immunofluorescence.   J. Exp. Med., *129*: 697, 1969.

56. Klein, G., Geering, G., Old, L. J., Henle, G., Henle, W., and Cliifford, P.   Comparison of the Anti-EBV Titer and the EBV-associated Membrane Reactive and Precipitating Antibody Levels in the Sera of Burkitt Lymphoma and Nasopharyngeal Carcinoma Patients and Controls.   Int. J. Cancer, *5*: 185, 1970.

57. Klein, G., and Harris, H.   Polyoma induced transplantation antigen in Cell hybrids.   Submitted for Publication.

58. Klein, G., Klein, E., and Clifford, P.   Search for Host Defenses in Burkitt Lymphoma: Membrane Immunofluorescence Tests on Biopsies and Tissue Culture Lines.   Cancer Res., *27*: 2510, 1967.

59. Klein, G., Klein, E., and Haughton, G.   Variation of Antigenic Characteristics between Different Mouse Lymphomas Induced by the Moloney Virus.   J. Nat. Cancer Inst., *36*: 607, 1966.

60. Klein, G., Pearson, G., Nadkarni, J. S., Nadkarni, J. J., Klein, E., Henle, G., Henle, W., and Clifford, P.   Relation between Epstein-Barr Viral and Cell Membrane Immunofluorescence of Burkitt Tumor Cells.   I. Dependence of Cell Membrane Immunofluorescence on Presence of EB Virus.   J. Exp. Med., *128*: 1011, 1968.

61. Klein, G., Sjögren, H. O., Klein, E., and Hellström, K. E.Demonstration of Resistance against Methylcholanthrene-induced Sarcomas in the Primary Autochthonous Host.   Cancer Res., *20*: 1561, 1960.

62. Macpherson, I.   The Characteristics of Animal Cells Transformed *in* vitro. Adv. Cancer Res., *13*: 169, 1970.

63. Manolov, G.   Personal communication.

64. Mathé, G.   Antigenicité Nouvelle (Demontrée par Isogreffe) D'un Fragment de Peau de Souris Infectée par un Virus Leucémogène.   Compt Rend. Acad. Scie., Paris, *264*: 2702, 1967.

65. Mathé, G.   Approaches to the Immunological Treatment of Cancer in Man.   Br. Med. J., *5674*: 7, 1969.

66. Meyer, M. G., Birg, F., and Bonneau, M. H.   Cinetique de l'Antigène de Membrane dans le Systeme Virus Polyome-hamster.   Compt Rend. Acad. Scie., Paris, *268*: 2848, 1969.

67. Mizell, M., Toplin, I., and Isaacs, J. J.   Tumor Induction in Developing Frog Kidneys by a Zonal Centrifuge Purified Fraction of the Frog Herpes-type Virus.   Science, *165*: 1134, 1969.

68. Mora, P. T., Brady, R. O., Bradley, R. M., and McFarland, V. W.   Gangliosides

in DNA Virus-transformed and Spontaneously Transformed Tumorigenic Mouse Cell Lines. Proc. Nat. Acad. Sci., *63*: 1290, 1969.

69. Muir, C. S., and Shanmugaratnam, K. Cancer of the Nasopharynx. UICC Monograph Series. pp. 1. Munksgaard, Copenhagen, 1967.

70. Möller, G. Demonstration of Mouse Isoantigens at the Cellular Level by the Fluorescent Antibody Technique. J. Exp. Md., *114*: 415, 1961.

71. Nadkarni, J. S., Nadkarni, J. J., Clifford, P., Manolov, G., Fenyö, E. M., and Klein, E. Characteristics of New Cell Lines Derived from Burkitt Lymphomas. Cancer, *23*: 64, 1969.

72. Nadkarni, J. S., Nadkarni, J. J., Klein, G., Henle, W., Henle, G., and Clifford, P. EB Viral Antigens in Burkitt Tumor Biopsies and Early Cultures. Int. J. Cancer, *6*: 10, 1970.

73. Ngu, V. A. The African Lymphoma (Burkitt Tumor): Survivals Exceeding Two Years. Brit. J. Cancer, *19*: 101, 1965.

74. Niederman, J. C., Evans, A. S., Subrahmanyan, L., and McCollum, R. W. Prevalence, Incidence and Persistence of EB Virus Antibody in Young Adults. New England J. Med., *282*: 361, 1970.

75. Nishioka, K., Tachibana, T., Klein, G., and Clifford, P. Complementological Studies on Tumor Immunity. Measurement of Cl Bound to Tumor Cells and Immune Adherence with Burkitt Lymphoma Cells. GANN Monograph, *7*: 49, 1968.

76. Old, L. J., and Boyse, E. A. Immunology of Experimental Tumors. Ann. Rev. Med., 15: 167, 1964.

77. Old, L. J., Boyse, E. A., Geering, G., and Oettgen, H. F. Serologic Approaches to the Study of Cancer in Animals and in Man. Cancer Res., *28*: 1288, 1968.

78. Old, L. J., Boyse, E. A., Oettgen, H. F., de Harven, E., Geering, G., Williamson, B., and Clifford, P. Precipitating Antibody in Human Serum to an Antigen Present in Cultured Burkitt's Lymphoma Cells. Proc. Nat. Acad. Sci., *56*: 1699, 1966.

79. Pasternak, G. Serologic Studies on Cells of Grafi Virus-induced Myeloid Leukemia in Mice. J. Nat. Cancer Inst., *34*: 371, 1965.

80. Pasternak, G. I. Antigens Induced by the Mouse Leukemia Viruses. Adv. Cancer Res., *12*: 1, 1969.

81. Pearson, G., Dewey, S., Klein, G., Henle, G., and Henle, W. Relation between Neutralization of Epstein-Barr Virus (EBV) and Antibodies to Cell-Membrane Antigens Induced by the Virus. J. Nat. Cancer Inst., *45*: 989, 1970.

82. Pearson, G., Klein, G., Henle, G., Henle, W., and Clifford, P. Relation between Epstein-Barr Viral and Cell Membrane Immunofluorescence in Burkitt Tumor Cells. IV. Differentiation between Antibodies Responsible for Membrane and Viral Immunofluorescence. J. Exp. Med., *129*: 707, 1969.

83. Pollack, R. E., Green, H., and Todaro, G. J. Growth Control in Cultured Cells: Selection of Sublines with Increased Sensitivity to Contact Inhibition and Decreased Tumor-producing Ability. Proc. Nat. Acad. Sci., *60*: 126, 1968.

84. Pope, J. H., Horne, M. K., and Scott, W. Identification of the Filtrable Leukocyte-transforming Factor of QIMR-WIL Cells as Herpes-like Virus. Int. J. Cancer, *4*: 255, 1969.

85. Rabinowitz, Z., and Sachs, L. The Formation of Variants with a Reversion of Properties of Transformed Cells. Virology, *40*: 193, 1970.

86. Rapp, F., Bubtel, J. S., Feldman, L. A., Kitahara, T., and Melnick, J. L. Differential Effects of Inhibitors on the Steps Leading to the Formation of SV40 Tumor and Viral Antigens. J. Exp. Med., *121*: 935, 1965.

87. Rich, M. A. Virus-induced Murine Leukemia. *In* Experimental Leukemia. North Holland Publishing Co., ed. by M. A. Rich. Amsterdam, 1968, p. 1.

88. Roizman, B. Herpes-viruses, Membranes, and the Social Behaviour of Infected Cells. Proc. of the Int. Symposium on Applied and Medical Virology. Fort Lauderdale, Florida, Dec. 1969.

89. Roizman, B., and Spring, S. B. Alteration in Immunologic Specificity of Cells Infected with Cytolytic Viruses. Proc. of the Conference on Cross Reacting Antigens and Neo-antigens, ed. by Trentin. Williams & Wilkins & Co., Baltimore, 1967, p. 85.

90. Rubin, H. A Virus in Chick Embryos Which Induces Resistance *in vitro* to Infection with Rous Sarcoma Virus. Proc. Nat. Acad. Sci., *46*: 1105, 1960.

91. de Schryver, A., Friberg, S., Jr., Klein, G., Henle, W., Henle, G., de Thé, G., Clifford, P., and Ho, H.-C. Epstein-Barr Virus-associated Antibody Patterns in Carcinoma of the Post-nasal Space. Clin. Exp. Immunol., *5*: 443, 1969.

92. de Schryver, A., Klein, G., and de Thé, G. Surface Antigens on Lymphoblastoid Cells Derived from Nasopharyngeal Carcinoma. Clin. Exp. Immunol., *7*: 161, 1970.

93. Sjögren, H. O. Transplantation Methods as a Tool for Detection of Tumor Specific Antigens. Progr. Exp. Tumor Res., *6*: 289, 1965.

94. Sjögren, H. O., and Hellström, I. Induction of Polyoma Specific Transplantation Antigenicity in Moloney Leukemia Cells. Exp. Cell Res., *40*: 208, 1965.

95. Skipper, H. E. Destruction of Leukemia Cells in Animals. Criteria Associated with Destruction of Leukemia and Solid Tumor Cells in Animals. Cancer Res., *27*: 2636, 1967.

96. Smith, R. T., Klein, G., Klein, E., and Clifford, P. Studies of the Membrane Phenomenon in Cultured and Biopsy Cell Lines from the Burkitt Lymphoma. *In* Advances in Transplantation, ed. by Dausset, Hamburger and Mathé, Vol. 779, p. 484, Copenhagen: Munksgaard, 1967.

97. Southam, C. M., Tanaka, S., Arata, T., Simkovic, D., Miura, M., and Peptiopules, S. F. Enhancement of Responses to Chemical Carcinogens by Nononcogenic Viruses and Antimetabolites. Progr. Exp. Tumor Res., *11*: 194, 1969.

98. Stjernswärd, J., Clifford, P., Sing, S., and Svedmyr, E. Indications of Cellular Immunological Reactions Against Autochthonous Tumor in Cancer Patients Studied *in vitro*. East African Med. J., *45*: 484, 1968.

99. Stück, B., Old, L. J., and Boyse, E. A. Antigenic Conversion of Established Leukemias by an Unrelated Leukaemogenic Virus. Nature, *202*: 1016, 1964.

100. Svedmyr, A., Demissie, A., Klein, G., and Clifford, P. Antibody Patterns in Different Human Sera against Intracellular and Membrane-antigens and Reutralization of EBV Infectivity. J. Nat. Cancer Inst., *44*: 595, 1970.

101. Svet-Moldavsky, G. J., Mkheidze, D. M., and Liozner, A. L. Phenomena Associated with Skin Grafting. Two Phenomena Associated with Akin Grafting from Tumor-bearing Syngeneic Donors. J. Nat. Cancer Isnt., *38*: 933, 1967.

102. Wiener, F., Klein, G., and Harris, H. The Analysis of Malignancy by Cell Fusion. III. Hybrids between Diploid Fibroblasts and Other Tumor Cells. J. Cell Science, *8*: 681, 1971.

103. Yata, J., and Klein, G. Some Factors Affecting Membrane Immunofluorescence Reactivity of Burkitt Lymphoma Tissue Culture Cell Lines. Int. J. Cancer, *4*: 767, 1969.

104. Yata, J., Klein, G., Hewetson, J., and Gergely, L. Effect of Metabolic Inhibitors on Membrane Immunofluorescence Reactivity of Established Burkitt Lymphoma Cell Lines. Int. J. Cancer, *5*: 394, 1970.

Immunological Studies on The Cell Membrane Receptors of Cultured Cells Derived from Nasopharyngeal Cancer, Burkitt's Lymphoma, and Infectious Mononucleosis

Kusuya Nishioka, Takehiko Tachibana, Takeshi Hirayama, G. de Thé, George Klein, Mitsuru Takada, and Akiyoshi Kawamura, Jr.

Virology Division and Epidemiology Division, National Cancer Center Research Institute, Tokyo, Japan [K. N., T. T., T. H.]; Biological Carcinogenesis Unit, International Agency for Research on Cancer, Lyon, France [G. T.]; Department of Tumor Biology, Karolinska Institute, Stockholm, Sweden [G. K.]; Department of Virology, Kitasato Institute, Tokyo, Japan [M. T.]; Department of Immunology, Institute of Medical Science, University of Tokyo, Tokyo, Japan [A. K.]

At present, more information on the nature of the cells carrying EB virus and on the biological activity of EB virus which could be detected by simple techniques is required to clarify the etiological problem of the virus. Concerning these two problems, we would like to present two new findings.

First, a method for the characterization and differentiation of the membranes of cultured cells of Burkitt's lymphoma from those of nasopharyngeal carcinoma or infectious mononucleosis was found.

Second, a new biological activity of EB virus was found in certain types of cells, capable of inducing a receptor that would bind sheep erythrocytes sensitized with IgG antibody.

New Immunocytological Cell Markers: Adherence of Immune Complex to Cell Receptors

Before the presentation of our experimental results, the immunocytological markers which have been employed in our experiments will be explained briefly.

They are the immune adherence (IA) receptor reacting with sheep erythrocytes sensitized with rabbit IgM antibody carrying the fourth and third components of complement [EA(IgM)C43], the IgG receptor reacting with sheep erythrocytes sensitized with rabbit IgG antibody [EA(IgG)], and the IgM receptor reacting with sheep erythrocytes sensitized with rabbit IgM antibody [EA(IgM)]. Adherence of EA(IgG) to the altered cell membrane, induced by infection with herpes simplex virus, was also noticed. Comparing these four kinds of receptors, either genetically determined by cell differentiation or induced by virus infection, the nature of the cell membrane reacting with each of these immune complexes can be differentiated.

IA receptor

The characteristics of the immune adherence receptor are shown in Table 1. Immune adherence (*23*) has been known as a phenomenon in which an antigen-antibody complex specifically attaches to the IA receptor of indicator cells only when the complex has been reacted with the first four components of complement, *i.e.*, C1, C4, C2 and C3 to form the antigen-antibody C1423 complex (*25*). Immune adherence essentially involves C3, as it can be shown that removal of C1 by EDTA treatment (*37*), C2 by prolonged incubation at 37°C (*25*), or C4 by pronase digestion (*32*) from the EAC1423 complex did not change its immune adherence characteristics. A similar phenomenon was shown to occur between human erythrocytes and tanned sheep erythrocytes coated with highly purified guinea pig C3 only, *i.e.*, without antibody, C1, C4, or C2 (*28*). These results indicate that the C3 bound on the antigen surface is the sole complement component reacting with the IA receptor of indicator cells.

The specific receptor site is present on primate erythrocytes or nonprimate platelets. On the other hand, evidence for the lack of the IA receptor in nonprimate erythrocytes and primate platelets has accumulated [see review (*20*)]. Recently more attention has been paid to the nature of the IA receptor of polymorphonuclear or mononuclear leucocytes. The presence of the IA receptor has

TABLE 1. Immune Adherence (IA) Receptor

Indicator	Detected on (+)	Species	Not detected on (−)
EA (IgM) C43	erythrocyte erythroblast platelet megakaryocyte	primate non-primate	platelet megakaryocyte erythrocyte erythroblast

	leucocytes
	  neutrophil
	  eosinophil
	macrophage
	monocyte in Blood
		primate
		and
		non-primate
			leucocytes
			  basophil
			
			peritoneal
			  mast cell

	reticular cell
	lymphocytes from
	lymph node, blood,
	spleen (10–25%)
			lymphocyte
			  from thymus
			  from lymph node
			  or blood (75–90%)
			plaque forming cell
			lymphoblast

	cultured NPC cells cultured IM cells	human	cultured BL cells

	chronic myelogenic
	  leukemia
		human	acute myelogenic &
			chronic lymphatic
			  leukemia

Destroyed by: trypsin, chymotrypsin, papain, tannic acid and formaldehyde, acetone and other organic solvents.

Not destroyed by: neuraminidase, periodate.

been demonstrated on both primate and nonprimate leucocytes (39). Since a distinction of the IA receptor from the IgG receptor which reacts with IgG in the absence of complement has been made (13), IgM antibody was used to make antigen antibody complement complex to detect the IA receptor. Employing these indicator cells, more clear-cut results on the distribution of the receptor on various cells were obtained. It was demonstrated on macrophages, blood monocytes, polymorphonuclear neutrophils, and eosinophils but was not detected on basophils or peritoneal mast cells. Ten to 25% of the lymphocytes taken from circulating blood, lymphnodes, or spleen showed the presence of IA receptors while none of the thymus lymphocytes showed any reactivity (16). A method for specific depletion of these EAC- reactive lymphocytes was devised after reacting EA(IgM)C43 followed by ultracentrifugation in a gradient of bovine serum albumin (2). More detailed information on these lymphocytes from mice as well as humans has been accumulating (18).

Mucoids or mucopeptides derived from human erythrocytes have been presumed to be IA receptors (22) but the yield and activity has not been high enough to convincingly identify these substances as IA receptors. Although the reactivity of normal human erythrocytes was found to be abolished by treatment with trypsin, tannic acid, papain, chymotrypsin, and formaldehyde (14, 21), and with acetone and other organic solvents (30), the physicochemical characterization of the IA receptor requires further experiment. Immunoglobulin G (IgG) from nonimmunized animals did not inhibit the interaction of the IA receptor and antigen-antibody complement complex while distinct inhibition was observed in the adherence of the antigen-antibody (IgG) complex with the IgG receptor (13). The inhibitory effects of EDTA vary according to the type of cells. Adherence of the EA(IgM)C complex to the IA receptor of certain types of cells [group (A)] was inhibited by the addition of EDTA; the other type of cells [group (B)] was not inhibited by EDTA. A requirement for Mg^{2+} was shown in the reaction of group (A) cells, such as mouse leucocytes (16, 44). Whether there is an essential difference between (A) type receptors and (B) type receptors, and if so, whether the cells of the (B) type contain (A) type receptor sites on the cells should be investigated further by more quantitative methods.

Employing these EA(IgM)C43 cells, the distribution of IA receptors on a variety of human cells was examined more quantitatively (24, 33, 44). On the average, 60% of peripheral erythrocytes from healthy adults and 90% of granulocytes and monocytes showed positive adherence. A similar distribution pattern was observed in erythrocytes and erythroblasts from a three month fetus. Leukemia cells obtained from chronic myelogenous leukemia showed a positive adherence pattern with EA(IgM)C43. On the other hand, those obtained from chronic lymphatic leukemia, acute lymphatic leukemia, and acute myelogenous leukemia did not react with EA(IgM)C43, indicating a lack of IA receptor.

IgG receptor and IgM receptor

Without participation of the complement system, antigen-antibody complexes adhere to a variety of cells. Depending upon the immunoglobulin class, the re-

TABLE 2.   IgG Receptor

Indicator	Detected on (+)	Species
EA (IgG)	monocytes	human, rabbit, guinea pig
"	macrophages	" " " "
"	neutrophils	human
EA (rabbit IgG)	neutrophils	rabbit
EA (g.p. IgG)	neutrophils	guinea pig (Henson)

Inhibited by :   normal IgG (Huber *et al.*)
Destroyed by :   iopoacetamide, *p*-chloromercury benzoate, formaldehyde, isothiocyanate, periodate, nitrite, lecithinase C (Howard *et al.*).
No inhibition by :   EDTA.
Not destroyed by :   trypsin, acetone, ethanol, phenol (Nishioka).

TABLE 3.   IgM Receptor

Indicator	Detected on (+)	Species
EA (rabbit IgM)	macrophages	rabbit
EA (mouse IgM)	macrophages	mouse
EA (rabbit IgM)	neutrophils	rabbit

Inhibited by :   EDTA : Ca^{2+} requiring.
No inhibition by :   IgG.
Not destroyed by :   trypsin (Lay *et al.*)

ceptors of these cells were classified as IgG receptors (*17*) and IgM receptors (*15*). Some characteristics of these two receptors are summarized in Tables 2 and 3.

For the detection of IgG receptors, sheep erythrocytes sensitized with the IgG fraction of antibody were most widely employed.   EA(IgG) was prepared by mixing sheep erythrocytes and optimal amounts of IgG antibody obtained from prolonged hyperimmunization, which gives the highest rate of rosette formation with target cells.   Adherence of EA(IgG) to neutrophils and macrophages or monocytes was observed.

As for the nature of the IgG receptor of neutrophils, much remained obscure. The receptor of macrophages or monocytes resembles the receptor for cytophilic antibodies (*1, 10*).   Human monocytes interact at least preferentially with IgG1 and IgG3, showing subclass specificity; the binding site of IgG for macrophages resides in the Fc fragment (*12*).   Ten μg/ml of free normal IgG could inhibit the reaction (*13*), but essentially no inhibition was observed after the addition of EDTA in the interaction of neutrophils and monocytes with EA(IgG) (*44*).   The IgG receptor site on guinea pig macrophages was removed or destroyed by treatment with   iodoacetamide,   *p*-chloromercury   benzoate,   formaldehyde,   isothiocyanate, periodate, nitrite, and lecithinase C.   From these results, it could be stated that free SH groups play an important part in the reactivity of the IgG receptor site peculiar to the macrophage surface membrane (*10*).   In contrast to the IA receptor, the IgG receptor could not be abolished by treatment with trypsin, organic solvent, or phenol (*26*).   The IgG receptor was uniformly lacking on lymphocytes, lymphoid cells, and lymphocytes stimulated with phytomitogens *in vitro*.   Huber *et al.* (*11*) proposed that IgG receptor could be an immunological marker for identification of mononuclear cells.   This has been utilized to distinguish monocyte or macrophage from lymphatic cells, and showed possibilities for use in pursuing the development cycle or differentiation pathway of cells of the monocyte-macrophage system.

The receptor for the EA(IgM) complex has been very recently described. When a large amount of IgM antibody of the same species of origin was used for the sensitization of E, EA(IgM) complex adhered to the rabbit macrophages or neutrophils and to mouse macrophage.   This reaction required Ca^{2+} and was not inhibited by the addition of IgG.   The receptor could not be destroyed by trypsin (*15, 44*).

Adherence of sensitized sheep erythrocytes after virus infection

A different type of adherence phenomenon of antigen-antibody (IgG) to the cell membrane infected with herpes simplex virus (HSV) has been described (*40*). As shown in Table 4, this phenomenon should be differentiated from the IA receptor, IgM receptor, and especially from the IgG receptor.   HeLa cells do not have IA or IgG receptors but, in an early stage after infection with herpes simplex virus, the adherence of EA(IgG) was observed and the adsorption was inhibited by anti-HSV antibody.

Development of profound alteration in the cell surface of HeLa cells was observed after HSV infection.   First, within one hr, the infected cells lost the ability to spread on the glass; this phenomenon was termed membrane paralysis (*41*).   Within 5 to 6 hr, virus antigen appeared at the cell surface and the cell acquired the ability to adsorb EA(IgG) complex.   Eight hr after infection, cell fusion and giant cell formation were observed (*4*).   Finally, infective virus appeared in 12 hr.   In this time table, hemadsorption coincided with the appearance of viral antigen on the cell surface.   From an inhibition study with actinomycin D and 5′-iodo-2 deoxyuridine, Watkins (*42*) explained the appearance of hemadsorption of EA(IgG) on the infected cell membrane as follows.   Infecting viral DNA codes for RNA, which in turn codes for the antigen that appears at the surface about an hr after the completion of DNA-directed RNA synthesis.   The synthesis of com-

TABLE 4.   Adherence of Sensitized Sheep Erythrocytes after Virus Infection

Indicator	Detected on (+)
EA(IgG)	cells infected with herpes simples virus (Watkins) cultured BL cells cultured host cells transformed by BL cell extract or NPC cell extract

Not destroyed by :   iodoacetamide, lecithinase C, *p*-chloromercury benzoate.
Destroyed by :   phenol, methanol (Yasuda).
No Inhibition by :   EDTA, normal IgG.

plete viral DNA is not necessary for this hemadsorption phenomenon but is required for cell fusion.

Hemadsorption of EA(IgG) to infected cells was not due to the appearance of cross-reacting antigen on the cell surface nor to the IgG receptor, since no inhibition was observed by anti-sheep E(IgM) antibody and normal IgG. Furthermore, some preliminary physicochemical characterization studies showed distinct differences. Treatment with iodoacetamide or *p*-chloromercury benzoate and lecithinase C had no effect, while mercaptoethanol, phenol, or methanol abolished the reactivity (*43*). These results show quite the reverse of the effects of these chemical treatments on the IgG receptor of monocytes and on the receptor of HSV infected cells for antigen-antibody (IgG) complex. Although much more quantitative analysis is required (*34*), antiglobulin affinity to the HSV-infected cells was differentiated from the IgG receptor by these experiments. The possibility that it might be analogous to the rheumatoid factor has been suggested by Milgrom (*43*).

MATERIALS AND METHODS

Cultured cell lines derived from nasopharyngeal cancer, Burkitt's lymphoma, and infectious mononucleosis

The establishment and maintenance of the cell lines from biopsies of nasopharyngeal cancer (NPC), Burkitt's lymphoma (BL), and peripheral leucocytes of infectious mononucleosis (IM) have been described in detail (*5, 19, 36, 38*). The following cell lines were used.

Cell lines derived from nasopharyngeal cancer: 204, 223, 306, and 307 are the cell lines obtained from three male NPC patients in Taiwan. Liang Kuang Seng, 55 yrs, male; and Fong Hui Tsai, 36 yrs, male respectively. Ly1, Ly2, Ly11, Ly17, Ly20, Ly23, Ly25, and Ly26 developed in Lyon from NPC biopsies provided by Dr. Ho in Hong Kong (*38*) were studied. Two other African NPC-derived lines were developed in Lyon; 9 were from male patients and 3 from females.

Cell lines from Burkitt's lymphoma: Twentyeight cell lines derived from biopsies of BL patients were employed. They were the P3HR1, P3HR1-X, and P3HR1-N cell lines cloned by Dr. Hinuma at Tohoku University (*9*); EB3 (*6*); Jijoye; Raji (*29*); Esther (NK-8) (*19*); Silfere (NK-9) (*19*); Daudi (NK-10) (*19*); Maku (NK-51) (*19*); and BT-1 derived from a Japanese BL patient (*27*). In addition to these established cell lines, newly cultured cell lines which had been established partly by Drs. J. S. and J. J. Nadkarni and partly by Dr. Bal Gothoskar were employed. They were the Wanyama Famba III, Onesmas, Penina (max), Penina (ova), Salim Mwalim III, Namalwa IV, Akinyi (ova), Margaret (abd.), David (mand.), Isabella (breast), Isabella (max.), Sulubu, M. Wekesa, W. Nyikande I, and W. Nyikande II cell lines which were cultured in the Department of Tumor Biology, Karolinska Institutet. Cell lines, Ly 45 and Ly 46, were developed in Lyon from BL biopsies obtained from Nairobi, by the country of Dr. P. Clifford. The biopsy patients were a 6 year old male and an 8 year old female.

Cell lines derived from peripheral leucocytes of infectious mononucleosis: Kaplan, Scherzer, IM 63, and IM 71, which have been isolated in Dr. Henle's laboratory and maintained in the IARC laboratory were used. The IMJI cell line was derived from the lymph nodes of an IM patient in Tokyo Teishin Hospital, a 7 year old male, and cultured by Takada at the Kitasato Institute.

All these cell lines were cultured in medium RPMI-1640 or Eagle's MEM supplemented with 20% fetal calf serum and were harvested on the day of the experiment and washed three times with 0.1% gelatin veronal buffered saline (pH 7.5) containing 0.15 mM $CaCl_2$ and 0.5 mM $MgCl_2$ (GVB^{2+}).

Sheep erythrocyte (E), rabbit antibody to sheep erythrocyte (A), EA(IgG), EA(IgM)C43

All these reagents were prepared according to the methods described in a previous paper (*26*). In the later experiments, EA(IgG) cells prepared after the method of Tachibana *et al.* (*34*) were employed to detect hemadsorption reactivity.

For the indicator cells to detect the IA receptor, EA(IgM)C43 cells were employed. In our laboratory, these cells were prepared first by sensitization of the optimal amount of IgM rabbit antibody against sheep E; 1,000 SFU of guinea pig C1, 300 SFU of human C4, 200 SFU of guinea pig C2, and 300 CIA50 of guinea pig C3 per sheep erythrocyte were added. Second, C1 and C2 are removed by EDTA and by prolonged incubation at 37°C.

Normal IgG fraction of rabbit serum, guinea pig macrophage, enzymes, and chemicals

These have been described in reference (*26*).

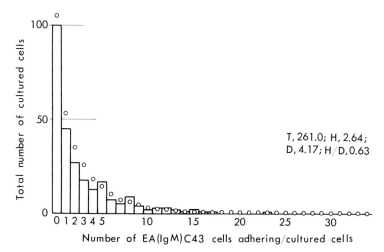

FIG. 1. Frequency distribution of EA(IgG)C43 cells adhering to single cultured cells derived from NPC(204).

	0	1	2	3	4	≥ 25
Found	100	45	27	18	13	58
Calculated	105.4	53.8	35.4	25.1	18.4	60.1

○ : Calculated from Pólya-Eggenberger distribution.

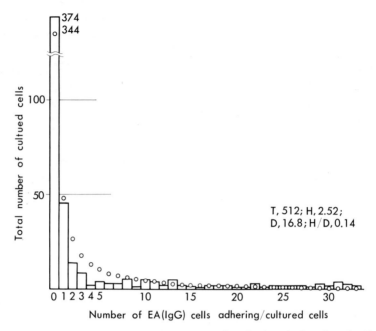

FIG. 2.   Frequency distribution of EA(IgG) cells adhering single cultured cells derived from Burkitt's lymphoma (P3HRI).

	0	1	2	3	4	≥ 5
Found	374	45	14	9	2	68
Calculated	344.0	48.5	26.3	17.8	13.2	77.2

○ : Calculated from Pólya-Eggenberger distribution.

Frequency distribution of EA(IgM)C43 cells or EA(IgG) cell adhering to single cultured cells

The cultured cells were washed and 5×10^6/ml of the cell suspension in 0.025 ml of GVB^{2+} was mixed with a equal volume of 1×10^8/ml EA(IgM)C43 cells or 1×10^8/ml of EA(IgG) in a U type microplate.   After incubation for 60 min at 37°C and 60 min at 20°C, the adherence pattern was read under a microscope.   In the later experiment with EA(IgG), the pattern was read after incubation at 25°C for 5 hr or more to obtain the maximum reactivity (*34*).   The number of EA(IgM) C43 cells adhering to each of the cultured cells of NPC origin was counted under a microscope and plotted diagramatically in Fig. 1.   The number of EA(IgG) cells attached to a single cell of the BL cell line is plotted in Fig. 2.   The distribution curve of both types of reactions, *i.e.*, EA(IgM)C43 with the NPC cell line and EA (IgG) with the BL cell line, showed patterns of Pólya-Eggenberger distribution rather than Poisson distribution as shown in both figures.   The calculated value and experimental data of adherence distribution are shown in the figures which both coincide very closely and show a single type of distribution as regards the interaction of these cell populations with EA(IgM)C43 or with EA(IgG).

As they proved to show a single type of distribution, the cultured cells were classified routinely according to the number of indicator cells [EA(IgMC43) or EA (IgG)] adhering to the cultured cell surface.

RESULTS AND DISCUSSION

Differentiation of NPC cell lines from BL cell lines with regard to the interaction with EA(IgM) C43 or EA (IgG).

A part of our experimental results are shown in Table 5 and Fig. 3. Three Burkitt's lymphoma cell lines (P3HR1, Raji, and Maku) showed no adherence of EA(IgM)C43 cells. Only a small percentage of these cells showed adherence patterns with one or, at most, two EA(IgM)C43 cells and typical rosette formation was not observed at all. On the other hand, all of the NPC cell lines [Lyll, 204 cells cultured in RPMI 1640 medium (204R) or in Eagle's MEM (204M)] showed a very strong reaction with EA(IgM)C43 cells. A large number of these NPC cell lines adhered to more than two EA(IgM)C43 cells, resulting in typical rosette formation.

The statistical analysis is shown in Fig. 3 by taking Lyll cells as the identified distribution (*3*), *i.e.*, average ridit 0.500. Average ridits of 204R and 204M were 0.554 (0.612–0.497) and 0.497 (0.55–0.439), respectively. On the other hand, those of the BL cell lines were 0.153 (0.210–0.095) for P3HR1, 0.147 (0.205–0.089) for Maku and 0.147 (0.205–0.095) for Raji. These statistical analyses confirmed the above observation and, from their ridit values, all these cell lines were classified into two groups. 1) Lyll, 204R, and 204M, which have IA receptors, and 2) P3HR1, Maku, and Raji, which lack IA receptors. The first three cell lines were of NPC origin and the second three cell lines originated from Burkitt's lymphoma.

Instead of EA(IgM)C43, EA(IgG) was reacted with these six cell lines. Here, none of the positive adherence pattern was observed with Lyll, 204M, and 204R cells, while a strong rosette formation was observed with P3HR1, Maku, and Raji cells. Ridit analysis was performed and the results, summarized in Table 5, showed

TABLE 5.   Percentage of Frequency Distribution of Number of EA (IgM) C43 Cells or EA (IgG) Cell Adhering to Cultured Cell Surface

Number of EA (IgM) C43/cells	0	1	2	3	4	≥5
NPC : Lyll	28	12	5	17	10	28
NPC : 204 R	15	14	6	19	15	30
NPC : 204 M	29	15	5	10	16	26
BL : P3HR1	94	5	1	0	0	0
BL : Raji	93	7	0	0	0	0
BL : Maku	97	2	1	0	0	0
Number of EA (IgG)/cell	0	1	2	3	4	≥5
BL : P3HR1	55	6	6	4	2	27
BL : Raji	43	11	5	4	3	34
BL : Maku	71	1	1	1	6	16
NPC : Lyll	93	6	1	0	0	0
NPC : 204 M	100	0	0	0	0	0
NPC : 204 R	98	1	0	1	0	0

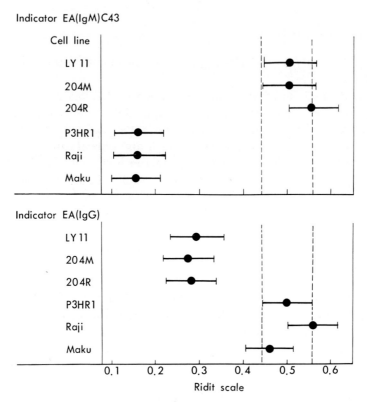

FIG. 3. Relative identified distribution of cultured cell line in reference to adherence of EA(IgM) C43 and EA(IgG).

that all three cell lines obtained from BL could be classified into one group which showed a positive adherence pattern to the EA(IgG) complex, while all three lines derived from NPC could be classified into the other group which did not show any positive adherence of EA(IgG) cells. The results described in the above experiments indicate that all three cell lines obtained from NPC patients showed a positive adherence pattern with EA(IgM)C43 and a negative pattern with EA(IgG). On the contrary, the three cell lines obtained from BL patients showed positive adherence of EA(IgG) but were negative with EA(IgM)C43, thus a method for differentiating cultured cell lines of NPC from those of BL was presented.

No positive reaction was observed in any of these BL and NPC cells when reacted with sheep erythrocytes (E), sheep erythrocytes sensitized with A(IgM) E(AIgM), EA(IgM)C14, or EA(IgM)C142 cells. Even when a 10 times greater concentration of A(IgM) was used for sensitization of sheep E, no adherence pattern was observed with these EA(IgM) cells.

Reactivity of cultured NPC cell lines with EA(IgM)C43 and EA(IgG)

Starting from these preliminary tests, the reactivity of 16 cultured cell lines with EA(IgM)C43 and EA(IgG) was examined. The average ridit values of all cell

TABLE 6. Reactivity of Cultured NPC Cell Lines with EA(IgM)C43 and EA(IgG)

Cell line	Place	Patient's name	Age	Sex	Ridit value reacting with EA(IgM)C43	EA(IgG)
204	TW	H.T.S.	42	M	0.500	0.269
223	TW				0.665	0.312
306	TW	L.K.S.	55	M	0.648	0.314
307	TW	F.H.T.	36	M	0.673	0.279
Ly1	HK	H.S.	43	M	0.443	0.318
Ly2	HK	T.S.	52	M	0.568	0.267
Ly11	HK	C.K.L.	40	M	0.666	0.319
Ly17	HK	P.F.L.	45	M	0.839	0.262
Ly20	HK	K.W.S.	64	F	0.806	0.264
Ly23	HK	T.S.S.	62	M	0.367	0.420
Ly25	HK	T.Y.K.	19	F	0.664	0.268
Ly26	HK	L.M.S.	72	M	0.677	0.264
Ly28	HK	N.Y.T.	38	M	0.763	0.269
Ly42	HK	F.S.Y.	35	M	0.640	0.318
Ly12	NB	S.C.	38	F	0.864	0.276
Ly13	NB	N.K.	35	M	0.719	0.277
Control cell line						
P3HR1	BL standard				0.367	0.500

TW: Taiwan; HK: Hong Kong; NB: Nairobi.

lines with reference to EA(IgM)C43 are shown in Table 6 in the first columm; those with reference to EA(IgG) are shown in the second columm of the same table.

As a representative of NPC cell lines, the 204 cell line was taken as an identified distribution, 0.500 with regard to its reactivity with EA(IgM)C43. As a prototype of BL cell lines, P3HR1 cells were taken as an identified distribution, 0.500, with regard to its reactivity with EA(IgG). From these figures, it was concluded that all four cell lines from Taiwan, and two lines from Nairobi showed high reactivity with EA(IgM)C43. One out of the ten cell lines obtained from Hong Kong, Ly 23, did not show a positive reaction with EA(IgM)C43 and Ly1 showed a weak reaction. The other 8 cell lines showed high reactivity with EA(IgM)C43.

On the contrary, except for one cell line, Ly23, all 15 cell lines showed essentially negative or very weak reaction with EA(IgG). The conclusion obtained in a preliminary experiment, that cultured NPC cell lines showed high reactivity with EA(IgM)C43 and low reactivity with EA(IgG), was confirmed with only the exception of Ly23.

As listed in Table 6, NPC cell lines taken from either Hong Kong, Taiwan, or Nairobi showed no differences.

As so far examined, the results supported the view that the hemadsorption activity of NPC cell lines with EA(IgM)C43 and not with EA(IgG) is predominantly determined by the the disease of origin, i.e., NPC. Any significant differences with reference to age, sex, race, or geographical distribution could not be observed.

The positive reaction of the NPC cell lines with EA(IgM)C43 was not inhibited by EDTA or normal IgG as described above (26). These observations indicate the

TABLE 7. Reactivity of Cultured IM Cell Lines with EA(IgM)C43 and EA(IgG)

Cell line	Isolated by	Ridit value reacting with	
		EA(IgM)C43	EA(IgG)
IMJI	Takada	0.706	0.261
Kaplan	Henle	0.662	0.263
IM 63	Henle	0.623	0.277
Scherzer	Henle	0.510	0.271
IM 71	Henle	0.490	0.269
Control cell line			
P3HR1	BL standard	0.367	0.500
204	NPC standard	0.500	0.269

lack of an IgG receptor or an IgM receptor on the surface of cell lines from NPC, since the IgG receptor is known to react with the EA(IgG) complex and is inhibited by IgG (13), and the IgM receptor is known to react with EA(IgM) in the presence of Ca^{2+} (15). On the contrary, when these cells were treated with trypsin or acetone, almost all of the reactivity with EA(IgM)C43 was lost. When the IA receptor were removed by trypsin (20) and acetone (31), no inhibition was observed with normal IgG (13); thus, the presence of the IA receptor on the surface of the cell lines from NPC was established. Since EDTA did not show any inhibition, the IA receptor present on cells from NPC was considered to be the B type (16), which was known to be present on primate erythrocytes and on a portion of lymph node cells, rather than the A type IA receptor, which was known to be present in nonprimate platelets or other cells requiring Mg^{2+} in the interaction with the EA(IgM)C complex (16).

Reactivity of cultured IM cell lines with EA(IgM)C43 and EA(IgG)

Five cell lines derived from peripheral leucocytes or lymph node biopsies of IM patients were examined. Taking the same identified distribution, it was shown that all of the five cell lines showed essentially no reaction with EA(IgG), while 4 cell lines (IMJI, Kaplan, Scherzer and IM 63) showed high reactivity with EA(IgM)C43, and the IM 71 cell line showed a rather low reactivity with EA (IgM)C43. As shown in Table 7, the patterns are similar with the reactivities of NPC cell lines and not with those of BL cell lines. Again, it was confirmed that the reactions of these cell lines were not inhibited by EDTA or IgG or removed after treatment by acetone or trypsin as examined by the previously described method (26).

Reactivity of cultured BL cell lines with EA(IgM)C43 and EA(IgG)

The same types of experiment as described above were carried out and the re-results, with 28 cell lines obtained from 27 cases of African BL and one case of Japanese BL, are shown in Table 8.

Taking the same standard as in the experiment with the NPC cell lines, it was demonstrated that (i) except for 5 cell lines [M. Wekesa, W. Nyikande I and

TABLE 8. Reactivity of Cultured BL Cell Lines with EA(IgM)C43 and EA(IgG)

Cell line and patients name		Age	Sex	KCC No.	Ridit value reactivity with	
					EA(IgM)C43	EA(IgG)
NK–8	Esther	11	F	674	0.384	0.359
NK–9	Silfere	6	F	732	0.378	0.341
NK–10	Daudi	16	M	750	0.363	0.797
NK–51	Maku	8	F	2076	0.366	0.430
BT–1		5	M	(Tokyo)	0.423	0.275
Ly45	O.W.	6	M	(Lyon)	0.458	0.396
Ly46	P.M.	8	F	(Lyon)	0.686	0.443
Akinyi	O.	7	F	1230	0.365	0.411
David	R.	13	M		0.379	0.338
Isabella	R. breast	15	M	1225	0.368	0.334
	max.				0.358	0.277
Margaret	N.	13	F	1223	0.378	0.341
Masafu	W.	6	F	1076	0.558	0.312
Namalwa	J. IV	5	F	976	0.363	0.415
Onesmas	N.	3	M	1041	0.357	0.572
Salim	M.	5	M	1040	0.553	0.456
Wanyama	F.	8	M	1046	0.381	0.589
Wekesa	N. I	7	F	1080	0.358	0.277
	II				0.373	0.291
Penina	M. max.	8	F	1140	0.369	0.532
	ova				0.418	0.431
Sulubu					0.386	0.323
Control cell lines (BL)						
P3HR1					0.367	0.500
P3HR1 X					0.359	0.448
P3HR1 N					0.362	0.409
Jijoye					0.469	0.538
EB3					0.364	0.467
Raji					0.352	0.554
Control cell line (NPC)						
204					0.500	0.269

II, Isabella (max.), and BT-1], the 23 cell lines derived from BL showed strong reactivity with EA(IgG). (ii) Ly 46, M. Wekesa and S. Mwalim III showed strong reactivity with EA(IgM)C43 and Ly 45, Jijoye, and Penia (ova) cell lines showed a weakly positive reaction with the same indicator cells. All the other 22 cell lines showed an essentialy negative reaction with EA(IgM)C43. Since in all the cell lines except for the P3HR1 cells, the cell lines were not yet cloned, some monocytes or lymphoreticular cells which show reactivity with EA(IgM)C43 might be present.

Considering these possibilities, in this case too, the high reactivity of most cultured BL cell lines with EA(IgG) and low reactivity with EA(IgM)C43 seem to be predominantly determined by their disease of origin, i.e., Burkitt's lymphoma.

As for the positive reaction of the cells from BL with EA(IgG), two possibilities were considered. First, it could be due to the presence of an IgG receptor on the BL cells or second, it could be due to an altered state of the membrane induced by infection with EBV, and analogous to the receptor induced by herpes simplex virus (HSV).   The IgG receptor was not digested by trypsin (*10*) and no inhibition was observed with the addition of EDTA (*13*).   However, acetone treatment or phenol treatment abolished the reactivity of BL cells with EA(IgG); no inhibition was observed with the addition of IgG as described in (*26*).   These results did not coincide with the IgG receptor so far known.   On the other hand, the hemadsorption activity which appeared on the cell membrane infected with HSV was removed by acetone or phenol (*8*) and IgG preparation did not inhibit the reaction.   Therefore, comparative studies by chemical modification were attempted.

Trypsin did not remove the reactivity of P3HR1, Raji, or guinea pig macrophages.   However, a distinct difference from the nature of the IgG receptor was observed when these P3HR1 or Raji cells were treated with acetone and phenol. Both reagents diminished the reactivity of these cells, while the IgG receptor present on guinea pig macrophage remained intact.   It is most plausible that the interaction of BL with EA(IgG) fits into the category of adherence of sensitized sheep erythrocytes after HSV-infection and not that of the IgG receptor or genetic cell marker, although both were reacted with EA(IgG).

In the case of herpes simplex virus infection, the virus particles are liberated and the host cells undergo lysis, resulting in lytic infection.   On the other hand, through the entire course of EBV-BL cell line interaction, no lytic infection occurred.   However, it is an important finding that these BL cell lines showed a similar reaction to EA(IgG) as the cells in the early stage of herpes simplex virus infection did.   It is most plausible that these reactions might be due to the manifestation of the biological activity of EBV harboring in BL cell lines.   We would like to emphasize here that not only the P3HR1 and other BL cells which have been known as typical EBV-producing cells, but a nonvirus-producing BL cell line, Raji, also showed hemadsorption of EA(IgG) and both were removed by acetone or phenol.   These findings are in line with the suggestion that an apparently virus-free line of Burkitt's tumor cells may contain DNA derived from the viral genome (*7*), indicating a similarity between EBV and known oncogenic DNA viruses.

Reactivity of transformed cells after addition of BL or NPC cell extract to fibroblastic cultured cell sheets of NPC origin

Finally, the authors would like to present one more experimental result supporting the view that adherence of EA(IgG) to BL cell lines is considered to be related to a newly discovered biological activity of EB virus.   Takada has reported (*35*) that they obtained T1, T3, and T4 cell lines which have been transformed by the addition of a millipore filtrate of P3HR1 cell extract or 204 cell extract to fibroblastic cultured cell sheets of nasopharyngeal origin.   T1 are transformed cells from an N12 mother cell sheet after the addition of extract of BL cell P3HR1 and T3 are transformed cell from the same mother cells by an extract of NPC cell line 204.   T4 are newly transformed cells from N27 mother cells after the addition of a millipore filtrate of 204 cell extract.   Both these filtrates have been considered to contain intact EB virus particles.   All these mother cells (N12 and N27) did not show any sign of floating or spontaneous transformation without

TABLE 9. Percentage of Frequency Distribution of Number of EA(IgG) Cell Adhering to Cells Transformed by BL or NPC Cell Extract

Origin	Infected with cell extract from	Cell line	Number of EA(IgG)/cell					
			0	1	2	3	4	≥ 5
BL	—	P3HR1	51.5	9.5	7.5	6.5	4.0	22.0
NPC	—	204	196.5	2.0	1.5	0	0	0
N12	(P3HR1)	T1	62.8	16.5	9.1	5.8	3.3	2.5
N12	(204)	T3	54.5	15.5	8.0	4.0	3.5	15.0
—	—	N27	196.5	3.5	0	0	0	0
N27	(204)	T4	57.0	17.0	9.0	4.0	1.0	17.0

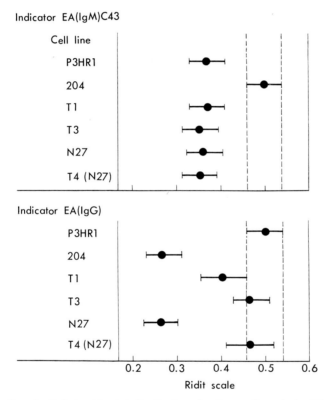

FIG. 4. Relative identied distribution of cells transformed by BL or NPC cell extract.

the addition of the cultured cell filtrate of 204 or P3HR1.

All these cell lines, T1, T3, T4, and the mother cells, N27, were examined for their reactivities with EA(IgM)C43 and EA(IgG). Regarding the 204 cell line as representative of the reactivity with EA(IgM)C43 and the P3HR1 cells as representative of the reactivity with EA(IgG), the corresponding reactivities of the transformed cells and their mother cells are shown in Table 9 and Fig. 4. Neither T1, T3, nor T4 showed any adherence of EA(IgM)C43 but all three of them showed adherence of EA(IgG) in a similar way as the P3HR1 cells did. In contrast, N27 cells, the uninfected mother cells of T4, did not show any adherence of EA(IgG) or of EA(IgM)C43.   Therefore, the adherence of EA(IgG) to T1, T3, and T4 cells is due to the manifestation of the viral genome of the EB virus derived from NPC or BL cell extract, as is demonstrated in the early stage of HSV-infection or in the persistent infection of EB virus in BL cell lines.   The adherence of EA(IgG) to cultured BL cells could be considered as the expression of the EB virus genome in a state of persistent infection.

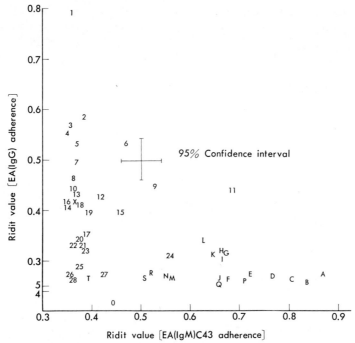

FIG. 5. Differentiation of cell lines derived from nasopharyngeal carcinoma, infections mononucleosis and Burkitt's lymphoma.

Burkitt's lymphoma		Burkitt's lymphoma		Nasopharyngeal carcinoma			Infectious mononucleosis	
1	Daudi (NK–10)	15	Ly45 NB	A	Ly12	N B	P	IMJI
2	Wanyama farba III	16	Namalwa IV	B	Ly17	H K	Q	Kaplan
3	Onesmas	17	Esther (NK–8)	C	Ly20	H K	R	IM63
4	Raji	18	Akinyi (ova)	D	Ly28	H K	S	Scherzer
5	Penina (max)	19	Silfere (NK–9)	E	Ly13	H K	T	IM71
6	Jijoye	20	Margaret (abd)	F	Ly26	H K		
7	P3HR1 K	21	David (mand)	G	307	T P		
8	EB3	22	Isabella (breast)	H	Ly11	H K		
9	S. Mwali III	23	Sulubu	I	223	T P		
10	P3HR1 X	24	M. Wekesa	J	Ly25	H K		
11	Ly46 NB	25	W. Nyikande II	K	306	T P		
12	Penina (ova)	26	Isabella (max)	L	Ly42	H K		
13	Maku (NK–51)	27	BT–1 TK	M	Ly 2	H K		
14	P3HR1 N	28	W. Nyikande I	N	204	T P		
				O	Ly 1	H K		
				X	Ly23	H K		

The reason why the NPC cell lines obtained from NPC biopsies did not show adherence of EA(IgG) must be clarified in further experiments. Two possibilities could be considered. First, *in vivo*, the target cells of EB virus in NPC patients might differ from those of BL patients. As a second alternative, it is possible that different kinds of EBV carrying cells become established *in vitro*, depending on some of the many different conditions by which NPC patients and their tumors differ from BL patients. The difference probably is due to the effect of age, the immunological maturity of the host or to other environmental or genetic reasons.

It is noteworthy, however, that both EB virus preparations derived from NPC and BL cells showed similar types of transformation of cultured cell sheets which have been attributed to the common character of the EB virus.

In summary, as shown in Fig. 5, the average ridit of each cell line with reference to EA(IgG) adherence was plotted in a vertical line and the average ridit with reference to EA(IgM)C43 in the horizontal line. P3HR1 and 204 cells were taken as an identified distribution, 0.500 representing the prototype of BL and NPC cells. As shown in this figure, 27 of the 28 Burkitt's cell lines showed a positive reaction with EAIgG; the negative line was M Wekesa. Fifteen out of sixteen NPC cell lines showed positive adherence with EAIgMC43. The one exception was Ly 23. All 5 cell lines of IM origin showed adherence of EA(IgM)C43 and were negative with EAIgG.

Except for one exceptional case of each, the BL lines and NPC lines were classified into two groups, that is, BL predominantly reacting with EA(IgG) and NPC predominantly reacting with EA(IgM)C43. IM cell lines showed a similar pattern to NPC cell lines.

The reactivity with EA(IgG) similar to the BL cell lines was observed in some kinds of proper host cells when these cells were infected and transformed with EB virus preparations derived from cell extracts of both NPC and BL.

SUMMARY

Based on phylogenetic or ontogenetic characteristics, immunocytological markers have recently been applied to the classification and characterization of a variety of cells which had been difficult to deal with by other cytological methods. They are the immune adherence (IA) receptor reacting with EA(IgM)C43, the IgG receptor reacting with EA(IgG), and the IgM receptor reacting with EA(IgM). Adherence of EA(IgG) to an altered cell membrane, induced by infection with herpes simplex virus, was also noticed by studying the four kinds of receptors, either genetically determined or induced by virus infection, the nature of the cell membrane reacting with each of these immune complexes can be differentiated.

Based on these immunochemical characteristics, differentiation was made between EBV-carrying blastoid cell lines derived from nasopharyngeal carcinoma (NPC), Burkitt's lymphoma (BL), and infectious mononucleosis (IM). The NPC and IM cell lines showed adherence with EA(IgM)C43 and the BL cell lines showed adherence of EA(IgG).

All the results examined so far indicate that the NPC and IM cell lines have

IA receptors. The cell lines derived from BL showed a reaction with EA(IgG) similar to the hemadsorption phenomenon observed in the early stage of herpes simplex virus infection, indicating that EBV may have a similar, previously unknown, biological activity.

Reactivity of transformed cells after the addition of BL or NPC cell extract to a fibroblastic cultured cell sheet of NPC origin was also examined. These floating cells showed high reactivity with EA(IgG) while fibroblastic cells before infection by BL or NPC did not. This indicated that the floating cells developed receptors for the adsorption reaction as a result of EBV-infection and, possibly, transformation.

The work of our group was supported by grants from the Ministry of Health and Welfare, Ministry of Education, Princess Takamatsu Fund for Cancer Research and the Society for Promotion of Cancer Research. The author wish to thank Drs. J. S. and J. J. Nadkarni and Dr. Gothoskar for their kindness in supplying the tissue culture cell lines used in this experiments.

REFERENCES

1. Berken, A., and Benacerraf, B. Properties of Antibodies Cytophilic to Macrophages. J. Exp. Med., *123*: 119–144, 1966.
2. Bianco, C. Patrick, R., and Nussenzweig, V. A Population of Lymphocytes Bearing a Membrane Receptor for Antigen-antibody-complement Complexes. J. Exp. Med., *132*: 702–720, 1970.
3. Bross, I. D. J. How to Use Ridit Analysis, Biometrics. Biometrics Society, *14*: 18–88, 1958.
4. Bungay, C., and Watkins, J. F. Observations on Polykaryocytosis in HeLa Cells Infected with Herpes Simplex Virus. Brit. J. Exp. Path., *45*: 48–55, 1966.
5. Diehl, V., Henle, W., and Kohn, G. Demonstration of a Herpes Group Virus in Cultures of Peripheral Leucocytes from Patients with Infectious Mononucleosis. J. Virol., *2*: 663–669, 1969.
6. Epstein, M. A., Barr, Y. M., and Achong, R. G. Studies with Burkitt's Lymphoma in Methodological Approaches to the Study of Leukemias. Wistar Inst. Sympos. Monograph, *4*: 69–79, 1965.
7. zur Hausen, H., and Schulte-Holthausen, H. Presence of EB Virus Nucleic Acid Homology in a " Virus Free " Line of Burkitt Tumor Cells. Nature, *227*: 245–248, 1970.
8. Hayashi, K. Membrane Changes of Cells Infected with Herpes Simplex Virus. Proceedings of The 1st International Symposium of the Princess Takamatsu Cancer Research Fund, pp. 139, University of Tokyo Press, Tokyo, 1971.
9. Hinuma, Y., and Grace, J., Cloning of Immunoglobulin Producing Human Leukemic and Lymphoma Cells in Long-term Cultures. Proc. Soc. Exp. Biol. Med., *124*: 107–111, 1967.
10. Howard, J. G., and Benacerraf, B. Properties of Macrophage Receptors for Cytophilic Antibodies. Brit. J. Exp. Path., *47*: 193–200, 1966.
11. Huber, H., Douglas, S. D., and Fudenberg, H. H. The IgG Receptor, an Immunological Marker for the Characterization of Mononuclear Cells. Immunology, *17*: 7–12, 1969.
12. Huber, H., and Fudenberg, H. H. Receptor Sites of Human Monocytes for IgG.

Int. Arch. Allergy, *34*: 18–31, 1968.

13. Huber, H., Polley, M. J., Linscott, W. D., Fudenberg, H., and Müller-Ebehard, H. J. Human Monocytes, Distinct Receptor Sites for the Third Component of Complement and for Immunoglobulin G. Science, *162*: 1281–1283, 1968.

14. Kourilsky, R., Pieron, R., Kourilsky, S., and Voisin, G. Recherches sur le Méchanisme du Phénomêne de L'immune-Adhérence. Ann. Inst. Pasteur, *89*: 273–279, 1955.

15. Lay, W., and Nussenzweig, V. Ca^{2+}-Dependent Binding of Antigen-19S Antibody Complexes to Macrophages. J. Immunol., *102*: 1172–1178, 1969.

16. Lay, W. H., and Nussenzweig, V. Receptors for Complement on Leukocytes. J. Exp. Med., *128*: 991–1007, 1968.

17. Lo Buglio, A. F., Contran, R. S., and Handle, J. H. Red Cells Coated with Immunoglobulin G. Binding and Sphering by Mononuclear Cells in Man. Science, *158*: 1582–1585, 1967.

18. Michlmar, G., and Huber, H. Receptor Sites for Complement on Certain Human Peripheral Blood Lymphocytes. J. Immunol., *105*: 670–676, 1970.

19. Nadkarni, J. S., Nadkarni, J. J., Clifford, P., Manolov, G., Fenyö, E. M., and Klein, E. Characteristics of New Cell Lines Derived from Burkitt Lymphomas. Cancer, *23*: 64–79, 1969.

20. Nelson, D. S. Immune Adherence. Advan. in Immunology, *3*: 131–180, 1963.

21. Nelson, D. S., and Nelson, R. A., Jr. On the Mechanism of Immune Adherence. Yale J. Biol. Med., *31*: 185–200, 1959.

22. Nelson, D. S., and Uhlenbruck, G. Studies on the Nature of the Immune Adherence Receptor. I. The Inhibition of Immune Adherence by Soluble Mucoids and Mucopeptides and by Human Erythrocyte Ghosts. Vox Sang., *12*: 43–67, 1967.

23. Nelson, R. A., Jr. The Immune Adherence Phenomenon. An Immunologically Specific Reaction between Microorganisms and Erythrocytes Leading to Enhanced Phagocytosis. Science, *118*: 733–737, 1963.

24. Nishioka, K. Complement and Tumor Immunology. Advan. Cancer Research, *14*: 231–293, 1971.

25. Nishioka, K., and Linscott, W. D. Components of Guinea Pig Complement, I. Separation of a Serum Fraction Essential for Immune Hemolysis and Immune Adherence. J. Exp. Med., *118*: 767–793, 1963.

26. Nishioka, K., Tachibana, T., Sekine, T., Inoue, M., Hirayama, T., Sugano, H., Yoshida, T. O., Takada, M., Kawamura, Jr., and Wang, C.-H. Immunocytological Studies on Cultured Cells Derived from Nasopharyngeal Carcinoma and Burkitt Lymphoma and an Improved Method of Immune Adherence Reaction. GANN Monograph, *10*: 265–279, 1970.

27. Oboshi, S., and Seido, T. Establishment of Cell Lines of Burkitt Lymphoma Origin. Igaku no Ayumi, *74*: 220–222, 1970 (in Japanese).

28. Okada, H., Kawachi, S., and Nishioka, K. Immune Adherence Reactivity by C3 Molecules without Antibody and Other Factors of the Complement System. Biochim. Biophys. Acta, *208*: 541–543, 1970.

29. Puvertaft, J. V. Cytology of Burkitt's Tumour (African Lymphoma). Lancet, *1*: 238–240, 1964.

30. Sekine, T. Personal communication, 1970.

31. Sekine, T. Personal communication, 1970.

32. Sekine, T., Mayumi, M., and Nishioka, K. Studies on the Mechanism of Immune Adherence. Japan. J. Allergology, *18*: 142, 1969 (in Japanese).

33. Sekine, T., Nishioka, K., Yoshida, T., and Imai, K.   Reaction of Phagocytes and Blood Cells with Antigen Antibody Complement Complex.   Immunobiology, *3*: 34–38, 1969 (in Japanese).

34. Tachibana, T., Nishioka, K., Hirayama, T., and Kawamura, A., Jr.   Immunological Analysis on Hemadsorption of Cultured   Cells Derived from Burkitt's Lymphoma. Proceedings of The 1st International Symposium of The Princess Takamatsu Cancer Research Fund, pp. 433, University of Tokyo Press, Tokyo, 1971.

35. Takada, M.   Kawamura, A., Jr., and Sugano, H. Biological Activities of Herpes Type Virus Derived from Nasopharyn geal Carcinoma and Burkitt's Lymphoma. Proceedings of the 1st International Symposium of The Princess Takamatsu Cancer Research Fund, pp. 189, University of Tokyo Press, Tokyo, 1971.

36. Takada, M., Lin, Y.-C., Shiratori, O., Sugano, H., Yang, C.-S., Hsu, M.-M., Lin, T.-C., To, S.-M., Chen, H.-C., Hamajima, K., Murata, M., Gotoh, A., Kawamura, A., Yoshida, T. O., Sato, T., and Ito, Y.   Cultivation *in vitro* of Cells Derived from Nasopharyngeal Carcinoma.   GANN Monograph, *10*: 149–161, 1970.

37. Tamura, N., and Nelson, R. A., Jr.   Three Naturally-occurring Inhibitors of Components of Complement in Guinea Pig and Rabbit Serum.   J. Immunol., *99*: 528–589, 1967.

38. de Thé, G., Ho, H.-C., Kwan, H.-C., Desgranges, C., and Favre, M. C.   Nasopharyngeal Carcinoma (NPC).   I. Types of Cultured Cells Derived from Tumour Biopsies and Non-tumourous Tissues of Chinese Patients with Special Reference to Lymphoblastoid Transformation.   Int. J. Cancer, *6*: 189–206, 1970.

39. van Loghem, and van der Hart.   Immune Adherence to the Surface of Leucocytes, Vox Sang., *7*: 539–544, 1962.

40. Watkins, J. F.   Adsorption of Sensitized Sheep Erythrocytes to HeLa Cells Infected with Herpes Simplex Virus.   Nature, *202*: 1364–1365, 1964.

41. Watkins, J. F.   Inhibition of Spreading of Hela Cells after Infection with Herpes Simplex Virus.   Virology, *23*: 436–438, 1964.

42. Watkins, J. F.   The Relationship of the Herpes Simplex Haemadsorption Phenomenon to the Virus Growth Cycle.   Virology, *26*: 746–753, 1965.

43. Yasuda, J., and Milgrom, F.   Hemadsorption by Herpes Simplex Infected Cell Cultures.   Int. Arch. Allergy, *33*: 151–170, 1968.

44. Yoshida, T. O., Imai, K., Ito, Y., Sekine, T., and Nishioka, K. Studies on IA Receptor of Hematopoetic Cells, Macrophages, Leukemic Cells and Suspension Cultured Cells in Humans.   Japan J. Allergology, *19*: 71, 1970 (in Japanese).

Discussion of Papers by Drs. G. Klein, and Nishioka

Dr. Takashashi: I would like to ask two questions of Dr. Nishioka. In your experiments with BL cell lines and EA(IgG), (1) which fragment of A(IgG), Fc, or Fab reacts with cultured cells? (2) Was the reaction of BL cells with EA(IgG) blocked by anti-EBV antibody or patients' sera?

Dr. Nishioka: (1) The Fc fragment of A(IgG) plays an essential role in the reaction of BL cells. (2) In general, patients' sera from NPC and Izumi fever showed a significant blocking effect, while BL patients' sera did not.

Dr. Nelson: You emphasized one of the differences between the cells of the macrophage family and lymphoblastoid cells. According to your table, the macrophage family has both an IA receptor and an IgG receptor, while lymphoblastoid cells may have either. From this point, you can't use these receptors as cell markers, although Fudenberg and his group used the IgG receptor as the marker for the macrophage family. Rather multipotent, uncommitted cells undergo changes such that virus from NPC has the capacity to cause the IA receptor to become unmasked or to be induced by the viral genome; do other viruses have other capacities? Perhaps what you started with is not transformation or a changing of the total cell population but a selection of the cells which have such potencies?

Dr. Nishioka: Lymphoblastoid cells did not show any adherence due to the IgG receptor. Lymphoblast-like cells derived from the BL cell line showed adherence of EA(IgG), but the reactivity was destroyed after acetone or phenol treatment, while the IgG receptor of the macrophage family was left unchanged after this chemical treatment. Lymphoreticular cells or cells derived from NPC or IM adhered to EA(IgM)C43 cells but they did not show any adherence to EA(IgG). It has also been described that both EA(IgG) and EA(IgM)C43 adhere to the surface of single cells of the macrophage family but that the sites were different. The first was blocked by normal IgG and the latter was removed by trypsin. In this way, there is no confusion in differentiating the macrophage family from lymphoblastoid cells and BL cells from NPC, IM, or other lymphoreticular cell lines.

As for the second question, the possibility you raised could be considered. At this moment, however, so far as we have examined, we could not see any evidence concerned with the difference between the IA receptor genetically determined and present in the macrophage family or in lymphoreticular cells and those present in

421

cultured cell lines from NPC or IM.   In this circumstance, we could not conclude whether the adherence of EA(IgG)C43 to NPC cells is related to the presence of the EB viral genome or if the EBV is just harbouring in host cells such as lymphoreticular cells, which have genetically determined IA receptors.

On the contrary, the adherence of EA(IgG) to BL cell lines could be considered to be an induced change or transformation of host cells due to the EBV genome; we have good evidence to support this view.

Dr. G. Klein: Cultured 204 cells derived from NPC adhere to EA(IgM)C43 and not to EA(IgG).   But T3 or T4 cells which were transformed by an extract of 204 cells showed adherence to EA(IgG).   How do you explain this?

Dr. Nishioka: Adherence of EA(IgG) to BL cells or to proper host cells, like N-12, could be considered as a common character of EBV, derived from either BL or NPC cultured cells when they transformed proper host cells.   In this meaning, 204 cells or other spontaneously floating NPC cell lines are not proper host cells for detecting this biological common character of EBV.

Dr. Epstein: I think a very important function of a meeting like this is to clear away the area of misunderstanding.   I think I detected just now an embryonic misunderstanding which we ought to avoid instantly.   Concerning the term transformation, we have malignant transformation; normal cells turned into malignant cells by known oncogenic viruses and transformation of lymphocytes into lymphoblasts under the influence of such transforming agents as phytohemagglutinin, for example.   We must not get confused because the possibility of the transformation of fibroblastic monolayer cells into lymphoid cells is so obscure.   This is the thing I pointed out; I think I detected the area of difficulties when Dr. Nelson was talking.

Dr. de Thé: I want to answer what Dr. Epstein just said concerning the term which has been accepted.   A few years ago, the American Association for Tissue Culturists proposed some terms.   For the word transformation, the definition was denaturation of tissue culture induced by foreign genetic material.   Under this condition, what do we have in our culture?   We have enough morphological alteration, that is, denaturation, which is induced by material foreign to the cells.   This term, transformation, is perfectly acceptable under the tissue culture terminology.

Dr. Epstein: If you could really say that you have alteration of cells, I would be absolutely with you.   The thing is, we have not definite information on such alteration.   The point is that you could very well have a very large number of rounded lymphoid cells present in your culture from the beginning which started to grow at the later stage.   Thus, the overall appearance of the culture is different but the cells have not changed.   At some stage, one population of the cells grows up instead of the others.

DR. NELSON: What I would like to suggest is that the virus did infect a selected population of cells and that they have the potential of possessing one or more of these cell markers. When they are selectively proliferated preferentially by the virus, then these cells with markers have a high population in culture. This is really no different from what you are calling transformation.

DR. E. KLEIN: I have had some small experience with Lyll cells of NPC origin which were supplied by Dr. de Thé. We have maintained both the so-called transformed lymphoblastoid cell line and the monolayer cultured line. I was carrying these cell lines for a while in our laboratory; they were behaving as they should. One was floating cells and the other was attached fibroblast-like cells. I mistreated the monolayer cells a little bit because I went on vacation. After I returned, when I looked at the monolayer cell line, I was surprised that the cells had started clumping and that round cells which looked exactly like floating cell lines had appeared. This cell line had for a long time been cultured as a monolayer culture.

DR. DE THÉ: I would like to mention here the results Dr. Paraf *et al.* recently published in the Proceedings of the National Academy of Science (Paraf, A., Moyne, M.A., Duplan, J.F., Scherrer, R., Stanislawski, M., Bettane, M., Lelievre, L., Rouze, P., and Dubert, J.M. Differentiation of Mouse Plasmocytomas *in vitro;* Two Phenotypically Stabilized Variants of the Same Cell. Proc. Nat. Acad. Sci. USA, *67:* 983–990, 1970). He observed the transformation of free-floating cell-cultures (derived from mouse plasmocytoma) in attached polygonal cells, taking the appearance of epithelial cells and *vice-versa.* These transformations were induced by changes in the tissue culture conditions, especially in serum concentration. Therefore, we cannot exclude the possibility that in our cultures, the free-floating cells might in fact derive from either the fibroblastoid elements, or even the epithelial cells.

Furthermore, in our cultures, the term ' transformation ' is correct, as it represents changes induced in the cell-cultures by the presence of a foreign genetic material, *i.e.,* the herpes-type virus DNA (American Tissue Culture Association. Proposed Usage of Animal Tissue Culture Terms. *In Vitro, 2:* 155–159, 1966).

DR. NISHIOKA: Considering the possibility that tissue cultured cells derived from NPC patients' biopsies would be more susceptible to EBV-infection than the cultured cells from nonpatients' material, Takada reported his successful transformation experiment employing fibroblastic cells derived from NPC as target host cells to EBV.

In the experiment with NPC cell extract or BL cell extract which transformed fibroblastic cell layer N-12 or N-27 cells into floating lymphoblastoid cells, we could present evidence of transformation such as wheat germ lipase or concanavalin agglutination, the appearance of FA-positive cells, and the increase in tritiated thymidine uptake. But the question raised is that the host cells derived from NPC patients, N-12, or N-27 might have been contaminated with lymphoblastoid cells. These cells might have appeared spontaneously without any addition of NPC or

BL cell extracts. Since we employed the attached fibroblastic cells derived from NPC patients, as host cells, such a possibility that floating lymphoblastoid cells appeared spontaneously after prolonged cultivation could hardly be excluded theoretically from the above evidence even if we had taken great pains in observing as many control tubes as possible to exclude spontaneous floating of the lymphoid cells. However, we could exclude this possibility based on our experimental results presented here. If we could obtain spontaneously floating cells from biopsy of NPC, they should show adherence of EA(IgM)C43 and not EA(IgG). All we got in the experiments with N-27 and probably in the case of the N-12 cells also, were the floating lymphoblastoid cells which appeared after the addition of NPC or BL cell extracts. These showed negative adherence of EA(IgM)C43 and positive adherence with EA(IgG), and have been considered to contain EB virus from both tumors. Therefore, the possibility that the contamination of lymphoid cells was present in tissue culture from the beginning and grew spontaneously in the later stage without action by the virus could be excluded. From this viewpoint, in the fibroblastic host cells of NPC origin, the characteristic change, that is, to adhere to EA(IgG), was induced by the EB virus present in the NPC or BL cell extract. Is there any other way but to call such induced alteration of cultured cells transformation?

DR. HO: I wonder how long can these lymphoblastic cells live? In the beginning do they divide very slowly and then exponentially build up and then appear as floating cells? Can they just stay in the position of mitotic division for long periods and then gradually grow up after a long period?

DR. G. KLEIN: I am afraid I don't know. I wish I knew.

DR. W. HENLE: Lymphocytes might survive within the culture for quite some time. When the cultures are maltreated, because of such an occasion as my vacation, they might loosen, die off, and liberate some cells; these cells might now transform and go on. I think this would be a possibility. Lymphocytes are known to survive for many, many months if not for a year.

Suppression of Antigen in Burkitt's Lymphoma and Human Melanoma Cells Grown in Selected Human Sera

Tadao Aoki*, Gayla Geering, Elke Beth, and Lloyd J. Old

Division of Immunology, Sloan-Kettering Institute for Cancer Research, New York, U.S.A.

In Burkitt's lymphoma, intracellular antigens demonstrable by the immunofluorescence of acetone-fixed cells have only rarely been found in cells obtained directly from patients, but antigens have become detectable after culture of the cells *in vitro* (*7, 10*). This suggests that intracellular antigens of this type may be masked *in vivo* or that their sythesis may be suppressed by antibody. This problem was further investigated *in vitro* with the Burkitt's lymphoma cell line, P3J (*3, 4*), and the human malignant melanoma cell line, SK-Mel 1 (*9*).

The P3J cells contained Burkitt herpes-type virus (EB virus) (*2*) and were rich in Burkitt's lymphoma (BL) antigens demonstrable by both immunofluorescence [intracellular antigens (*3, 8*) and cell-surface antigens (*4, 5*)] and immunoprecipitation (*6, 8, 11*) with a reference serum from a patient with carcinoma of the nasopharynx. This serum was used throughout the experiments to test for the variation of BL antigens by both tests. When P3J cells were grown in Eagle's Minimal Essential Medium (EMEM) containing 15% serum obtained from a selected healthy donor [previously shown to have antibody (Burkitt-positive human serum) to cell-surface and intracellular antigens by immunofluorescence and immunoprecipitation tests], the level of intracellular BL antigens demonstrable in acetone-fixed P3J cells by immunofluorescence tests sharply decreased during one passage. The immunofluorescence test remained negative as long as the Burkitt-positive human serum was included in the medium, but after replacing this serum with the serum from a healthy donor shown to lack BL antibody, or with fetal bovine serum (FBS), the BL antigens gradually returned to the original level (Fig. 1). Cells grown in EMEM containing either of the latter sera showed no loss of the BL antigens throughout the experiments (controls). In the same experiments the variation of cell-surface BL antigens was also examined by immunofluorescence of viable cells with the re-

---

* Present address: Viral Leukemia and Lymphoma Branch, National Cancer Institute, NIH, Bethesda, Maryland 20014, U.S.A.

425

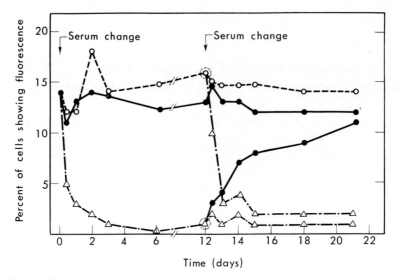

Fig. 1. Suppression of Burkitt's lymphoma antigen (BL antigen) in P3J cells cultured in human serum containing antibody from a healthy donor; (Feeding with serum was carried out every 3 days); immunofluorescence test. ●, fetal bovine serum; ○, human serum, antibody-negative; △, human serum, antibody-positive.

ference Burkitt-positive serum; a parallel correlation was found between intracellular and cell-surface BL antigens in both suppression and reappearance, although the suppression of cell-surface BL antigens was partial. Since some surface antigen remained, however, antibody-blocking also took place as reported by Klein in this symposium. The disappearance or decrease of BL antigens seems to be attributable to the suppression of antigen synthesis, rather than to blocking of BL antigen sites by unlabeled antibody in the culture medium, because cells grown in the Burkitt-positive human serum did not react with the fluorescent anti-human immunoglobulin G(γG) reagent used in the test. Moreover, the disappearance of intracellular BL antigen was confirmed by negative immunoprecipitation tests performed with the same P3J cells used for immunofluorescence (Table 1). Antigenic suppression, however, was not complete; at least 1% of the cells contained intracellular BL antigen demonstrable by the immunofluorescence test. This may be ascribed to a difference

TABLE 1. Suppression of Burkitt's Lymphoma (BL) Antigens Demonstrable by the Immunofluorescence and Immunoprecipitation Tests in the P3J Cell Line by Growth in the Serum Containing Antibody

Serum added to the culture medium	Intracellular BL antigens demonstrable by immunofluorescence	BL antigens demonstrable by immunoprecipitation
Fetal bovine serum	+(approx. 15%)[c]	+
Burkitt-negative serum[a]	+(approx. 18%)	+
Burkitt-positive serum[b]	−(1–3%)	−

[a] A human serum lacking antibody.
[b] A selected antibody-positive human serum.
[c] % cells showing positive fluorescence.

TABLE 2. Burkitt's Lymphoma (BL) Antigens in P3J Cells Detected by Immunofluorescence and Immunoprecipitation Tests with a Positive Human Serum

	Immunofluorescence titer[a]	Immunoprecipitation test[b]	
Human serum used in tests for BL antigens	1/160	B++	P++
Human serum used for P3J cell culture	1/160	B+	P−

[a] Intracellular antigens.

[b] The two major precipitin bands observed with strongly reactive human sera are designated as B and P lines (6). −, negative; +, weak positive; ++, strong positive.

between the two Burkitt-positive human sera used; the reference Burkitt-positive serum detected two major distinct soluble antigens of P3J cells by immunoprecipitation (B and P; see Table 2), but the other serum used in the culture medium detected only one antigenic specificity (B) (6). It appears, therefore, that at least one of the two BL antigens was suppressed by the positive serum from the healthy donor. Immunoprecipitation tests, however, showed antigen suppression of *both* BL soluble antigens. This suggests either that the immunofluorescence test was more sensitive in revealing one of the two specific BL antigens which was not detected by immunoprecipitation, or that both major antigens associated with the precipitation reaction were suppressed and a third BL antigen remained expressed, one not represented in the positive serum used in cultures. Antigenic suppression of cell-surface BL antigens " antigenic purging " was observed by Klein and his colleagues (13) following incubation of cultured Burkitt cells in human serum containing BL antibody.

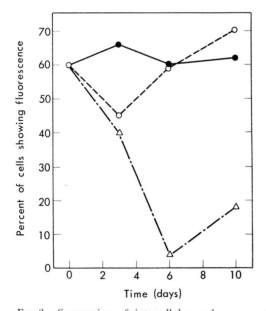

FIG. 2. Suppression of intracellular melanoma antigen in SK–Mel 1 melanoma cells shown in serum from a patient with malignant melanoma (Feeding with serum was carried out every 3 days); immunofluorescence test. ●, fetal bovin serum; ○, human serum, antibody-negative; △, human serum, antibody-positive.

We were not able to ascertain the effect of antibody on the production of EB virus because only few EB virus particles were present in cultured P3J cells fed with serum every 3 days.

In a line of pigment-producing cells (SK-Mel 1), originally isolated from the thoracic duct of a patient with malignant melanoma, specific intracellular antigen was demonstrated by the indirect immunofluorescence test on acetone-fixed cells (9). In this case suppression of antigen was also observed during culture of the cells in human serum containing antibody (Fig. 2).

What is the mechanism? Direct reaction of antibody with intracellular antigens seems unlikely. Possibly antibody reaching the cell-surface and reacting with surface antigens may thus indirectly suppress formation of (other) viral antigens or virus-induced cellular antigens. In terms of cell-surface antigens, there is some similarity between BL antigen suppression and TL antigenic modulation (1, 12). The latter suggests repression of the cellular *Tla* locus, which itself has been suspected of being a viral genome. By this somewhat tenuous analogy, certain BL antigens may be specified by an integrated viral genome (14).

This work was supported by grants from the National Cancer Institute (CA 08748), the John A. Hartford Foundation, Inc., and the New York Cancer Research Institute, Inc.

REFERENCES

1. Boyse, E. A., and Old, L. J.   Some Aspects of Normal and Abnormal Cell Surface Genetics.   Ann. Rev. Genetics, *3*: 269–290, 1969.
2. Epstein, M. A., Achong, B. G., and Barry, Y. M.   Virus Particles in Cultured Lymphoblasts from Burkitt's Lymphoma.   Lancet, *1*: 702–703, 1964.
3. Henle, G., and Henle, W.   Immunofluorescence in Cells Derived from Burkitt's Lymphoma.   J. Bacteriol., *91*: 1248–1256, 1966.
4. Klein, G., Clifford, P., Klein, E., and Stjernsward, J. Search for Tumor Specific Immune Reactions in Burkitt Lymphoma Patients by the Membrane Immunofluorescence Reaction.   Proc. Natl. Acad. Sci. U.S., *55*: 1628–1635, 1966.
5. Klein, G., Clifford, P., Klein, E., Smith, R. T., Minowada, J., Kourilsky, F. M. and Burchenal, J.   Membrane Immunofluorescence Reactions of Burkitt Lymphoma Cells from Biopsy Specimens and Tissue Culture.   J. Natl. Cancer Inst., *39*: 1027–1044, 1967.
6. Klein, G., Geering, G., Old, L. J., Henle, G., Henle, W., and Clifford, P.   Comparison of the Anti-EBV Titer and the EBV-associated Membrane Reactive and Precipitating Antibody Levels in the Sera of Burkitt Lymphoma and Nasopharyngeal Carcinoma Patients and Controls.   Int. J. Cancer, *5*: 185–194, 1970.
7. Nadkarni, J. S., Nadkarni, J. J., Klein, G., Henle, W., Henle, G., and Clifford, P. EB Viral Antigens in Burkitt Tumor Biopsies and Early Cultures.   Int. J. Cancer, *6*: 10–17, 1970.
8. Oettgen, H. F., Aoki, T., Geering, G., Boyse, E. A., and Old, L. J.   Definition of an Antigenic System Associated with Burkitt's Lymphoma.   Cancer Res., *27*: 2532–2533, 1967.
9. Oettgen, H. F., Aoki, T., Old, L. J., Boyse, E. A., de Harven, E., and Mills, G. M.

Suspension Culture of a Pigment-Producing Cell Line from a Human Malignant Melanoma.   J. Natl. Cancer Inst., *41*: 827–843, 1968.

10. Old, L. J., Boyse, E. A., Geering, G., and Oettgen, H. F.   Serologic Approaches to the Study of Cancer in Animals and in Man.   Cancer Res., *26*: 1288–1299, 1968.

11. Old, L. J., Boyse, E. A., Oettgen, H. F., de Harven, E., Geering, G., Williamson, B., and Clifford, P.   Precipitating Antibody in Human Serum to an Antigen Present in Cultured Burkitt's Lymphoma Cells.   Proc. Natl. Acad. Sci. U.S., *56*: 1699–1704, 1966.

12. Old, L. J., Stockert, E., Boyse, E. A., and Kim, J. H.   Antigenic Modulation, Loss of TL Antigen from Cells Exposed to TL Antibody.   Study of the Phenomenon *in Vitro*. J. Exp. Med., *127*: 523–539, 1968.

13. Smith, R. T., Klein, G., Klein, E., and Clifford, P.   Studies of the Membrane Phenomenon in Cultured and Biopsy Cell Lines from the Burkitt Lymphoma.   Advance in Transplantation, Dausset, Hamburger, & Mathé, eds. Munksgard, Copenhagen, *779*: 483–493, 1967.

14. zur Hausen, H., and Schulte-Holthausen, H. Presence of EB Virus Nucleic Acid Homology in a " Virus-Free " Line of Burkitt Tumour Cells.   Nature, *227*: 245–248, 1970.

IMMUNOLOGICAL INTERACTION OF HOST AND EBV CARRYING CELLS

Chairmen:

David S. Nelson, Yorio Hinuma

Immunological Analysis of Hemadsorption of Cultured Cells Derived from Burkitt's Lymphoma

Takehiko Tachibana, Kusuya Nishioka, Takeshi Hirayama, and Akiyoshi Kawamura, Jr.

Virology Division, and Epidemiology Division, National Cancer Center Research Institute, Tokyo, Japan [*T. T., K. N., T. H.*]; *Department of Immunology, Institute of Medical Science, University of Tokyo, Tokyo, Japan* [*A. K.*]

The adherence of sheep erythrocytes sensitized with rabbit anti-sheep erythrocyte serum on cultured cells derived from Burkitt's lymphoma (BL) has been reported (*9, 10*). In those papers, it was pointed out that the adherence of sensitized sheep erythrocytes on cultured BL cells resembled the attachment of sensitized erythrocytes to the IgG receptor of monocytes and macrophages, but the receptor for sensitized erythrocytes on cultured BL cells was distinguished from the IgG receptor of monocytes or macrophages by the different stabilities of the receptors of both types of cells after a variety of chemical treatments.

In this study, some immunological analyses of this phenomenon were attempted in order to clarify the mechanism of the adherence of sensitized sheep erythrocytes [EA(IgG)] and the character of the receptor for EA(IgG) on cultured BL cells.

Kinetics of The EA(IgG) Adherence of Cultured BL Cell Lines

To begin with, the optimal conditions for this EA(IgG)-adherence phenomenon were determined. The number of cells having two or more erythrocytes were scored as positive cells out of the 200 cells counted and expressed as positive percent. As shown in Fig. 1, the temperature of the reaction was optimal at 25 to 30°C rather than at 37°C. The time required to reach a plateau was approximately 5 hr after the addition of sensitized sheep erythrocytes to the target cells, regardless of the reactivity of the target cells.

Blocking of The EA(IgG) Adherence of Cultured BL Cell by Polymerized Human IgG

Since it has been reported that the attachment of sensitized erythrocytes to the IgG receptor of monocytes was inhibited by low concentrations of IgG in the fluid phase (*6*), the effect of IgG on the EA(IgG) adherence of cultured BL cells was

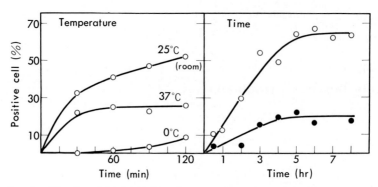

FIG. 1.   Kinetics of the EA(IgG) adherence reaction of cultured BL cells.   ◯, Daudi cells ;
●, Raji cells.

TABLE 1.   Blocking Effect of Human IgG and Rabbit anti-H-chain Specificities on the EA(IgG) Adherence
of Daudi Cells

		Final concentration of IgG and its derivatives		
		2,250	750	250 μg/ml
	Human IgM monomer	54.7[a]	58.2	64.3
	Human IgM polymer	5.6	43.2	34.5
Exp. Ia		8,000	2,700	900 μg/ml
	Human IgG 5S fragment, polymerized	72.4	77.9	74.4
		67	—	μg/ml
	Human IgG monomer	24.6		
Exp. II	Human IgG polymer	9.8		
	No addition		28.6	
		Dilution of antiserum		
		1 : 4.5	1 : 40.5	
	Rabbit normal serum	62.1	72.2	
	Rabbit anti-γ	1.0	1.4	
Exp. Ib	Rabbit anti-α	0.0	3.7	
	Rabbit anti-μ	1.0	2.4	
	Rabbit anti HSV	58.4	65.6	

[a] Percentage of cells having two or more erythrocytes.   One drop (0.025 ml) of target cell suspension (5 ×
10⁶/ml) was added to 0.05 ml of diluted IgG fraction or serum.   After incubation at 37°C for 60 min, the
cells were washed three times and resuspended in 0.025 ml of medium.   One drop of sensitized erythrocytes
(1 × 10⁸/ml) was added to the cell suspension.   After standing at 25°C for 5 hr, the percentage of cells
having two or more erythrocytes was evaluated by counting 200 cells.

tested.   Cultured BL cells were treated with human IgG fraction or rabbit normal
serum at 37°C for 60 min.   After washing three times, sensitized erythrocytes were
added to the washed cultured cells.   In this experiment, Daudi cells, an established
lymphoblastoid BL cell line which was obtained through the courtesy of Dr. G.
Klein, were used as the target cells, because this cell line showed the highest reactivity with EA(IgG).   As seen in Table 1, human IgG fraction and normal rabbit
serum showed a slight inhibition at an extremely high concentration.   On the other

hand, polymerized IgG, prepared by treatment of 6 M urea (4) showed a remarkable blocking effect. However, polymerized 5S IgG, which was prepared by pepsin digestion followed by treatment with 6 M urea, did not show any blocking effect at all, even when used in concentration as high as 8,000 μg per ml (Exp. Ia). When a preparation of Daudi cells showing low reactivity was used, a lower concentration of polymerized IgG, 67 μg per ml, showed strong blocking, but untreated IgG fraction did not (Exp. II). From these data, it is obvious that the Fc part of antibody or immunoglobulin molecules plays a role in EA(IgG) adherence, and the arrangement of the Fc parts of antibody molecules on sheep erythrocytes make up a suitable conformation for the attachment to the receptor of target cells. Of course, it was confirmed that free rabbit anti-sheep erythrocyte antibodies did not block this phenomenon at all. Huber, Douglas, and Fudenberg (6) recently reported that approximately 95 per cent of the IgG receptor on human monocytes and macrophages was inhibited with free IgG at 10 μg per ml, when they used IgG anti-Rh_0 antibody-coating erythrocytes. It is, of course, not adequate to compare their results with the above results directly, but it is very likely that the receptor of BL cells is different, to some extent, from normal IgG receptors.

Effects of Antisera against Human Immunoglobulin Chain Specificities on The Adherence of Cultured BL Cell Lines

Since Klein and her collaborators (8) have demonstrated that Daudi cells have antigenic materials on the cell surfaces reacting with anti-μ and anti-κ antibodies, an experiment was performed to see whether anti-μ antiserum inhibits EA(IgG) adherence or not. Two other anti-H chain specificities were used as a control. These reagents were purchased from Behringwerke, West Germany. As shown in Table 1, Exp. Ib, rabbit normal serum and anti-herpes simplex virus antiserum did not give a significant inhibition, but a striking inhibition with all three rabbit antisera against γ, α and μ was observed. A more unexpected result was that an approximately 1 to 40 dilution of all antisera still inhibited strongly to the same degree. It is indeed a very interesting observation in connection with the EA (IgG) adherence of HSV-infected HeLa cells that they were also equally inhibited by pre-treatment with anti-γ, -α, and -μ antisera, as reported by Hayashi (3).

It is less probable that this inhibition is caused by contaminating antibodies to the other two H-chain specificities in an antiserum reagent, because a higher dilution of all three antisera evenly inhibited EA(IgG) adherence. If the antigenic moieties similar to the H-chain of immunoglobulin are associated with the receptor structure, the principle of the above specific inhibition with anti-H-chain antibodies, and probably with anti-L-chain antibodies as well, should be applicable to the other cultured BL cell lines.

Three different cell lines, Daudi, Raji, and P3HR-1, were treated with rabbit anti-γ, -α, and -μ, and horse anti-κ and anti-λ antisera before the addition of EA (IgG). The results were evaluated by ridit analysis and are summarized in Fig. 2. The effects of these antisera on the EA(IgG) adherence of cultured BL cell lines were not even. Again, the EA(IgG) adherence of Daudi cells was strongly blocked

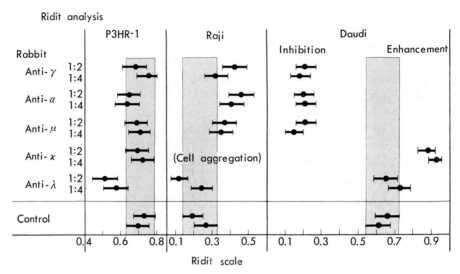

FIG. 2.   Effect of anti-immunoglobulin specificities on the EA(IgG) adherence in cultured BL cell lines.   ●, indicates average ridit; |——|, indicates 95% confidence interval.

by pretreatment of all these anti-H-chain specificities.   But, horse anti-κ antiserum unexpectedly enhanced EA(IgG) adherence.   In this case, more than 80 per cent of the positive cells were surrounded by erythrocytes to make rosettes.   Anti-λ antiserum had no influence at all.   On the contrary, all anti-H-chain antisera enhanced the EA(IgG) adherence of Raji cells.   Anti-κ antiserum formed massive aggregates of target cells so that the effect of this reagent on EA(IgG) adherence could not be analyzed.   Anti-λ blocked that of Raji cells.   On P3HR-1 cells, all antisera showed no reaction with the exception of anti-λ serum which showed inhibition.   The question of why the antiserum which inhibits the EA(IgG) adherence of one cell enhances that of the other cells is not easily answered.   Perhaps an allosteric effect of antiserum might be considered at this point.   From these results, however, it would, generally, be possible to say that all cultured BL cell lines tested here have some antigenic determinants cross-reacting with anti-immunoglobulin antisera.

Effects of Alloantisera on The EA(IgG) Adherence of Cultured BL Cell Lines

To get further proof for the aforementioned antigenicity of cultured BL cell lines, the effect of alloantisera on EA(IgG) adherence was tested.   It had been previously observed that multiple transfused sera strongly blocked the EA(IgG) adherence of a cultured BL cell line or of all cultured BL cell lines tested.   Two alloantisera, #3 and #5 which were obtained from the Blood Transfusion Service of Tokyo University Hospital, strongly blocked the EA(IgG) adherence of all BL cell lines.   It has been confirmed that these sera contain a high level of anti-leucocytes and anti-platelet antibodies.   Now, it was thought that they also might contain alloantibodies against human IgG.   To confirm this idea, an immunoad-

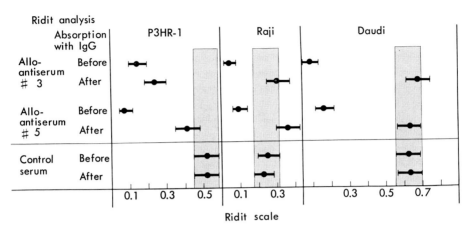

FIG. 3.   Effect of alloantisera on the EA(IgG) adherence of cultured BL cell lines before and after absorption of sera with insoluble IgG complex.   ●, indicates average ridit; |———|, indicates 95% confidence interval.

sorbent of human IgG was prepared with glutaraldehyde (1).   After several washings to remove free IgG, packed immunoadsorbent was added to the alloantisera and mixed well.   After 1 hr of incubation at room temperature, a clear supernatant was obtained by centrifugation.   The blocking effect of alloantisera was determined before and after the absorption with insoluble IgG complex.   As shown in Fig. 3, the strong blocking effect of alloantisera was almost completely diminished after absorption.

These results indicate that the alloantisera used here contained anti-IgG activities in addition to anti-cellular components such as anti-leucocytes and anti-platelets.   Only antibodies against IgG were related to the blocking activity of alloantisera on the EA(IgG) adherence of cultured BL cell lines.   In other words, anti-cellular component antibodies did not interfere the reaction even if they remained in the sera after absorption and reacted on the cell surfaces.   The data suggest that antigenic determinants similar to those of immunoglobulin are closely associated with or identical to the antigenic structure of the receptor for EA(IgG) on cultured BL cell lines.

Effects of Metabolic Inhibitors on The EA(IgG) Adherence of Cultured BL Cell Lines

Next, a preliminary experiment which was concerned with the effect of metabolic inhibitors on the EA(IgG) adherence of cultured BL cell lines was carried out.   Yata, Klein, Hewetson and Gergely (12) have reported the enhancing effect of metabolic inhibitors on the membrane immunofluorescence (MIF) reactivity of BL cell lines.   Klein also showed these results togather with other interesting results on early antigens in the same line (7).   In the experiment described below, only given concentrations of inhibitors were used.   These were: 10 ng of mitomycin C per ml, 1 ng of actinomycin D per ml, 50 ng of cytosine arabinoside per ml, and 200 ng of puromycin per ml, respectively.   Cells were cultured in the presence

TABLE 2. Effect of Metabolic Inhibitors on the EA(IgG) Adherence of Cultured BL Cell Lines

Cells (Intial conc.)	Treatment	Cell increment in 4 days	Viability (%)	No. of EA(IgG)/BL cell						Total
				0	1	2	3	4	≥5	
P3HR–1	Mitomycin C, 10 ng/ml	5.7	90.2	28	7	15	18	19	113	200
1.5×10^5/ml	Actinomycin D, 1 ng/ml	3.4	84.4	12	0	9	10	2	167	200
	Cytosine arabinoside, 50 ng/ml	1.9	82.1	13	8	8	5	13	163	200
	Puromycin, 200 ng/ml	0.5	24.2	112	7	8	4	5	64	200
	Control	5.7	94.0	33	24	35	16	11	81	200
Daudi	Mitomycin C, 10 ng/ml	4.6	90.1	45	14	30	27	27	57	200
3×10^5/ml	Actinomycin D, 1 ng/ml	3.0	88.0	10	10	7	24	31	118	200
	Cytosine arabinoside, 50 ng/ml	2.2	80.7	20	19	17	20	27	97	200
	Puromycin, 200 ng/ml	0.2	23.9	143	19	13	5	4	20	200
	Control	9.3	94.0	21	8	16	24	30	101	200
Raji	Mitomycin C, 10 ng/ml	2.7	60.9	143	22	12	1	7	15	200
2×10^5/ml	Actinomycin D, 1 ng/ml	2.3	53.3	184	7	6	1	1	1	200
	Cytosine arabinoside, 50 ng/ml	1.2	43.1	115	18	8	2	5	52	200
	Puromycin, 200 ng/ml	0.2	8.4	180	8	5	0	2	2	200
	Control	2.0	59.1	98	27	13	2	4	56	200

of the inhibitors in Eagle's MEM, containing 20% fetal calf serum for 4 days. Initial concentration of cells, increment of cell numbers, and viability are shown in Table 2.

As seen in Table 2, the concentrations of the metabolic inhibitors were not adequate for evaluation of the relationship between EA(IgG) adherence reactivity and the DNA synthesis system, because the cells were still growing and the viabilities of the cells were also high, except in the case of puromycin. But the EA(IgG) adherence reactivities of cultured BL cell lines were influenced in various ways. Figure 4 shows the ridit analysis of the distribution of negative and positive cells. Positive cells were scored as numbers of cells attached to one, two, three, four, and

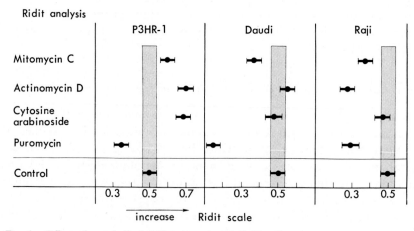

FIG. 4. Effect of metabolic inhibitors on the EA(IgG) adherence of cultured BL cell lines. ●, indicates average ridit; |——|, indicates 95% confidence interval.

five or more erythrocytes separately, as shown in Table 2. Reactivity of P3HR-1 cells was increased by the addition of mitomycin C, actinomycin D, and cytosine arabinoside; that of Daudi cells was decreased by mitomycin C; and reactivity of Raji cells was decreased by mitomycin C and actinomycin D. Puromycin decreased the reactivities of all BL cell lines, and the viabilities of the cells also dropped. It is of interest that the increasing effect of these inhibitors on the P3HR-1 cells which produce many viruses and contain more VCA (virus capsid antigen), resemble the tendencies of MIF reactivity of heavily virus carrying Maku cells (12). In their experiments, all inhititors inhibited cell growth, while in the present experiment, it must be noted that all inhibitors except puromycin permit cells to grow. The data obtained so far seem to suggest that the receptor for EA(IgG) of cultured BL cells would be induced by virus infection, but further investigation should be carried out to clarify an association of virus with the appearance of the receptor in BL cultured cell lines.

A Tentative Hypothesis on The Role of EBV in The Development of Nasopharyngeal Cancer

Finally, it would be worthwhile to discuss a possible role for EB virus in Burkitt's lymphoma and nasopharyngeal carcinoma (NPC) from the viewpoint of the immunological cell markers of floating cultured cells obtained so far.

Before proceeding with the subject, it is useful to note that two major situations for oncogenesis by virus have been elucidated in the field of experimental tumor immunology in the last decade. As illustrated in Fig. 5, the first situation is that an oncogenic virus induces tumor directly. The second situation is that the impairment of the immune surveillance system by oncogenic agents causes an increasing incidence of tumor. The amount of the antigen and the developmental stage when it is induced appear to be of importance, together with genetic factors, in influencing the character of the immune response of the host. In addition, immunosuppression by the oncogenic agent and by an aging effect may also play a role. Full tolerance was only found when a viral oncogen was introduced into a fetal or newborn host.

To return, floating cultured cells derived from BL and NPC biopsies are virus carrying cells indeed. What kind of cell is the target for virus proliferation *in vivo?* Our hypothesis is as follows: When the cells which are carrying virus *in vivo* are brought to tissue culture, such cells may selectively continue to proliferate *in vitro;* Pope has demonstrated continuous proliferation of normal human leucocytes after *in vitro* infection with EB virus (11). So if this is the case, floating cultured cell lines carrying virus will be the target cells for virus infection *in vivo.* Now, we were able to differentiate the floating cultured cells derived from BL biopsies from those derived from NPC biopsies by means of their different immunological cell markers. The former has a receptor for EA(IgG), but not an IA receptor, while the latter has an IA receptor but not receptor for EA(IgG) (9, 10). The cytological figures of both cultured cells are closely similar, but it seems fair to say from these cell markers that the cells derived from BL are lymphoblastoid cells and the cells derived from NPC are reticular cells. In addition, the latter were positive to the supravital

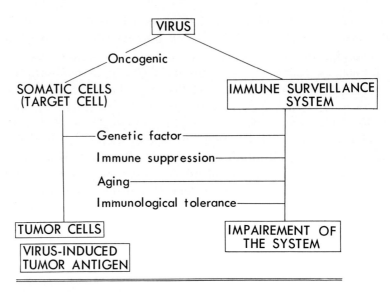

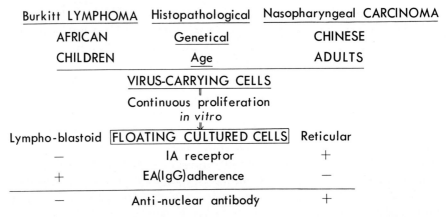

FIG. 5.   Possible roles of EB virus in Burkitt's lymphoma and nasopharyngeal carcinoma.

staining test, even though it was weak.   The cultured cells derived from infectious mononucleosis and even from lymphoid tissue of normal healthy persons also belong to the category of those derived from NPC.   Therefore the cells in this category will, in general, be the real target cells for virus infection.   But BL cultured cells are an entirely different kind of cells.

With this in mind, when one considers the other facts so far obtained, it is evident that BL is of lymphoblastic origin and NPC is of epithelial origin, as Chen has clearly demonstrated (2).   Genetically, BL appears in Africans and NPC in Chinese. This point was shown by Ho (5).   And lymphoma appears in children, while carcinoma appears in adults.   So if we consider the aforementioned two major situations of oncogenesis in these malignant diseases, we could understand the possibility that Burkitt's lymphoma may be induced by EB virus even though some other factor, such as malaria might be concerned, but the same possibility is not suitable for the understanding of nasopharyngeal carcinoma. It is conceivable that the alteration of the immune surveillance system may play another important role in the development of nasopharyngeal cancer. In connection with this assumption, it is of interest and of significance that anti-nuclear antibodies are demonstrated in NPC patients' sera at relatively high frequency, but not in BL patients' sera (*13*).

This study was supported by grants from the Ministry of Health and Welfare, the Ministry of Education, the Princess Takamatsu Fund for Cancer Research, and the Society for Promotion of Cancer Research.

REFERENCES

1. Avrameas, S., and Ternynck, T. The Cross-linking of Proteins with Glutaraldehyde and Its Use for the Preparation of Immunoadsorbents. Immunochemistry, *6*: 53–66, 1969.
2. Chen, H.-C., Shu Yeh, Tu, S.-M., Hsu, M.-M., Lynn, T.-C., and Sugano, H. Anaplastic Carcinoma of the Nasopharynx. Proceedings of The 1st International Symposium of The Princess Takamatsu Cancer Research Fund, pp. 237, University of Tokyo Press, Tokyo, 1971.
3. Hayashi, K. Membrane Changes of Cells Infected with Herpes Simplex Virus. Proceedings of The 1st International Symposium of The Princess Takamatsu Cancer Research Fund, pp. 139, University of Tokyo Press, Tokyo, 1971.
4. Hirose, S.-I., and Osler, A. G. Interaction of Rabbit Anti-human H Chain Sera with Denatured Human γ-Globulin. J. Immunol, *98*, 618–627, 1967.
5. Ho, H.-C. Genetic and Environmental Factors in Nasopharyngeal Carcinoma. Proceedings of The 1st International Symposium of The Princess Takamatsu Cancer Research Fund, pp. 275, University of Tokyo Press, Tokyo, 1971.
6. Huber, H., Douglas, S. D., and Fudenberg, H. H. The IgG Receptor: An Immunological Marker for the Characterization of Mononuclear Cells. Immunology, *17*: 7–21, 1969.
7. Klein, G. Membrane Antigen Changes in Burkitt's Lymphoma Cells. Proceedings of The 1st International Symposium of The Princess Takamatsu Cancer Research Fund, pp. 379, University of Tokyo Press, Tokyo, 1971.
8. Klein, E., Klein, G., Nadkarni, J. S., Nadkarni, J. J., Wigzell, H., and Clifford, P. Surface IgM-kappa Specificity on a Burkitt Lymphoma Cell *in vivo*. Cancer Res., *28*: 1300–1310, 1968.
9. Nishioka, K. Tachibana, T., Hirayama, T., de Thé, G., Klein, G., Takada, M., and Kawanura, A., Jr. Immunological Studies on the Cell Membrane Receptors of Cultured Cells Derived from Nasopharyngeal Cancer, Burkitt's Lymphoma, and Infectious Mononucleosis. Proceedings of The 1st International Symposium of The Princess Takamatsu Cancer Research Fund, pp. 401, University of Tokyo Press, Tokyo, 1971.
10. Nishioka, K., Tachibana, T., Sekine, T., Inoue, M., Hirayama, T., Sugano, H., Yoshida, T. O., Takada, M., Kawamura, A., Jr., and Wang, C.-H. Immunological Studies on Cultured Cells Derived from Nasopharyngeal Carcinoma and Burkitt Lymphoma and an Improved Method of Immune Adherence Reaction. GANN Monograph, *10*: 265–281, 1971.

11. Pope, J. H.   EB Virus as a Biologically Active Agent.   Proceedings of The 1st International Symposium of The Princess Takamatsu Cancer Research Fund, pp. 177, University of Tokyo Press, Tokyo, 1971.

12. Yata, J., Klein, G., Hewetson, J., and Gergely, L.   Effect of Metabolic Inhibitors on Membrane Immunofluorescence Reactivity of Established Burkitt Lymphoma Cell Lines.   Int. J. Cancer, 5: 394–403, 1970.

13. Yoshida, T. O.   High Incidence of Antinuclear Antibodies in the Sera of Nasopharyngeal Cancer Patients.   Proceedings of The 1st International Symposium of The Princess Takamatsu Cancer Research Fund, pp. 443, University of Tokyo Press, Tokyo, 1971.

High Incidence of Antinuclear Antibodies in The Sera of Nasopharyngeal Cancer Patients

Takato O. Yoshida

Laboratory of Viral Oncology, Aichi Cancer Center Research Institute, Nagoya, Japan

Virological and immunological studies on Burkitt's lymphoma (BL) have been carried out intensively at serveral laboratories since Epstein *et al.* (*1*) revealed the association of EB virus (EBV) particles with cultured BL cells as demonstrated by the electron microscope. Subsequently, Henle *et al.* (*3*) showed EB virus antigen in cells derived from BL by the immunofluorescence technique, and Klein *et al.* (*9, 10*) demonstrated the membrane specific antigens on the surface of BL biopsy cells and cultured cells derived from BL biopsy materials, employing the membrane immunofluorescence technique. These data all point toward the fact that BL patients possess high titers of anti-EB virus antibody. The antibody related to EB virus has also been demonstrated in infectious mononucleosis (*4*).

The antigens located on the membrane surface of BL cells and in the BL cells have been reported to be related to and expressed by the EB virus (*11, 13*).

Furthermore, anti-EBV antibody levels in the sera of patients with other neoplastic diseases have been investigated by the immunofluorescence technique and the agar-diffusion method. It has been reported that nasopharyngeal cancer (NPC) patients in particular possessed high titers of the anti-EBV antibody in their sera against EBV-carrying BL cultured cells (*6, 8*) and EBV antigen-extracted BL cultured cells (*14*).

Yoshida *et al.* (*23*) have reported that the sera of NPC patients in Taiwan showed high titers of antibody against the membrane surface antigens of BL cultured cells and P3HR-1, as indicated by the fluorescence index (F. I.). Klein *et al.* (*12*) have reported that the anti-membrane surface antigen(s) antibody-conjugated FITC in the serum of BL patients (Mutua) was strongly blocked by the sera of NPC patients in Africa on the surface membrane of BL cultured cells as indicated by the blocking index (BI).

On the other hand, NPC cells carried viral antigens and the tumor cell-specific antigens have not yet been definitely detected by autoantibodies based at the autochthonous level (*19, 21, 22, 24*).   During the course of the studies using this tumor immunological approach, antinuclear antibodies (ANA) against monolayer cultured cells derived from NPC biopsy materials have been found in the sera of NPC patients acting as autoantibodies and isoantibodies.   It was confirmed that these ANA were heterophilic by testing with the nuclei of other cultured cell lines including human cells, *i.e.*, Raji, embryonic lung cells, normal omemtum cells, HeLa and SiHa, and animal cultured cells, *i.e.*, rat fibroblast, mouse fibroblast, rabbit skin cells, rabbit Shope papilloma cells (Sp-8), and monkey kidney cells (*25*).

The purposes of the present studies were to examine 1) whether further findings of ANA in the sera of NPC patients could be made, specifically in the nuclei of NPC cells derived from biopsy materials, other human cultured cells, and animal cultured cells, by the indirect immunofluorescence technique; 2) whether ANA could be demonstrated in the sera of other tumor patients, particularly focusing on BL; 3) whether there was a correlation between ANA titer and anti EBV titer; 4) what the nature of the antigen was in the nuclei; and 5) what immunoglobulin classes of ANA were in the sera.

Also to be discussed in these studies is the production of heterophilic antinuclear antibodies in cancer patients, which appeared to be one of the impairments of immunological surveillance in tumor-bearing hosts.

MATERIALS AND METHODS

Cells

a) Cultured human cells—(1) Cultures of cells derived from NPC biopsy materials: NPC–4, –12, –13, –19, –25B, –27, –31A, –34, –35, –79B, and –82 (*16, 18*) were started at the National Taiwan University, and have been maintained at Taiwan University, Aichi Cancer Center, University of Tokyo, and the Shionogi Co.   They were grown in Eagle's minimum essential medium (MEM) supplemented with 20% fetal calf serum.   The cells between the 4th and 10th transfer generation were used for this experiments.

(2) Human embryo cells: Monolayer cultures of fibroblastic cells derived from the lung of a 6 month-old human embryo were used.   The cells between the 3rd and 14th transfer generation were employed for the experiment.   Human embryo kidney (HEK) cultured cells were also used.

(3) Burkitt's lymphoma cells: Two cell lines, P3HR-1 and Raji, derived from Burkitt's lymphoma biopsy material, were employed.

(4) Human cell lines: HeLa, and SiHa (*2*), both derived from carcinoma of the uterus, were used as the established cell lines.

b) Cultured animal cells—(1) Rat fibroblast: The fibroblastic monolayer cells derived from rat embryo and from the muscle of newborn Wistar King A strain rats were used.

(2) Mouse fibroblast: The fibroblastic monolayer cells derived from mouse embryo and from the muscle of newborn C57BL/10J strain mice were employed.

(3) Rabbit Shope papilloma cells: Sp-8 cells (*15*) (130th transfer generation) were used.

(4) Cottontail rabbit cells: NCR cells (*5*) (22nd transfer generation) were used.

(5) Monkey kidney cells: The epitheloid cells derived from the kidneys of adult monkeys were used.

It was confirmed that none of the cells of these cell lines possessed any detectable amount of SV40 T-antigen, adenovirus 12 T-antigen, or EBV antigen when checked by the direct immunofluorescence technique.

Deoxyribonucleic acid (DNA)

DNA type 1 (sodium salt, highly polymerized) isolated from calf thymus (Sigma Chemical Co.) was used in phosphate butter saline (PBS).

Histone

Histones (G. R.) purified from calf thymus nuclei (Sigma Chemical Co.) were used in PBS.

Protamine

Protamine sulfate (Lot 22M) made by the Seikagaku Kogyo Co., Ltd., was used in PBS.

Sera

NPC—Sera from 147 Chinese patients with NPC were collected at the National Taiwan University Hospital, Taipei, Taiwan, Republic of China. Sera from 15 Japanese patients were collected at the Aichi Cancer Center Hospital and at the Kobe University Hospital.

Lymphoma and lymphosarcoma

Sera from 15 Chinese patients with lymphoma and lymphosarcoma were collected at the National Taiwan University Hospital.

Leukemia

Sera from 15 Chinese patients with leukemia were collected at the National Taiwan University Hospital. Sera from 38 Japanese patients with leukemia were collected at the Aichi Cancer Center Hospital.

Burkitt's lymphoma

Sera from 41 African patients with Burkitt's lymphoma were kindly supplied by Dr. George Klein, Karolinska Institute, Sweden.

Other cancers

Sera from 9 Japanese patients with esophageal carcinoma; from 62 Japanese patients with gastric carcinoma; from 10 Japanese patients with colonic carcinoma; from 10 Japanese patients with hepatoma; from 10 Japanese patients with lung carcinoma; from 25 Japanese patients with mammary carcinoma; and from 18

Japanese patients with uterine carcinoma were collected at the Aichi Cancer Center Hospital.

Normal healthy subject

Sera from 50 normal healthy Chinese people were collected at the National Taiwan University Hospital. Sera from 30 normal healthy Japanese people were collected at the Aichi Cancer Center Research Institute, and at a primary school, as controls.

Immunofluorescence tests

The cultured cells grown on a cover-slip in a small square bottle were washed 3 times with phosphate buffer saline (PBS), dried rapidly with a dryer, and fixed with acetone. Acetone was finally selected from several fixatives such as methanol, ethanol, acetone, methyl alcohol, ethyl alcohol, carbon tetrachloride, 4% formaldehyde in PBS, 2.5% glutaraldehyde in 0.05 M PB, 2% glutaraldehyde and 2% paraformaldehyde solution in PBS, and the acetone-fixed monolayer cultured cells thus prepared were used, or stored at −20°C. The acetone-fixed monolayer cultured cells thus prepared were used as the target cells. The test serum was diluted 1:5 with 0.1% sodium azide PBS and was routinely used.

The indirect immunofluorescence procedure was performed to detect ANA in the test sera using suitably diluted fluorescein isothiocyanate-conjugated goat anti-human globulin. A specimen mounted with 10% carbonate buffered glycerol was examined under ultraviolet illumination (Osram HBO 200W lamp) with a Tiyoda immunofluorescence microscope (FM 200A).

Immunoglobulin classes of ANA were determined by the indirect immunofluorescence procedure using goat anti-human IgG globulin conjugated with fluorescein (Hyland, Lot No. 2201HOO2A1) and goat anti-human IgM globulin conjugated with fluorescein (Hyland, Lot No. 2211HOO2A1). These fluorescein labeled antibodies were prepared by the absorption of acetone powder of rabbit embryos and human liver, and were suitably diluted for use.

RESULTS

The first observation of ANA, in April 1969, detected by the immunofluorescence procedure, was performed utilizing 10 established cell lines: NPC-4, -12, -13, -19, -25B, -27, -31A, -31B, -34, and -35, derived from NPC biopsy materials the sera collected from same patients at the National Taiwan University Hospital, our standard NPC serum (anti EBV titer 1/2,560), Burkitt's lymphoma patient Mutua serum (anti EBV titer 1/2,560) kindly supplied by Dr. George Klein for detection of EBV antigens and other antigens, and normal healthy control serum (anti EBV titer 1/40). The serum of the NPC—12 patient was unique in the sense that the γ-globulin in the serum reacted with the nuclei of all 10 cultured cell lines tested for autoantibodies and isoantibodies. The fluorescence staining pattern "Speckled", pattern 4 in Table 1 and Fig. 3 was clearly shown in the nuclei of cultured cells. The other sera have not shown any specific reactions in the nuclei.

TABLE 1. Summary of the Results of Tests for Antinuclear Antibodies in the Sera of Nasopharyngeal Cancer Patients Who Came to the Clinic for Their Initial Treatment

Case \ Pattern in nucleus	1	2	3	4	5	6	Positive cases / Total cases (%)		
Positive	3	11	3	1	2⌣1⌣6		Chinese	26/97	28
							Japanese	1/15	7
Weak positive	4	12	3	0	0	0	Chinese	17/97	18
							Japanese	2/15	13
Total	7	23	6	1	2⌣1⌣6		Chinese	43/97	45
							Japanese	3/15	20
Healthy control	0	0	0	0	0	0	Chinese	0/50	0
							Japanese	0/30	0

Six staining patterns have been observed within the nuclei of monolayer cultured cells detected by indirect fluorescent antibody technique.

Later, it was confirmed that none of the cells of all these cell lines possessed any detectable amount of SV40 T-antigen, adenovirus 12 T-antigen, or EBV antigen when checked by the direct immunofluorescence technique (25).

The cultured cells, human embryo lung, NPC-12, NPC-27, NPC-79B, and Raji were also selected as target cells for the detection of ANA in the sera of NPC patients. The results of the experiments are summarized in Table 1 (25). The definite positive cases of ANA were found in 26 out of 97 Chinese cases with NPC, all patients who came to National Taiwan University Hospital for their initial treatment, and in 1 out of the 15 Japanese cases with NPC at the Aichi Cancer Center

TABLE 2. Summary of the Results of Tests for Antinuclear Antibodies in the Sera of Nasopharyngeal Cancer Patients Who Have Been Treated at the Clinic

Case \ Pattern in nucleus	1	2	3	4	5	6	Positive cases / Total cases (%)		
Positive	1	1	7	5	1	5	Chinese	20/50	40
Weak positive	0	1	4	0	0	1	"	6/50	12
Total	1	2	11	5	1	6	"	26/50	52

Hospital and at the Kobe University Hospital. Seventeen out of the 97 Chinese cases and 2 out of the 15 Japanese cases with NPC showed weak positive reactions to the nuclei of the selected cultured cells. Fifty randomly eslected Chinese and 30 normal healthy Japanese sera did not show any specific reactions within the nuclei of the cultured cells.

Six patterns have been observed within the nuclei of NPC-27, 79B, human fibroblastic cells derived from the omemtum tissue of gastric cancer patients, and human embryo lung cultured cells at a resting stage as shown in Tables 1 and 2. The various nuclear stainings were usually " diffuse " (pattern 1), " dotted " (pattern 2, Fig. 1), " speckled " (pattern 3, Fig. 2, pattern 4, Fig. 3), " nucleolar " (pattern 5) and " nucleolar combined with speckled " (pattern 6, Figs. 4, and 5) in Tables 1, and 2.

In a small percentage of the cells of patterns 3, 4, and 6, there was accompanying peripheral staining of the nuclei (Fig. 6).

These sera positive to the nuclei have also been tested with the nuclei of other cultured cell lines, including human cells, *i.e.*, HeLa and SiHa derived from uterine cancer, and animal cultured cells, *i.e.*, rat fibroblast, mouse fibroblast, rabbit skin cells (NCR), rabbit Shope papilloma cells (Sp-9), and monkey kidney cells. The results suggested that the ANA in the sera of NPC patients were really heterophilic (*25*).

Table 2 summarizes the ANA in the sera of 50 patients with NPC, who had been treated in the clinic at the National Taiwan University Hospital. Twenty out of 50 cases with NPC showed a positive reaction and 6 out of 50 cases showed a

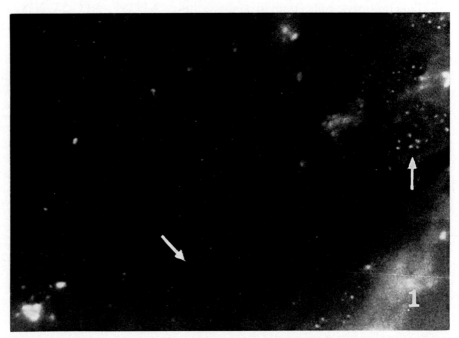

FIG. 1.   Fluorescence of photomicrograph of pattern 2, " dotted " staining with the serum of on NPC patient in the nuclei of human embryo lung fioroblastic cells.   × 400.

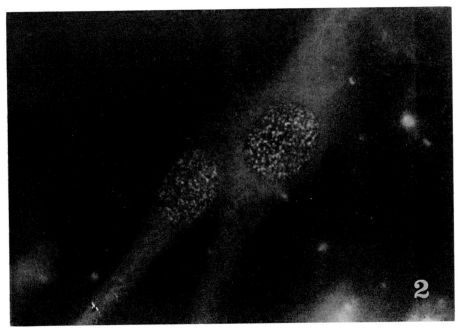

Fig. 2.   Fluorescence of photomicrograph of pattern 3, " speckled " staining with the serum of an NPC patient.   The specks filled homogeneously in the nuclei of human embryo lung fibroblastic cells.   × 400.

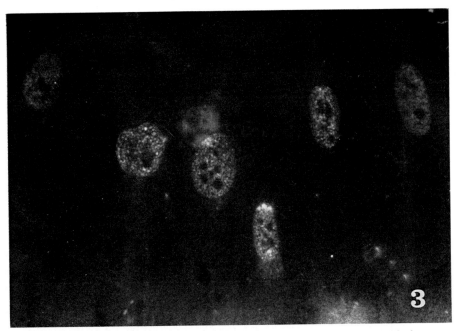

Fig. 3.   Fluorescence of photomicrograph of pattern 4, " speckled " staining with the serum of an NPC patient, except for the nucleolar regions, in the nuclei of human embryo lung fibroblastic cells.   × 400.

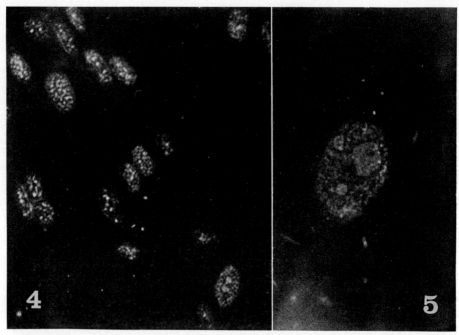

FIGS. 4 and 5.   Fluorescence of photomicrograph of pattern 6, " nucleolar combined with speckled " staining with the serum of an NPC patient in the nuclei of human embryo lung fibroblastic cells.   × 100, × 400.

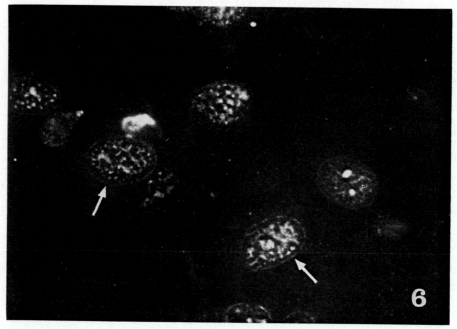

FIG. 6.   The arrows indicate the peripheral staining of the nuclei with the sera of NPC patients, which sera showed patterns 3, 4, and 6.   × 400.

weak positive reaction.   The percentage of definite ANA positive cases increased and the percentage of ANA weak positive cases decreased in the NPC patients who had been treated as compared with ANA positive cases in the sera of NPC patients who came to the clinic for their first visit.   Simultaneously, checks were made for LE cells in the smear specimens prepared from the clotted blood of the 50 cases with NPC, in cooperation with Dr. Wang at the Department of Hematology, National Taiwan University.   LE cells were not found, but nucleo-phagocytes were found in the specimens (20).

A high incidence of heterophilic ANA in NPC patients was found during the immunological investigation of NPC.

No evidence so far has been observed at the NPC clinic of the National Taiwan University Hospital that the NPC patients combine antinuclear antibody producing autoimmune diseases, such as systemic lupus erythematosus (SLE), scleroderma (SD), rheumatoid arthritis, juvenile rheumatoid arthritis (JRA) lupoid hepatitis, Sjögren's syndrome, periarteritis nodosum, and infectious monucleosis.   No clinical findings of autoimmune diseases were observed in NPC patients, according to Prof. Tu, Dr. Hsu, and other staff members at the Department of Otolaryngology, National Taiwan University (25).

No histopathological evidence of autoimmune diseases was found in NPC biopsy materials or the limited number of 20 autopsy cases with NPC according to Prof. Yeh and Prof.Chen at the Department of Pathology, National Taiwan University (25).

The results of the tests for ANA in the sera of other cancer patients, particularly focusing on BL, are shown in Table 3.   No definite ANA was detected in 41 African cases with BL, and 2 out of the 41 cases showed a very weak positive reaction.   In 15 Chinese cases with lymphoma and lymphosarcoma, there were no definite positive cases, and just one very weak positive case.   In 15 Chinese cases with leukemia, there was only one definite positive case.   In Japanese cases with other cancers at Aichi Cancer Center Hospital, there was one definite positive case out of 9 cases with esophageal cancer, 10 definite positive and 7 weak positive cases out of 62

TABLE 3.   Results of Tests for Antinuclear Antibodies in the Sera of Other Tumor Patients

Tumor		Test cases	Positive	Weak positive	%
Burkitt's lymphoma	African	41	0	2?	
Lymphoma Lymphosarcoma	Chinese	15	0	1?	
Leukemia	,,	15	1	0	
Esophageal Ca.	Japanese	9	1	0	
Gastric Ca.	,,	62	10	7	27.3
Colonic Ca.	,,	10	0	0	
Hepatoma	,,	10	0	0	
Lung Ca.	,,	10	1	0	
Breast Ca.	,,	25	3	2	20.0
Uterine Ca.	,,	18	3	1	22.2
Leukemia	,,	38	1	4	13.2

cases with gastric cancer, 1 definite positive case out of 10 cases with lung cancer, 3 definite positive and 2 weak positive cases out of 25 cases with breast cancer, 3 definite positive and 1 weak positive cases out of 18 cases with unterine cancer, 1

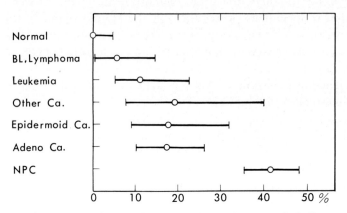

FIG. 7.   Percent of antinuclear antibody-positive cases, including weak positive cases, in tumor patients.   BL, Burkitt's lymphoma ; NPC, nasopharyngeal cancer.

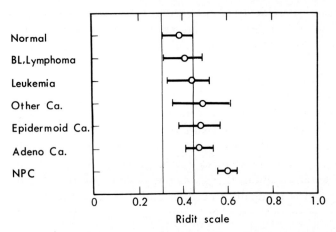

FIG. 8.   A comparison of the results of the antinuclear antibody test for selected tumors by ridit analysis.

No. of case		P	WP	Ng	Average ridit	95% Confidence interval
Normal	80	0	0	80	0.389	0.454–0.325
BL, Lymphoma	58	0	3	54	0.412	0.487–0.336
Leukemia	53	2	4	47	0.442	0.521–0.363
Other Ca.	21	4	0	17	0.492	0.618–0.366
Epidermoid Ca.	40	4	3	33	0.476	0.567–0.384
Adeno Ca.	82	8	6	68	0.474	0.537–0.410
NPC	201	56	28	117	0.600	0.641–0.559

BL, Burkitt's lymphoma ;   NPC, nasopharyngeal cancer ;   P, positive ;   WP, weak positive ; Ng, negative.

definite positive and 4 weak positive cases out of 38 cases with leukemia, and no positive reaction cases out of 10 cases with colonic cancer and 10 cases with hepatoma (20).

TABLE 4. χ^2 Matrix on the Results of the Antinuclear Antibody Test for Selected Tumors

	Normal	Malignant neoplasm of haematopoietic organs	Cancer	NPC
Normal		6.87[a]	15.75[b]	47.69[b]
Malignant neoplasm of haematopoietic organs			8.29[a]	40.92[b]
Cancer				22.85[b]
NPC				

[a] Significant at 5% level under 2 degrees of freedom.
[b] Significant at 1% level under 2 degrees of freedom.
NPC : nasopharyngeal cancer.

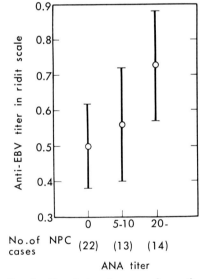

FIG. 9.   Correlation between the antinuclear antibody titer and the anti-EBV titer in sera of nasopharyngeal cancer patients.

Anti-EBV titer	ANA titer		
	0	5–10	20≦
<40	0	0	0
40	1	0	1
160	5	2	0
640	10	7	3
2,560	6	4	10
Total	22	13	14

$\chi^2 = 12.75$; $N = 5$; $P < 0.05$.

A statistical analysis of the frequency of ANA positive cases, including weak positive cases, in the sera of tumor patients was made by several methods, including percentage, ridit analysis, and χ^2-matrix, with the kind cooperation of Dr. T. Hirayama, National Cancer Center, Tokyo. The percent of ANA positive cases, including weak positive cases, in tumor patients is shown in Fig. 7. Tumors were classified into groups of: BL and lymphoma, leukemia, other cancer (unspecified), epidermoid carcinoma, adeno-carcinoma, and NPC. A comparison of the results of the ANA test for tumors made by ridit analysis showed a statistically significant difference from the normal controls in the presence of ANA in tumor sera, as shown in Fig. 8. The χ^2-matrix also showed this statistically significant difference, expressed numerically in Table 4. Among these, NPC was by far the highest, and the next group was other cancers. The cases with malignant neoplasm of haematopoietic organs were very low.

A slight correlation between ANA titer and EBV titer in the sera of NPC patients was observed as shown in Fig. 9.

The results of the investigation of the immunoglobulin classes of ANA in 27 cases with NPC and 4 cases with other cancers are shown in Fig. 10. Eleven cases

IgG   11 cases

IgM   2 cases

IgG,IgM 18 cases   ——   IgG≑IgM 9 cases
                                    IgG>IgM 1 cases
                                    IgG≫IgM 6 cases
                                    IgG<IgM 2 cases

FIG. 10. Immunoglobulin classes of antinuclear antibodies in 27 cases with nasopharyngeal cancer and 4 cases with other cancers.

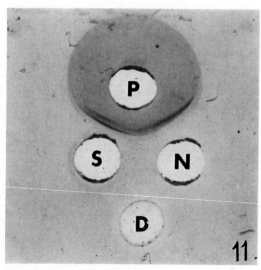

FIG. 11. Precipitin reaction of NPC serum and SLE serum with protamine in agar. P, protamine; N, NPC serum; S, SLE serum; D, DNA.

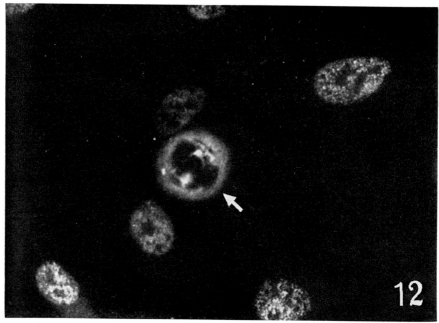

FIG. 12.   The arrows indicate the fluorescence of a spindle-like fiber in the nucleus at metaphase stained with serum as shown in pattern 4.   ×400.

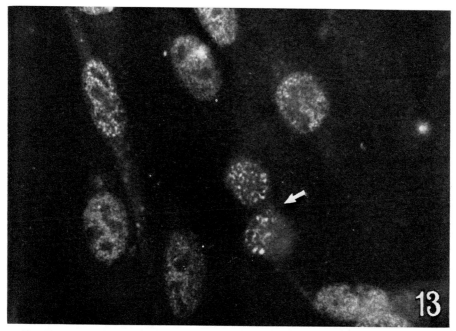

FIG. 13.   The arrows indicate the fluorescence of another pattern staining in the nucleus at terophase with the serum shown in pattern 4.   ×400.

showed IgG only, 2 cases showed IgM only, and 18 cases showed both IgG and IgM.

Preliminary attempts to find substances having antigenicity have been made using purified DNA, histones, and protamine.   The ANA of NPC patients was able to adsorb with histones and protamine, but was not able to adsorb with DNA. The ANA of one typical SLE patient was able to adsorb with DNA, histones, and protamine.   The protamine (sulfate solution) reacted with the ANA and could make a precipitation line in agar as shown in Fig. 11.   It was found that the ANA shown in patterns 4 and 6 in the nuclei of resting cultured cells did not react with chromosomes at the metaphase, but did react with a spindle-like fiber as observed by the indirect immunofluorescent technique in Fig. 12, and the same ANA showed another staining pattern in the nuclei of terophase cultured cells in Fig. 13.

DISCUSSION

During the course of the studies of tumor immunological approaches, heterophilic ANA in the sera of NPC patients was found first, and later was also found in the sera of other cancer patients.   A statistical analysis of ANA positive cases including weak positive cases in the sera of tumor patients showed that the cases with NPC were by far the highest, other cancer cases showed the next highest incidence, and cases with malignant neoplasma of haematopoietic organs were very low.

Many question can be raised pertaining to the present observation.   How do NPC and other cancer patients produce ANA, is ANA related in any way to the hypothetical infectious agent or agents which may induce malignant transformation and subsquently provide stimulus for autoantibody formation in autoimmune disorders?   It is conceivable that immunological surveillance may have been impaired in tumor-bearing hosts, and as a result, the heterophilic ANA has appeared in patients.   Another conceivable possibility is that antibodies against tumor-specific antigens also show the nature of heterophilic antibodies.

The evidence is that heterophilic ANA in cancer patients may indicate a special condition of the tumor-bearing host, and may take one of several abnormal directions, which direction may be related to cachexia.   This phenomenon could be understood as an impairment of immunological surveillance in cancer patients. The production of heterophilic antinuclear antibodies in cancer patients may seem more surprising to cancer researchers than to tumor immunologists.   But it seems clear that here is a new immunological concept now introduced into the cancer research field, and the immunological relationship between tumor and host has to be reconsidered and clarified on the basis of this new concept, together with the many recent advances in human tumor biology and immunology in man.

Kaplan and Tan (7) have reported that ANA, cryoproteins in infectious mononucleosis, appeared in the clinical course of patients with infectious mononucleosis, and very recently Henle et al. (4) have found EBV to be a causative agent of infectious mononucleosis.   Therefore, the sera must be carefully investigated in the clinical course of BL patients, because the investigation of ANA in the limited number of sera of BL patients shown in Table 3 showed very weak positive results in just

2 out of 41 cases.   Further investigation of ANA in the sera of cancer patients has to be carefully made in the clinical course of patients undergoing various kinds of treatment.

Six patterns have been observed within the nuclei of cells of a human embryo fibroblastic cell line derived from embryonic lungs, and NPC cell lines derived from NPC biopsy materials, as shown in Tables 1, and 2.   When the ANA in the sera was tested with HeLa and SiHa cells, it showed a different pattern, having big dots scattered in the nuclei; the patterns were not specifically classified with various ANA.   Also unclassified were the various patterns in the lymphoid cell lines, Raji and P3HR-1.   Tan (17) described the different patterns of immunofluorescent nuclear staining in the nuclei of a whole mouse kidney snap-frozen section produced by sera from patients with SLE, they were correlated with the precipitating antibodies, i.e., the nuclear rim and internuclear fibrillar staining were shown to be produced by the antibody to DNA and the antibody to soluble nucleo-protein. Speckled nuclear staining was produced by the antibody to Sm antigen, a saline-soluble component of the nucleus devoid of nucleic acids or histones, and homogeneous nuclear staining was produced by an antibody reacting with particulate nucleoprotein.   Therefore, attempts to show nuclear-staining patterns in the frozen tissue section of mouse liver and kidney, and in human liver, with ANA in the sera of NPC patients, have been made several times, but such clear staining patterns as shown in Figs. 1, 2, 3, 4, 5, 6, 12, and 13 were never obtained.

The staining patterns of ANA will be important in biochemical studies of antigenic substances in nuclei related to infectious agents and malignant transformation.   It may be immunologically possible to identify the various antigens in nuclei by a blocking test of the direct immunofluorescence technique.

In this study, varying sizes and forms of the specks or dots in speckled staining patterns with various sera of cancer patients on the same monolayer cultured cell sheet have been observed, especially, as previously described (25), patterns 3, 4, 5, and 6.   One of the pattern 6 sera showed small specks filling the nucleolus, but for the most cases nucleoli were homogeneously stained.   The ANA in the selected sera of NPC patients shown to be patterns 3, 4, and 6 was observed to be able to adsorb with the histones and the protamine, but not with the DNA.

Chromosomes of cells at the metaphase were not stained with ANA, which could normally be adsorbed with the histones and the protamine, but instead, the spindle-like fibers were clearly stained with the ANA-positive sera as shown in Fig. 12.   This was strikingly interesting in substances such as antigens in the nuclei at various phases of cell growth.   The localization of antigenic substances has been investigated with an electron microscope, using an indirect peroxidase antibody technique, in cooperation with Dr. Ohashi and Dr. Y. Kato at the University of Nagoya; further electron microscopic studies of the localization of antigenic substances will be made.   The biochemical analysis of antigenic substances and their localization in the nuclei must be comparatively observed simultaneously.

As concerns the relation of the treatment of cancer patients, particularly blood transfusions and radiation to the production of ANA, almost none of the patients in the Aichi Cancer Center had received blood transfusions and radiation at the time of the serum collection. The sera of the 97 Chinese cases with NPC in Table 1 who came to the National Taiwan University Hospital for their first visit were also collected before treatment, and the other 50 cases with NPC in Table 2 had received radiotherapy or chemotherapy. Other cases with lymphoma, leukemia, and other cancers were unknown. Therefore, it is not strongly conceivable that the existance of ANA in patients was related to radiotherapy or chemotherapy.

The correlation of the appearance of ANA in cancer patients with EBV infection and other viral infections must be carefully investigated in the future.

SUMMARY

A high incidence of heterophilic antinuclear antibodies in patients with nasopharyngeal cancer was found within the nuclei of human and animal cultured cells during immunological studies on nasopharyngeal cancer; later, heterophilic antinuclear antibodies were also found in the sera of other tumor patients. A statistical analysis of antinuclear antibody-positive cases in tumor patients showed that the cases with nasopharyngeal cancer were by far the highest, the cases with malignant neoplasma of haematopoietic organs were very low, and the cases with other cancer were at a level between nasopharyngeal cancer and haematopoietic neoplasma. Clinically, these nasopharyngeal patients have not encountered complications with the well-known antinuclear antibody-producing autoimmune diseases. The various patterns of nuclear staining in the immunofluorescence procedure have been observed within the tissue culture cells as diffuse, speckled, nucleolar, and nucleolar combined with speckled. By contrast, normal healthy sera did not show any specific immunoreaction within the nuclei of the cultured cells.

The immunoglobulin classes, IgG only, IgM only, and both IgG and IgM, of antinuclear antibodies in the sera of the patients were observed. A slight correlation between antinuclear antibody titer and EBV titer in the sera of nasopharyngeal patients was statistically observed. Impairment of immunological surveillance was discussed with respect to the evidence of antinuclear antibodies in cancer patients, which may be related to cachexia.

This work was supported in part by grants from the Ministry of Health and Welfare, the Princess Takamatsu Cancer Research Fund, and the Ministry of Education, Government of Japan.

The author is greatly indebted to Drs. M. Takada, C.-S. Yang, S.-M. Tu, C.-H. Liu, C.-H. Wang, M.-M. Hsu, Mr. Y.-C. Lin, Drs. K. R. Utsumi, G. Klein, K. Imai, T. Suchi, and Mr. Akaza for their valuable cooperation; and to Drs. Y. Ito, A. Kawamura, K. Nishioka, T. Hirayama, and T. Tachibana for their encouragement and valuable suggestions; and to Miss M. Kajiyama for technical assistance.

REFERENCES

1. Epstein, M. A., Achong, B. G., and Barr, Y. M. Virus Particles in Cultured Lymphoblasts from Burkitt's Lymphoma. Lancet, *1*: 702–703, 1964.
2. Friedl, F., Kimura, I., Osato, T., and Ito, Y. Studies on a New Human Cell Line

(SiHa) Derived from Carcinoma of the Uterus. I. It's Establishment and Morphology. Proc. Soc. Exp. Biol. & Med., *135*: 543–545, 1971.

3. Henle, G., and Henle, W. Immunofluorescence in Cells Derived from Burkitt's Lymphoma. J. Bacteriol., *91*: 1248–1256, 1966.

4. Henle, G., Henle, W., and Diehl, V. Relation of Burkitt's Tumor-associated Herpes-type Virus to Infectious Mononucleosis. Proc. Natl. Acad. Sci., U.S.A., *59*: 94–101, 1968.

5. Ishimoto, A., Oota, S., Kimura, I., Miyake, T., and Ito, Y. *In vitro* Cultivation and Antigenicity of Cottontail Rabbit Papilloma Cells Induced by the Shope Papilloma Virus. Cancer Research, *30*: 2598–2605, 1970.

6. Ito, Y., Takahashi, T., Tu, S.-M., and Kawamura, A., Jr. High Anti-EB Virus Titer in Sera of Patients with Nasopharyngeal Carcinoma: A Small Scaled Seroepidemiological Study. GANN, *60*: 335–340, 1969.

7. Kaplan, M. E., and Tan, E. M. Antinuclear Antibodies in Infectious Mononucleosis. Lancet, *1*: 561–563, 1968.

8. Kawamura, A., Jr., Takada, M., Gotoh, A., Hamajima, K., Sanpe, T., Murata, M., Ito, Y., Takahashi, T., Yoshida, T. O., Hirayama, T., Tu, S.-M., Liu, C.-H., Yang, C.-S., and Wang, C.-H. Seroepidemiological Studies on Nasopharyngeal Carcinomas by Fluorescent Antibody Technique with Cultured Burkitt Lymphoma Cells. GANN, *61*: 55–71, 1970.

9. Klein, G., Clifford, P., Klein, E., Smith, R. T., Minowada, J., Kourilsky, F. M., and Burchenal, J. H. Membrane Immunofluorescence Reactions of Burkitt Lymphoma Cells from Biopsy Specimens and Tissue Cultures. J. Nat. Cancer Inst., *39*: 1027–1044, 1967.

10. Klein, G., Clifford, P., Klein, E., and Stjernswärd, J. Search for Tumor-specific Immune Reaction in Burkitt Lymphoma Patients by the Membrane Immunofluorescence Reaction. Proc. Natl. Acad. Sci., U.S.A., *55*: 1628–1635, 1966.

11. Klein, G., Pearson, G., Henle, G., Henle, W., Diehl, V., and Niederman, J. C. Relation between Epstein-Barr Viral and Cell Membrane Immunofluorescence in Burkitt Tumor Cells. II. Comparison of Cell and Sera from Patients with Burkitt's Lymphoma and Infectious Mononucleosis. J. Exp. Med., *128*: 1021–1030, 1969.

12. Klein, G., Pearson, G., Henle, G., Henle, W., Goldstein, G., and Clifford, P. Relation between Epstein-Barr Viral and Cell Membrane Immunofluorescence in Burkitt Tumor Cells. III. Comparison of Blocking of Direct Membrane Immunofluorescence Anti-EBV Reactivities of Different Sera. J. Exp. Med., *129*: 697–705, 1969.

13. Klein, G., Pearson, G., Nadkarni, J. S., Nadkarni, J. J., Klein, E., Henle, G., Henle, W., and Clifford, P. Relation between Epstein-Barr Viral and Cell Membrane Immunofluorescence of Burkitt Tumor Cells. I. Dependence of Cell Membrane Immunofluorescence on Presence of EB Virus. J. Exp. Med., *128*: 1011–1028, 1968.

14. Old, L. J., Boyse, E. A., Oettgen, H. F., de Hakven, E., Geering, G., Williamson, B., and Clifford, P. Precipitating Antibody in Human Serum to an Antigen Present in Cultured Burkitt's Lymphoma Cells. Proc. Natl. Acad. Sci., U.S.A., *56*: 1699–1704, 1966.

15. Shiratori, O., Osato, T., Utsumi, R., and Ito, Y. Growth and Other Characteristics of a Cell Line (Sp-8) Established from Shope Virus-induced Cutaneous Papilloma of Domestic Rabbit. Proc. Soc. Exp. Biol. & Med., *128*: 12–18, 1968.

16. Takada, M., Lin, Y.-C., Shiratori, O., Sugano, H., Yang, C.-S., Hse, M.-M., Lin, T.-C., Tu, S.-M., Chen, H.-C., Hamajima, K., Murata, M., Gotoh, A., Kawamura,

A., Jr., Yoshida, T. O., Osato, T., and Ito, Y.   Cultivation *in vitro* of Cells Derived from Nasopharyngeal Carcinoma.   GANN Monograph, No. 10, 149–161, 1970.

17. Tan, E. M.   Relationship of Nuclear Staining Patterns with Precipitating Antibodies in Systemic Lupus Erythematosus.   J. Lab. and Clin. Med., *70*: 800–812, 1967.

18. Utsumi, K. R., and Yoshida, T. O.   A Chromosome Survey on Tissue Culture Cells Derived from Nasopharyngeal Cancer.   GANN Monograph, No. 10, 291–293, 1970.

19. Yoshida, T. O.   Further Evidence of Immunologic Reaction against Methylchrolanthrene-induced Autochthonous Tumors.   Japan J. Exp. Med., *35*: 115–124, 1965.

20. Yoshida, T. O., Hsu, M.-M., Wang, C.-H., Lin, Y.-C., and Kajiyama, M.   Further Findings of Antinuclear Antibodies in the Sera of Nasopharyngeal Cancer Patients and Other Tumor Patients.   To be published.

21. Yoshida, T. O., and Imai, K.   Auto-antibody to Human Leukemic Cell Membrane as Detected by Immune Adherence.   Europ. J. Clinic. and Biol. Research, *15*: 61–65, 1970.

22. Yoshida, T. O., Imai, K., and Sugiyama, T.   Auto-antibody to 7, 12-Dimethylbenz(a)anthracene-induced Leukemic Cells in Rats as Detected by Immune Adherence.   Int. J. Cancer, *3*: 720–726, 1968.

23. Yoshida, T. O., Liu, C.-H., Yang, C.-S., and Ito, Y.   Membrane Immunofluorescence Reaction of Burkitt Lymphoma Cell (P3HR-1) Exposed to Sera of Tumor Patients and Healthy Normal Subjects: with Particular Reference to the Action of Sera of Nasopharyngeal Cancer Patients.   GANN Monograph, No. 7, 211–214, 1969.

24. Yoshida, T. O., and Southam, C. M.   Attempts to Find Cell Associated Immune Reaction against Autochthonous Tumors.   Japan J. Exp. Med., *33*: 369–383, 1963.

25. Yoshida, T. O., Takada, M., Kawamura, A., Jr., Yang, C.-S., Tu, S.-M., Liu, C.-H., and Ito, Y.   Anti-Nuclear Antibodies in the Sera of Nasopharyngeal Cancer Patients.   GANN Monograph, No. 10, 283–289, 1970.

Discussion of Papers by Drs. Tachibana, and Yoshida

Dr. Takahashi: Did you use a direct immunofluorescent technique to demonstrate anti-nuclear antibodies and did you try a blocking test?

Dr. Yoshida: I hope to do so, but I do not have sufficient ANA positive sera to conjugate directly with fluorescein. I tried absorption of sera with purified DNA, histones, and protamine, after which they were tested by the indirect immunofluorescent technique. The ANA of selected sera (patterns 4 and 6 from NPC patients) was removed by absorption with histones and protamine, but the titers did not change after absorption with DNA. The ANA of a patient with typical systemic lupus erythematosus was removed by absorption with DNA, histones, and protamine.

Dr. G. Klein: Could these interesting findings of Drs. Tachibana and Yoshida be related to the theory proposed by Dr. Tachibana that EBV acts by decreasing immunological surveillance? I could not quite understand your thinking on this point: could you explain it further, please? Also, is there a difference in the incidence of ANA between Chinese and Japanese? And are Africans like Japanese in this respect?

Dr. Tachibana: I simply interpreted the presence of antinuclear antibodies as reflecting an altered immunological state in nasopharyngeal cancer. Of course, no one can argue that antinuclear antibodies directly imply decreasing immunological surveillance. But thinking of the alteration of the immune surveillance mechanism with the natural occurrence of tumor, the high incidence of antinuclear antibody in this cancer is very interesting, because of the little information we now have of the presence of antinuclear antibody in the cancerous stage. However, the precise immunological significance of antinuclear antibody awaits clarification.

Dr. Yoshida: Dr. Klein's question raises serveral points about the relationship between area, race, and the host response to the antigens. The incidence of ANA in NPC patients in Taiwan was over 40%, in Japan 20%, and in Africa about 25%.

Dr. E. Klein: I wonder whether, considering the number of cases, a difference in incidence is responsible for the fact that ANA was missed through the years when the sera were tested by the Henle method for anti-EBV antibody; the technique for

461

detection is much the same. I wonder whether it was not seen on the first attempts to look for anti-EBV antibodies?

DR. YOSHIDA: The sera tested contained antibodies to EBV antigen. The target cell monolayers did not have EBV or other viral antigens, as checked by direct immunofluorescence.

DR. W. HENLE: We have seen ANA in some sera but the observation did not " connect." Of course the ANA is present in rather low titer and would often be diluted out and so missed in the usual test for anti-EBV antibodies. I wanted to ask Dr. Yoshida whether the ANA-positive sera were all from untreated patients and whether there appeared to be any relationship to the stage of disease, to treatment, and so on?

DR. YOSHIDA: Sera were collected from patients with NPC who were on their first visit to the National Taiwan University Hospital. About half the patients were at the early stage, the rest being at the moderate to advanced and late stages. In the cases at Aichi Cancer Center Hospital the sera were collected mostly just before operation. The stomach and mammary cancer patients were not at the advanced stage. Almost none of the patients had received any special treatment such as blood transfusion, radiation, etc. We are now planning to study ANA activities in relation to the clinical course and stages of NPC and other diseases.

DR. G. HENLE: Have you checked any animal sera for ANA activity? We had some experience when looking for cross-reactions between Marek's disease and Burkitt's lymphoma using pooled chicken sera. With Marek's disease sera we observed the strongest antinuclear reaction we had ever seen—completely solid staining whether the cells were infected or non-infected. Have you any experience with animal sera?

DR. YOSHIDA: Thank you. I want to find out more about this phenomenon in animals.

DR. HO: May I ask Dr. Yoshida how he differentiates between lymphoblasts and reticular cells? Are they from cultures of cells described as lymphoblastoid?

DR. YOSHIDA: I take it you are thinking of immature *versus* mature cells, and cells of the lymphoid group *versus* other types of cells. I have tried to stain peripheral white blood cells with ANA positive sera. The nuclei of lymphocytes could be stained in the same way as those of cultured lymphoblastoid cells, but the staining of polymorphonuclear cell nuclei was unremarkable. It seems to me that lymphoblasts and lymphocytes are not different in this respect, and I am interested in finding out why polymorphonuclear cells are different. Further studies of staining patterns in different cell types should be done.

DR. CHANG: In many of the so-called auto-immune diseases, such as systemic lupus erythematosus and rheumatoid arthritis, there is a very high incidence of anti-nuclear antibody. Is this different from the anti-nuclear antibody in NPC, or are they the same biologically or clinically?

DR. YOSHIDA: I can't determine the differences now. I think that with further studies we may be able to say that the conformation of some nuclear materials (as antigens) changes after infection with some agents, or transformation by some chemical carcinogens, or chemotherapy.

DR. AOKI: Regarding Dr. Henle's question about animal systems: we have screened many mice of different strains, especially NZB and NZW, for ANA. We found no special differences from other strains which have no auto-immune disease, such as C57Bl. They produce a lot of ANA with increasing age, so we found no special significance in the incidence of ANA. However, NZB and NZW mice infected with lymphocytic choriomeningitis virus produced much more ANA.

In humans with melanoma and leukaemia we found a high incidence of ANA. In such cases there is difficulty in distinguishing nonspecific ANA from antobodies to tumor-specific nuclear antigens.

IMMUNOGLOBULIN PRODUCTION OF EBV CARRYING CELLS

Chairmen:

Yorio Hinuma, David S. Nelson

Immunoglobulin Production in Cultured Human Lymphoid Cells Derived from Burkitt's Lymphoma and Other Malignancies

Morinobu Takahashi

Department of Molecular Immunology, Cancer Institute, Kanazawa University, Kanazawa, Japan

A number of human lymphoblastoid lines have been established from tumor tissues of patients with Burkitt's lymphoma. Similar lymphoblastoid cells have been obtained as continuous suspension cultures from the buffy coat of the peripheral blood of healthy or diseased individuals. The majority of these culture lines were shown to produce various types of immunoglobulin or its component polypeptide chains (*3–6, 9, 13, 15, 17, 27, 28*). The availability of these immunoglobulin producing clones greatly aids the study of the regulatory and biosynthetic processes of immunoglobulin in human lymphocytoid cells. On the other hand, the study of the production of immunoglobulin in these culture lines will serve, in turn, to identify the lymphoid culture lines and to understand the origin of cultured lymphoid cells. The formation of immunoglobulins by cultured cells has been successfully demonstrated by several methods and studies have been developed in different directions.

General Characterization of Immunoglobulin Production in Human Lymphoblastoid Cells in Continuous Culture

Studies of a number of culture lines by several laboratories including ours can be summarized as follows.

1) Most culture lines of lymphoid appearance produce immunoglobulin.

2) Some lines produce several classes of immunoglobulin, while other lines produce only one type of immunoglobulin or its component chains. Detection of different types of heavy chains and light chains in some culture lines raised a question as to whether more than one type of immunoglobulin is synthesized in individual cells or whether these lines consist of more than one clone, each producing a single type of immunoglobulin. The double immunofluorescence method has been particularly useful in studying the immunoglobulin production in individual cells and was used to

467

answer this question.   By this method, the presence of two different heavy chains was confirmed in a significant number of cells of several culture lines (5, 23, 25). Therefore, structural genes for two different classes of heavy chains appear to be expressed in individual cells in these cell lines.   This is a rather extraordinary finding, because all studies to date have indicated that malignant plasma cells and lymphoid cells *in vivo* synthesize only one class of heavy chain and one type of light chain (for review, see ref. *8*).

3)   The immunoglobulin produced by culture cells are of relatively restricted molecules as judged by electrophoretic mobility, suggesting their monoclonal nature.

4)   Synthesized molecules appear normal in terms of size, antigenicity, and gross polypeptide chain composition.

5)   The ability of a given culture line to produce its biosynthetic product appears very stable, although fluctuation of cell populations, each producing a different type of immunoglobulin was observed, probably due to selection.

6)   Immunoglobulin synthesis occurs in a very limited period of the cell life cycle. This conclusion was reached in a study of synchronized cultures.   Two culture lines, one RPMI. 4666 lines, which produces IgA of the κ-type, the other a Burkitt's lymphoma line, NK-9a, which produces IgM of the λ-type, were synchronized at the boundary of the Gl and S phase by two sequential exposures to excess thymidine. The content of immunoglobulin in the cells harvested at different times was measured by an immunocytochemical method.   With these two lines, the cellular immunoglobulin level reached its peak in the early part of the DNA synthetic phase, then decreased gradually throughout the late S and G2 periods and reached its lowest level in the the mitotic period (*26*).   Essentially the same result has been reported by Buell and Fahey with synchronized cultures of two other lymphoid lines, WiL 2 line and IM-4 line (*2*).   The restricted expression of genes for immunoglobulins implies a limited period of gene transcription.   Sequential gene transcription during the cell life cycle has been demonstrated for bacterial and yeast enzyme synthesis, tyrosine aminotransferase induction in hepatoma cells, histone synthesis in HeLa cells, and coordinated transcriptional and translational events prior to mitosis represent similar phenomena in mammalian cells.   Our observation indicates that limited gene transcription is also characteristic of the genes for immunoglobulins in human lymphoid cells.   The elucidation of the mechanisms controlling immunoglobulin synthesis in culture lines should lead to an understanding of similar events during active immune responses.

7)   Herpes-like virus particles have been found in a number of culture lines.   In the work of several laboratories, no correlation was found between the presence or absence of virus and the characterization of immunoglobulin synthesized.   Similarly, we found no correlation between the diagnosis of the donor from which the cultures were derived with the type of immunoglobulin synthesized, or with the number of different immunoglobulins produced by individual cells.

8)   The capability of lymphoblastoid clones in the production of immunoglobulin appeared to be very stable.   In the repeated examinations over the years of a number of culture lines, no change in the type of immunoglobulin produced was found with any culture line.

The Site of Immunoglobulin Synthesis in Lymphoblastoid Cells

In recent years, the importance of membrane-bound polyribosomes in the synthesis of secreted proteins has been brought to light. Biochemical studies on antibody forming plasma cells have suggested that immunoglobulin is probably formed by the mebrane-bound polysome (for review, see ref. *1*). The site of immunoglobulin synthesis within lymphoblastoid cells is a subject of particular interest, because those lymphoblastoid cells in continuous culture are morphologically quite distinct from cells of a plasmacytic series, especially in the arrangement of polyribosomes. The development of endoplasmic reticulum in the lymphoblastoid cells of continuous culture is significantly lower than in antibody-producing plasma cells. In contrast to plasma cells, free polysomes apparently outnumber the membrane-bound polysomes in cultured lymphoid cells. In order to elucidate the function of various types of polysome in the synthesis of immunoglobulin, we used immunocytochemistry with electron microscopy. Electron microscopic immunocytochemistry utilized enzyme-labeled antibodies, each monospecific to component polypeptide chains of human immunoglobulin molecules (*22*, *24*). Purified antibody was coupled with horseradish peroxidase, following the method of Nakane and Pierce (*16*). The enzyme-labeled antibody method was first successfully applied to the ultrastructural localization of immunoglobulin within cells of the RPMI. 4666 line. This line was derived from peripheral leucocytes of a patient with chronic myelogeneous leukemia. In extensive immunochemical and immunohistological study in Dr. Pressman's laboratory, it was revealed that individual cells of this line synthesize and secrete IgA of the κ-type along with free κ-chain (*10*). Intracellular distribution was demonstrated within significant number of RPMI. 4666 cells when fixed cells were treated either with peroxidase-conjugated anti-a or with peroxidase-conjugated anti-κ antibody. By this method, free polysomes as well as membrane-bound polysomes were identified as the subcellular organelles engaged in the synthesis of immunoglobulin. Free polysomes were reactive with peroxidase-conjugated anti-α antibody more strongly than with peroxidase-conjugated anti-κ antibody, suggesting that the α-chain was primarily synthesized on the free polysomes within lymphoblastoid cells (*20*). Our finding was the first to present evidence that free polysomes are capable of the synthesis of exportable proteins.

In the present work, a similar type of study was extended to lymphoblastoid cells of a Burkitt's lymphoma line, P3J (*18*). The development of endoplasmic reticulum in P3J cells is much lower than in other lymphoid cells of non-Burkitt's origin such as RPMI. 4666 cells (Fig. 1). In contrast, free polysomes were abundant over the whole cytoplasm. In addition to the general characteristics of primitive lymphoblasts shared by other culture cells of Burkitt's lymphoma origin, P3J cells were distinguished from cells of other lymphoid lines by the frequent occurrence of an extraordinary arrangement of polysomes (helical polysomes, *19*, see Fig. 2). Drastic alteration in the ratio of polysomes of helical arrangement versus polysomes of rosette form was observed when P3J cells were subjected to antigenic stimulation (*19*). This culture line was shown to produce IgM of the κ-type. Procedures for

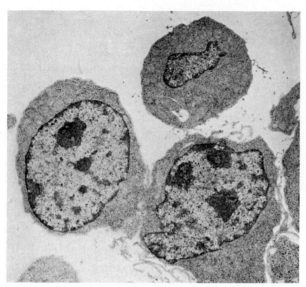

Fig. 1. Electron micrograph of lymphoid cells of a Burkitt's lymphoma line (P3J). These cells show the appearance of primitive lymphoblasts. Fixation with glutaraldehyde; lead and uranium. ×5,000.

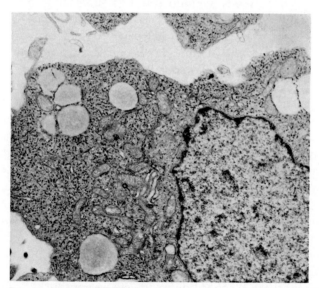

Fig. 2. A part of a P3J cell. This electron micrograph reveals very scarce endoplasmic reticulum and a large number of free polysomes within the cell. Note that numerous helical polysomes coexist with abundant polysomes of rosette form. Fixation with glutaraldehyde; lead and uranium. ×8,000.

ultrastructural localization of IgM (μ, κ) closely followed the method of Nakane and Pierce with minor modifications (16, 20). P3J cells were washed with phosphate buffered saline (PBS), pH 7.4, and then fixed with a mixture of 2.5% glutaraldehyde and 2% formaldehyde in PBS. After washing with PBS containing 4.5%

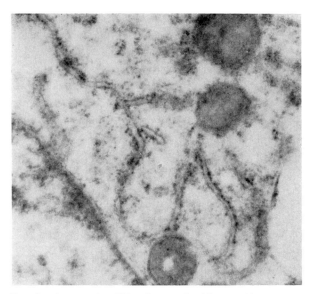

FIG. 3. A part of a P3J cell treated with peroxidase-conjugated anti-κ antibody. A positive reaction is demonstrated as fine electrondense deposits on the endoplasmic reticulum and polysomes bound to the ergastoplasmic membrane. Since the ultrathin section was photographed without lead and uranium double staining, all the electrondense granules became inconspicuous except for the electrondense deposits arising from the peroxidase reaction. Fixation with glutaraldehyde ; no electron staining. × 35,000.

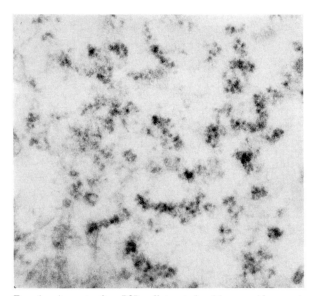

FIG. 4. A part of a P3J cell treated with peroxidase-conjugated anti-κ antibody. Note electrondense reaction products on many, but not all free polysomes. Both the helical polysome and rosette polysomes were reacted with the peroxidase conjugate. Fixation with a mixture of glutaraldehyde and paraformaldehyde ; no electron staining. × 40,000.

sucrose, the fixed cells were exposed to peroxidase-labeled antibody (anti-κ or anti-μ) (22, 24).   Details of subsequent cytochemical reactions and procedures for electron microscopic observation closely followed the method already published (20).   Electron staining with lead citrate and uranyl acetate was usually excluded, because such treatment obscured positive reaction by intensifying the electron density of many osmiophilic granules.   When electron staining with lead and uranium was omitted, the electron dense background almost completely disappeared and only electron dense deposits arising from the peroxidase reaction persisted as shown in Figs. 3 and 4. Figures 3 and 4 show a part of a P3J cell reacted with peroxidase conjugated anti-κ antibody.   The electron micrographs photographed without electron staining show some positive reactions on the endoplasmic reticulum, as well as on the free polysome of the rosette form and of the helical form.   Similar experiments using peroxidase conjugated anti-μ antibody gave essentially the same result.   These findings suggest that not only the endoplasmic reticulum, but the polysomes of the rosette form or the polysomes of helical arrangement are also engaged in the synthesis of immunoglobulin components in P3J cells of Burkitt's lymphoma origin.   All the P3J cells, treated either with peroxidase labeled normal goat globulin or with peroxidase alone or with substrate alone showed no comparable electrondense deposits.   Comparison of intact positive cells and intact negative cells, often observed side by side, sets aside non-specific absorption of peroxidase.   In order to confirm this result, the incorporation of radioactive amino acid into nascent polypeptide chains on polysomes of various types was studied.

Details of the isolation procedures of the polysomes of P3J cells were published elsewhere (21). In brief, 5×10^7 to 15×10^7 cells were resuspended in 1–3 ml Ca^{2+}-Tes (Good's buffer) and were allowed to stand for 8 min in an ice bath.   Cell disruption was accomplished by gentle strokes (5 to 8 times) with a Dounce glass homogenizer. The nuclear fraction was removed by cold centrifugation at 2,000 rpm for 10 min. One ml each of supernatant fraction (cytoplasmic extract) was layered on 28 ml of sucrose (10–40% gradient in TKM containing 0.01% heparin).   Ultracentrifugation was performed at 25,000rpm for 165 min in a Spinco SW 25.1 rotor at 2°C. A 1 ml fraction was collected and the absorption at 254 mμ was measured on an ISCO gradient fractionator.   Incorporation of a ^{14}C amino acid mixture (protein hydrolysate) was carried out under the following conditions: 15×10^7 P3J cells were resuspended in 60 ml of medium RPMI. 1640 (14) containing 1/100 the standard concentrations of amino acids.   After preincubation at 37°C for 15 min, cells were exposed to 75μCi of ^{14}C-protein hydrolysate (1.25 μCi/ml) at 37°C for 5 min. Cytoplasmic extract was obtained as described above.   Subsequent ultracentrifugation on a sucrose gradient and fractionation in an ISCO fractionator were also performed under the same conditions.   After 0.1 ml of 0.25% bovine serum albumin was added to each fraction as carrier protein, 1 ml of 20% trichloracetic acid was mixed with each fraction and the mixture was allowed to stand at room temperature for 10 min.   Insoluble fractions were collected on a Whatman glass fiber filter and their radioactivity was measured with a Packard liquid scintillation counter.   A typical polysome pattern obtained by these fractionation procedures is shown in Fig. 5.   Peaks designated as S,L, and Mo represent a small ribosomal subunit,

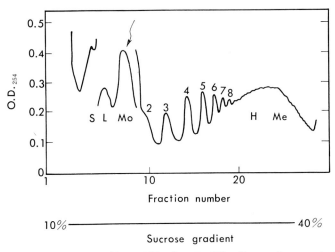

FIG. 5. Polysome profiles of P3J cells. 5×10^7 cells were homogenized and the cytoplasmic extract was centrifuged on a 10–40% (w/v) sucrose gradient for 165 min at 25,000 rpm in a SW 25.1 Spinco rotor. Fractionation and measurement of the optical density at 254 mμ were performed on an ISCO gradient fractionator. The arrow indicates the measurement on the 2.5 scale instead of the 0.5 scale. S, small subunit; L, large subunit; Mo, monomer; R, polysomes of rosette form; H, helical polysomes; Me, membranous components. Arabic numerals on each peak indicate the numbers of ribosomes comprising the polysome.

a large ribosomal subunit, and a monomer, respectively. The peak of the dimer appeared as a shoulder of a peak representing the monomer. Fractions containing polymers of 3, 4, 5, 6, 7, 8, and 9 ribosomes (free polysomes of rosette form) were separated as distinct peaks as shown in Fig. 5. The last broad peak was found to contain both helical polysomes and membranous structures. The first half of this broad peak largely consisted of helical polysomes; the second half corresponded to the membrane fraction. This conclusion was reached by electron microscopic examination and by testing the sensitivity of these fractions to treatment with detergents or ribonuclease. Electron microscopic examination of each fraction outlined by negative stains confirmed their nature. Treatment of cytoplasmic extract with a mixture of 0.5% DOC and 0.5% Triten X for 15 min in an ice bath resulted in the decrease of the broad peak, notably of its second half which contained membranous components (second row of Fig. 6). When the cytoplasmic extract was treated with pancreatic ribonuclease (2.5 μg/ml) for 15 min in an ice bath and was then subjected to ultracentrifugation on a sucrose gradient, the peaks corresponding to free polysomes of the rosette form almost completely disappeared (the third row of Fig. 6). It was also noted that the broad peak, particularly its first half (fractions of helical polysomes) significantly decreased, suggesting that ribosomes of helical structures are connected by a substance sensitive to ribonuclease. The fractions containing membranous components apparently remained after RNase treatment.

^{14}C-amino acid was incorporated largely into the helical polysomes and membranous components. Incorporation was also observed on the free polysomes (rosette form) of larger size. As shown in Fig. 6, proteins are synthesized more actively

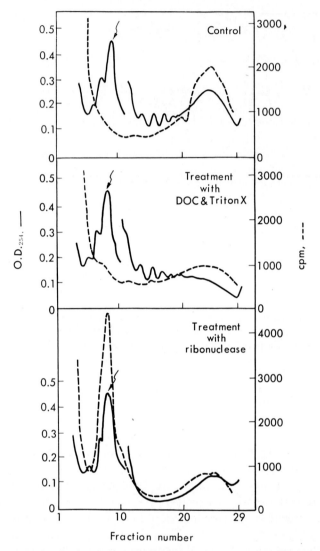

FIG. 6. Incorporation of radioactivity into nascent polypeptide chains on various types of polysomes in P3J cells after pulse exposure (5 min) to 1.25 μCi/ml ^{14}C-protein hydrolysate. The cytoplasmic extract was divided into 3 portions. After treated either with detergents (0.5% DOC and 0.5% Trition X), or with pancreatic ribonuclease (2.5 μg/ml), or with buffer only (control), the cytoplasmic extract was subjected to fractionation on a sucrose gradient centrifugation and on an ISCO gradient fractionator (see legends for Fig. 5). Radioactivity (dotted line) was demonstrated on free polysomes (rosettes of larger size and polysomes of helical form) and membranous components (see text). The arrows indicate the measurement on the 2.5 scale instead of the 0.5 scale.

on the helical polysomes and membranous components than on free polysomes of rosette form. We are now attempting to identify the proteins synthesized on the various types of polysomes.

Origin of Lymphoblastoid Cells in Established Culture Line

One of the most important questions about the cultured lymphoid cells concerns their origin and their function *in vivo*. This question is difficult to resolve at the present time. Since a number of cell lines were originally developed from patients with malignant diseases as part of the studies of human neoplasm, they were thought to be derived directly from malignant cells like leukemic cells. However, morphological and immunocytological studies, along with chromosome analysis, seem to have minimized this possibility. The general morphology of lymphoid cells, their capacity of producing immunoglobulin, and the fact that several weeks were required for the establishment of a lymphoid culture suggest that these lymphoid cells may have arisen by the blastformation of small lymphocytes in a similar manner as the stimulation of small lymphocytes by phytohemagglutinin. Based on the study of immunoglobulin production, particularly from the analyses of immunoglobulin produced by the culture lines, most cell lines appear to be " normal," except for two cases. One of these exceptional cases is the RPMI. 8226 line derived from the peripheral leucocytes of a patient with multiple myeloma (*9, 11, 12*). Extensive immunochemical analyses of the immunoglobulin light chain purified from culture fluids showed that this protein is identical with the Bence-Jones protein found in the urine of the original donor. Actually, the amount of light chain secreted by the cells of this culture was found to be 5–10 times greater than that secreted by other lymphoid cultures (*10*). These findings suggest that RPMI. 8226 cells originated directly from the myeloma cells present in the circulation of the original donor suffering from multiple myeloma. The other case is the cell lines derived from Burkitt's lymphoma. Most cell lines derived from Burkitt's lymphoma produce IgM. In most cases, IgM molecules appear to be of 7S subunits rather than 19S macromolecules (*28*). Furthermore, the ammount of immunoglobulin produced by most Burkitt's lymphoma lines is significantly smaller than that of other culture lines, although extensive comparative study is to be done to draw a definite conclusion on this subject. Based also on the electron microscopic observation that cells of Burkitt's lymphoma lines appear more " primitive " in their general morphology, it may be assumed that most Burkitt's lymphoma lines have been derived from a cell population quite distinct from the cell group from which other " normal " lymphoid lines have originated. Recently, Imamura *et al.*, revealed that cell lines derived from Burkitt's lymphoma have higher plating efficiency on semisolid agar than other lymphoblastoid lines (*7*). Furthermore, we found that the generation time of Burkitt's lymphoma lines, which ranges from 16–18 hr, is considerably shorter than the generation time of other lymphoid lines (24–30 hr). If the two parameters cited above (plating efficiency and generation time) can be considered as the measure of the growth capacity of culture cells, these two lines of evidence further support the assumption that culture cells derived from Burkitt's lymphoma are of malignant origin.

This work was partly supported by grants from the Naito Foundation (the Naito Research grants for 1970) and from the Ministry of Education, Government of Japan.

REFERENCES

1. Askonas, B. A., and Williamson, A. R.   Biosynthesis and Assembly of Immunoglobulin G.   Cold Spring Harbor Symposium, *32*: 223–231, 1967.
2. Buell, D. N., and Fahey, J. L.   Limited Period of Gene Expression in Immunoglobulin Synthesizing Cells.   Science, *164*: 1524–1526, 1969.
3. Fahey, J. L., Finegold, I., Rabson, A. S., and Manaker, R. A.   Immunoglobulin Synthesis *in vitro* by Established Human Cell Lines.   Science, *152*: 1259–1260, 1966.
4. Finegold, I., Fahey, J. L., and Granger, H.   Synthesis of Immunoglobulins by Human Cell Lines in Tissue Culture.   J. Immunol., *99*: 839–848, 1967.
5. Finegold, I., Fahey, J. L., and Dutcher, T. K.   Immunofluorescent Studies of Immunoglobulins in Human Lymphoid Cells in Continuous Culture.   J. Immunol., *101*: 366–373, 1968.
6. Hinuma, Y., and Grace, J. T., Jr.   Cloning of Immunoglobulin-producing Human Leukemic and Lymphoma Cells in Long-term Cultures.   Proc. Soc. Exp. Biol. Med., *124*: 107–109, 1967.
7. Imamura, T., Huang, C.-C., Minowada, J., Takahashi, M., and Moore, G. E.   Cloning of Human Hematopoietic Cell Lines.   J. Nat. Cancer Inst., *44*: 845–854, 1970.
8. Lennox, E. S., and Cohn, M.   Immunoglobulins.   Ann. Rev. Biochem., *36*: Pt. 1, 365–385, 1967.
9. Matsuoka, Y., Moore, G. E., Yagi, Y., and Pressman, D.   Production of Free Light Chains of Immunoglobulin by a Hematopoietic Cell Line Derived from a Patient with Multiple Myeloma.   Proc. Soc. Exp. Biol. Med., *125*: 1246–1250, 1967.
10. Matsuoka, Y., Takahashi, M., Yagi, Y., Moore, G. E., and Pressman, D.   Synthesis and Secretion of Immunoglobulins by Established Cell Lines of Human Hematopoietic Origin.   J. Immunol., *101*: 1111–1120, 1968.
11. Matsuoka, Y., Yagi, Y., Moore, G. E., and Pressman, D.   Isolation and Characterization of Free λ-chains of Immunoglobulin Produced by an Established Cell Line of Human Myceloma Cell Origin.   1. λ-chain in Culture Medium.   J. Immunol., *102*: 1136–1143, 1969.
12. Matsuoka, Y., Yagi, Y., Moore, G. E., and Pressman, D.   Isolation and Characterization of Free λ-chains of Human Immunoglobulin Produced by an Established Cell Line of Human Myeloma Cell Origin.   II. Identity of λ-chains in Cells and in Medium.   J. Immunol., *103*: 962–969, 1969.
13. Minowada, J., Klein, G., Clifford, P., Klein, E., and Moore, G. E.   Studies of Burkitt's Lymphoma Cells.   Cancer, *20*: 1430–1437, 1967.
14. Moore, G. E., Gerner, R. E., and Franklin, H. A.   Culture of Normal Human Leukocytes.   J. Amer. Med. Assoc., *199*: 519–524, 1967.
15. Nadkarni, J. S., Nadkarni, J. J., Clifford, P., Manolov, G., Fenyö, E. M., and Klein, E.   Characteristics of New Cell Lines Derived from Burkitt's Lymphomas.   Cancer, *23*: 64–79, 1969.
16. Nakane, P. K., and Pierce, G. B., Jr.   Enzyme-labelled Antibodies for the Light and Electron Microscopic Localization of Tissue Antigens.   J. Cell Biol., *33*: 307–318, 1967.
17. Osunkoya, O., McFarlane, H., Luzatto, L., Udeozo, I. O. K., Mottram, F. C., Williams, A. I. O., and Ngu, V. A.   Immunoglobulin Synthesis by Fresh Biopsy

Cells and Established Cell Lines from Burkitt's Lymphoma. Immunology, *14*: 851–860, 1968.

18. Pulvertaft, R. J. V.   Cytology of Burkitt's Tumor (African Lymphoma).   Lancet, *1*: 238–240, 1964.

19. Suzuki, I., Kamei, H., and Takahashi, M.   Ultrastructural Study on the Ribosome Helix and Its Change after Antigenic Stimulation in P3J Cells.   Exp. Mol. Path., *11*: 28–37, 1968.

20. Suzuki, I., Takahashi, M., Kamei, H., and Yamamoto, T.   Intracellular Distribution of Immunoglobulin Heavy and Light Chains within Tissue Culture Cells of Human Lymphoid Origin Detected by Electron Microscopy.   J. Immunol., *104*: 907–917, 1970.

21. Suzuki, I., Takahashi, T., Kamei, H., and Takahashi, M.   Helical Polysomes in the P3J Cell Line.   Symposia for Cell Biol., *21*: 41–55, 1971 (in Japanese).

22. Takahashi, M., Yagi, Y., and Pressman, D.   Preparation of Fluorescent Antibody Reagents Monospecific to Heavy Chains of Human Immunoglobulin.   J. Immunol., *100*: 1169–1175, 1968.

23. Takahashi, M., Tanigaki, N., Yagi, Y., Moore, G. E., and Pressman, D.   Presence of Two Different Immunoglobulin Heavy Chains in Individual Cells of Established Human Hematopoietic Cell Lines.   J. Immunol., *100*: 1176–1183, 1968.

24. Takahashi, M., Yagi, Y., and Pressman, D.   Preparation of Fluorescent Antibody Reagents Monospecific to Heavy Chains of Human Immunoglobulin.   J. Immunol., *102*: 1268–1273, 1968.

25. Takahashi, M., Yagi, M., Moore, G. E., and Pressman, D.   Pattern of Immunoglobulin Production in Individual Cells of Human Hematopoietic Origin in Established Culture.   J. Immunol., *102*: 1274–1283, 1969.

26. Takahashi, M., Yagi, Y., Moore, G. E.   and Pressman, D.   Immunoglobulin Production in Synchronized Cultures of Human Hematopoietic Cell Lines.   J. Immunol., *103*: 834–843, 1969.

27. Tanigaki, N., Yagi, Y., Moore, G. E., and Pressman, D.   Immunoglobulin Production in Human Leukemic Cell Lines.   J. Immunol., *97*: 634–646, 1966.

28. Wakefield, D. J., Thorbecke, G. J., Old, L. J., and Boyse, E. A.   Production of Immunoglobulins by Established Cell Lines from Leukemia and Burkitt's Lymphoma. J. Immunol., *99*: 308–319, 1967.

Immunoglobulin Production of Lymphoid Cells

Eva KLEIN

Department of Tumor Biology, Karolinska Institutet, Stockholm, Sweden

Synthesis and Secretion of Immunoglobulin (as a Trait of Burkitt's Lymphoma)

Some of the lymphoblast culture lines of different origins are known to synthesize and secrete immunoglobulins (*4, 5*).   In a comparison of the profile of immunoglobulin secretion of a number of Burkitt biopsies and culture lines, we have found that among the biopsies taken from thirty five patients, twenty one cases were positive.   The study was performed by autoradiography of the immuno-electrophoretic patterns of cell suspension cultures in a medium containing radioactive amino acids.   In 12 cases we were able to compare the biopsies with the culture lines developed from them.   Identical patterns were obtained in nine cases, and in the two cases the culture cell line was found to be producing additional immunoglobulin chains (*6*).   This may have been due either to selection of a cell type representing a minority in the biopsy or to the better performance of the established lines during the 48 hr incubation period when compared to the biopsy cells.   The good correspondence of the immunoglobulin secretion pattern indicates that the cells of established lines can be considered to represent the *in vivo* tumor cell population.

Cell Membrane Associated Immunoglobulin Moieties (in Burkitt's Lymphoma, Malignant and Normal Lymphoid Populations)

Also, several biopsies from Burkitt's lymphoma cases were found to have cell membrane-associated immunoglobulin moieties (*13*).   In all cases examined, the reaction with anti-immunoglobulin reagents indicated the presence of IgM with or without a kappa light chain.   Derived culture lines maintained this trait, showing that the immunoglobulin is a cell product, and not merely due to antibody coating *in vivo*.

In Table 1 are summarized the reactivities of those biopsies from which culture lines could be established.

TABLE 1.   Reactivity[a] of Burkitt's Lymphoma Biopsy Cells on Single or Repeated Occasions; from These Biopsies Culture Lines Were Established

	No. of patients	Number of reactive cases with				IgM pos. culture line
		Anti-IgG	Anti-IgA	anti-κ	anti-λ	
No. reactivity with anti IgM serum	10/36 28%	0	0	0	0	0
Intermediate reactivity with anti IgM serum	17/36 47	4	0	3	0	0
Strong reactivity with anti-IgM serum	9/36 25		0	5	0	5

[a] This evaluation is based on the brilliance and extent of the reactivity.

The cell membrane-bound immungloblin was initially detected when viable cells were exposed to fluorescein-conjugated anti-IgM antibodies. As expected, the reaction was inhibited by the addition of soluble IgM (*13*). The staining could also be blocked by pretreatment of the cells with unlabeled antibody of the same specificity. However, anti-lymphocyte serum did not block, proving that its receptors are distinct from the immunoglobulin moieties. The mu and kappa structures could be demonstrated by cytotoxicity, and also by agglutination, using the relevant antibodies. In these cells no intracellular immunoglobulin could be detected by comparing the absorbing efficiency of viable and killed (by freezing and thawing three times) cells or by immunofluorescent staining of fixed cells (*12*).

A search for this trait in other lymphoid malignancies revealed that it can be found in chronic lymphocytic leukemia and lymphocyte-lymphoblast lymphoma

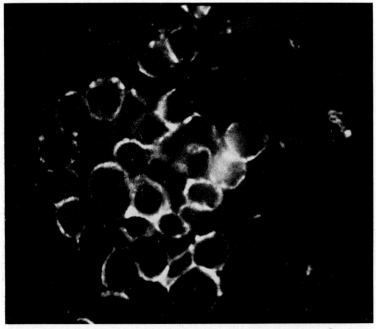

FIG. 1.   Chronic lymphatic leukemia cells from peripheral blood (patient T. P.) fixed in acetone and exposed to conjugated goat anti-human IgM serum diluted 1 : 15 (× 4,000).

TABLE 2. Reactivity of Lymphoid Malignancies with Fluorescein-Conjugated Anti-IgM Serum

Diagnosis and source of cells	Reactivity with anti-IgM serum[a]			Total no. of patients
	Absent or weak	Inter-mediate	Strong	
1. Chronic lymphocytic leukemia and lymphocyte-lymphoblast lymphoma				41
a) leukemia cells from peripheral blood	10 37%	12 39%	9 24%	
b) leukemia cells from bone marrow or lymph nodes	5	4	1	
2. Chronic granulocytic leukemia				2
a) leukemia cells from peripheral blood	1			
b) leukemia cells from bone marrow	1			
3. Undifferentiated leukemia				6
a) leukemia cells from peripheral blood	2			
b) leukemia cells from bone marrow or lymph nodes	4			
4. Polycythemia vera				1
a) normal granulocytes from peripheral blood	1			
5. Plasmacell tumors				2
a) leukemia cells from peripheral blood (multiple myeloma)	1			
b) plasmacells from cutaneous lesion	1			
6. Hodgkin's disease				1
a) cells from lymph node lesion	1			
7. Essential monoclonal IgG Proteinemia				1
a) normal lymphocytes from peripheral blood	1			
8. Tuberculosis				1
a) cells from lymph node lesion	1			

[a] The evaluation is based on the brilliance and extent of the reactivity.

(Fig. 1, Table 2) (9, 10). In these cases, also judged from the intensity of the fluorescence reaction with the anti-IgM serum, the amount of IgM was found to be variable in cells from different patients; but it was similar in different samples taken during the course of the disease and was present in almost all cells in the cases in which the reactivity was strong. Cells of this type—lymphoblast with strong membrane reactivity with anti-μ and anti-κ serum—were found to occur in normal cell populations derived from the bone marrow, thymus, and liver of human fetuses, indicating that the membrane bound immunoglobulin is not connected with the malignant transformation but may represent a state of differentiation, maintained in the tumor. Organs from two human fetuses at a gestation period of 4 months were examined by staining viable cell suspensions. In one of the thymus preparations, 1/400 cells reacted with anti-IgM serum; the reactivity was weak and had a dotted pattern. This suspension was not studied with anti-κ serum. In the other thymus, with the anti-κ reagent, 3/90 cells were found to be intensely stained on the whole cell membrane; 18/90 cells had no confluent but clear brilliant aggregates on the cell surface; the latter cells were larger. No reactive cells were seen with either anti-λ or anti-IgA serum. In the liver cell population typical surface staining of (4/144) round lymphoblast-like cells was seen with anti-IgM serum. It was not possible to estimate the real frequency because of the heterogeneity of the cell population. Also, anti-κ serum stained some cells. In the bone marrow suspension, 11/ 674 cells reacted with anti-IgM serum; no stained cells were seen with the anti-IgA and anti-λ sera.

Also, two cell suspensions derived from adult bone marrow contained IgM reactive cells. These cells showed mainly fluorescent aggregates and dots of varying intensity; 45/780 and 8/309 reactive cells were counted in the two samples stained with anti-IgM and 23/250 and 8/245 with anti-κ serum.

It is probable that a number of the IgM reactive cells detected previously in fixed preparations of liver, spleen, thymus, and peripheral blood of human fetuses were those with cell surface-bound immunoglobulins (5, 7). The significance of this finding from the point of view of Burkitt's lymphoma is the relationship to chronic lymphatic leukemia in spite of the dissimilarity in the clinical course and age of onset, and furthermore, in the possibility of identification of the common cell type which is the target for the neoplastic transformation.

The evidence that normal lymphoid cells synthesize and accumulate immuno-globulin structures in the cell membrane is also provided by other experiments in which anti-immunoglobulin antibodies were observed to bind to the surface of lymphoid cells or influence the immunological performance of such cells (for review see 14). In these and in our studies, only the antigen determinants corresponding to the various parts of serum immunoglobulin molecules have been detected on the surface of the lymphoid cells. There is, however, scanty additional information on the relationship of the structures to serum immunoglobulins and about the nature of their location in the cell membrane. As the tumor cells may be regarded as a malignant clonal outgrowth of immunoglobulin carrying normal lymphocytes main-taining their product of differentiation, they provide a good tool for studies of these problems. The present status of our knowledge will be shortly summarized.

Quantitation and Characterization of Immunoglobulin Structures on The Cell Membrane

Determinations of the average absolute amount of immunoglobulin structures on cells were achieved by comparing their ability to bind anti-mμ and anti-κ antibodies with that of known amounts of purified IgM. The residual activity was evaluated by visual observation of immunofluorescence on reactive lymphoma (T.P.) cells, by agglutination of IgM-coated formalinized sheep red blood cells (passive hemagglutination), or by the cytotoxic effect on cells of a reactive Burkitt culture line (Daudi). Similar results were obtained with the three methods (12).

Two cell populations, Daudi and T.P., were among the strongest reactive ones when stained with fluorescein conjugated reagents; also, their absorbing efficiency was highest. Calculations based on these experiments indicated that 10^9 cells were equivalent to mu and kappa structures in 25 μg of serum IgM. The other cells tested, in accordance with their lower reactivity in immunofluorescence and cyto-toxicity tests, were found to contain lower amounts.

In order to characterize the mu and kappa structures in more detail, they were liberated from the T.P. lymphoma cells by homogenization (3, 11). After cen-trifugation of the homogenate at 1,000 g max. for 10 min, which was sufficient to sediment nuclei and unbroken cells, the supernatant was found to contain mu and kappa structures.   The amount of liberated mu structures was equivalent to the amount on viable cells.   Immunoglobulin structures bound to cellular particles were thereafter sedimented by ultracentrifugation for two hr at 100,000 g max.   The supernatant contained mu structures, but the amount was reduced by about 50 per cent.

The size of the liberated immunoglobulin structures was determined by sucrose density gradient ultracentrifugation and gel filtration on Sephadex G-200.   Before use, the supernatant was concentrated about 10 times.   Iodine-labeled 7S rabbit gamma-globulin was added to the supernatant as the reference substance.   19S IgM was also used as a reference by running normal human serum added to iodine-labeled 7S rabbit gamma-globulin in a parallel tube.   The fractions obtained after ultracentrifugation or gel filtration were analyzed for μ and κ structures by inhibition of passive hemagglutination.   In both types of experiments all the μ and some of the κ activity coincided with the peak radio activity of 7S rabbit γ-globulin.   Some kappa structures were apparently of smaller size, as the sedimentation was slower and the elution delayed compared to the 7S rabbit gamma-globulin.   We concluded that the mu and some of the kappa chains were linked to form 7S IgM-molecules, while some κ chains were free.   7S IgM has previously been found in small quantities in normal serum and intracellularly in a mouse plasma cell tumor secreting 19S IgM.   7S IgM is also found when 19S IgM is reduced, and the subunits consist of two mu and two light (κ and λ) chains and have a molecular weight of about 180,000.

If the IgM immunoglobulin moieties are thus present on the cell surface in the form of 7S subunits, the average number of such molecules would be approximately 80,000/cell (assuming 25 μg/10^9 cells).   According to the pattern of fluorescence staining, the distribution is uneven, thus the density is different on different parts of the cell surface.

While—as it was mentioned before—repeated samples of leukemia cells from the same patient showed the same intensity of immunofluorescence, the Daudi tissue culture cells seemed to vary depending on the culture conditions.   This was confirmed when quantitations were performed daily in the growing cultures (11).   It was found that, after an initial rise, the amount of mμ structures declined as the culture aged.   The decline was also reflected by resistance to the cytolytic effect of anti-mμ antibodies.   Preliminary results indicate that the immunoglobulin is shed bound to cell membrane fragments in the aging cells (3).

Membrane antigen components, such as genetically determined H-2 antigens and certain virally determined surface antigens as well, have been found to undergo cyclic variation during the growth cycle (1), with maximum expression during the G1 phase, decreasing during the S phase, and minimum expression in the course of G2 and mitosis.   In synchronized cultures the surface bound immunoglobulin, judged by the intensity and extent of reactivity with fluorescein-labeled antiserum, was parallel to the reactivity with isoantiserum.   Thus its expression coincided with the synthesis of other, essential constituents of the cell membrane (2).

Cells from the Daudi culture line were hybridized with A9 (L cell variant sub-

line) mouse fibroblasts.   The hybrid nature of the cells was confirmed by chromosomal examination and the expression of mouse and human specific cell surface
antigens.   No immunoglobulin was detected on the surface of the hybrid cells (8).

This work was performed in collaboration with Drs. T. Eskeland, B. Johansson, R.
van Furth, M. Inoue, J. J. and J. S. Nadkarni, and P. Clifford.

This work has been supported by grants from the Swedish Cancer Society, the Cancer
Society of Stockholm, Contract No. 69–2005 within the Special Virus-Cancer Program
of the National Cancer Institute, NIH, PHS, the Medical Research Council, and the Jane
Coffin Childs Memorial Fund for Medical Research.

REFERENCES

1. Cikes, M., and Friberg, S.   Expression of H-2 and Moloney Leukemia Virus-de-
    termined Cell Surface Antigens in Synchronized Cultures of a Mouse Cell Line.
    Proc. Nat. Acad. Sci., 566–569, 1971.
2. Cikes, M., and Klein, E. unpublished.
3. Eskeland, T., Klein, E.   Inoue, M., and Johansson, B. J. exp. Med. *134*: 265, 1971.
4. Fahey, J. L., Finegold, I., Rabson, A. S., and Manaker, R. A.   Immunoglobulin
    Synthesis *in vitro* by Established Human Cell Lines.   Science, *152*: 1259–1261, 1966.
5. van Furth, R.   The Formation of Immunoglobulins by Circulating Lymphocytes.
    Seminars of Hematology, *6*: 84–103, 1969.
6. van Furth, R., Gorter, H., Nadkarni, J. S., Nadkarni, J. J., Klein, E., and Clifford,
    P.   Immunology, in press.
7. van Furth, R., Schuit, Henrica R. E., and Hijmans, W.   The Immunological De-
    velopment of the Human Fetus.   J. Exp. Med., *122*: 1173–1188, 1965.
8. Harris, H., Wiener, F., Klein, G., and Klein, E.   To be published.
9. Johansson, B., and Klein, E.   Cell Surface Localized IgM–kappa Immunoglobulin
    Reactivity in a Case of Chronic Lymphocytic Leukaemia.   Clin.   Exp. Immunol.,
    6: 421–428, 1970.
10. Johansson, B.,   To be published.
11. Klein, E., and Eskeland, T.   Surface IgM on Lymphoid Cells.   Proceedings of the
    3rd Sigrid Juselius Symposium, pp. 91, Academic Press. 1971.
12. Klein, E., Eskeland, T., Inoue, M., Strom, R., and Johansson, B.   Surface Immuno-
    globulin-moieties on Lymphoid Cells.   Exp. Cell Res., *62*: 133–148, 1970.
13. Klein, E., Klein, G., Nadkarni, J. S., Nadkarni, J. J., Wigzell, H., and Clifford, P.
    Surface IgM–kappa Specificity on a Burkitt Lymphoma Cell *in vivo* and in Derived
    Culture Lines.   Cancer Res., *28*: 1300–1310, 1968.
14. Singhal, S. K., and Wigzell, H.   Cognition and Recognition of Antigen by Cell
    Associated Receptors.   Progress in Allergy, *15*, in press.
15. Takahashi, M., Tanigaki, N., Yagi, Y., Moore, G. E., and Pressman, D.   Presence
    of Two Different Immunoglobulin Heavy Chains in Individual Cells of Established
    Human Hemapoietic Cell Lines.   J. Immunol., *100*: 1176–1183, 1968.

Discussion of Papers by Drs. Takahashi, and E. Klein

Dr. W. Henle: Did you study any infectious mononucleosis cell lines for these components?

Dr. E. Klein: I have studies three or four cell lines obtained from you; all were negative.

Dr. Nelson: An increasing amount of evidence from studies of both human myeloma and macroglobulinaemia and mouse myeloma shows that a high proportion of the monoclonal proteins produced have antibody activity, for example, immunological specificity for dinitrophenol (DNP). Dr. Klein, has IgM on the cell membrane of your cloned cell line any antibody-like activity?

Dr. E. Klein: I have tested one cell line (Daudi) for binding of DNP but It did not show a higher reactivity than lines which do not have surface IgM. Obviously, the first thing I thought of was antibody activity of the surface IgM against EB virus. However, these Daudi cells can be infected with EBV, just as Raji cells can, so it is very improbable that the surface IgM has antibody directed against EBV. I dont' know about other antigens—so far we have only negative evidence about antibody activity.

Dr. Epstein: May I ask the immunologists how immunoglobulins are released from cells? I am particularly interested in Burkitt cells which have very little endoplasmic reticulum and abundant free ribosomes. Presumably a large amount of new protein is being made by these ribosomes; this has been demonstrated very beautifully in the preceding papers. If this is the case, is it known how this large molecule of protein gets out of the cell?

Dr. E. Klein: This is the question we are facing. This is why a comparison of our surface immunoglobulin cell line with immunoglobulin-secreting cell lines is a good problem for study.

Dr. Nelson: Isn't it true that mouse myeloma cells secreting macroglobulins show a rather long lag between synthesis of immunoglobulin chains and either assembly or release? Could this be blocked in your cells?

DR. E. KLEIN: Yes. The lag period between the synthesis of protein chains and secretion is probably the time when the sugar components are put on. I can't tell you, but I hope to find out whether the sugar component is put on this protein molecule.

IMMUNO-ELECTRON MICROSCOPY STUDY

Chairmen:

David S. Nelson, Yorio Hinuma

Characterization of Antibodies Emerging in Epsein-Barr Virus-associated Disease by Immuno-electron Microscopy

Ikuo Suzuki, and Munemitsu Hoshino

Laboratory of Ultrastructure Research, Aichi Cancer Center Research Institute, Nagoya, Japan

Burkitt's lymphoma has attracted the interest of many oncologists, because of its possible viral etiology. The fact that herpes-like virus particles (Epstein-Barr virus: EBV) were found in most culture cell lines established from the tumor tissues is now well known (5). Furthermore, various serological surveys, including immunofluorescence, detected a high titer of serum antibody reactive with Burkitt's lymphoma cells in most patients suffering from this malignancy (9, 13, 24). These serological tests, however, did not allow any definite conclusion as to whether the serum antibody thus found was really directed against virus particles (EBV) detectable in Burkitt's lymphoma cultures, or was directed against cellular antigens other than the structural antigen of the virus.

On the other hand, Old and his associates (24) were the first to report that the high antibody reactivity directed against antigen in Burkitt's lymphoma cells (P3J) was associated with nasopharyngeal cancer (NPC) in a very high incidence. The authors suggested also a possible viral etiology of this neoplasm and its close relationship to Burkitt's lymphoma. These facts encourage the search for virus similar to that found in Burkitt's lymphoma cell lines. Indirect immunofluorescence tests have also detected a frequent occurrence of antibody reactive against Burkitt's lymphoma (anti-EBV) in nasopharyngeal cancer sera of Africa and North America (9). The observation on the high incidence of this malignancy among Chinese people, along with the high titer of serum antibody directed against Burkitt's lymphoma cells (10, 12, 22), has caused renewed interest in the etiology of this disease. Recently, herpes-like virus particles very similar to EBV have been detected by electron microscopy in lymphoblastoid cells established during the culture of tumor tissue from nasopharyngeal cancer (28).

Considering the electron microscopic and serological studies on Burkitt's lymphoma cells and the discrepancy between the rather high percentage of immunofluorescence positive cells, which often amount to 30%, and the very low incidence of

489

cells having morphologicaly demonstrable virus particles (EBV), which are usually detectable in less than 1% of the observed cells, raised a question about the correlation of these different parameters.   Besides, these serological and electron microscopic findings raised an important question as to the relationship between these two clinically and histopathologically distinct diseases: Burkitt's lymphoma (BL) and nasopharyngeal carcinoma (NPC).   De Schryver *et al.* (*26*) revealed the multiple nature of anti-EBV in Burkitt's lymphoma and nasopharyngeal cancer sera; some of the antibody population was directed against EBV itself.   It is particularly noteworthy that they have demonstrated the crossreactivity of anti-EBV antibodies contained in Burkitt's lymphoma and nasopharyngeal cancer sera, suggesting their common etiology.

The present study has attempted to explore some facets of the etiology of Burkitt's lymphoma and the relationship between Burkitt's lymphoma and nasopharyngeal cancer by elucidating the nature of the EBV-related antigen in the cells of Burkitt's lymphoma origin which react with the so-called anti-EBV antibody emerging in the sera of patients with Burkitt's lymphoma and nasopharyngeal cancer, using the peroxidase conjugated antibody method with electron microscope.

MATERIALS AND METHODS

1)   Serum

Four serum specimens with high anti-EBV titers were selected from African patients with Burkitt's lymphoma: Mutua, Kenya Cancer Council (KCC) No. 454, Nakamicha, KCC No. 856; Opasa, KCC No. 766; and Isaac, KCC No. 788. Nine serum specimens with high anti-EBV titers were also selected from eight Chinese patients with a diagnosis of nasopharyngeal carcinoma (Exps. No. 106, 111, 119, 120, 201, 202, 203, and 204) and one with a diagnosis of lymphosarcoma (Exp. No. 108). In addition to these cases, one serum specimen with a high anti-EBV titer from an African patient with nasopharyngeal carcinoma, Apondy, was also examined. Their anti-EBV titer measured by indirect immunofluorescence was $640 \times$ to $2560 \times$ (*12*).

2)   Target cell

A Burkitt's lymphoma culture line, P3HR-1, which has been shown to harbor EBV and to be immunofluorescence positive, was used for test cells throughout the experiment.   A suspension culture was maintained in stationary flasks.   The medium used for culture was RPMI-1640 (*21*) supplemented by 10% calf serum and antibiotics (penicillin and streptomycin).   The cell concentration was maintained at 5 to 15×10^5/ml by the daily addition of fresh medium.   Only cultures exceeding 95% in viability as judged by the trypan blue exclusion test were employed.   As a control, several lymphoid cell lines of human origin, including the Raji line derived from the tissue of Burkitt's lymphoma, were used.   The maintainence conditions for these cell lines were similar to those for the P3HR-1 line.   Table 1 shows the cell lines used in this experiment.

TABLE 1. Culture Lines Used for Immuno-electron Microscopic Studies

Cell line	Diagnosis of donor	Source of tissue
P3HR-1	Burkitt's lymphoma	tumor tissue
Raji	Burkitt's lymphoma	tumor tissue
RPMI 4666	Chronic myelogen leukemia	peripheral leucocytes
RPMI 8335	Chronic myelogen leukemia	peripheral leucocytes
RPMI 8226	Multiple myeloma	peripheral leucocytes
RPMI 3236	Hodgkin's disease	peripheral leucocytes
RPMI 41	Osteosarcoma	peripheral leucocytes

3) Electron microscopic immunocytochemistry
a) Conjugation of antibody with peroxidase—The antibody IgG fraction separated from patients sera was coupled to horseradish peroxidase (C.F. Boehringer and Sohne, Germany) according the method of Avrameas (*1*).   40 mg of γ-globulin from each patient's serum, dissolved in 3 ml of 0.1 M phosphate buffer, pH 7.0, was mixed with 40 mg of peroxidase.   Then, 0.1 ml of 1% glutaraldehyde solution was added to the mixture.   The reaction was continued at room temperature for 2 hr with gentle stirring.   Enzyme conjugated antibody and unreacted antibody were separated from unreacted peroxidase by 50% saturation with ammonium sulfate.   The ammonium sulfate was removed by dialysis.

b) Electron microscopy—The procedure for staining and electron microscopic observation principally followed the method of Nakane and Pierce (*23*).   Fixation of cell sediment was carried out at 4°C for 30 min using a mixture of 2.0% paraformaldehyde and 2.5% glutaraldehyde in 0.05 M phosphate buffer, pH 7.2, instead of glutaral dehyde alone, since it was confirmed that the antigenicity in glutaraldehyde-fixed cells reduced the reactivity with peroxidase-conjugated antibody.   Fixed cell sediment was washed overnight at 4°C with several exchanges of phosphate buffer containing 4.5% surcose (washing solution).   For the reaction of the direct method, fixed cell sediment was exposed to peroxidase-conjugated antibody at a concentration of about 0.7 mg/ml at 4°C for 8 to 12 hr.   For the reaction of the direct method, the cell sediment was exposed to unconjugated patient serum at 4°C for 8 to 12 hr and was washed with washing solution for 8 to 12 hr at 4°C, then was exposed to peroxidase conjugated goat anti-human IgG serum at 4°C for 8 to 12 hr.   The cell sediments for both the direct and indirect methods were washed overnight at 4°C in the washing solution, then fixed again with a mixture of paraformaldehyde and glutaraldehyde for 2 hr to assure firm binding.   The fixative was washed off with the buffer overnight and the cells were placed in Karnovsky's solution (*7*) without peroxide at room temperature for 30 min, then in complete Karnovsky's solution (*7*) at room temperature for 20 to 30 min.   The cell sediment was washed three times with distilled water for 30 min respectively, and was finally fixed in 2% OsO_4 in phosphate buffer for 1 hr, dehydrated, and embedded in Epon (*19*).   This sections, cut on an LKB Ultratome at a thickness of 500 to 600 Å, were examined under the electron microscope with or without uranyl acetate and lead citrate double staining (*25*).

In the experiment for detection of the antigenicity of EBV itself, two procedures, that is, fixation with the mixture of paraformaldehyde and glutaraldehyde and omission of fixation with those, were both performed.

Control experiments were carried out from three sides; that is, from the antigenic side, from the antibody side and from the side of the cytochemical process. The details are given in the following section.

OBSERVATION

The reaction products resulting from the antigen-antibody complex within the cells were precipitated as electron dense regions at the site of the antigen in the cell. The percentage of positive cells differed from one serum to another, and good parallels with the results of the immunofluorescence test (11) were found. Essentially, no difference was observed in the results by the direct and indirect peroxidase-conjugated antibody methods in the present system; furthermore, no difference was found between the results obtained from the sera of patients with Burkitt's lymphoma and nasopharyngeal cancer ruling out several specific cases. From the result of experiments using the sera of patients with Burkitt's lymphoma, nasopharyngeal cancer, and healthy donors, the staining patterns were classified as follows:

1. cytoplasmic pattern
2. nuclear pattern

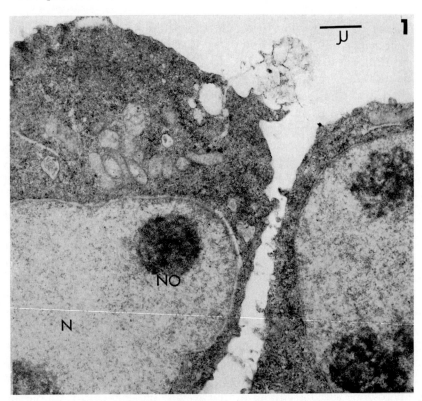

Fig. 1. Two parts of P3HR-1 cells reacted with Burkitt's lymphoma serum (peroxidase conjugated γ-globulin from Nakamicha's serum). Positive reaction was diffusely noted in cytoplasm, especially cytoplasmic polysomes, and nucleolus. Fixation with glutaraldehyde and paraformaldehyde. No electron staining. ×11,000.

3.   pattern of plasma membrane
4.   EBV particle.

1) Cytoplasm

The positive reaction usually appeared in the cytoplasm of about 10–30% of P3HR-1 cells in experiments with almost all test sera.   The distribution patterns of the reaction product in the cytoplasm were further classified as to two types, one was the diffuse type and the other was mainly positive in the protein synthesizing organelles, such as the endoplasmic reticulum, nuclear envelope, and free cytoplasmic polysomes.   These two staining types frequently co-existed in one cell.   Figure 1 shows an electron micrograph of a positive cell which was reacted with Nakamicha's serum (BL).   In this case, the positive reaction was diffusely distributed over the whole cytoplasm, especially the cytoplasmic free ribosomes.   As shown in Fig. 2, a positive reaction on various cell organelles, especially protein synthesizing organelles such as the endoplasmic reticulum, nuclear envelope, ribosomes lining the endoplasmic reticulum, and free cytoplasmic polysomes, was observed as the most com-

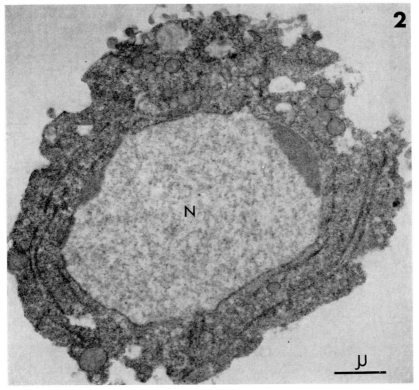

FIG. 2. A P3HR-1 cell reacted with peroxidase conjugated serum (Nakamicha).   Note the positive reaction in the cytoplasmic organelles (endoplasmic reticulum and cytoplasmic polysomes).   Negativity of the nucleus is obvious when compared with the electron dense cytoplasm.   Fixation with glutaraldehyde and paraformaldehyde.   No electron staining. × 14,000.

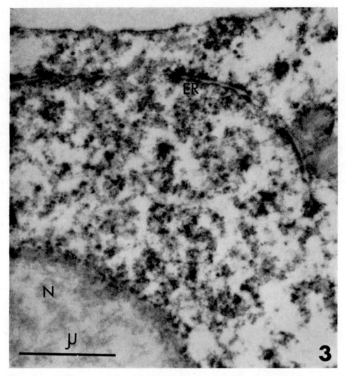

Fig. 3. A electron micrograph of large magnification showing a part of a P3HR-1 cell reacted with peroxidase-conjugated serum (nasopharyngeal cancer, Exp. No. 120). Reaction products of peroxidase-conjugates are clearly observed on the endoplasmic reticulum, cytoplasmic polysomes, and plasma membrane. Fixation with glutaraldehyde and paraformaldehyde. No electron staining. × 26,000.

mon pattern. It was noted that without electron staining with uranium and lead, the electron-dense precipitates arising from the peroxidase reaction were clearly shown, whereas other osmiophilic granules were completely invisible. Reactivity in cytoplasm with conjugates was detected in almost all sera tested from patients with both Burkitt's lymphoma and nasopharyngeal cancer. Figure 3 shows a large magnification electron micrograph of P3HR-1 cells reacted with conjugated serum from a patient with nasopharyngeal cancer (Exp. No. 120).

2) Nucleus

With the sera from both Burkitt's lymphoma and nasopharyngeal cancer, various nuclear regions of P3HR-1 cells were observed as the positive sites. Four different positive sites associated with the nucleus were classified in the nuclei of P3HR-1 cells. As shown in Fig 4, the whole nucleus of the P3HR-1 cell on the left side was strongly positive with conjugated Nakamicha's serum. On the other hand, a P3HR-1 cell on the right side showed a positive reaction primarily in the cytoplasm, and a degenerative cell in the upper part also showed a positive reaction in the nucleus. Actually, the staining patterns of these two intact cells were representative. Cells reacted with conjugates and unreacted cells were usually observed side by side.

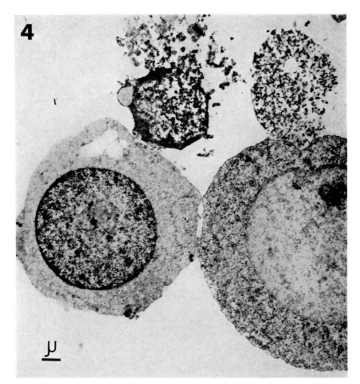

Fig. 4. A electron micrograph showing P3HR-1 cells reacted with peroxidase conjugated Nakamicha's serum. A strongly positive reaction was observed in the whole nucleus of a cell shown on the left side. In a cell shown on the right side, a positive reaction is seen on the cytoplasmic polysomes and nucleolus, and, conversely, the nucleus is obviously negative. A degenerative cell in the upper part shows a positive reaction in the nucleus, especially the chromatin. Fixation with glutaraldehyde and paraformaldehyde. No electron staining. × 4,800.

Although cytoplasmic staining was more frequently encountered, nuclear reaction was not rare with the same conjugates, and the ratio of cytoplasmic and nuclear staining seemed to vary from one harevst to another in the same culture stock.

The staining pattern of the whole nucleus was closely similar to that of the anti-nuclear antibody which appeared in the serum of a patient with systemic lupus erythematosus (20). The second staining pattern of the nucleus was observed in the nuclear chromatin of a P3HR-1 cell reacted with the serum of an African patient (Apondy) with nasopharyngeal cancer. As shown in Fig. 5, the perinuclear chromatin was obviously stained with conjugated Apondy serum. This serum contains an antibody highly reactive with nuclear components along with antibody directed against the cytoplasm. In the metaphase stage of P3HR-1, not only chromatin, but also virus like particles which were irregularly distributed in the metaphase chromatin structure, were stained. A similar pattern was observed in the interphase nucleus of P3HR-1 cells reacted with the conjugated serum from a Chinese patient with nasopharyngeal cancer, serum Exp. No. 108. As shown in Fig. 6, in addition to the positive reaction of the cytoplasm, particles regularly arranged in the perinu-

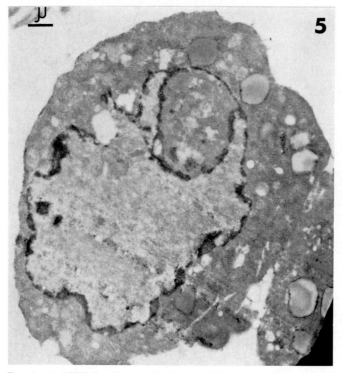

Fig. 5.   A P3HR-1 cell reacted with peroxidase conjugated serum (African nasopharyngeal cancer, Apondy).   Strong reactivity is definitely located on the nuclear chromatin.   Fixation with glutaraldehyde and paraformaldehyde.   No electron staining.   × 6,500.

clear chromatin were strongly stained.   By the examination of electron micrographs of higher magnification, they were shown to be spherically shaped inclusions whose size varied from 200 Å to 800 Å (Fig. 7).   The positive reaction in the nucleolus, as shown in Fig. 1, was also frequently encountered accompanying the cytoplasmic diffuse patern.   Except for the positive pattern of the nucleolus, the other two nuclear staining patterns, *i.e.*, whole nucleus and nuclear chromatin, were observed only in limited cases as mentioned above.

3) Plasma membrane

The plasma membrane was one of the representative sites of positive reaction. Reactivity directed against the cell surface membrane was observed in sera including Burkitt's lymphoma, nasopharyngeal cancer, and even in healthy donors.   Figure 8 shows a positive reaction on the plasma membrane of a P3HR-1 cell reacted with serum from a Chinese patient with nasopharyngeal cancer, serum Exp. No. 119; Fig. 9 also shows reactivity on the plasma membrane accompanying a positive pattern of cytoplasmic protein synthesizing organelles in serum from a healthy donor whose serum was known to contain a low titer of so-called anti-EBV antibody, but had immunoadherence reactivity.

In general, the sites of EBV-related cellular antigen revealed by peroxidase

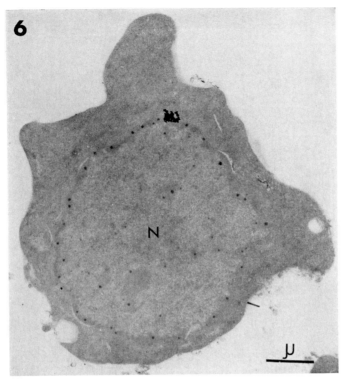

Fig. 6.   A P3HR-1 cell reacted with peroxidase conjugated serum (nasopharyngeal cancer, Exp.. No 108).   The regular arrangement of virus-like particles which are positively stained in the nucleus along the chromatin is noteworthy.   Fixation with glutaraldehyde and para-formaldehyde.   No electron staining.   × 13,000.

conjugated globulin were analogous to those presented by immunofluorescence with FITC conjugates in the experiments using sera of both Burkitt's lymphoma and nasopharyngeal cancer.   Concerning the sera of healthy donors, however, two reactivities, on cytoplasm and plasma membrane, were presented.   Besides, sera showing these two reactivities were observed only in the case in which the serum had immunoadherence reactivity.   Conversely, sera from healthy donors having relatively high titered so-called anti-EBV antibody showed only cytoplasmic positive patterns.

4)   EBV particle
    EBV-like particles were usually very rare in the P3J or its subline cultures pro-pagated in our laboratry and were detected only in less than 1% of cells.   The stainability of the EBV, rarely found in P3HR-1 cells, was not reproducible;   some particles seemed to be stained, but some particles were negative.   Therefore, the isolated virus preparations were used to decide whether the so-called anti-EBV antibody was directed against EBV virion or not.   The virus particles, in a concen-trated preparation, were outlined by a negative staining method (Fig. 10).   The preparation contained 1) enveloped virion, 2) virus capsid with nucleoid but without envelope, 3) capsid without envelope and nucleoid.   The immuno-electron

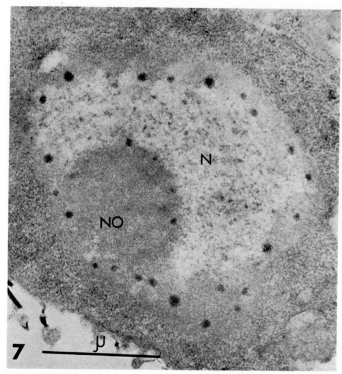

FIG. 7. A large magnification of an electron micrograph showing the same pattern as Fig. 6. The size of the particles varies. It is confirmed that the particles locate in the nucleus along the chromatin and nucleolus. Fixation with glutaraldehyde and paraformaldehyde. No electron staining. × 32,000.

microscopic examination was performed with four selected sera: Nakamicha (Burkitt's lymphoma), Exp. No. 120 (Chinese nasopharyngeal cancer), Apondy (African nasopharyngeal cancer), and healthy donor (the anti-EBV titer was measured as × 40).

In the experiment in which the virus preparation was pretreated with the same fixative used to fix cells throughout the present experiment, EBV particles were definitely unstained by any of the conjugates used. It was noted that the contaminated cell debris, which seemed to have been derived from endoplasmic reticulum and polysome, was positively stained. The succeeding reaction was carried out between an unfixed virus preparation and the conjugates. In the experiment using an unfixed virus preparation, reaction products showing the site of the antigen were observed clearly on the virus envelopes (Figs. 11–13). Figure 11 shows three virus particles coated with electron dense reaction products on their envelopes after reacting with conjugated serum (Nakamicha). Furthermore, it was also clearly observed that three virus particles without envelopes on the opposite side of this figure were definitely negative. Besides, as shown in Fig. 12, the viral capsid and core were definitely not stained, notwithstanding the fact that the surrounding ruptured envelope was strongly stained. Experiments by the indirect method using the same sera gave essentially the same result.

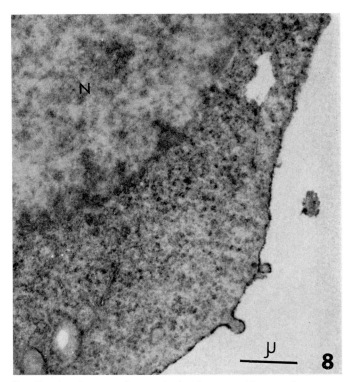

FIG. 8.   An electron micrograph showing a positive reaction on a portion of the plasma membrane of a P3HR-1 cell reacted with peroxidase conjugated serum (nasopharyngeal cancer, Exp. No. 119).   Fixation with glutaraldehyde and paraformaldehyde.   No electron staining.   × 15,000.

5)   Control

a)   As a control on the antigenic side, various lymphoblastoid cells, as indicated in Table 1, were used.   These cells were never stained with any of the conjugated sera used in the present study with the immuno-electron microscopic procedure performed under the same conditions.   Figure 14 shows a cell of an EBV-free Burkitt's lymphoma line, Raji, after reacting with conjugated Nakamicha's serum without lead or uranium staining.   The general ultrastructure of the cell remained unclear.

b)   In reference to the specificity of test sera, two experiments were performed. P3HR-1 cells treated with peroxidase-conjugated rabbit or goat globulin, and P3HR-1 cells pretreated with unconjugated test sera, then treated with conjugated sera, were both definitely negative.

c)   As a control for cytochemical specificity, two experiments were also carried out.   Complete cytochemical procedure was applied to untreated P3HR-1 cells in order to detect the endogenous peroxidase, and no reactivity was detected.   P3HR-1 cells reacted with conjugated test sera were treated without 3-3′-diaminobenzidine in the course of the cytochemical process, and no reaction products were observed.

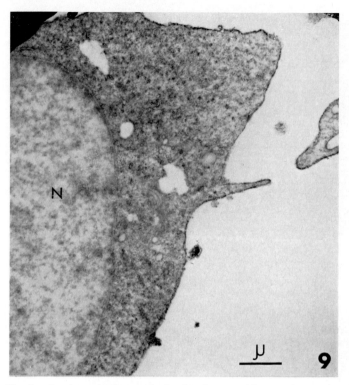

FIG. 9.   An electron micrograph also showing a positive reaction on the plasma membrane of a P3HR-1 cell treated with peroxidase conjugated serum from a healthy donor.   Fixation with glutaraldehyde and paraformaldehyde. No electron staining.   × 11,000.

DISCUSSION

The results of this investigation showed the ultrastructural sites of EB virus related antigen in the cells of the P3HR-1 line which has been known as an abundant EB virus containing cell line.   Various sites of the P3HR-1 cell, such as the whole nucleus, nucleolus, nuclear chromatin, virus-like particles in the perinuclear chromatin, whole cytoplasm, cytoplasmic polysomes, plasma membrane, and virus envelope, were stained positively with various sera from patients with Burkitt's lymphoma and patients with nasopharyngeal cancer.

Reactivity in the whole nucleus was observed in the reaction with the serum of Burkitt's lymphoma.   The patterns of positive reaction in the whole nucleus were very similar to those of the anti-nuclear antibody which appeared in the serum of systemic lupus erythematosus, which is known as auto-immune disease (20).   The occurrence of anti-nuclear antibody in the sera of patients with nasopharyngeal cancer has been reported as having been detected by immunofluorescence (30).   The positive pattern of the whole nucleus present in the P3HR-1 cell with the serum of Burkitt's lymphoma seems to be the same phenomenon as that shown by immunofluorescence in the sera of nasopharyngeal cancer.   Nevertheless, although the

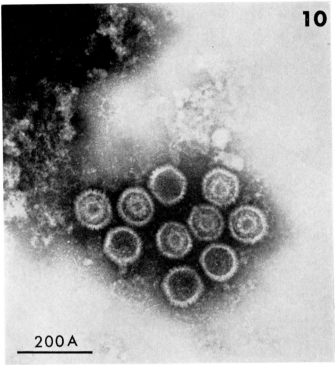

FIG. 10.   An electron micrograph of negatively stained virus particles isolated from P3HR-1 cells.   Virus particles of different appearance are seen.   × 100,000.

meaning of this is not clear at present the analogy between these two distinct diseases seems to be significant.   Concerning this pattern, the positivity in the nuclear chromatin with the serum of an African nasopharyngeal cancer patient, Apondy, may be supposed to represent one kind of anti-nuclear antibody.

The reactivity on the plasma membrane of P3HR-1 cells was clearly observed in the reaction with the sera of not only Burkitt's lymphoma patients and nasopharyngeal cancer patients but also healthy donors.   This reactivity on the surface membrane of P3HR-1 demonstrates by the peroxidase conjugated antibody method was thought to coincide with the membrane immunofluorescence which was revealed by Klein et al. (14).   Klein et al. (16) reported that the membrane immunofluorescence of cultured Burkitt's lymphoma cells depended on the presence of EB virus, but that there was no constant relationship between the number of cells containing virus and the number of cells showing membrane fluorescence.   In addition, they reported that approximately 10 times more cells showed membrane fluorescence than contained EB virus antigen.   The results presented here also show that the membrane fluorescence depends on the presence of EB virus, because the control cell lines, including the Raji line which was derived from the biopsy material of Burkitt's lymphoma but did not contain virus particle, showed no reactivity.   However, the percentage of cells showing a positive reaction on the plasma membrane did not coincide with the percentage of cells containing the EB virus antigen, but

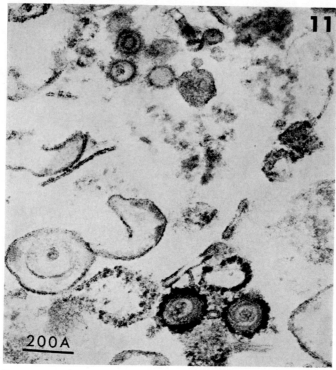

F<small>IG</small>. 11.   Virus particles treated with peroxidase-conjugated serum (Nakamicha).   Strongly positive reaction products are definitely observed on the surface of virus envelopes.   No reactivity was seen on the virus particles without envelopes on the opposite side.   No fixation with glutaraldehyde and paraformaldehyde.   No electron staining.   ×70,000.

rather depended on the serum.   The cells containing demonstrable EB virus particles were less than 1% among the total population of the P3HR-1 line propagated in our laboratory at the time of sampling, and the percentage of cell showing a positive reaction on the plasma membrane was obviously greater than 10% of the total population, varying with the sera used.   Furthermore, the reactivity on the plasma membrane was always accompanied by the reactivity of the cytoplasm, notwithstanding the reactivity of the cytoplasm was not always accompanied with surface positivity.   The serum from a healthy donor, having a low titer of the so-called anti-EBV antibody, ×40, but having immuneadherence reactivity, clearly showed a positive reaction on the membrane of P3HR-1 cells.   In contrast with this serum, sera from healthy individuals having a high titer of anti-EBV antibody measured by indirect immunofluorescence, but no immuneadherence, reactivity showed no reactivity on the plasma membrane of P3HR-1 cells.   Klein *et al.* also reported that sera from 12 healthy Swedish blood donors did not react with cells from Burkitt's lymphoma biopsy specimens in membrane immunofluorescence (*15*).   The discrepancy between the results might be accounted for by the cell type used, namely, fresh tumor cells and cells from culture, and a difference in the serum from the healthy donors used.   The results of our investigation showed that 1) surface antigen was presented only in EB-virus containing cells, but no correlation was observed bet-

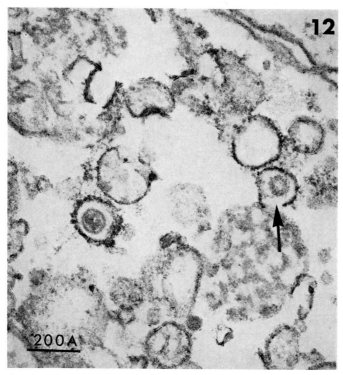

FIG. 12. Virus particle with ruptured envelope (arrow). The reaction products located only on the virus envelope, even in the virion with a partially ruptured envelope. No fixation and no electron staining. × 70,000.

ween the percentage of demonstrable virus particle containing cells and surface antigen containing cells, 2) antibody directed against surface antigen was detected in test sera from patients with Burkitt's lymphoma and masopharyngeal cancer, and even in sera from healthy individuals, but in sera from healthy individuals, the antibody directed against surface antigen was detected in only limited cases, 3) surface antigen detected by the peroxidase conjugated antibody method was always accompanied by cellular antigen detected by the same method. These results were mainly in agreement with the report of Dunkel and Ziegel (4).

The cytoplasmic pattern of reactivity was thought, in the main, to correspond to positive immunofluorescence by light microscopy. In this pattern, the main reactive site was always cytoplasmic polysomes. This might mean that the reaction products on the polysomes were not produced by the reaction with the between polysomes themselves and conjugates, but between nascent proteins synthesized on polysomes and conjugates. It has been reported that the antibody produced on polysomes in lymphocytes was stained with peroxidase conjugate after hyperimmunization (2, 3, 17). The staining pattern in both cases was closely similar, and furthermore, the cytoplasmic diffuse pattern of positivity in the present experiment was also analogous to the localization of antibody in lymphocytes (3, 17). On the other hand, the staining pattern of cytoplasm in the present experiment is also analogous to that of neoantigen in an other system studied by the same method (18,

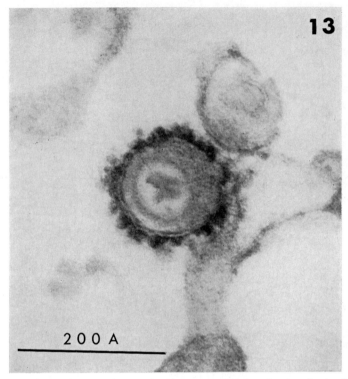

Fig. 13.   A electron micrograph of large magnification showing the details of the reactive site on an EB virion.   The virus capsid and core are both clearly negative.   × 200,000.

29).   It assumes that if these nascent polypeptides on polysomes are viral antigen and a disturbance of the particle assembly mechanism occurs, the demonstrable virus particles ought to be stained also with peroxidase-conjugates.   Therefore, it is natural to suppose that the nascent polypeptides on the polysome differ from viral antigen.   From these points of view, the reactivity on polysomes represents the neoantigen (T antigen) which generally appears in viral infection or viral transformation.   Furthermore, it was also supposed that the cytoplasmic diffuse pattern of reactivity represented the pooled neoantigen detached from cytoplasmic polysomes.

It was revealed that three antibodies, anti-nuclear antibody, antibody directed against surface antigen, and antibody directed against neoantigen, were contained in the sera of patients with both Burkitt's lymphoma and nasopharyngeal cancer. Some parts of the antibodies directed against these antigens are contained in the serum of healthy individuals.

The most important purpose of the present experiments were, however, to obtain direct evidence as to whether the serological reactivity in patient serum is specific for EB virus antigen, notably a morphologically demonstrable virus.   Electron microscopically demonstrable virus particles in P3HR-1, as mentioned above, did not show reactivity by peroxidase-conjugated method.   It was suspected that the result was presumably caused by the infrequency of virus particles in P3HR-1

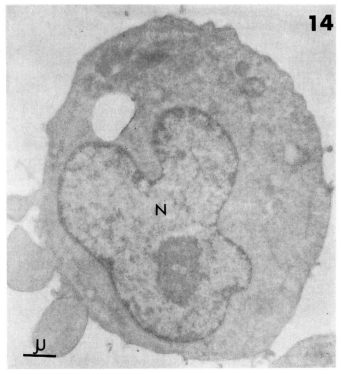

FIG. 14. An EBV-free Burkitt's lymphoma cell, Raji, reacted with peroxidase-conjugated serum (Nakamicha). No electron dense reaction precipitate is observed. Fixation with glutaraldehyde and paraformaldehyde. No electron staining. × 8,400.

cells propagated in our laboratory, and consequently by the difficulty of suitable fixation in an immuno-cytochemical reaction. This disadvantage was removed by the use of isolated EB virus preparation instead of P3HR-1 cells. Experiment using a virus preparation with the same procedure as used at the cell level, however, did not show any positive reaction with the EB virion, although contaminating cell debris, such as endoplasmic reticulum and polysomes, was stained positively, presumably indicating neoantigen. Repeated experiments were carried out using unfixed virus preparation. A positive reaction was definitely observed on the envelope of the EB virus. The experiments were performed using several sera, such as serum from a patient with Burkitt's lymphoma, Nakamicha; serum from a patient with nasopharyngeal cancer, Exp. No. 120; sera from two healthy donors, one having a low anti-EBV titer but a high immuno-adherence reactivity and the other having both low anti-EBV titer and a low level of immuneaherence reactivity. The reaction precipitates on the envelope were only observed in the sera from Burkitt's lymphoma and nasopharyngeal cancer, and the two sera from healthy donors brought a definitely negative result. Both direct and indirect peroxidase conjugated antibody methods were applied in the experiment, and the same results were confirmed.

The results indicated that the so-called anti-EBV antibody in patients sera contained antibody directed against the envelope of the EB virus and did not contain antibody directed against the viral capsid or core.

So far, the direct proof as to whether the antibody emerging in the sera of patients with Burkitt's lymphoma and nasopharyngeal cancer was directed against the EB virion has not yet been developed.

Virus particles are detectable only by electron microscopy, and furthermore, immuno-electron microscopic methods, such as immunoferritin and immuno-peroxidase techniques, would presumably be able to reveal the direct relationship between a morphologically evident virus and serological specificity. Comparing these two methods, the immunoferritin method was thought to be difficult to use in detecting the intracellular antigen, because ferritin-conjugated antibody has a large molecular weight, and therefore, it is very difficult for it to penetrate into the cell. It was thought, however, that the immunoferritin method would be excellent for the detection of surface antigen.

Sugawara and Osato (27) reported the direct correlation between the EB virion and γ-globulin of patient serum by the immunoferritin technique. They mentioned that specific ferritin tagging was clearly evident not only with the EB virus particles but also in the nuclear matrix and on the surface membrane of the virus containing cell.

Hampar et al. (8) have also reported on the relationship between the EB virion and the so-called anti-EBV antibody, carrying out a parallel examination using herpes simplex virus (HSV), rabbit anti-EBV hyperimmune serum and rabbit anti-HSV hyperimmune serum. They showed that the ferritin tagging of the EBV capsid, reacted with conjugated human EBV-positive globulins following the reaction of the cells with unconjugated rabbit anti-EBV hyperimmune serum, was present on the antibody coat rather than on the capsid membrane. They concluded that EBV and HSV did not share a common or cross-reacting capsid surface antigen. In their experiment, cell preparations contained too few enveloped particles to permit determination as to whether these sera also contained antibodies against EBV envelope antigens. Comparing the results of our study to that of Sugawara and Osato, both results are analogous, as a whole. A difference was found with reference to the virus particle. On this point, the results presented by Hampar et al. were of interest, because they observed that ferritin tagging was present on the antibody coat surrounding the virus capsid rather than on the capsid membrane. Generally, as mentioned above, the cells used in the immunoferritin technique had to be partially ruptured in order to permit the conjugates to enter. The difference between the present study and studies carried out by both of those groups presumably was caused by a difference in techniques. On the other hand, Gerber and Goldstein (6) reported that surface antigens on EBV-transformed lymphoid cell and on cultured Burkitt's lymphoma cells were closely related or identical, and that antibodies reacting with these membrane antigens were specific for the EBV envelope. They suggested, therefore, that these membrane antigens shared components with the viral envelope material. Furthermore, they mentioned that EBV capsid specific anti-serum failed to react in the indirect membrane immunofluorescence test, did not block the direct membrane immunofluorescence, and had no detectable EBV neutralizing antibodies directed against envelope and capsid.

With respect to the identification of the antigenicity of the envelope and surface antigens on the plasma membrane in our study, antibody directed against the plasma membrane of EBV infected cells was observed not only in patient sera but also in sera from healthy donors, and conversely, antibody directed against the virus envelope was detected only in patients sera.   This fact strongly suggests that these two antigens, *i.e.* surface antigen and EBV envelope antigen, are distinct.

It was concluded from the present study that,
1)   So-called anti-EBV antibody emerging in sera of patients with malignant tumors, such as Burkitt's lymphoma and nasopharyngeal cancer, and even in the sera of healthy individuals, contains polyvalent antibodies,
2)   Burkitt's lymphoma and nasopharyngeal cancer are closely related or identical serologically by the immunoperoxidase electron microscopic method, and
3)   The most significant difference in the so-called anti-EBV antibody in the sera of patients with Burkitt's lymphoma or nasopharyngeal cancer and in healthy individuals was the evidence that the anti-EBV envelope antibody exists only in the former.

We are greatly indebted to Dr. M. Takahashi, Department of Molecular Immunology, Cancer Institute, Kanazawa University, Kanazawa, Japan, and Dr. T. Takahashi, Laboratory of Biochemistry, Aichi Cancer Center Research Institute, Nagoya, Japan, for their continued advice and help during this study.   We are also indebted to Dr. Nishioka, National Cancer Inst., Tokyo, Japan, for his continued interest and for sending the sera of Burkitt's lymphoma patients, kindly supplied through Dr. G. Klein, Karolinska Inst., Sweden; to Dr. Kawamura, University of Tokyo, Tokyo, Japan, for sending the sera of nasopharyngeal cancer patients, kindly supplied through Dr. Hi-chin, National Taiwan University, Taiwan, China ; to Dr. Hinuma, Tohoku University, Sendai, Japan for sending the cells of the P3HR-1 line ; and to Dr. Ito, Aichi Cancer Center Research Institute, Nagoya, Japan, for sending the EB virus preparation which was supplied through SCVP, U.S.A.

We gratefully acknowledge the excellent techniqal assistance by Miss S. Suno, and Miss T. Yamaguchi.

This work was partly supported by a grant from the Ministry of Education, Government of Japan.

REFERENCES

1.   Avrameas, S.   Coupling of Enzymes to Proteins with Glutaraldehyde.   Use of the Conjugates for the Detection of Antigens and Antibodies.   Immunochemistry, *6*: 43, 1969.
2.   Avrameas, S., and Bouteille, M.   Ultrastructural Localization of Antibody by Antigen Label with Peroxidase.   Exptl. Cell Res., *53*: 166, 1968.
3.   Avrameas, S., and Leduc, E. H.   Detection of Simultaneous Antibody Synthesis in Plasma Cells and Specialiled Lymphocytes in Rabbit Lymph Nodes.   J. Exptl. Med., *131*: 1137, 1970.
4.   Dunkel, V., and Zeigel, R.   Studies on the Relation of Membrane Immunofluorescence to Epstein-Barr Virus Infection.   J. Nat. Cancer Inst., *44*: 133, 1970.

5. Epstein, M. A., Achong, B. G., and Barr, Y. M.   Virus Particles in Cultured Lymphoblasts from Burkitt's Lymphoma.   Lancet, *1*: 702, 1964.

6. Gerber, P., and Goldstein, G.   Relationship of Epstein Barr Virus-induced Membrane Antigens in Lymphoid Cells to Viral Envelope Antigens.   J. Immunol., *105*: 793, 1970.

7. Graham, R. C., and Karnovsky, M. J.   The Early Stages of Injected Horseradish Peroxidase in the Proximal Tubules of Mouse Kidney: Ultrastructural Cytochemistry by a New Technique.   J. Histochem. Cytochem., *14*: 291, 1965.

8. Hampar, B., Gerber, P., Hsu, K.-C., Martos, L. M., Walker, J. L., Sigüenza, R. F., and Wells, G. A.   Immunoferritin and Immunofluorescent Studies with Epstein-Barr Virus and Herpes Simplex Virus by Use of Human Sera and Hyperimmune Rabbit Sera.   J. Nat. Cancer Inst., *45*: 75, 1970.

9. Henle, G., Henle, W., and Diehl, V.   Relation of Burkitt's Tumor-associated Herpes-type Virus to Infectious Mononucleosis.   Proc. Nat. Acad. Sci. U.S.A., *59*: 94, 1968.

10. Ito, Y., Takahashi, T., Kawamura, A., Jr., and Tu, S.-M.   High Anti-EB Virus Titer in Sera of Patients with Nasopharyngeal Carcinoma: A Small Scaled Seroepidemiological Study.   GANN, *60*: 335, 1969.

11. Kawamura, A., Hamajima, K., Murata, M., Goto, A., Takada, M., Nishioka, K., Hirayama, T., Yoshida, T., Yang, C., Wang, C.-S., Tu, S.-M., Liu, C.-H., and Lin, T.-M. Studies on Nasopharyngeal Carcinoma and Burkitt Lymphoma by Immunofluorescence. Anal. N.Y. Acad. Sci., in press.

12. Kawamura, A., Jr., Goto, A., Takada, M., Hamajima, K., Sanpe, T., Murata, M., Ito, Y., Yoshida, T. O., Takahashi, T., Hirayama, T., Tu, S.-M., Liu, C.-T., Yang, C.-S., and Wang, C.-H.   Seroepidemiological Studies on Nasopharyngeal Carcinoma by Fluorescence Antibody Techniques with Cultured Burkitt's Lymphoma Cells. GANN: *61*, 55, 1970.

13. Klein, G., Clifford, P., Klein, E., Smith, R. T., Minowada, J., Kourilsky, F. M., and Burchenal, J. H.   Membrane Immunofluorescence Reactions of Burkitt Lymphoma Cells from Biopsy Specimens and Tissue Cultures. J. Nat. Cancer Inst., *39*: 1024, 1967.

14. Klein, G., Clifford, P., Klein, E., and Stjernsward, J.   Search for Tumor-specific Immune Reactions in Burkitt Lymphoma Patients by the Membrane Immunofluorescence Reaction.   Proc. Nat. Acad. Sci. U.S.A., *55*: 1628, 1966.

15. Klein, G., Clifford, P., Klein, E., and Stjernsward, J.   Search for Tumor Specific Immune Reactions in Burkitt Lymphoma Patients by the Membrane Immunofluorescence Reactions, *In* " Treatment of Burkitt's Tumour ", p. 209, (UICC Monograph, vol. 8) J. H. Burchenal and D. P. Burkitt eds., Springer-verlag Berlin Heidelberg, 1967.

16. Klein, G., Henle, G., and Henle, W.   Relation between Epstein-Barr Viral and Cell Membrane Immunofluorescence of Burkitt Tumour Cells.   I. Dependence of Cell Membrane Immunofluorescence on Presence of EB Virus.   J. Exp. Med., *128*: 1011, 1968.

17. Leduc, E. H., Scott, G. B., and Avrameas, S.   Ultrastructural Localization of Intracellular Immune Globulins in Plasma Cells and Lymphoblasts by Enzyme-labeled Antibodies.   J. Histochem. Cytochem., *17*: 211, 1969.

18. Leduc, E., Wicker, R., and Avrameas, S.   Ultrastructural Localization of S.V40 T Antigen with Enzyme-labelled Antibody.   J. Gen. Virology, *4*: 609, 1969.

19. Luft, J. H.   Improvements in Epoxy Resin Embedding Methods.   J. Biophys. Biochem. Dytol., *9*: 409, 1961.

20. Machida, M., and Hoshino, M.   The Ultrastructural Localization of Antigens in

Ehrlich Ascites Tumor Cells against Antinuclear Factors in Lupus Erythematosus Sera by Peroxidase-labelled Antibody Method. Experientia, *27*: 201, 1971.

21. Moore, G. E., Gerner, R. E., and Franklin, H. A. Culture of Normal Human Leukocytes. J. A. M. A., *199*: 519, 1967.

22. Muir, C. S., and Shaumgaratnam, K. The Incidence of Nasopharyngeal Cancer in Singapore, *In* " Cancer of Nasopharynx," pp. 47, (UICC Monograph, vol. 1) C. S. Muir and Shaumgaratnam eds., Munksgaard, Copenhagen, 1967.

23. Nakane, P. K., and Pierce, G. B., Jr. Enzyme-labeled Antibodies for the Light and Electron Microscopic Localization of Tissue Antigens. J. Cell Biol., *33*: 307, 1967.

24. Old, L. J., Boyse, E. A., Oettgen, H. F., de Harven, E., Geering, G., Williamson, B., and Clifford, P. Precipitating Antibody in Human Serum to an Antigen Present in Cultured Burkitt's Lymphoma Cells. Proc. Nat. Acad. Sci. U.S.A., *56*: 1699, 1966.

25. Sato, T. A Modified Method for Lead Staining of Thin Sections. J. Electron Microsc., *16*: 193, 1967.

26. de Schryver, A., Friberg, S., Jr., Klein, G., Henle, W., Henle, G., de Thé, G., Clifford, P., and Ho, H.-C. Epstein-Barr Virus (EBV)-associated Antibody Patterns in Carcinoma of the Post-nasal Space. Clin. Exp. Immunol., *5*: 443, 1969.

27. Sugawara, K., and Osato, T. An Immunoferritin Study of a Burkitt Lymphoma Cell Line Harboring EB Virus Particles. GANN, *61*: 279, 1970.

28. de Thé, G., Ambrosioni, J. C., Ho, H.-C., and Kwan, H.-C. Lymphoblastoid Transformation and Presence of Herpes-type Viral Particles in a Chinese Nasopharyngeal Tumour Cultured *in vitro*. Nature, *221*, 770, 1969.

29. Wicker, R., and Avrameas, S. Localization of Virus Antigens by Enzyme-labelled Antibodies. J. Gen. Virology, *4*, 465, 1969.

30. Yoshida, T. O. Anti-nuclear Antibodies in Sera of Nasopharyngeal Cancer Patients. Proceedings of The 1st International Symposium of The Princess Takamatsu Cancer Research Fund, pp. 443. University of Tokyo Press, 1971.

Discussion of Paper by Dr. Suzuki

DR. NELSON: Dr. Suzuki, I understood that you said the antigens you detected were different from EBV antigens, because you got positive staining with your cell lines which were negative for EA, VCA, or membrane antigens. Did you in fact get positive staining, by immunoelectron microscopy, with EBV-negative cell lines?

DR. SUZUKI: We tested the Raji cell line. This is the only cell line we tried and EB virus particles could not be detected.

DR. AOKI: How did you determine the specificity of this method? Did you try blocking tests? For example, in the direct test, did you run a blocking test with unconjugated anti-serum? If you used a different species of serum, was it absorbed with human cells and then reacted with these cells or with another negative control?

DR. SUZUKI: We tried all bolcking tests both from the antigen side and the antibody side. All the blocking controls were negative.

DR. NELSON: The papers and discussions in this session have covered rather a lot of ground and I shall not attempt to summarize everything that has been said. They seem to me to have involved particularly three areas in which much good and exciting work is being done and in which we might expect interesting advances in the near future.

The first is the discovery of immunological markers, other than putatively tumor-specific and/or virus-determined antigens, on lymphoblastoid cell lines. Not only do some cell lines synthesize immunoglobulins, but they may also carry one or more of a variety of receptors for immune complexes.

Second, the immunoglobulin-synthesizing cell lines provide very useful tools for analyzing the synthesis, assembly, and release of human immunoglobulins *in vitro*. It may not be too far-fetched to speculate that some of the lines which synthesize, but do not release, protein with IgM-specificity may represent malignant clones of thymus-derived or T-cells analogous to plasmacytomas which may be viewed as malignant clones of bone marrow-derived or B-cells.

Third, the finding that the sera of some patients with NPC and other malignancies contain antibodies reactive with very widely distributed nuclear constituents is highly intriguing. There is little doubt that many centers will wish to pursue this findings. With the accumulation and analysis of more data the implications, at present speculative, may turn out to be quite far-reaching.

PROBLEMS OF CELL-MEDIATED AND HUMORAL IMMUNITY IN CANCER

Chairmen:

Chester M. Southam, Kusuya Nishioka

Cross-reacting Antibody in Cellular Immunity

Genshichiro Fujii, Shunji Goto, Tetsuro Nishihira, and Yukio Ishibashi

Department of Surgery, Institute of Medical Science, University of Tokyo, Tokyo, Japan

Since immunological reactions which require the participation of living lymphoid cells have been recognized, many workers have been studying the mechanism of cell-mediated immunity. Cell-bound antibody (also called cellular antibody) has been a hypothetical antibody or antibody-like substance(s) which was proposed to explain the refined specificity of delayed hypersensitivity and transplantation reactions. The binding of labeled antigen by lymphocytes from animals (*10*) or humans (*3*) with delayed hypersensitivity suggests the recognition of antigen by antibody-like molecules on the lymphocytes surface. It has been found that gamma globulin antibody in the supernatant of sonically disrupted sensitized lymphoid cells is capable of destroying, in accelerated fashion, skin homografts (*4*), and that 19S antibody extracted from the cellular membrane of sensitized lymphocytes destroys allogeneic target cells in the presence of complement (*8*). These findings support the hypothetical concept of cell-bound " antibody." However there has been little information on the origin and the function of the " antibody."

In 1961, Nelson (*13*) introduced the concepts of immunological cross-reaction and antibody transfer to explain the immunological mechanism functioning in homograft rejection. After an exchange of tissue between individuals of the same species, antibody would be produced with a specificity for the donor antigens but would react also with antigens in the recipient tissues. This would be an expression of an immunochemical cross-reaction of structural groups on molecules possessed by the donor and by the recipient.

After the formation of cross-reacting antibody-antigen complexes on the cell surface, the antibody would recognize the antigens of the donor graft cells and transfer from the cross-reacting antigens on the host's cells, such as lymphocytes, to the donor antigens responsible for immunization.

Many previous studies have indicated a close immunochemical cross-reaction of the antigen isolated from sheep red blood cells (SRBC) and those isolated from tissues of guinea pigs, horses, and other animal species (2, 5).   From the hypothesis described above, it would be anticipated that the exchange of tissue among xenogeneic species possessing Forssman antigens would result in the formation of an antibody which would sensitize certain tissues of the recipient.   It would be expected that this antibody would not appear in the serum under ordinary circumstances. Based on the standpoint described above, immunization and transplantation between various species of animals that share the heterophile Forssman antigens would be a model of allotransplantation immunity.

Fujii and Nelson (7) have reported previously that guinea pig lymph node cells and kidney cells and horse kidney cells cross-reacted with rabbit antibody to SRBC-stromata.   The dissociation of the cross-reacting antibody from a cross-reacting antigen and its preferential reassociation with a more closely related antigen were also observed.

In previous assays for hemolytic antibody produced in guinea pigs following injection with SRBC, no inhibition was observed with Forssman antigen (7).   Fujii et al. (6) could also demonstrate that γ-globulin dissociated from the lymph node cells and platelets of guinea pigs following injection with SRBC was inhibited by Forssman antigen.   These previous results indicate that guinea pigs produce two types of antibodies.   One, in the serum, is predominantly of the " isophile " or non-Forssman-type and the other, bound to the cells, is of the " heterophile " or Forssman-type antibody.   It was also shown that the antibody dissociated from the lymph node cells was sensitive to 0.1 M 2-mercaptoethanol.

Based on these results in the model experiments using a Forssman antigen-antibody system, similar experiments were made to determine cell-bound antibody on the lymph node cells of mice following skin allotransplantation.   The results indicated that γ-globulin dissociated from the sensitized regional lymph node cells possessed cytotoxic activity in the presence of guinea pig complement and was also sensitive to 2-mercaptoethanol.   In these experiments, however, it was still uncertain where the antibody was located.

The experiments presented here were designed to show the cross-reacting cell-bound antibodies on the surface of the sensitized lymph node cells in a model using the Forssman system, in skin allotransplantation and tumor isotransplantation in mice.   For the purpose of determing the class of the immunoglobulin of the cell-bound antibodies, radio-iodine-labeled antibodies to mouse IgG and IgM were employed.

MATERIALS AND METHODS

Animals

C3H/He Jms and (DDD × C3H/He Jms) Fi hybrid adult female mice, weighing 20±2 g, were used as recipients, and female C57BL/6 Jms mice as donors, of skin grafts.

Tumor

A mouse ascites tumor MM2, which originated as a spontaneous mammary carcinoma in a female C3H/He Jms mouse, was established as an ascites tumor in the Department of Oncology of this Institute and had been carried intraperitoneally through serial passages in female C3H/He/jms mice.

Sheep red blood cells (SRBC)

Blood from a sheep was mixed with two volumes of Alsever's solution and refrigerated until use. For immunization of mice a sample was washed three times with normal saline, and then adjusted to 3% in volume.

Crude methanol extract of SRBC

As Forssman antigen particles, a crude methanol extract of SRBC-stromata was prepared as outlined by Rapp (16) and Fujii and Nelson (7). For antibody transfer experiments the extract in absolute methanol was mixed with two volumes of normal saline in order to insolubilize the Forssman antigen. A few coarse particles were removed by centrifugation at 1500 rpm for 10 min. The fine particles were washed three times in normal saline by centrifugation at 40,000 rpm for 30 min and resuspended to the original volume.

Skin transplantation

A circular full-thickness skin graft of 11 mm in diameter was placed on a suprapannicular graft bed prepared on the midline of the back of the recipient.

Guinea pig and mouse lymph node cell suspension

Axillary and femoral lymph nodes were collected from sensitized or non-sensitized animals. After the removal of adhesive fat tissue, the nodes were teased in gelatin-veronal buffer containing 0.2 g potassium chloride and 1.0 g glucose per liter, designated as K-GVB (7). In later experiments with mouse lymph node cells, Eagle's medium containing 4 fold amino acids and vitamins was employed. The suspension was filtered through glass wool, and washed three times by low speed centrifugation; i.e., 800 rpm, for 10 min at 0°C, with cold diluent. Any cells which agglutinated during the washings were removed by allowing the suspension to stand for 5 min. The concentration of cells was determined by counts in a hemocytometer.

Rabbit anti-mouse IgG and IgM anti-mouse IgG sera

The rabbit antisera against mouse IgG and IgM were prepared as described by Nariuchi (12). In brief, healthy white rabbits approximately 6 months old were injected into the four foot pads and intramusculaly in the back with an antigen-antibody precipitate of mouse IgG or IgM, obtained by immunoelectrophoresis, and Freund's complete adjuvant. Three weeks later the animals were injected intravenously or intraperitoneally with approximately the same amount of specific precipitate used in the first injection without Freund's adjuvant. The animals were bled between the 8th and 24th day after the last injection, and the serum obtained was tested by immuno-electrophoresis. The sera, which gave a single precipitation line of IgG, was stored at −20°C.

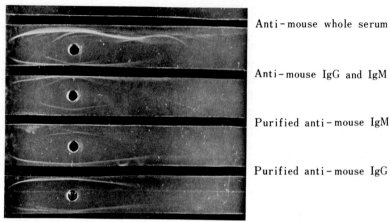

Anti-mouse whole serum

Anti-mouse IgG and IgM

Purified anti-mouse IgM

Purified anti-mouse IgG

FIG. 1. Immunoelectrophoresis of rabbit antisera to mouse IgG and IgM.

The rabbit antisera obtained by immunization with mouse IgM-rabbit anti-mouse globulin serum were absorbed at room temperature for 1 hr with a 1/10 volume of newborn mouse serum. After the absorption, the serum gave a single IgM precipitation line in immunoelectrophoresis.

Purification and radio-iodinelabeling of antisera

The rabbit antiserum to mouse IgG or mouse IgM was specifically purified by employing insolubilized mouse gamma globulin as the immunoadsorbent as described by Avrameas and Ternynck (*1*).

Each of the specifically purified rabbit antisera showed single precipitation lines of IgG and IgM in immunoelectrophoresis as shown in Fig. 1. The specifically purified antibodies were labeled with ^{125}I or ^{131}I after the method described by Masouredis *et al.* (*11*). Normal rabbit γ-globulin labeled with ^{131}I was used as the control.

Assays for antibodies bound to lymph node cells of mice immunized with SRBC

Five adult female C3H/He Jms mice were intradermally injected into the four foot pads with a total dose of 0.4 ml of 3% SRBC suspension and Freund's complete adjuvant on day −14 and on day −6. On day 0 the immunized mice and 5 normal C3H/He Jms mice were sacrificed and the lymph nodes were collected from the axillary and inguinal regions. Lymph node cell suspensions, 5×10^6 cells/ml, 2.5×10^6 cells/ml, and 1.25×10^6 cells/ml, in Eagle's medium containing 4-fold amino acids and vitamins were prepared as described above. The lymph nodes and the cell suspension were kept at 0°C during the procedure. A test was performed by mixing samples of 1.0 ml of the lymph node cells with 0.5 ml of a 1/10 dilution of radioiodine-labeled rabbit antibodies to mouse IgG or IgM at 0°C for 1 hr. After the incubation, the reactin mixtures were centrifuged at 800 rpm for 10 min and the sedimented cells were washed four times with cold Eagle's medium by additional centrifugation. Finally, the radioactivity of the radioiodine-labeled antibodies bound to the lymph node cells in each Wasserman tube was measured by a well-type scintillation counter.

The transfer of antibodies to crude Forssman antigen from the lymph node cells of mice immunized with SRBC

A number of lymph nodes of (DDD × C3H/He Jms) F1 mice immunized with SRBC were excised carefully and, after washing thoroughly in cold K-GVB, were adjusted to 1.5×10^8 per ml. Transfer of antibodies was performed by mixing 1.0 ml of a crude methanol extract of SRBC with 5.0 ml of a sensitized lymph node cell suspension, 1.5×10^8 per ml, at 37°C. After 3 hr the reaction mixture was centrifuged at 1,000 rpm for 10 min to remove the cells. The supernatant fluid containing crude Forssman antigen particles was kept at 4°C overnight, then centrifuged at 40,000 rpm for 30 min. The sedimented crude Forssman particles were washed three times with the cold diluent by ultracentrifugation and resuspended in 7 ml of cold diluent.

The assay for the transferred antibodies was performed by mixing the washed crude Forssman particles which would associate with antibodies dissociated from lymph node cells with 0.5 ml of a 1/10 dilution of the ^{131}I-labeled antibody to mouse IgG or IgM at room temperature for 60 min. After the incubation, the crude Forssman particles in the reaction mixture were washed four times with 10 ml of cold diluent by ultracentrifugation at 40,000 rpm for 30 min. The radioactivity of the radio-iodine labeled antibody, reacted with Forssman antigen particles, was measured by a well-type scintillation counter.

Crude liver tissue and tumor antigen particles

For tissue transplantation antigens in the antibody transfer experiment, fractions of C3H/He/Jms liver cells and MM2 ascites tumor cells were prepared as described by Nishioka *et al.* (*15*). In brief, 5 ml of packed cells was mixed with an equal volume of 0.2% sodium deoxycholate (DOC) (Difco) in veronal buffer containing 5 mM $MgCl_2$. After homogenization with a Teflon homogenizer, extraction was continued for 4 hr at 0°C. Then the homogenate was centrifuged at $10,000 \times g$ for 30 min. The supernatant fluid was dialysed against 0.15M NaCl for 48 hr in the cold, and was centrifuged at $105,000 \times g$ for 60 min. The precipitate was resuspended in 5 ml of 0.15 M NaCl and homogenized with a Teflon homogenizer. The homogenate was centrifuged at $120 \times g$ for 10 min to remove the coarse aggregates formed during the procedures.

RESULTS

Antibodies bound to the lymph node cells of mice immunized with SRBC

Preliminary study indicated that C3H/He Jms mice injected intradermally into the four foot pads with SRBC and Freund's complete adjuvant demonstrated a positive reaction in the foot pad test, which is a type of delayed reaction, as described by Nelson (*14*). In this experiment, an attempt was made to establish the presence of γ-globulin antibodies bound to the surface of the regional lymph node cells and the classes of the immunoglobulins. Adult female C3H/He Jms mice were intradermally injected into the four foot pads with a total dose of 0.4 ml of 3% SRBC suspension and Freund's complete adjuvant. The lymph node cells collected on day

6 and on day 14 were mixed with radioiodine-labeled rabbit antibodies to mouse IgG and IgM at 0°C for 1 hr. Uptake of the labeled antibodies by the lymph node cells indicated the presence of IgG or IgM immunoglobulins bound to the cells.

The radioactivity (cpm) given by each of the three concentration of lymph node cells; *i.e.*, 5, 2.5, and 1.25×10^6 cells, is shown in Fig. 2. A significant increase

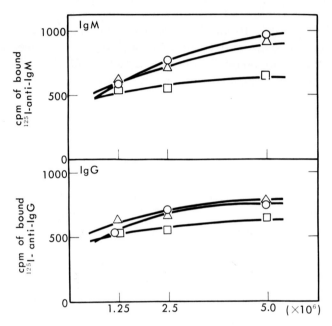

Fig. 2. Antibodies bound to lymph node cells of mice immunized with sheep red cells. ○, 14 days; △, 6 days; □, 0 day.

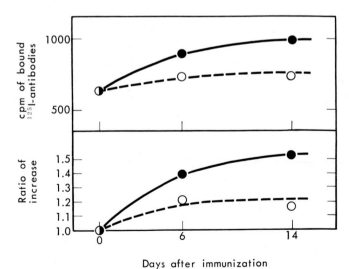

Days after immunization

Fig. 3. Antibodies bound to lymph node cells of mice immunized with sheep red cells. ●, IgM; ○, IgG.

in cpm by labeled anti-mouse IgM occurred with the sensitized lymph node cells collected on day 6 and on day 14, and an approximately maximal increase was observed with 5×10^6 cells.

A comparison of the rate of increase in cpm between IgM and IgG bound to the lymph node cells was made by plotting the cpm of 5×10^6 cells against the time after immunization (Fig. 3).   It was evident that there was a significant increase in the bound IgM with an increase ratio of 1.53 on day 14.   Whereas only a slight increase of bound IgG was observed, with a ratio of increase of only 1.15.   Thus, it may be indicated that after immunization, regional lymph node cells of mice bind more IgM and less IgG on the cells, while the immunological specificity of the antibody bound to the lymph node cells was not clarified in this experiment.

The transfer of antibodies to crude Forssman antigen from the sensitized lymph node cells

The present experiment was designed to demonstrate the transfer of antibodies bound to the lymph node cells shown in the previous experiment to Forssman antigen, and to determine the specificity of the antibodies which would cross-react with the Forssman antigen of mouse lymph node cells.   C3H/He Jms mice were injected with SRBC and on day 15 the second injection was performed as described previously.   From the radioactivity (cpm) of the crude Forssman antigen particles to which antibodies would be transferred from the lymph node cells collected on day 4, and on day 7, after primary injection, and on day 4, after the boosting, the ratio of these cpm to the cpm on day 0 was calculated.   The ratios of transferred antibody were plotted against time after immunization (Fig. 4).   As shown in Fig. 4, the ratio of transferred IgM antibody increased significantly after the immunization with a maximal ratio of 1.2 on day 7, while the ratio of transferred IgG antibody slightly increased only after the booster injection.   Since radioiodine-labeled normal rabbit γ-globulin showed no increase in the ratio during the period observed, the increased ratio herein was attributed to the transfer of antibody produced after the immunization.

Antibodies bound to lymph node cells of mice immunized with skin allograft

In a previous report (7), we demonstrated γ-globulin antibody dissociated, with

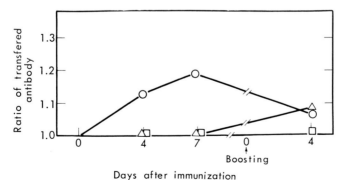

FIG. 4.   Transfer of lymph node cell-bound antibody to Forssman antigen.   ○, IgM ; △, IgG ; □, control.

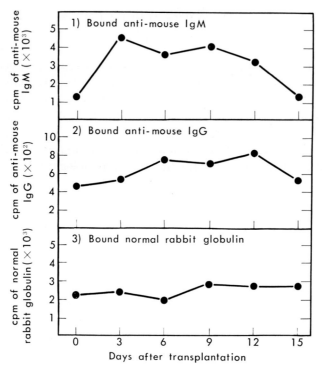

FIG. 5. Antibodies bound to regional lymph node cells after skin allotransplantation.

hypertonic saline, from lymph node cells of mice immunized with skin allografts. The dissociated γ-globulin was cytotoxic against lymphoid cells of the donor's mouse strain in the presence of complement, and was inactivated by treatment with 0.1 M 2-mercaptoethanol at 37°C for 30 min. In this experiment, an attempt was made to demonstrate antibody on the cell surface of mice transplanted with skin allograft using the technique described in the previous experiment. The axillary and inguinal lymph node cells were collected from the (DDD × C3H/He Jms) Fl mice on days 3, 6, 9, 12, and 15 after skin grafting from C57BL/6 Jms mice. A lymph node cell suspension of preimmune (DDD × C3H/He Jms) Fl mice was used as a control. The thoroughly washed cells (2 × 10⁶ cells) were incubated with 0.5 ml of ^{131}I-labeled rabbit antibodies to both mouse IgM and IgG at 0°C for 1 hr. The radioactivity (cpm) of the radio-iodine labeled anti-IgM that was bound to the lymph node cells collected on six different days is shown in Fig. 5–1. Such a plot demonstrates that the IgM antibody bound to the lymph node cells increases in an early stage with a peak between 3 and 9 days after transplantation. Figure 5–2 shows that IgG antibody bound to the lymph node cells also increases by the stimulation of skin allografting. The increase of the bound IgG is in the later stage with a peak on day 12 and the ratio of cpm at the peak to that of preimmune cells is lower than the ratio of increase of bound IgM. Figure 5–3 demonstrates that there were no changes in the level of nonspecific binding of normal rabbit γ-globulin by the lymph node cells tested.

The transfer of antibodies to donor's tissue antigen from the lymph node cells of mice transplanted with skin allograft

The previous results indicated the occurrence of antibodies bound to the surface of the lymph node cells of the mice sensitized with skin allograft.   The present experiment was undertaken to show the formation of an immune complex by an allotransplantation antibody and the antigen on the recipient's own node cells.   For this purpose, the procedures were designed to show the selective transfer of antibodies from the sentitized lymph node cells to the donor's tissue antigen particles as was done in the previous experiment.   The test was performed by mixing 3.0 ml of the thoroughly washed sensitized lymph node cells of C3H/He Jms mice, $1.2-1.5 \times 10^8$ cells per ml, with 1.0 ml of either C57BL/6 Jms antigen as the donor's tissue antigen or C3H/He Jms antigen as the recipient's own tissue antigen at 37°C for 3 hr.   After the incubation, the reaction mixture was divided equally.   To one aliquot, radio-labeled anti-mouse IgM was added and to the other, radio-labeled anti-mouse IgG. Percent transferred antibody was calculated from the radioactivity (cpm) of the tissue antigen particles on which transferred antibody-radio-labeled antibody complexes were formed and the radioactivity (cpm) of the dose of lymph node cells used in this antibody transfer experiment.   Significant transfer of antibody to the donor's tissue antigen was observed in both IgM and IgG antibody as shown in Table 1. The maximal percent of transfer of IgM antibody was 19.5 and that of the transfer of IgG antibody, 18.7, on day 15.   No significant transfer of antibody to the recipient own tissue antigens was seen in either IgM or IgG.

The results may indicate the formation of cross-reacting cell-bound antibody and the specific transfer of antibody, either IgM or IgG, to the donor's tissue antigen from the cross-reacting antigen-antibody complex on the lymph node cells.

TABLE 1.   Transfer of Cross-reacting Antibody to Donor Tissue Antigen

Antibody on lymph node cells	Transferred to	Percent antibody transferred				
		Days after skin grafting				
		0	4	7	10	15
IgM	Donor: C57BL	0	8.1	6.1	8.6	19.5
	Recipient: (DDD×C3H) F1	0		2.2		0
IgG	Donor: C57BL	0	7.6	6.2	8.0	18.7
	Recipient: (DDD×C3H) F1	0		1.8		5.8

Antibodies bound to lymph node cells of mice resistant to isogeneic tumor

The previous experiments indicated the formation of cross-reacting immune complexes on the lymph node cells by immunization of mice with heterophile Forssman antigen as a model of allotransplantation and also with skin allotransplantation. Similar experiments were performed in mice which were immunized with an isogeneic tumor.   Aliquots of a suspension of an antigen of MM2 tumor extracted with sodium deoxycholate were injected intraperitoneally into forty adult female C3H/He/ Jms mice as follows: 0.5 ml of DOC extract at increasing concentrations, 1/100,

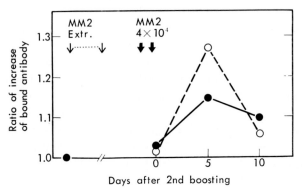

Fig. 6. Antibodies bound to lymph node cells in mice resistant to isogeneic tumor. ●, IgM ; ○, IgG.

1/100, 1/100, 1/50, 1/50, 1/50, 1/20, 1/20, 1/20, and 1/10 dilutions, every other day for a total 10 times (9).

On day 17 the animals were challenged with an intraperitoneal injection of MM2 tumor cells, 4×10^4. Thirty-five of the mice rejected the inoculated MM2 tumor cells and the remainder died due to the growth of the MM2 tumor. The second challenge was made for each group of ten mice on days 22 and 27 with 4×10^4 cells of MM2 tumor. All animals tolerated the second challenge without any signs of growth of the ascites tumor. On day 32 all the mice were sacrificed, and the lymph node cells were collected from the mesenterial, inguinal, and axillary nodes. Antibodies bound to the lymph node cells were assayed by using radio-iodine-labeled antibodies to mouse IgG and IgM and the ratio of the bound antibodies of the immunized animals to that in preimmune animals was calculated.

As shown in Fig. 6, without the second challenge only a very slight increase of IgG and IgM antibodies bound to the lymph node cells was observed. After the second boosting, however, a rapid increase of the bound antibodies occurred in both IgG and IgM antibodies with a peak on day 5. In contrast to the greater increase in IgM in the previous two experiments, the IgG antibody increased more than did the IgM antibody in these mice treated by hyperimmunization with isogeneic tumor cells.

The transfer of antibodies to tumor antigen from the lymph node cells of mice immunized with the tumor

Specific release and reassociation of antibodies bound to the lymph node cells with the MM2 tumor antigen particles was examined by the antibody transfer technique as described above. For the antibody transfer, 1.0 ml lymph node cell suspension, 1×10^8 per ml, was mixed with 1.0 ml of a DOC extract of the MM2 tumor, prepared as described previously, at 37°C for 3 hr. The procedure for the assay of the transferred antibodies was the same as those in the previous experiments. As shown in Table 2, on day 17, after the first challenge, radioactivities (cpm) of 532 and 625 were shown by transferred IgM and IgG antibodies, respectively. On days 5 and 10 after the second challenge, the lymph node cells, which had

TABLE 2.   Tranfer of Antibodies Bound to Lymph Node Cells to Tumor Antigen

Group	Days after		cpm of ^{125}I-antibodies	
	1st challenge	2nd challenge	IgM	IgG
A	0		0	0
B	17	0	532	625
C		5	NT	703
D		10	NT	750

revealed the increared levels of IgG antibodies on the surface of the cells in the previous experiments, denonstrated antibody transfer with a slight increase in cpm. Although the transfer of IgM antibody after the second challenge could not be accomplished, the results obtained herein may indicate that the cross-reacting cell-bound antibodies of both IgG and IgM are formed on the surface of the lymph node cells in mice immunized with isogeneic tumor cells. The rate of specific release and reassociation of the bound antibodies does not always appear to be parallel with the amounts of the antibodies bound to the lymph node cells. No explanation for this was apparent.

DISCUSSION

Allotransplantation is an exchange of tissue between individuals of the same species who share a similar, but not identical, chemical structure of antigens in the tissues. After the allotransplantation, antibody would be produced with a specificity for the donor antigen but would react also with antigens in the recipient's tissue. Thus the allotransplantation immunity would be an expression of an immunoche-mical cross-reaction of structural groups on molecules possessed by the donor and by the recipient as described by Nelson (7, 13). The antibody which cross reacts with antigens on the recipient cells would be a type of so-called cell-bound antibody.

The concept of the cross-reactivity of antigens shared by the individuals of the same species would apply equally well to individuals of species which share chemi-cally similar antigens. The so-called Forssman antigen is shared by several species. From the hypothesis described above it would be anticipated that the exchange of tissue among xenogeneic species possessing Forssman antigens would be a model of allotransplantation.

In the previous paper (Fujii and Nelson) (7), a close immunochemical rela-tionship of Forssman-type antigens in cells or in a methanol extract of guinea pig kidney, lymph nodes, and platelets, of horse kidneys, and of sheep erythrocytes was demonstrated. The dissociation of the antibody from these cross-reacting complexes and reassociation with antigens of sheep red blood cells used for immunization was also infered.

In the initial assays for antibody produced in guinea pigs following injection with sheep red blood cells, it was assumed that the antibody in the serum was pre-dominantly of the " isophile " or non-Forssman-type. Fujii et al. (6) demonstrated later two types of antibody in the guinea pigs injected with sheep red blood cells.

TABLE 3. Humoral and Cell-bound Antibodies of Guinea Pigs Immunized with Sheep Erythrocyte Stromata

Material	Percent inhibition	Type of antibody	
Serum	0	non-Forssman	humoral
Globulin on lymph node cells	44.0	mixed	
Globulin on platelet	86.9	Forssman	cell-bound

As shown in Table 3, hemolytic antibody in the serum could not be absorbed or inhibited by large amounts of a methanol extract of sheep red blood cell stromata. The globulin fractions dissociated from the lymph node cells showed hemolytic activity in the presence of guinea pig complement, and the antibody was absorbed by the methanol extract of sheep red blood cell stromata. As described in the previous initial experiment, it was assumed that the antibody in the serum was of a non-Forssman-type and that the other antibody, on the cells, was of a Forssman-type which cross-reacted with the Forssman antigens on the lymph node cells and platelets.

In the skin allotransplantation in guinea pigs, the initial evidence indicating the cross-reacting antibody on the recipient lymph node cells had been demonstrated by the immune adherence technique (13). We could also show an increase in the number of Cl molecules per lymph node cell in mice with a peak on day 5 after skin allotransplantation, by using a very sensitive technique of the transfer of Cl. The result indicated also the occurrence of a cross-reacting cell-bound antibody on the lymph node cells in allotransplantation.

In an attempt to extract the antibody bound to the lymph node cells of mice immunized with skin allograft, it was shown that the γ-globulin dissociated from the sensitized lymph node cells was specifically cytotoxic against the donor's lymphoid cells in the presence of complement, and that the cytotoxic activity was inactivated by treatment with 0.1 M 2-mercaptoethanol at 37°C for 30 min.

In the present study, the experiments were designed to establish the presence of the cross-reacting cell-bound antibody and the preferential transfer of the antibody from the antigen antibody complexes on the lymph node cells to the donor's cells. Employing radio-iodine labeled rabbit antibodies to mouse IgG and IgM, the identification of the class of the antibodies was also performed. The results obtained in the experiments using this sensitive method confirmed the formation of cross-reacting antibodies on the regional lymph node cells following skin allotransplantation. It was of very great interest that, when mice were sensitized by multiple injections of isogeneic tumor, similar cross-reacting antibodies were indicated.

The class of the immuno-globulin of the antibodies was found to be not only IgM but also IgG. Concerning the functions of the cross-reacting cell-bound antibody in the rejection of allograft and tumor isograft, little is known. However, this antibody, as a type of so-called cell-bound antibody, would be expected to serve as an antigen-recognition receptor of the sensitized lymphoid cells to sensitize or destroy the target cells.

SUMMARY

Nelson (1961) proposed a theory that cell-bound antibody could be an expression of an immunological cross-reaction of structural groups on molecules possessed by a recipient and donor that have a similar, but not identical, chemical structure of antigens in the tissues.   It was postulated that the antibody would dissociate or transfer from the cross-reacting antigens on the host's cells to the antigens on the donor graft cells responsible for immunization.

The present experiments were designed to confirm the cross-reacting cell-bound antibody demonstrated previously by us and to establish the presence and the class of the γ-globulin of the cross-reacting antibody on the surface of the sensitized lymph node cells in skin allotransplantation and tumor isotransplantation in mice.   The lymph node cells of mice sensitized with skin allografts or tumor isografts bound much more radio-iodinated anti-mouse IgG and anti-mouse IgG antibodies than the preimmune lymph node cells did.   It was also demonstrated that the antibodies bound to the cells were transferred in vitro to the graft antigens.   These observations indicate that IgG and IgM antibodies bound to the surface of the sensitized lymph node cells are the antibodies cross-reacting with the recipient's own cells.   Based on the hypothesis described above, it is postulated that the cross-reacting cell-bound antibody would be a type of cell-bound antibody functioning in cell-mediated immunity.

This work has been supported by research grants from the Ministry of Education, Japan.   The authors would like to thank Dr. R. A. Nelson, Jr. and Dr. K. Nishioka for the initiation of these studies.   The authors are grateful to Prof. T. Matsuhashi, Department of Allergology, and Dr. I. Kato, Department of Physical Biochemistry, of this institute for the preparation and radio-isotope-labelling of the rabbit antisera to mouse immunoglobulin.

REFERENCES

1. Avrameas, S., and Ternynck, T.   The Cross-linking of Proteins with Glutaraldehyde and Its Use for the Preparation of Immunoadsorbents.   Immunochem., 6: 53–66, 1969.
2. Buchbinder, L.   Heterophile Phenomena in Immunology.   Arch. Path., 19: 841–880, 1935.
3. Cruchaud, S., and Frei, P. C.   Demonstration of Specific Antibodies on Human Circulating Lymphocytes by a New Technique.   Int. Arch. Allergy, 31: 455–464, 1967.
4. Feldman, J. D., and Najarian, J. S.   Skin Homograft Destruction by "Antibody" Derived from Sensitized Lymphoid Cells.   Ann. N.Y. Acad. Sci., 120: 21–25, 1964.
5. Forssman, J.   Die Herstellung hochwertiger spezifischer Schafhämolysine ohne Verwendung von Schafblut.   Biochem. Z., 37: 78–115, 1911.
6. Fujii, G., Hirose, Y., Goto, S., Kozawa, T., and Ishibashi, Y.   Studies on Humoral and Cell-bound Antibodies in Allotransplantation Immunity.   Japan. J. Allergy, 16: 821–831, 1967.

7. Fujii, G., and Nelson, R. A. The Cross-reactivity and Transfer of Antibody in Transplantation Immunity. J. Exp. Med., *118*: 1037–1058, 1963.
8. Hanaoka, M. On the Nature of the Cellular Antibody of Lymphocytes in Homo-transplantation Immunity. Acta Haem. Japon, *27*: 155–165, 1964.
9. Irie-Furuse, R., Nishioka, K., Tachibana, T., and Takeuchi, S. Immunological Studies on Mouse Mammary Tumors. IV. Extraction and Solubilization of Transplantation Antigen of Mouse Mammary Tumor. Int. J. Cancer, *4*: 150–158, 1969.
10. Martin, A. B., Moore, W. D., Dickinson, J. B., and Raffel, S. Cellular Activities in Hypersensitive Reactions. III. Specifically Reactive Cells in Delayed Hypersensitivity: Tuberculin Hypersensitivity. J. Immunol., *93*: 953–959, 1965.
11. Masouredis, S. P., Melcher, L. R., and Kablick, D. C. Specificity of Radioiodinated (^{131}I) Immune Globulin as Determined by Quantitative Precipitin Reaction. J. Immunol., *66*: 297–302, 1951.
12. Nariuchi, H. Preparation of Rabbit Anti-mouse γ-globulin. Japan. Transplantation J., *2*: 44–46, 1968.
13. Nelson, R. A. Immunologic Mechanisms for Homograft and Heterograft Reactions. In 2nd Int. Symposium on Immunopathology (P. Graber and P. Miescher, editors), pp. 223, Basel, V. B. Schwabe and Co., 1961.
14. Nelson, D. S., and Mildenhall, P. Studies on Cytophilic Antibodies. 1. The Production by Mice of Macrophage Cytophilic Antibodies to Sheep Erythrocytes: Relationship to the Production of Other Antibodies and the Development of Delayed-type Hypersensitivity. Aust. J. Exp. Biol. Med. Sci., *45*: 113–130, 1967.
15. Nishioka, K., Irie-Furuse, R., Kawana, T., and Takeuchi, S. Immunological Studies on Mouse Mammary Tumors. III. Surface Antigens Reacting with Tumor-specific Antibodies in Immune Adherence. Int. J. Cancer, *4*: 139–149, 1969.
16. Rapp, H. J. Purification and Immunochemical Characterization of the Heat-stable, Alcohol-soluble Hemolytic Antibody Inhibitor of the Sheep Erythrocyte. Thesis, School of Hygiene & Public Health, Johns Hopkins University, 1953.

Humoral Factors in Cell-mediated Immunity

David S. NELSON

Department of Bacteriology, The University of Sydney, Sydney, Australia

There is now abundant evidence linking cell-mediated immune processes to tumor-specific immunity. In experimental animals, cell-mediated immunity (CMI) is of major importance in immunological resistance to syngeneic or autologous tumors induced by chemical carcinogens (*1, 101*) and oncongenic viruses (*3, 107*). In man there is increasing evidence that cell-mediated immune responses are mounted against autologous tumors (*79, 80*) and that such responses bear some relationship to the clinically apparent resistance of patients to their tumors (*52, 53, 87*). Information about the mechanisms involved in the induction and expression of CMI is therefore relevant to the problems of tumor immunity in man.

It has been usual to define as cell-mediated those immunological reactions occurring *in vivo* and having both of the following characteristics: (1) that reactivity can be conferred upon non-immunized animals by means of lymphoid cells from actively immunized animals; and (2) that reactivity can *not* be conferred upon non-immunized animals by means of serum from actively immunized animals. This definition stems from the classical and frequently confirmed work of Landsteiner and Chase (*34, 106*) on the passive transfer of contact sensitivity and of delayed cutaneous reactivity to tuberculin in guinea pigs. This in turn followed indirectly from the demonstration by Zinsser (*230*) and Zinsser and Mueller (*231*) that " bacterial allergies " (*i.e.*, delayed-type hypersensitivity) were different in kind from antibody-mediated anaphylactic reactions.

In the light of some of the evidence to be discussed in this paper, this definition may be too rigid. A broader definition should take into account the possible role, in some reactions, of cytophilic antibodies and related factors, or of conventional immunoglobulins, with or without complement, acting in conjunction with lymphoid cells. In this twilight zone outside the area of classically defined CMI may be found some reactions of considerable importance in tumor immunity. In this discussion I shall consider as CMI those reactions in which: (1) the critical, immunologically specific step is the reaction of antigen with a specific receptor, either antibody or antibody-like, at the surface of a mononuclear cell (lymphocyte or macrophage); and/or (2) mononuclear cells (lymphocytes or macrophages), whose behaviour may have been changed as a result of an immunologically specific reaction, are essential components.

There is little disagreement about many of the reactions which may be included in the category of CMI. Those occurring *in vivo* include: the skin reactions characteristic of delayed-type hypersensitivity (DTH); some forms of allograft rejection; some (probably most) forms of tumor isograft rejection; some auto-immune diseases, clinical and experimental; acquired cellular resistance to infection; the systemic tuberculin reaction; and the macrophage disappearance reaction; (reviewed in *153, 204, 205*). Those which can be observed and studied *in vivo* have aroused more interest in recent years as they are more susceptible to experimental analysis. They include: target cell destruction by lymphocytes (reviewed in *168*) and macrophages (*68*) from specifically sensitized hosts; most examples of lymphocyte stimulation by antigens (*141, 165*); macrophage migration-inhibition (*22, 43, 58*); some examples of macrophage chemotaxis (*215*); macrophage aggregation (*115*); inhibition of macrophage spreading (*45*); macrophage activation (*124*) and mitosis (*57, 121*) (the activation of and induction of mitosis in macrophages are more readily achieved *in vivo* than *in vitro* but the alterations in the cells are easily seen on subsequent culture *in vitro*); and pyrogen production (*11, 92*) (demonstration of pyrogen production obviously requires the testing of the pyrogen in intact animals).

In this paper the role of a variety of humoral factors in the development or expression of CMI will be examined, with particular reference to those factors which may be relevant to tumor immunity. This is not intended as a complete review of the subject and the examples used will be taken, as dictated by convenience, from among any of the phenomena listed above.

Specific Depression of Cell-mediated Immunity

Passively administered antibody can specifically inhibit or abolish an active cell-mediated immune response, just as it can specifically inhibit active antibody production (*207, 208*). This is most notable in the case of tumor allografts. The immunological enhancement of such grafts by anti-serum may be sufficient to allow the tumor to grow progressively until it causes the death of the host (*95*). Passive enhancement probably involves both a central effect (on the cells which would otherwise have engaged in the cellular response) and a peripheral effect (on the transplanted cells, protecting the putative target cells against damage by those specifically sensitized cells which are produced). Depression of CMI by passive antibody has also been reported for allografts of normal tissues (*149, 194*), for delayed-type hypersensitivity (*12, 40*) and for tumor isografts (*82*).

In vitro studies have shown in a clear-cut fashion that certain antibodies to antigens of tumor cells can protect against the cytotoxic effects of lymphocytes (*29, 76–78, 81*). This phenomenon, which is probably of major importance in determining the outcome of the host's immune responses to an autologous tumor, is dealt with by the Hellströms elsewhere in this Symposium.

The effect of antigen in modulating cell-mediated immune responses deserves some comment.   Of the greatest interest in relation to tumor immunity is the effect of the mode of presentation of antigen on the development of CMI.   Active enhancement of the growth of tumor allografts can be produced by appropriate pre-immunization of the recipient with donor antigen, especially lyophilized tumor or tumor extract (95).   Guinea pigs generally develop delayed-type hypersensitivity to protein antigens or sheep erythrocytes only when the antigens are incorporated in Freund's complete adjuvant.   Pre-immunization with antigen alone or in Freund's incomplete adjuvant causes immune deviation (reviewed in 8).   The animals develop antibodies of the γG_1 class but on subsequent challenge with antigen in Freund's complete adjuvant fail to develop delayed-type hypersensitivity or high levels of γG_2 antibodies (including cytophilic antibodies) (157).   A similar phenomenon occurs in mice (39, 41) and rats (12).   Experimental autoimmune diseases may be similarly abrogated (91, 187) and immune deviation may play a part in the active enhancement of tumor allografts in mice (137).

It is conceivable that something akin to immune deviation contributes to the failure of animals to make an effective immune response to their own primary chemically-induced tumors.   There may be some histological signs of an immune response while the tumor is present (105, 181).   Only when the tumor has been removed, however, is a response mounted of a type and intensity sufficient to cause resistance to an autograft of the same tumor (2, 102, 136, 198, 214).

In other circumstances, however, the maintenance of effective CMI towards a tumor may require the presence of antigen in the form of the tumor itself.   The hamster lymphomas studied by Gershon, Carter, and their colleagues provide an interesting example.   One of the tumors normally failed to metastasize.   Resistance to a second isograft of this tumor could be demonstrated while a first isograft was in place.   Such resistance was specific and was passively transferable by peritoneal cells.   If the original isograft was removed the hosts became susceptible to rechallenge, their peritoneal cells could no longer transfer resistance, and metastases from the original tumor appeared (59–61).

These radically different situations indicate that the effects of tumor antigens on the response to autologous tumors may be extremely varied and that considerable caution should be exercised in extrapolating to the human situation observations made on a single animal model.

Injection of soluble antigen may also temporarily depress the capacity of an animal to express previously induced CMI, not only delayed skin reactivity (8) but also antigen-induced lymphocyte transformation (104).   Exposure to antigen in vitro may also depress the capacity of lymphoid cells from an actively immunized animal to transfer delayed-type hypersensitivity to a normal animal (9).   As with immune deviation the mechanism of desensitization is unknown, but could be an additional factor in the late and extensive growth of demonstrably immunogenic tumors.

Non-specific Depression of Cell-mediated Immunity

A wide variety of immunologically non-specific factors can affect the general capacity of an animal to develop or express a cell-mediated immune response. Chief among those which might be termed physiological is the presence or absence, at the appropriate stage of development, of a thymus, both in experimental animals (*7, 64, 138, 139, 216*) and in man (see *113*). The thymus may fulfil its function mainly by supplying specialized lymphocytes capable of engaging in these responses (see *135*). However, the earlier work of Miller and Osoba (*140, 166*) on the restorative capacity of thymus grafts in cell-impermeable Millipore chambers suggested that the defect in neonatally thymectomized mice was at least partly due to a deficiency of a thymus hormone. This possibility has been confirmed by Stutman *et al.* (*195*) using grafts of either functional non-lymphoid thymomas or normal thymuses in cell-impermeable diffusion chambers. The period after thymectomy at which the thymus humoral factor was effective was, however, limited; after 30 to 50 days only free grafts were effective (*196*).

Glucocorticoids presumably play a physiological role in CMI, if only because of their central role in all metabolic activities. Large doses of glucocorticoids are part of the transplantation physician's standard immunosuppressive armamentarium to prolong allograft survival. Experimentally, large doses also inhibit delayed skin reactions (*38*), depress reticulo-endothelial activity (*211*) and depress cell-mediated resistance to infection (*54, 98*). Tuberculin shock is more severe in adrenalectomized, and less severe in corticosteroid-treated hypersensitive mice than in untreated mice (*73*). Thyroid hormone levels also affect the degree of cell-mediated resistance to infection (*98, 99*) especially to tuberculosis (*120*). In females, variations in resistance to infection and in reticuloendothelial activity may be related to variations in the levels of estrogens and progestational hormones during menstrual or estrous cycles and in pregnancy (*160*). All these hormones may exert their effects on lymphocytes and/or macrophages (*153, 199*). More recently, evidence has been presented that deficiency in pituitary hormones, especially growth hormone, can depress CMI (*172, 173*). So far as human tumor immunity is concerned, the possible risk of an increased incidence of other malignant diseases in conditions associated with marked alterations in hormone levels is generally masked by the risk of death from the primary disease, or abolished by teratment of the primary disease. However, there does appear to be an increased risk of malignant disease in renal allograft recipients on prolonged immunosuppressive therapy, which almost always includes corticosteroids (*125, 226*).

Histamine may also depress CMI. Patients with hay fever do not normally give delayed skin reactions to the allergens responsible. Their lymphocytes may, however, transform *in vitro* in response to the allergen, suggesting the existence of CMI to the allergen. This was confirmed when patients were skin-tested while receiving anti-histamine drugs: in these circumstances delayed skin reactions could be elicited (*26, 110*). It is difficult to relate these findings to human malignant disease, since among patients with malignant disease, there appears to be a lower, rather than a higher, incidence of "allergic" histories (56, 209).

Apart from congenital immunological deficiencies, impairment of CMI is being recognized in a growing number of human diseases. This has been shown *in vivo* as a decrease in the incidence or intensity of delayed skin reactions to common microbial antigens or contact sensitizers; or *in vitro* as a depressed response of lymphocytes to specific or non-specific mitogens. In some of these diseases depression of the *in vitro* response has been attributable, at least in part, to factors present in the patients' sera, which may depress the response of normal lymphocytes to mitogens. Conditions in which such factors have been reported to occur include: Hodgkin's disease (167, 203); secondary syphilis (111); lepromatous leprosy (30, 158); idiopathic steatorrhoea and some forms of cirrhosis (223); hepatitis and carriage of hepatitis-associated antigen (133, 134); and carcinoma of various types (188), although this has not been confirmed (63). The origin, nature, and general significance of these factors is unknown. We have suggested that they may not be new disease-specific factors, but may reflect the excessive production of factors which normally play a homeostatic role in CMI (158).

Some naturally occurring substances depress CMI either *in vivo* or *in vitro*. Kamrin (96) described the ability of an alpha-globulin fraction from normal serum to prolong the life of skin allografts when administered to rats. Mowbray (145) and Mannick and Schmid (130) also found that serum or plasma alpha-globulin preparations would prolong allograft survival. The factor responsible, though so far not purified, has been referred to as immuno-regulatory alpha-globulin (IRA) by Cooperband et al. (36, 37), who have carried out extensive studies on its action *in vitro*. In relatively large doses it has been shown to depress mitogen-induced lymphocyte transformation and to depress antigen-induced macrophage migration inhibition. Its action appeared to be upon the earliest events in the expression of CMI, *i.e.*, upon the interaction of mitogen or antigen with lymphocytes. The existence of alphaglobulins depressing lymphocyte transformation has been confirmed by Burrow and Forbes (31) and a somewhat similar factor has been isolated from bovine thymus (32). A crude aqueous extract of pig lymph nodes has also been reported to depress the response of human lymphocytes to PHA (144). In perhaps the most extreme situation, whole normal homologous serum has been reported to depress the response of chicken cells in mixed lymphocyte cultures (217). The biological significance of these factors is not yet known. They may be truly immuno-regulatory, playing a part in controlling the level of a cell-mediated response. In excess, they may be responsible for the depressive effect of certain pathological sera on lymphocyte transformation. The whole field of homeostasis of CMI has been insufficiently explored and further studies on these immuno-regulatory factors will be of considerable importance.

Closely intertwined with these investigations has been the study of the immuno-suppressive effect of ribonucleases. Jankovic and Dvorak (90) reported that RNAase treatment of sensitized rabbit lymph node cells inhibited their capacity to give an immune lymphocyte transfer reaction. Mowbray and Scholand (146) attributed to RNAase the capacity of alpha-globulins to depress humoral antibody production. Others have found only inconsistent depression of humoral antibody production by

RNAase (*33, 44, 176*).   However, Mowbray *et al.* (*147*) reported a dramatic inhibitory effect of polymerized RNAases on the response of lymphocytes to mitogens *in vitro*.   The suggestion that some cells carry RNA at their surface (*132*) increases the interest of these reports.   RNAases appeared not to be involved in the depressive effects of either alpha-globulins or pathological whole sera, since in neither case was a correlation found between RNAase activity and depressive activity (*37, 158*).

Non-specific Humoral Co-factors in Cell-mediated Immunity

In humoral immunity many effector mechanisms involve not only antibodies but also complement.   Homoral co-factors may also be involved in the expression of CMI.   A role for complement was suggested by the finding of Neveu and Biozzi (*159*) that delayed skin reactivity was reduced in rats de-complemented by the injection of aggregated gamma-globulin.   They pointed out, however, that factors other than those of the complement system could have been removed by this treatment.   The role in CMI of complement components, as defined in the conventional hemolytic system, remains unclear, especially as rabbits and mice deficient in individual components can express quite normally various manifestations of CMI (*62*).

Components of the blood coagulation system, or substances closely related to them, may act as co-factors in delayed-type hypersensitivity.   Heparin inhibits delayed ocular reactions to tuberculin (*225*), delayed skin reactions to tuberculin and other antigens (*35, 151*), and the macrophage disappearance reaction (*151*).   Warfarin and fumopimaric acid, both of which have a different mode of anticoagulant action from that of heparin, similarly inhibit delayed skin reactions (*55, 151*).   Heparin appears to act at some stage subsequent to the interaction of antigen with sensitized cells (*35*) and the action of anticoagulants is unrelated to any action they may have on complement (*151*).   The nature of the hypothetical co-factors affected remains otherwise unknown.

Reactions Mediated by Lymphocytes in The Presence of Specific Humoral Factors

Since the work of Govaerts (*66*), it has been repeatedly and consistently demonstrated *in vitro* that target cells are killed when incubated with lymphocytes from specifically immunized donors (*168*).   For this reaction neither specific humoral factors nor complement components are necessary.   One of the very elegant systems devised for the study of this type of reaction involves the use, as target cells, of mouse (DBA/2) mastocytoma cells labelled with ^{51}Cr; the degree of damage can be quantitatively assessed by measuring ^{51}Cr release after incubation with specifically sensitized lymphocytes, *e.g.*, from C57 mice immunized with DBA/2 tissues (*27, 28, 131*).   In this system humoral alloantibodies directed against antigens on the target cells protect them from the damaging effect of sensitized lymphocytes (*27*)–a machanism probably involved in immunological enhancement, as described above.

There is probably little doubt in the minds of most workers that models such as this provide a valid picture of the most common forms of lymphocyte—target cell interaction in the expression of CMI to allografts or tumor isografts.   Other modes of interaction *in vitro* have also been described and intensively investigated. The cytotoxic potential of non-specifically stimulated normal lymphocytes is considered below. Of additional and special interest is the capacity of nonimmune lymphocytes to destroy target cells sensitized by antibody specific to those target cells. This has been described by Möller (*142*) using mice and by MacLennan *et al.* (*128*) using human cells.

Recently MacLennan and his colleagues have presented a detailed investigation of this phenomenon using rats immunized with Chang cells (*126, 127*). The antibody responsible differed from complement-dependent IgM cytotoxic antibody, being found in the second (IgG containing) peak from Sephadex G-150. It was active at extremely high dilutions. Some activity was also found in the third peak, containing albumin and lower molecular weight proteins; although its activity was not investigated in depth, it may prove to be of interest in relation to lymphokines and cytophilic antibodies which have low molecular weights and/or migrate with albumin (see below). The cytotoxicity of lymphocytes from specifically immunized rats differed from that caused by antibody plus normal lymphocytes in two major respects. First, specific antibody actually inhibited the cytotoxicity of specifically immune cells, an effect similar to that already noted. Second, inhibitors of protein synthesis, such as Puromycin, inhibited their cytotoxic effect, whereas Puromycin did not inhibit the cytotoxic effect of lymphocytes on antibody-coated target cells.

Yet another mechanism of target cell damage is the cytotoxic effect of non-immune human lymphocytes on target cells (chicken erythrocytes) carrying antibody and the first seven components of complements (*169*).

The biological significance, especially for human tumor immunology, of the last two mechanisms of target cell damage by non-immune lymphocytes is not clear. They may represent reserve or accessory mechanisms supplementing the more commonly occurring cytotoxicity mediated by specifically sensitized lymphocytes. They may also be invoked to explain the occurrence of auto-immune thyroiditis which has the histological hallmarks of cell-mediated damage but is apparently dependent on thyroid auto-antibodies. This occurs in certain circumstances in rabbits injected with anti-thyroid antibodies (*148*) and spontaneously in the obese (OS) strain of chickens, in which its occurrence is, like humoral antibody production, bursa-dependent and thymus-independent (*219*).

Reactions Mediated by Macrophages: The Role of Cytophilic Antibodies

Macrophages from immune animals are capable of producing some reactions quite specifically in the absence of either immune lymphocytes or immune serum. It seems unavoidable to attribute the specificity of these reactions to cytophilic antibodies carried on the macrophages, since the cells appear themselves unable to produce antibodies (*153*). These reactions form the subject of this section. Those in which the interaction of lymphocytes and antigen appear to be of major importance, but which can be mimicked by the interaction of antigen with macrophages carrying cytophilic antibodies, are considered in the next section.

The properties of antibodies cytophilic for macrophages have been surveyed in recent reviews (114, 153, 155). Some of these properties, particularly those which affect their detection *in vitro*, deserve renewed emphasis. Cytophilic antibodies exist in a state of dynamic equilibrium between the macrophage surface, the environment (serum, plasma, or culture medium) and, probably, the cell interior. Macrophages, derived from appropriately immunized animals, which are carrying cytophilic antibodies, may rapidly lose them from their surface when cultured or even handled *in vitro*. This loss is more marked at 37°C than at lower temperatures and is very marked when the medium to which they are exposed includes normal serum. In such circumstances a greater uptake of antigen may be shown by normal macrophages cultured, washed, and then exposed *in vitro* to serum from immunized animals, than by those same animals' own macrophages cultured and washed *in vitro* before the addition of antigen. Cytophilic antibodies are physico-chemically heterogeneous. For guinea pigs they are found almost entirely among the γG_2 immunoglobulins but some may be found in chromatographic fractions containing alpha-globulins. In mouse serum they are found in the γG_2 and (with some antigens) the γM immunoglobulins; they may also be found in fractions containing albumin and a fast alpha-globulin. The different classes of mouse cytophilic antibodies attach to different receptors on macrophages. The receptors themselves, and antibodies attached to them, have different susceptibilities to trypsin (Full references and experimental justification for these statements may be found in references 86, 153, 154). Considering the readiness with which macrophages lose their cytophilic antibodies *in vitro* and the possibility that those appearing in serum may be an overflow from those already attached to cells *in vivo*, one may find it quite surprising that macrophages taken from immune animals have ever been shown to exert specific immunological activities. Such activities have, however, been demonstrated.

One of the most clear-cut is the destruction of allogeneic target cells *in vitro* described by Granger and Weiser (67–69, 86). This was shown to be effected by pure populations of immune macrophages and to depend on the presence of a cytophilic antibody on the macrophage surface. In the course of the reaction, macrophages, as well as target cells, were damaged or killed. This appears to be the counterpart *in vitro* of that mode of tumor allograft rejection *in vivo* in which macrophages appear to be the main effector cells (13, 65, 93); or in which isolated macrophages or macrophage-rich exudates from immune animals manifest tumor-suppressive activity when injected into non-immune hosts (4, 17, 164). There may be a requirement for a change in the macrophages additional to their acquistition of cytophilic antibodies, as macrophages obtained from normal mice and passively sensitized *in vitro* did not appear to be cytotoxic (67, 68, 86). Perhaps the metabolic changes of macrophage activation (see below) are required for the macrophages to become " killer cells " and cytophilic antibodies are responsible only for the first and immunologically specific step of the reaction.

The extensive studies of Takeda and his colleagues (198) have also indicated a role for macrophages as major effector cells in specific acquired immunity to autologous or syngeneic chemically-induced sarcomas in rats. Macrophages appeared to be considerably more effective than lymphocytes in destroying tumor cells *in vitro* and *in vivo*, both free in the peritoneal cavity and in diffusion chambers. Although no cytophilic antibodies were directly demonstrated, perhaps because of some of the difficulties outlined above, their presence may be tentatively inferred: (a) because macrophages from immune animals could effect an immunologically specific reaction in the absence of immune serum or lymphocytes; and (b) because tumor cells are destroyed when placed with normal macrophages in cell-impermeable diffusion chambers, the chambers themselves being placed within specifically pre-immunized rats.

Another example of macrophage-mediated immunity to tumor isografts is provided by the work of R. Evans, J. G. Hall, I. Parr and others on the lymphoma L5178Y of DBA/2 mice (J. G. Hall, personal communication). Mice immunized with irradiated tumor cells became resistant to challenge with viable cells. *In vitro*, macrophages from immune animals were cytotoxic to the lymphoma cells, but neither serum nor lymphocytes from the same animals were cytotoxic. Macrophages from non-immune mice could be rendered specifically cytotoxic by incubation with spleen cells from immune mice. This was associated with the appearance of mouse immunoglobulin on the surface of the macrophages. However, serum from immune animals did not render the cells cytotoxic, perhaps because cytophilic antibodies were present only in small quantities in the serum and/or perhaps because additional metabolic activation of the macrophages was required.

Acute graft-versus-host reactions have also been produced by macrophages from immunized animals. Weiser *et al.* (*218*) induced disease in A strain mice by means of intraperitoneal injections of purified macrophages from C57 mice immunized with an A strain tumor. With a large enough cell inoculum, mortality reached almost 100%. Death appeared to be due to acute pancreatitis and the donor macrophages were seen to penetrate the pancreas. The reaction was immunologically specific and it seems reasonable to attribute the specificity to a cytophilic antibody.

There is some evidence that the formation and release of a pyrogen in the systemic tuberculin reaction may be a property of macrophages carrying cytophilic antibodies. A pyrogen could be specifically released by alveolar macrophages incubated *in vitro* with tuberculin (*11*) and passive transfer of reactivity could be achieved by means of mononuclear cells of various types, including alveolar macrophages, as well as by plasma or serum (*72*).

Effector Substances Produced by Lymphocytes; Lymphocyte-macrophage Interactions

When antigen is incubated with lymphocytes from animals having specific CMI to that antigen, there appear in the culture fluid factors having a variety of biological effects related to the expression of CMI. In many cases these factors have been shown to exert their effects independently of antigen and to differ from classical antibodies; they have been given the generic name " lymphokines " (*47*). A comprehensive review of this rapidly growing field would be impossible here. A brief survey of some problems in the study of phenomena apparently mediated by lymphokines is, however, an essential part of this essay.

The most extensively investigated phenomenon is macrophage migration-inhibition. As studied with guinea pig cells, this reaction is very clearly an *in vitro* correlate of delayed-type hypersensitivity (*22, 43*). Several workers have described the appearance of migration-inhibition factor(s) (MIF) in the medium in which antigen and lymphocytes from specifically sensitized animals have been cultured (*19, 21, 22, 42, 43, 47, 191*). In some cases MIF has been shown to act on macrophages independently of antigen, *e.g.*, by fractionation of the culture supernatants in such a way that a very large proportion of the antigen is removed, the remaining MIF being active in the absence of additional antigen; or by dialysis to remove low molecular weight antigens such as DNP-oligolysines (*23, 47*; J. R. David, personal communication). In such circumstances MIF has been characterized as an acidic protein with alpha-globulin mobility, possessing neuraminic acid groups, of low molecular weight (<70,000), and apparently unrelated to conventional immunoglobulins (*23, 47, 178*). It has been reported to act on a trypsin-sensitive receptor on macrophages (*15*). MIF appears to lack species specificity, as sensitized human lymphocytes cultured with antigen generate a factor which can inhibit the migration of normal guinea pig macrophages (*179, 180, 202*). Lymphocytes from sensitive humans and rats can also be inhibited in their migration by specific antigens (*16, 51, 189, 200, 227*) and this type of reaction may also involve the release of a MIF (*50*). Both MIF release from human lymphocytes and human lymphocyte migration-inhibition are expected to be useful techniques in the study of tumor immunity in man.

Most of the experiments so far cited have produced results strongly suggesting antigen-independence of MIF. Other work has given almost equally clear-cut results suggesting that migration-inhibition can be produced in alternative or additional way by antigen-specific factors. Dumonde (*46*) reported that normal macrophages passively sensitized with serum from guinea pigs with delayed-type hypersensitivity to sheep erythrocytes failed to migrate normally in the presence of intact sheep erythrocytes (although soluble antigen did not inhibit their migration). Amos *et al.* (*6*) found that the specific soluble antigen would inhibit the migration of normal guinea pig macrophages carrying cytophilic antibodies to tuberculin-PPD or B-lactoglobulin. Spitler *et al.* (*193*) induced migration-inhibition by means of antigen-antibody complexes. They later reported briefly (*191*) that normal guinea pigs injected with relatively large amounts of serum from donors with delayed-type hypersensitivity could furnish macrophages whose migration was specifically inhibited by antigen. Heise *et al.* (*75*) found that alveolar macrophages from BCG-immunized guinea pigs showed migration-inhibition in the presence of PPD; that reactivity could be abolished by trypsin treatment and restored by exposure to immune serum or heat-eluates from immune macrophages; and that such serum or eluates would confer reactivity upon normal alveolar macrophages. The production of antigen-dependent MIF has also been demonstrated in some experiments. Bennett and Bloom (*18*) reported that supernatants from cultures of lymphocytes which had been mixed with antigen, then washed free of antigen before incubation, had a greater inhibitory effect on macrophage migration when specific antigen was added again than in the absence of specific antigen. A marked potentiating effect of added antigen on MIF activity was also found by Svejcar *et al.* (*197*) when lymphocytes had been cultured with very small doses of antigen. Amos and Lachmann (*5*) incubated specifically sensitized lymphocytes with antigen coupled to an insoluble carrier and found that the supernatants inhibited macrophage migration only in the presence of added (soluble) antigen. This report is of particular interest in that the immunologically specific factor was found in a Sephadex G-100 fraction containing albumin and alpha-globulin (*cf. 154*). In a slightly different vein, Barnet *et al.* (*14*) reported that a factor inducing the specific ingestion of sheep erythrocytes by macrophages was produced in cultures containing sheep erythrocytes and lymph node cells from rabbits immunized with sheep erythrocytes.

These sets of findings are probably best viewed, not as irreconcilable or even conflicting, but as reflecting a variety of mechanisms by which lymphocytes and macrophages can interact in this particular phenomenon. The peritoneal macrophage disappearance reaction, which may be an *in vivo* counterpart of macrophage migration-inhibition, can also be passively transferred both by pure peritoneal lymphocytes from actively sensitized guinea pigs and by normal peritoneal cells treated with serum from sensitized donors (*152, 156*). The existence of different mechanisms for the production of these reactions conceivably represents a means of amplification of biologically important reactions.

One may view in a similar light the production by antigen-stimulated immune lymphocytes of factors causing blastogenesis in non-immune lymphocytes (*129, 224*). Again there are apparently conflicting results regarding the action of the lymphokine released, Valentine and Lawrence (*210*) reporting antigen-dependence, and Spitler and Fudenberg (*192*) reporting antigen-independence. The study of secondary lymphocyte stimulation is complicated by the findings that unstimulated lymphocytes release a blastogenic factor (*97*) and that stimulated lymphocytes produce an apparently different factor which potentiates the response of immune lymphocytes to specific antigen (*89*).

Several groups of workers have investigated the production of cytotoxic factors *in vitro* by antigen-stimulated lymphocytes from specifically sensitized animals. Ruddle and Waksman (*183–185*) used rats with delayed-type hypersensitivity to various antigens and showed that antigen-induced production of cytotoxic factors was immunologically specific and correlated with skin reactivity. Both syngeneic and allogeneic cultured fibroblasts were affected, but damage was slow, being first apparent at 48 hr. Cytotoxicity was shown to be caused by a soluble factor released from lymphocytes, rather than by contact of lymphocytes with target cells to which antigen had been passively adsorbed. Likewise, Granger *et al.* (*70*) demonstrated the release of a lymphotoxin when antigen (PPD) was incubated with lymphocytes from the spleens of specifically sensitized mice or guinea pigs or from peripheral blood of tuberculin-sensitive humans. Similar findings were reported by Dumonde *et al.* (*47*) using lymph node cells from guinea pigs sensitive to protein antigens. The lymphotoxin studied by Granger and his colleagues produced target cell damage rather slowly (*220*) and different target cells varied in their susceptibilities (*222*). Lymphotoxin was also produced by PHA-stimulated human lymphocytes (*221*) and spontaneously by many permanent human lymphoblastoid cell lines (which also produced MIF) (*71*). Lymphotoxin production seems a most plausible explanation of the cytotoxic effects of lymphocytes stimulated in a variety of ways—not only by PHA (*84, 85, 168, 221*) but also by allogeneic lymphocytes (*84*), anti-lymphocyte serum (*118, 119*) and heterologous antigen-antibody complexes (*20, 143*). If what we have termed above as secondarily stimulated lymphocytes also produce lymphotoxin, this may be a useful form of biological amplification of target cell killing by lymphocytes. Further amplification may be provided by the release of cytotoxic factors from appropriately stimulated macrophages (*74, 174, 175*). The relevance of lymphotoxins or similar factors to tumor-specific immunity is illustrated by the experiments of Kikuchi *et al.* (*100*) using a mouse sarcoma and peritoneal cells from specifically immunized syngeneic mice. These were unusual in that the stimulating cells (which were also the target cells) were separated from the immune cells by a Millipore membrane. Destruction of the target cells was apparent in 48 to 72 hr and could be attributed to a soluble factor diffusing back across the membrane.

The changes in macrophages associated with acquired cellular resistance to infection (*122, 124*) may be conveniently referred to as activation. Once macrophages have been activated following appropriate immunization there is little specificity in their increased microbicidal power. Mackaness (*123*) has, however, provided strong evidence that their activation, in mice, involves an immunologically specific reaction between sensitized lymphocytes and antigens of the immunizing organism. This was achieved *in vivo* and there is no evidence concerning the nature of the activating factor(s), in particular whether or not they are antigen-dependent. Other studies suggest that cytophilic antibodies may play a part in acquired cellular resistance to infection (*177, 182*). Preliminary experiments by some workers indicate that macrophages can be activated *in vitro* by the products of stimulated lymphocytes (personal communications from J. R. David and R. J. W. Rees). Mitosis of macrophages appears to precede their activation *in vivo* (*162, 163*); it can be immunologically induced *in vivo* and easily quantitated *in vitro* (*57, 121*; D. S. Nelson and D. More, unpublished results). Further investigation of macrophage mitogenic factors *in vitro* may be a useful tool in the analysis of macrophage activation.

The classical and most extensively studied examples of CMI are the skin reactions characteristic of delayed-type hypersensitivity. They are slow in onset, reaching a maximum at about 24 hr, tending to persist, and characterized histologically by mononuclear cell infiltration. The conventional picture of the mechanism of their induction is derived from extensive studies by histological, passive transfer, and cell-labeling techniques (for review see *153, 190, 204, 206, 213*). According to this view, the reactions are initiated by the interaction of antigen with specifically sensitized lymphocytes. As a result, other mononuclear cells accumulate at the site. The specifically sensitized cells are thymus-derived or thymus-dependent, long-lived, and relatively radio-resistant, and form only a small proportion of the ultimate cell population at the test site. The majority of the cells at the site are derived from rapidly dividing radiosensitive precursors in the bone marrow and a high proportion of them are of the monocyte/macrophage class (*25, 112, 116, 117, 212*). Once within the lesion the monocyte/macrophage may show signs of activation, including mitosis (*103, 190*).

Specifically sensitized guinea pig lymphocytes incubated *in vitro* with antigen were found to release a lymphokine (" skin-reactive factor ") which, on intradermal injection into normal guinea pigs, induced a reaction having some of the characteristics of a delayed hypersensitivity reaction (*19, 47, 170*). There was substantial mononuclear infiltration but the reactions differed in their timecourse, being of much more rapid onset. More rapid reactions could also be induced by the injection of antigens into sites (in specifically sensitized animals) in which a mononuclear exudate had already been induced by a non-specific stimulus (*83*). It is possible, therefore, that delayed reactions are mediated by lymphokines released from lymphocytes on contact with antigen; and that the usually slow development of these reactions is due to the initially infrequent contact between antigen and cell. When the lymphokines are pre-formed, or a larger number of cells are initially available for contact, the reaction would proceed much faster. Again, there is further opportunity for biological amplification if secondary lymphocyte stimulation occurs at the site, as non-specific mitogens also cause the release of skin-reactive factors (*171, 186*).

The mode of action of skin-reactive factors is unknown. They could cause the accumulation of monocyte/macrophages both by immobilizing them in the course of their normal passage through the tissues (*150*), perhaps in a fashion analogous to migration-inhibition *in vitro*; and by chemotactic attraction of the cells from the circulation (*215*).

The antigen-dependence or independence of skin-reactive factors has not been investigated in detail (*170*). Some reports, however, indicate that cytophilic antibodies may sometimes mediate skin reactions resembling, or even identical with, those of classical delayed-type hypersensitivity. Hulliger *et al.* (*88*) produced such reactions in guinea pigs by local injection of sheep erythrocytes with normal peritoneal exudate cells coated with specific cytophilic antibody; reactions to soluble antigens could not, however, be similarly produced. Asherson and Zembala (*10*) transferred contact sensitivity in mice by means of peritoneal macrophages from immunized mice. They also transferred sensitivity by means of peritoneal macrophages from non-immune mice which had carried in their peritoneal cavities millipore chambers filled with lymphocytes from specifically immunized mice; in these circumstances cytophilic antibodies could be implicated in the transfer. We have observed delayed reactions in the footpads of normal mice following local injection of sheep erythrocytes treated with immune serum in which the only detectable antibody was a cytophilic alpha-globulin (*154*).

In general, attempts to transfer delayed skin reactivity by means of serum or plasma from immunized animals have been unsuccessful or, if successful, not reproducible (*153*). Recently, however, Dupuy *et al.* (*48, 49*) succeeded in producing specific delayed skin reactivity in normal guinea pigs by passive transfer of plasma from BCG-immunized donors which had been X-irradiated. The plasma factor was cytophilic for spleen cells, as spleen cells exposed to active plasma and then washed, could also transfer reactivity. The factor had fast alphaglobulin mobility (*cf. 154*) and was clearly distinct from conventional immunoglobulins.

As with other examples of CMI, these observations are perhaps best interpreted as indicating additional or alternate pathways, rather than being in conflict with the bulk of evidence indicating the great importance of lymphocyte-antigen interactions.

The role of macrophages in some forms of target cell destruction has already been considered. Some recent experiments suggest the potential importance of lymphocyte-macrophage interaction in the expression of tumor-specific immunity. The injection into the skin of normal recipient guinea pigs of mixtures of syngeneic target tumor cells and immune peritoneal exudate cells induced delayed skin reactions in which the tumor cells were killed. The immunological specificity of this reaction was attributable to lymphocytes but there was evidence that the extreme efficiency of target cell destruction was at least partly attributable to macrophages accumulating at the site of the reaction (228, 229). On the other hand, Nomoto et al. (161) using a hamster lymphoma (59) could demonstrate a major role only for specifically immune cells. The design of their experiments included the use of irradiated and thymectomized recipients, with or without bone marrow grafts, and the use of unfractionated peritoneal exudate cells. Because of these factors, and because rejection of the tumor in actively immunized animals is accompanied by intense macrophage activity (60) they were unwilling to conclude that macrophages did not normally play an important part in rejection, perhaps under the direction of lymphocytes.

Transfer Factor

Although strictly outside the scope of this paper, the transfer factor of Lawrence (108, 109) must be mentioned. This is a low molecular weight substance extractable from leucocytes, resistant to DNAase and RNAase, capable of conferring long-lasting specific CMI on an unimmunized recipient. Its mode of action is unknown. Its importance for tumor immunity lies in the obvious potential for transferring, from resistant donors to non-resistant recipients, CMI to those human tumors which may have common tumor-specific antigens. It remains to be seen whether similar transfers will be possible with RNA extracts from lymphoid cells, which have also been reported to transfer CMI *in vitro* (24, 94, 201).

REFERENCES

1. Alexander, P., and Fairley, G. H. Cellular Resistance to Tumours. Brit. Med. Bull., *23*: 86–92, 1967.
2. Alexander, P., Bensted, J., Delorme, E. J., Hall, J. G., and Hodgett, J. The Cellular Immune Response to Primary Sarcomata in Rats. II. Abnormal Responses of Rodes Draining the Tumour. Proc. Roy. Soc. B., *174*: 229–236, 1969.
3. Allison, A. C. Cell-mediated Immune Response to Virus Infections and Virus-induced Tumours. Brit. Med. Bull., *23*: 60–65, 1967.
4. Amos, D. B. Host Response to Ascites Tumours. *In* P. Grabar and P. Miescher (eds.) Mechanism of Cell and Tissue Damage Produced by Immune Reactions. II. International Symposium on Immunopathology, pp. 210–222, Basel: Schwabe, 1967.

5. Amos, H. E., and Lachmann, P. J.   The Immunological Specificity of a Macrophage Inhibition Factor.   Immunology, *18*: 269–277, 1970.

6. Amos, H. E., Gurner, B. W., Olds, R. J., and Coombs, R. R. A.   Passive Sensitization of Tissue Cells.   II. Ability of Cytophilic Antibody to Render the Migration of Guinea Pig Peritoneal Cells Inhibitable by Antigen.   Int. Arch. Allergy, *32*: 496–505, 1967.

7. Arnason, B. G., Jankovic, B. D., Waksman, B. H., and Wennersten, C.   Role of the Thymus in Immune Reactions in Rats.   II. Suppressive Effect of Thymectomy at Birth on Reactions of Delayed (Cellular) Hypersensitivity and the Circulating Small Lymphocyte.   J. Exp. Med., *116*: 177–206, 1962.

8. Asherson, G. L.   Antigen-mediated Depression of Delayed Hypersensitivity.   Brit. Med. Bull., *23*: 24–29, 1967.

9. Asherson, G. L., and Stone, S. H.   Desensitization *in vitro*—the Specific Inhibition, by Antigen, of the Passive Transfer of Delayed Hypersensitivity by Peritoneal Exudate Cells.   Immunology, *13*: 469–475, 1967.

10. Asherson, G. L., and Zembala, M.   Contact Sensitivity in the Mouse.   IV. The Role of Lymphocytes and Macrophages in Passive Transfer and the Mechanism of Their Interaction.   J. Exp. Med., *132*: 1–15, 1970.

11. Atkins, E., Bodel, P., and Francis, L.   Release of an Endogenous Pyrogen *in vitro* from Rabbit Mononuclear Cells.   J. Exp. Med., *126*: 357–383, 1967.

12. Axelrad, M., and Rowley, D. A.   Hypersensitivity: Specific Immunosuppression of the Delayed Type.   Science, *160*: 1465–1467, 1968.

13. Baker, P., Weiser, R. S., Jutila, J., Evans, C. A., and Blandau, R. J.   Mechanism of Tumour Homograft Rejection: the Behaviour of Sarcoma I Ascites Tumour in the A/J and the C57 B1/6K Mouse.   Ann. N.Y. Acad. Sci., *101*: 46–62, 1962.

14. Barnet, K., Pekarek, J., and Johanovsky, J.   Demonstration of Specific Induction of Erythrocyte Phagocytosis by Macrophages from Normal, Non-sensitized Rabbits by a Factor Released from Lymph Node Cells of Immunized Rabbits.   Experientia, *24*: 948–949, 1968.

15. Bartfelt, H., and Atoynatan, T.   Cytophilic Nature of Migration Inhibitory Factor Associated with Delayed Hypersensitivity.   Proc. Soc. Exp. Biol. Med., *130*: 497–501, 1969.

16. Bendixen, G., and Søborg, M.   Comments on the Leukocyte Migration Technique as an *in vitro* Method for Demonstrating Cellular Hypersensitivity in Man.   J. Immunol., *104*: 1551–1552, 1970.

17. Bennett, B.   Specific Suppression of Tumour Growth by Isolated Peritoneal Macrophages from Immunized Mice.   J. Immunol., *95*: 656–664, 1965.

18. Bennett, B., and Bloom, B. R.   Studies on the Migration Inhibitory Factor Associated with Delayed Type Hypersensitivity: Cytodynamics and Specificity.   Transplantation, *5*: 996–1000, 1967.

19. Bennett, B., and Bloom, B. R.   Reactions *in vivo* and *in vitro* Produced by a Soluble Substance Associated with Delayed-type Hypersensitivity.   Proc. Nat. Acad. Sci. (Wash.), *59*: 756–762, 1968.

20. Bloch-Shtacher, N., Hirschhorn, K., and Uhr, J. W.   The Response of Lymphocytes from Non-immunized Humans to Antigen-antibody Complexes.   Clin. Exp. Immunol., *3*: 889–899, 1968.

21. Bloom, B. R., and Bennett, B.   Mechanism of a Reaction *in vitro* Associated with Delayed-type Hypersensitivity.   Science, *153*: 80–82, 1966.

22. Bloom, B. R., and Bennett, B.   Migration Inhibitory Factor Associated with De-

layed-type Hypersensitivity. Fed. Proc., *27*: 13–20, 1968.

23. Bloom, B. R., and Bennett, B.   Relation of the Migration Inhibitory Factor (MIF) to Delayed-type Hypersensitivity Reactions.   Ann. N.Y. Acad. Sci., *169*: 258–265, 1970.

24. Bondevik, H., and Mannick, J. A.   RNA-mediated Transfer of Lymphocyte vs. Target Cell Activity.   Proc. Soc. Exp. Biol. Med., *129*: 264–268, 1968.

25. Bosman, C., and Feldman, J. D.   Composition, Morphology, and Source of Cells in Delayed Skin Reactions.   Am. J. Pathol., *58*: 201–218, 1970.

26. Brostoff, J., and Roitt, I.   Cell-mediated (Delayed) Hypersensitivity in Patients with Summer Hay Fever.   Lancet, *2*: 1269–1272, 1969.

27. Brunner, K. T., Mauel, J., Cerottini, J.-C., and Chapuis, B.   Quantitative Assay of the Lytic Action of Immune Lymphoid Cells on ^{51}Cr-labelled Allogeneic Target Cells *in vitro*; Inhibition by Isoantibody and by Drugs.   Immunology, *14*: 181–196, 1968.

28. Brunner, K. T., Mauel, J., Rudolf, H., and Chapuis, B.   Studies of Allograft Immunity in Mice.   I. Induction, Development and *in vitro* Assay of Cellular Immunity.   Immunology, *18*: 501–515, 1970.

29. Bubenik, J., Perlmann, P., Helmstein, K., and Moberger, G.   Cellular and Humoral Immune Responses to Human Urinary Bladder Carcinomas.   Int. J. Cancer, *5*: 310–319, 1970.

30. Bullock, W. E.   Impairment of Phytohaemagglutinin (PHA) and Antigen-induced DNA Synthesis in Leukocytes Cultured from Patients with Leprosy.   Clin. Res., *16*: 328, 1968.

31. Burrow, D. D., and Forbes, I. J.   Depression of the Primary Immune Response by Serum Protein Fractions.   Proc. Aust. Soc. Med. Res., *2*: 292, 1969.

32. Carpenter, C. B., Phillips, S. M., Boylston, A. W., and Merrill, J. P.   Immunosuppressive Alpha Globulin from Bovine Thymus: Mechanism of Action.   Third International Congress of the Transplantation Society, Abstracts, pp. 247, The Hague, 1970.

33. Chakrabarty, A. K., and Friedman, H.   Nucleases in Immunity. II.   Ineffectiveness of Exogenous RNAase on the Antibody Plaque Response of Immunized Mice. Clin. Exp. Immunol., *6*: 619–625, 1970.

34. Chase, M. W.   The Cellular Transfer of Cutaneous Hypersensitivity to Tuberculin.   Proc. Soc. Exp. Biol. Med., *59*: 134–135, 1945.

35. Cohen, S., Benacerraf, B., McCluskey, R. T., and Ovary, Z.   Effect of Anticoagulants on Delayed Hypersensitivity Reactions.   J. Immunol., *98*: 351–358, 1967.

36. Cooperband, S. R., Bondevik, H., Schmid, K., and Mannick, J. A.   Transformation of Human Lymphocytes: Inhibition by Homologous Alpha Globulin.   Science, *159*: 1243–1244, 1968.

37. Cooperband, S. R., Davis, R. C., Schmid, K., and Mannick, J. A.   Competitive Blockade of Lymphocyte Stimulation by a Serum Immuno-regulatory Alpha Globulin (IRA).   Transplantation Proc., *1*: 516–523, 1969.

38. Crowle, A. J.   Tuberculin Skin Reactions in Mice Hypersensitized by Vaccination with Living Avirulent Tubercle Bacilli.   Am. Rev. Respir. Dis., *81*: 893–903, 1960.

39. Crowle, A. J., and Hu, C. C.   Split Tolerance Affecting Delayed Hypersensitivity and Induced in Mice by Pre-immunization with Protein Antigens in Solution.   Clin. Exp. Immunol., *1*: 323–335, 1966.

40. Crowle, A. J., and Hu, C. C.   Specificity of Inhibition by Antiserum of the Development of Immediate and Delayed Hypersensitivities in Mice.   Proc. Soc. Exp. Biol.

Med., *127*: 190–193, 1968.

41. Crowle, A. J., and Hu, C. C.   Studies on the Induction and Time Course of Repression of Delayed Hypersensitivity in the Mouse by Low and High Doses of Antigen. Clin. Exp. Immunol., *6*: 363–374, 1970.

42. David, J. R.   Delayed Hypersensitivity *in vitro* : Its Mediation by Cell-free Substances Formed by Lymphoid Cell-Antigen Interaction.   Proc. Nat. Acad. Sci., (Wash.), *56*: 72–77, 1966.

43. David, J. R.   Macrophage Migration.   Fed. Proc., *27*: 6–12, 1968.

44. Davis, R. C., Cooperband, S. R., and Mannick, J. A.   Evaluation of the Immunosuppressive Properties of Ribonuclease Complexes.   J. Immunol., *103*: 1029–1037, 1969.

45. Dekaris, D., Fauve, R. M., and Raynaud, M.   Delayed Hypersensitivity and Inhibition of Macrophage Spreading : *in vivo* and *in vitro* Studies of Tuberculin and Streptococcal Hypersensitivities in Guinea Pigs.   J. Immunol., *103*: 1–5, 1969.

46. Dumonde, D. C.   The Role of the Macrophage in Delayed Hypersensitivity.   Brit. Med. Bull., *23*: 9–14, 1967.

47. Dumonde, D. C., Wolstencraft, R. A., Panayi, G. S., Matthew, M., Morley, J., and Howson, W. T.   " Lymphokines " : Non-antibody Mediators of Cellular Immunity Generated by Lymphocyte Activation.   Nature, *224*: 38–42, 1969.

48. Dupuy, J.-M., Perey, D. Y. E., and Good, R. A.   Passive Transfer with Plasma of Delayed Allergy in Guinea Pigs.   Lancet, *1*: 551–553, 1969.

49. Dupuy, J.-M., Kalpaktosoglou, P., and Good, R. A.   Transfer with a Plasma Fraction of Delayed Hypersensitivity to PPD in Guinea Pigs.   J. Immunol., *104*: 1384–1387, 1970.

50. Falk, R. E., Collste, L., and Möller, G.   Release of Migration Inhibitory Factors from Immune Rat Lymphocytes Confronted with Histocompatibility Antigens. Nature, *224*: 1206–1207, 1969.

51. Falk, R. E., Collste, L., and Möller, G.   *In vitro* Detection of Transplantation Immunity ; the Inhibition of Migration of Immune Spleen Cells and Peripheral Blood Leukocytes by Specific Antigen.   J. Immunol., *101*: 1287–1292, 1970.

52. Fass, L., Herberman, R. B., and Ziegler, J.   Delayed Cutaneous Hypersensitivity to Burkitt-lymphoma Cells.   New England J. Med., *282*: 776–780, 1970.

53. Fass, L., Herberman, R. B., Ziegler, J. L., and Kiryabwire, J. W. M., Cutaneous Hypersensitivity Reactions to Autologous Extracts of Malignant Melanoma Cells. Lancet, *1*: 116–118, 1970.

54. Fauve, R. M., Pierce-Chase, C. H., and Dubos, R.   Corynebacterial Pseudotuberculosis in Mice.   II. Activation of Natural and Experimental Latent Infections.   J. Exp. Med., *120*: 283–304, 1964.

55. Feinman, L., Cohen, S., and Becker, E. L.   The Effect of Fumopimaric Acid on Delayed Hypersensitivity and Cutaneous Forssman Reactions in the Guinea Pig.   J. Immunol., *104*: 1401–1405, 1970.

56. Fisherman, E. W.   Does the Allergic Diathesis Influence Malignancy?   J. Allergy, *31*: 74–78, 1960.

57. Forbes, I. J.   Mitosis in Mouse Peritoneal Macrophages.   J. Immunol., *96*: 734–743, 1966.

58. George M., and Vaughan, J. H.   *In vitro* Cell Migration as a Model for Delayed Hypersensitivity.   Proc. Soc. Exp. Biol. Med., *111*: 514–521, 1962.

59. Gershon, R. K., Carter, R. L., and Kondo, K.   On Concomitant Immunity in Tumour Bearing Hamsters.   Nature, *213*: 674–676, 1967.

60. Gershon, R. K., Carter, R. L., and Lane, N. J. Studies on Homotransplantable Lymphomas in Hamsters. IV. Observations on Macrophages in the Expression of Tumour Immunity. Am. J. Pathol., *51*: 1111–1133, 1967.

61. Gershon, R. K., Carter, R. L., and Kondo, K. Immunologic Defenses Against Metastases: Impairment by Excision of an Allotransplanted Lymphoma. Science, *159*: 646–648, 1968.

62. Gewurz, H., Clark, D. S., Finstad, J., Kelly, W. D., and Varco, R. L. Role of the Complement System in Graft Rejections in Experimental Animals and Man. Ann. N.Y. Acad. Sci., *129*: 673–713, 1966.

63. Golob, E. K., Israsena, T., Quatrale, A. C., and Becker, K. L. Effect of Serum from Cancer Patients on Homologous Lymphocyte Cultures. Cancer, *23*: 306–308, 1969.

64. Good, R. A., Dalmasso, A. P., Martinez, C., Archer, O. K., Pierce, J. C., and Papermaster, B. W. The Role of the Thymus in Development of Immunologic Capacity in Rabbits and Mice. J. Exp. Med., *116*: 773–796, 1962.

65. Gorer, P. A. Some Recent Work on Tumour Immunity. Adv. Cancer Res., *4*: 149–186, 1956.

66. Govaerts, A. Cellular Antibodies in Kidney Homotransplantation. J. Immunol., *85*: 516–522, 1960.

67. Granger, G. A., and Weiser, R. S. Homograft Target Cells: Specific Destruction *in vitro* by Contact Interaction with Immune Macrophages. Science, *145*: 1427–1429, 1964.

68. Granger, G. A., and Weiser, R. S. Homograft Target Cells: Contact Destruction *in vitro* by Immune Macrophages. Science, *151*: 97–99, 1966.

69. Granger, G. A., Rudin, J., and Weiser, R. S. The Role of Cytophilic Antibody in Immune Macrophage-target Cell Interaction. J. Reticuloendothelial Soc., *3*: 354, 1966.

70. Granger, G. A., Shacks, S. J., Williams, T. W., and Kolb, W. P. Lymphocyte *in vitro* Cytotoxicity: Specific Release of Lymphotoxin-like Materials from Tuberculin-Sensitive Lymphoid Cells. Nature, *221*: 1155–1157, 1969.

71. Granger, G. A., Moore, G. E., White, J. G., Matzinger, P., Sundsmo, S., Shupe, S., Kolb, W. P., Kramer, J., and Glade, P. R. Production of Lymphotoxin and Migration Inhibitory Factor by Established Human Lymphocyte Cell Lines. J. Immunol., *104*: 1476–1485, 1970.

72. Hall, W. J., Francis, L., and Atkins, E. Studies on Tuberculin Fever. IV. The Passive Transfer of Reactivity with Various Tissues of Sensitized Donor Rabbits. J. Exp. Med., *131*: 483–498, 1970.

73. Han, S.-H., and Weiser, R. S. Systemic Tuberculin Sensitivity in Mice. III. The Effects of Adrenalectomy and Treatment with Anti-anaphylactic Agents. J. Immunol., *98*: 1163–1166, 1967.

74. Heise, E. R., and Weiser, R. S. Factors in Delayed Sensitivity: Lymphocyte and Macrophage Cytotoxins in the Tuberculin Reaction. J. Immunol., *103*: 570–576, 1969.

75. Heise, E. R., Han, S.-H., and Weiser, R. S. *In vitro* Studies on the Mechanism of Macrophage Migration Inhibition in Tuberculin Sensitivity. J. Immunol., *101*: 1004–1015, 1968.

76. Hellström, I., and Hellström, K. E. Studies on Cellular Immunity and Its Serum-mediated Inhibition in Moloney-virus-induced Mouse Sarcomas. Int. J. Cancer, *4*: 587–600, 1969.

77. Hellström, I., and Hellström, K. E. Colony Inhibition Studies on Blocking and Non-blocking Serum Effects on Cellular Immunity to Moloney Sarcomas. Int. J. Cancer, *5*: 195–201, 1970.

78. Hellström, I., Evans, C. A., and Hellström, K. E. Cellular Immunity and Its Serum-mediated Inhibition in Shope-virus-induced Rabbit Papillomas. Int. J. Cancer, *4*: 601–607, 1969.

79. Hellström, I., Hellström, K. E., Pierce, G. E., and Yang, J. P. S. Cellular and Humoral Immunity to Different Types of Human Neoplasms. Nature, *220*: 1352–1354, 1968.

80. Hellström, I. E., Hellström, K. E., Pierce, G. E., and Bill, A. H. Demonstration of Cell-bound and Humoral Immunity Against Neuroblastoma Cells. Proc. Nat. Acad. Sci. (Wash.), *60*: 1231–1238, 1968.

81. Hellström, I., Hellström, K. E., Evans, C. A., Heppner, G. H., Pierce, G. E. and Yang, J. P. S. Serum mediated Protection of Neoplastic Cells from Inhibition by Lymphocytes Immune to Their Tumour-specific Antigens. Proc. Nat. Acad. Sci. (Wash.), *62*: 362–368, 1969.

82. Hellström, K. E., and Möller, G. Immunological and Immunogenetic Aspects of Tumour Transplantation. Progr. Allergy, *9*: 158–245, 1965.

83. Hill, W. C. The Influence of the Cellular Infiltrate on the Evolution and Intensity of Delayed-hypersensitivity Reactions. J. Exp. Med., *129*: 363–370, 1969.

84. Holm, G., and Perlmann, P. Cytotoxic Potential of Stimulated Human Lymphocytes. J. Exp. Med., *125*: 721–736, 1967.

85. Holm, G., and Perlmann, P. Quantitative Studies on Phytohaemagglutinin-induced Cytotoxicity by Human Lymphocytes Against Homologous Cells in Tissue Culture. Immunology, *12*: 525–536, 1967.

86. Hoy, W. E., and Nelson, D. S. Studies on Cytophilic Antibodies. V. Alloantibodies Cytophilic for Mouse Macrophages. Aust. J. Exp. Biol. Med. Sci., *47*: 525–539, 1969.

87. Hughes, L. E., Kearney, R., and Tully, M. A Study in Clinical Cancer Immunotherapy. Cancer, *26*: 269–278, 1970.

88. Hulliger, L., Blazkovec, A. A., and Sorkin, E. A Study of the Passive Cellular Transfer of Local Cutaneous Hypersensitivity. IV. Transfer of Hypersensitivity to Sheep Erythrocytes with Peritoneal Exudate Cells Passively Coated with Antibody. Int. Arch. Allergy, *33*: 281–291, 1968.

89. Janis, M., and Bach, F. H. Potentiation of *in vitro* Lymphocyte Reactivity. Nature, *225*: 238–239, 1970.

90. Jankovic, B. D., and Dvorak, H. F. Enzymatic Inactivation of Immunologically Competent Lymph Node Cells in the " Transfer Reaction ". J. Immunol., *89*: 571–581, 1962.

91. Jankovic, B. D., and Flax, M. H. Alterations in the Development of Experimental Allergic Thyroiditis Induced by Injection of Homologous Thyroid Extract. J. Immunol., *90*: 178–184, 1963.

92. Johanovsky, J. Production of Pyrogenic Substances in the Reaction of Cells of Hypersensitive Guinea Pigs with Antigen *in vitro*. Immunology, *3*: 179–189, 1960.

93. Journey, L. J., and Amos, D. B. An Electron Microscope Study of Histiocyte Responses to Ascites Tumour Homografts. Cancer Res., *22*: 998–1001, 1962.

94. Jureziz, R. E., Thor, D. E., and Dray, S. Transfer with RNA Extracts of the Cell Migration Inhibition Correlate of Delayed Hypersensitivity in the Guinea Pig. J. Immunol., *101*: 823–829, 1968.

95. Kaliss, N. Immunological Enhancement and Inhibition of Tumour Growth: Relationship to Various Immunological Mechanisms. Fed. Proc., *24*: 1024–1029, 1965.

96. Kamrin, B. B. Successful Skin Homografts in Mature Non-littermate Rats Treated with Fractions Containing Alpha-globulins. Proc. Soc. Exp. Biol. Med., *100*: 58–61, 1959.

97. Kasakura, S. Production and Specificity of a Blastogenic Factor in Mixed Leukocyte Cultures from Twin Sisters. Nature, *225*: 507–508, 1970.

98. Kass, E. H. Hormones and Host Resistance to Infection. Bact. Rev., *24*: 177–185, 1960.

99. Kass, E. H., and Finland, M. Adrenocortical Hormones in Infection and Immunity. Ann. Rev. Microbiol., *7*: 361–388, 1953.

100. Kikuchi, K., Reiner, J., and Southam, C. M. Diffusible Cytotoxic Substances and Cell-mediated Resistance to Syngeneic Tumours : *in vitro* Demonstration. Science, *165*: 77–79, 1969.

101. Klein, G. Tumour-specific Transplantation Antigens. Cancer Res., *28*: 625–635, 1968.

102. Klein, G., Sjögren, H. O., Klein, E., and Hellström, K. E. Demonstration of Resistance Against Methylcholanthrene-induced Sarcomas in the Primary Autochthonous Host. Cancer Res., *20*: 1561–1572, 1960.

103. Kosunen, T. U., Waksman, B. H., Flax, M. H., and Tihen, W. S. Radioautographic Study of Cellular Mechanisms in Delayed Hypersensitivity. I. Delayed Reactions to Tuberculin and Purified Proteins in the Rat and Guinea Pig. Immunology, *6*: 276–290, 1963.

104. Kreth, H. W., Thiessen, G., and Deicher, H. The Effect of Antigen Given Intravenously on Specific Antigen-sensitive Lymphocytes of Peripheral Blood in Man. Clin. Exp. Immunol., *7*: 109–114, 1970.

105. Kruger, G., Morphologic Studies of Lymphoid Tissues During the Growth of an Isotransplanted Mouse Tumour. J. Nat. Cancer Inst., *39*: 1–15, 1967.

106. Landsteiner, K., and Chase, M. W. Experiments on Transfer of Cutaneous Sensitivity to Simple Compounds. Proc. Soc. Exp. Biol. Med., *49*: 688–690, 1942.

107. Law, L. W. Studies of the Significance of Tumor Antigens in Induction and Repression of Neoplastic Diseases. Cancer Res., *29*: 1–21, 1969.

108. Lawrence, H. S. Transfer Factor. Adv. Immunol., *11*: 195–266, 1969.

109. Lawrence, H. S. Transfer Factor and Cellular Immune Deficiency Disease. New England J. Med., *283*: 411–419, 1970.

110. Leading Article: Cell-mediated Immunity in Hay Fever. Lancet, *1*: 27, 1970.

111. Levene, G. M., Turk, J. L., Wright, D. J. M., and Grimble, A. G. S. Reduced Lymphocyte Transformation Due to a Plasma Factor in Patients with Active Syphilis. Lancet, *2*: 246–247, 1969.

112. Lidén, S. The Mononuclear Cell Infiltrate in Allergic Contact Dermatitis. 2. Selective Accumulation of Cells from the Bone Marrow. Acta Pathol. et Microbiol. Scand., *70*: 58–66, 1967.

113. Lischner, H. W., and Di George, A. M. Role of the Thymus in Humoral Immunity. Observations in Complete or Partial Congenital Absence of the Thymus. Lancet, *2*: 1044–1049, 1969.

114. Lokaj, J., Zellaffine Antikörper und Ihre Biologische Bedeutung. Z. Bakt I Referate, *217*: 923–946, 1969.

115. Lolekna, S., Dray, S., and Gotoff, S. P. Macrophage Aggregation *in vitro* : a Cor-

relate of Delayed Hypersensitivity. J. Immunol., *104*: 296–304, 1970.

116. Lubaroff, D. M., and Waksman, B. H. Bone Marrow as Source of Cells in Reactions of Cellular Hypersensitivity. I. Passive Transfer of Tuberculin Sensitivity in Syngeneic Systems. J. Exp. Med., *128*: 1425–1435, 1968.

117 Lubaroff, D. M., and Waksman, B. H. Bone Marrow as Source of Cells in Reactions of Cellular Hypersensitivity. II. Identification of Allogeneic or Hybrid Cells by Immunofluorescence in Passively Transferred Tuberculin Reactions. J. Exp. Med., *128*: 1437–1449, 1968.

118. Lundgren, G., and Möller, G. Non-specific Induction of Cytotoxicity in Normal Human Lymphocytes *in vitro*: Studies of Mechanism and Specificity of the Reaction. Clin. Exp. Immunol., *4*: 435–452, 1969.

119. Lundgren, G., Collste, L., and Möller, G. Cytotoxicity of Human Lymphocytes: Antagonism between Inducing Processes. Nature, *220*: 289–291, 1968.

120. Lurie, M. B. The Reticuloendothelial System, Cortisone, and Thyroid Function: Their Relation to Native Resistance to Infection. Ann. N. Y. Acad. Sci., *88*: 83–98, 1960.

121. Mackaness, G. B. The Behaviour of Microbial Parasites in Relation to Phagocytic Cells *in vitro* and *in vivo*. *In* H. Smith and J. Taylor (eds.), Microbial Behaviour '*in vivo*' and '*in vitro*', 14th Symposium of the Society for General Microbiology, pp. 213–240. Cambridge, Cambridge University Press, 1964.

122. Mackaness, G. B. The Relationship of Delayed Hypersensitivity to Acquired Cellular Resistance. Brit. Med. Bull., *23*: 52–54, 1967.

123. Mackaness, G. B. The Influence of Immunologically Committed Lymphoid Cells on Macrophage Activity *in vivo*. J. Exp. Med., *129*: 973–992, 1969.

124. Mackaness, G. B., and Blanden, R. V. Cellular Immunity. Progr. Allergy, *11*: 89–140, 1967.

125. McKhann, C. F. Primary Malignancy in Patients Undergoing Immunosuppression for Renal Transplantation. Transplantation, *8*: 209–212, 1969.

126. MacLennan, I. C. M., and Harding, B. The Role of Immunoglobulins in Lymphocyte-mediated Cell Damage, *in vitro*. II. The Mechanism of Target Cell Damage by Lymphoid Cells from Immunized Rats. Immunology, *18*: 405–412, 1970.

127. MacLennan, I. C. M., Loewi, G., and Harding, B. The Role of Immunoglobulins in Lymphocyte-mediated Cell Damage, *in vitro*. I. Comparison of the Effects of Target Cell Specific Antibody and Normal Serum Factors on Cellular Damage by Immune and Non-immune Lymphocytes. Immunology, *18*: 397–404, 1970.

128. MacLennan, I. C. M., Loewi, G., and Howard, A. A Serum Immunoglobulin with Specificity for Certain Homologous Target Cells Which Induces Target Cell Damage by Normal Human Lymphocytes. Immunology, *17*: 887–910, 1969.

129. Maini, R. N., Bryceson, A. D. M., Wolstencroft, R. A., and Dumonde, D. C. Lymphocyte Mitogenic Factor in Man. Nature, *224*: 43–44, 1969.

130. Mannick, J. A., and Schmid, K. Prolongation of Allograft Survival by an Alpha Globulin Isolated from Normal Blood. Transplantation, *5*: 1231–1238, 1967.

131. Mauel, J., Rudolf, H., Chapuis, B., and Brunner, K. T. Studies of Allograft Immunity in Mice. II. Mechanism of Target Cell Inactivation *in vitro* by Sensitized Lymphocytes. Immunology, *18*: 517–535, 1970.

132. Mayhew, E., and Weiss, L. Ribonucleic Acid at the Periphery of Different Cell Types, and Effect of Growth Rate on Ionogenic Groups in the Periphery of Cultured Cells. Exp. Cell Res., *50*: 441–453, 1968.

133. Mella, B., and Lang, D. J. Chromosomal Aberrations and Suppression of Leuko-

cyte Mitosis Induced *in vitro* by a Circulating Factor Associated with Acute Infectious Hepatitis. Ann. N.Y. Acad. Sci., *155*: 880–887, 1968.

134. Mella, B., and Taswell, H. F. Suppression of Leukocyte Mitosis by Sera of Hepatitis Implicated Donors. Am. J. Clin. Path., *53*: 141–144, 1970.

135. Metcalf, D. The Thymus. Its Role in Immune Responses, Leukaemia Development and Carcinogenesis. Berlin, Heidelberg and New York, Springer-Verlag, 1966.

136. Mikulska, Z. B., Smith, C., and Alexander, P. Evidence for an Immunological Reaction of the Host Against Its Own Actively Growing Primary Tumor. J. Nat. Cancer Inst., *36*: 29–35, 1966.

137. Mildenhall, P., and Nelson, D. S. Serological Responses of Mice During Active Enhancement of Tumour Allografts. Brit. J. Exp. Path., *49*: 170–178, 1968.

138. Miller, J. F. A. P. Immunological Functions of the Thymus. Lancet, *2*: 748–749, 1961.

139. Miller, J. F. A. P. Effect of Neonatal Thymectomy on the Immunological Responsiveness of the Mouse. Proc. Roy. Soc. B., *156*: 415–428, 1962.

140. Miller, J. F. A. P., and Osoba, D. The Role of the Thymus in the Origin of Immunological Competence. *In* Wolstenholme, G. E. W., and Knight, J. (eds.), The Immunologically Competent Cell, Ciba Foundation Study Group No. 16, pp. 62–70. London, J. and A. Churchill, 1963.

141. Mills, J. A. The Immunological Significance of Antigen Induced Lymphocyte Transformation *in vitro*. J. Immunol., *97*: 239–247, 1966.

142. Möller, E. Contact-induced Cytotoxicity by Lymphoid Cells Containing Foreign Iso-antigens. Science, *147*: 873–879, 1965.

143. Möller, G. Induction of DNA Synthesis in Normal Human Lymphocyte Cultures by Antigen-antibody Complexes. Clin. Exp. Immunol., *4*: 65–82, 1969.

144. Moorhead, J. F., Paraskova-Tchernozenska, E., Pirrie, A. J., and Hayes, C. Lymphoid Inhibitor of Human Lymphocyte DNA Synthesis and Mitosis *in vitro*. Nature, *224*: 1207–1208, 1969.

145. Mowbray, J. F. Inhibition of Immune Responses by Injection of Large Doses of a Serum Glycoprotein Fraction. Fed. Proc., *22*: 441, 1963.

146. Mowbray, J. F., and Scholand, S. Inhibition of Antibody Production by Ribonuclease. Immunology, *11*: 421–426, 1966.

147. Mowbray, J. F., Boylston, A. W., Milton, J. D., and Weksler, M. Studies on the Mode of Action of Immunosuppressive Ribonucleases. Antibiot. et Chemother., *15*: 384–392, 1969.

148. Nakamura, R. M., and Weigle, W. O. Transfer of Experimental Autoimmune Thyroiditis by Serum from Thyroidectomized Donors. J. Exp. Med., *130*: 263–285, 1969.

149. Nelson, D. S. Immunological Enhancement of Skin Homografts in Guinea Pigs. Brit. J. Exp. Path., *43*: 1–11, 1962.

150. Nelson, D. S. Reaction to Antigen *in vivo* of the Peritoneal Macrophages of Guinea Pigs with Delayed-type Hypersensitivity. Effects of Anticoagulants and Other Drugs. Lancet, *2*: 175–176, 1963.

151. Nelson, D. S. The Effects of Anticoagulants and Other Drugs on Cellular and Cutaneous Reactions to Antigen in Guinea Pigs with Delayed-type Hypersensitivity. Immunology, *9*: 219–234, 1965.

152. Nelson, D. S. Local Passive Transfer of Reactivity of Peritoneal Macrophages to Antigen: Possible Role of Cytophilic Antibody in one Manifestation of Delayed-

type Hypersensitivity. Nature, *212* : 259–261, 1966.

153. Nelson, D. S. Macrophages and Immunity. Amsterdam, North-Holland Publishing Company, 1969.

154. Nelson, D. S. Studies on Cytophilic Antibodies. A Mouse Serum "Antibody" Having an Affinity for Macrophages and Fast Alpha-globulin Mobility. Aust. J. Exp. Biol. Med. Sci., *48* : 329–341, 1970.

155. Nelson, D. S., and Boyden, S. V. Macrophage Cytophilic Antibodies and Delayed Hypersensitivity. Brit. Med. Bull., *23* : 15–20, 1967.

156. Nelson, D. S., and Kossard, S. The Peritoneal Macrophage Disappearance Reaction in Guinea Pigs with Delayed-type Hypersensitivity. Proc. XI Congr. Int. Soc. Blood Transfusion, Sydney, 1966. Bibl. Haemat. No. 29, Part 2, pp. 643–652, Basel, Karger, 1968.

157. Nelson, D. S., and Mildenhall, P. Studies on Cytophilic Antibodies. II. The Production by Guinea Pigs of Cytophilic Antibodies to Sheep Erythrocytes and Human Serum Albumin ; Relationship to the Production of Other Antibodies and the Development of Delayed-type Hypersensitivity. Aust. J. Exp. Biol. Med. Sci., *46* : 33–49, 1968.

158. Nelson, D. S., Nelson, M., Thurston, J. M., Waters, M. F. R., and Pearson, J. M. H. Phytohaemagglutinin-induced Lymphocyte Transformation in Leprosy. Clin. Exp. Immunol., *9*, 33, 1971.

159. Neveu, T., and Biozzi, G. The Effect of Decomplementation on Delayed-type Hypersensitive Reactions to a Conjugated Antigen in Rats. Immunology, *9* : 303–309, 1965.

160. Nicol, T., and Vernon-Roberts, B. The Influence of the Estrus Cycle, Pregnancy and Ovariectomy on RES Activity. J. Reticuloendothelial Soc., *2* : 15–29, 1965.

161. Nomoto, K., Gershon, R. K., and Waksman, B. H. Role of Non-immunized Macrophages in the Rejection of an Allotransplanted Lymphoma. J. Nat. Cancer Inst., *44* : 739–749, 1970.

162. North, R. J. Cellular Kinetics Associated with the Development of Acquired Cellular Resistance. J. Exp. Med., *130* : 299–314, 1969.

163. North, R. J. The Mitotic Potential of Fixed Phagocytes in the Liver as Revealed During the Development of Cellular Immunity. J. Exp. Med., *130* : 315–326, 1969.

164. Old, L. J., Boyse, E. A., Bennett, B., and Lilly, F. Peritoneal Cells as an Immune Population in Transplantation Studies. *In* B. Amos, and H. Koprowski (eds.), Cell-bound Antibodies, pp. 89–98. Philadelphia, The Wistar Institute Press, 1963.

165. Oppenheim, J. Relationship of *in vitro* Lymphocyte Transformation to Delayed Hypersensitivity in Guinea Pigs and Man. Fed. Proc., *27* : 21–28, 1968.

166. Osoba, D. The Effects of Thymus and Other Lymphoid Organs Enclosed in Millipore Diffusion Chambers on Neonatally Thymectomized Mice. J. Exp. Med., *122* : 633–650, 1965.

167. Pappas, A., and Scheurlen, P. G. Untersuchungen über den Einflusz von Plasma Hodgkin Kranker auf die Phytohämagglutinin Transformation Normaler Lymphocyten. Verhandl. Dtsch. Gesellsch. Inn. Med., *74* : 1254–1256, 1968.

168. Perlmann, P., and Holm, G. Cytotoxic Effects of Lymphoid Cells *in vitro*. Adv. Immunol., *11* : 117–193, 1969.

169. Perlmann, P., Perlmann, H., Müller-Eberhard, H. J., and Manni, J. A. Cytotoxic Effects of Leukocytes Triggered by Complement Bound to Target Cells. Science, *163* : 937–939, 1969.

170. Pick, E., Krejci, J., Cech, K., and Turk, J. L. Interaction between " Sensitized Lymphocytes " and Antigen *in vitro*. I. The Release of a Skin-reactive Factor. Immunology, *17*: 741–767, 1969.

171. Pick, E., Krejci, J., and Turk, J. L. Release of Skin Reactive Factor from Guinea Pig Lymphocytes by Mitogens. Nature, *225*: 236–238, 1970.

172. Pierpaoli, W., and Sorkin, E. Hormones and Immunologic Capacity. I. Effect of Heterologous Anti-growth Hormone (ASTH) Antiserum on Thymus and Peripheral Lymphatic Tissue in Mice. Induction of a Wasting Syndrome. J. Immunol., *101*: 1036–1043, 1968.

173. Pierpaoli, W., Baroni, C., Fabris, N., and Sorkin, E. Hormones and Immunological Capacity. II. Reconstitution of Antibody Production in Hormonally Deficient Mice by Somatotropic Hormone, Thyrotropic Hormone and Thyroxin. Immunology, *16*: 217–230, 1969.

174. Pincus, W. B. Formation of Cytotoxic Factor by Macrophages from Normal Guinea Pigs. J. Reticuloendothelial Soc., *4*: 122–139, 1967.

175. Pincus, W. B. Cell-free Cytotoxic Fluids from Tuberculin-treated Guinea Pigs. J. Reticuloendothelial Soc., *4*: 140–150, 1967.

176. Pullar, D. M., James, K., and Naysmith, J. D. The Effect of an Alpha-globulin Preparation and of Polyribonuclease Complexes on Humoral Antibody Formation. Clin. Exp. Immunol., *3*: 457–461, 1968.

177. Ralston, D. J., and Elberg, S. S. Serum-mediated Immune Cellular Responses to *Brucella melitensis* Rev. 1. III. Infection of Macrophages Fixed-to-glass. Brit. J. Exp. Path., *49*: 586–596, 1968.

178. Remold, H. G., and David, J. R. Cellular Hypersensitivity: Characterization of Migration Inhibitory Factor (MIF) by Enzymatic Treatment. Fed. Proc., *29*: 305, 1970.

179. Rocklin, R. E., Meyers, O. L., and David, J. R. An *in vitro* Assay for Cellular Hypersensitivity in Man. J. Immunol., *104*: 95–102, 1970.

180. Rocklin, R. E., Rosen, F., and David, J. R. *In vitro* Lymphocyte Response of Patients with Immunological Deficiency Diseases: Correlation of Production of Macrophage Inhibitory Factor with Delayed Hypersensitivity. New England J. Med., *282*: 1340–1343, 1970.

181. Rosenau, W., and Moon, H. D. Cellular Reactions to Methylcholanthrene-induced Sarcomas Transplanted to Isogenic Mice. Lab. Invest., *15*: 1212–1224, 1966.

182. Rowley, D., Turner, K. J., and Jenkin, C. R. The Basis for Immunity to Mouse Typhoid. 3. Cell-bound Antibody. Aust. J. Exp. Biol. Med. Sci., *42*: 237–248, 1964.

183. Ruddle, N. H., and Waksman, B. H. Cytotoxicity Mediated by Soluble Antigen and Lymphocytes in Delayed Hypersensitivity. I. Characterization of the Phenomenon. J. Exp. Med., *128*: 1237–1254, 1968.

184. Ruddle, N. H., and Waksman, B. H. Cytotoxicity Mediated by Soluble Antigen and Lymphocytes in Delayed Hypersensitivity. II. Correlation of the *in vitro* Response with Skin Reactivity. J. Exp. Med., *128*: 1255–1265, 1968.

185. Ruddle, N. H., and Waksman, B. H. Cytotoxicity Mediated by Soluble Antigen and Lymphocytes in Delayed Hypersensitivity. III. Analysis of Mechanism. J. Exp. Med., *128*: 1267–1279, 1968.

186. Schwartz, H. J., Leon, M. A., and Pelley, R. P. Concanavalin A-induced Release of Skin Reactive Factor from Lymphoid Cells. J. Immunol., *104*: 265–268, 1970.

187. Shaw, C.-M., Fahlberg, W. J., Kies, M. W., and Alvord, E. C., Jr., Suppression of Experimental "Allergic" Encephalomyelitis in Guinea Pigs by Encephalitogenic Proteins Extracted from Homologous Brain. J. Exp. Med., *111*: 171–180, 1960.

188. Silk, M. Effect of Plasma from Patients with Carcinoma on *in vitro* Lymphocyte Transformation. Cancer, *20*: 2088–2089, 1967.

189. Søborg, M., and Bendixen, G. Human Lymphocyte Migration as a Parameter of Hypersensitivity. Acta Med. Scand., *181*: 247–256, 1967.

190. Spector, W. G. Histology of Allergic Inflammation. Brit. Med. Bull., *23*: 35–38, 1967.

191. Spitler, L. E., and Fudenberg, H. H. Serum Transfer of a "Cellular Immune Response". Fed. Proc., *29*: 305, 1970.

192. Spitler, L. E., and Fudenberg, H. H. Products of Interaction of Antigen-sensitized Leukocytes and Antigen: Further Characterization of the Mitogenic Factor. J. Immunol., *104*: 544–549, 1970.

193. Spitler, L. E., Huber, H., and Fudenberg, H. H. Inhibition of Capillary Migration by Antigen-antibody Complexes. J. Immunol., *102*: 404–411, 1969.

194. Stuart, F. P., Saitoh, T., Fitch, F. W., and Spargo, B. H. Immunologic Enhancement of Renal Allografts in the Rat. Surgery, *64*: 17–24, 1968.

195. Stutman, O., Yunis, E. J., and Good, R. A. Carcinogen-induced Tumours of Thymus. III. Restoration of Neonatally Thymectomized Mice With Thymomas in Cell-impermeable Chambers. J. Nat. Cancer Inst., *43*: 499–508, 1969.

196. Stutman, O., Yunis, E. J., and Good, R. A. Carcinogen-induced Tumours of the Thymus. IV. Humoral Influences of Normal Thymus and Functional Thymomas and Influence of Post-thymectomy Period on Restoration. J. Exp. Med., *130*: 809–819, 1969.

197. Svejcar, J., Pekárek, J., and Johanovský, J. Studies on Production of Biologically Active Substances Which Inhibit Cell Migration in Supernatants and Extracts of Hypersensitive Lymphoid Cells Incubated with Specific Antigen *in vitro*. Immunology, *15*: 1–11, 1968.

198. Takeda, K. Immunology of Cancer, with Special Reference to Tumour Immunity in the Primary Autochthonous Host. Sapporo, Hokkaido University School of Medicine, 1969.

199. Thompson, J., and Van Furth, R. The Effect of Glucocorticoids on the Kinetics of Mononuclear Phagocytes. J. Exp. Med., *131*: 429–442, 1970.

200. Thor, D. E. Human Delayed Hypersensitivity: an *in vitro* Correlate and Transfer by an RNA Extract. Fed. Proc., *27*: 16–20, 1968.

201. Thor, D. E., and Dray, S. The Cell-migration Inhibition Correlate of Delayed Hypersensitivity. Conversion of Human Nonsensitive Lymph Node Cells to Sensitive Cells with an RNA Extract. J. Immunol., *101*: 469–480, 1968.

202. Thor, D. E., Jureziz, R. E., Veach, S. R., Miller, E., and Dray, S. Cell Migration Inhibition Factor Released by Antigen from Human Peripheral Lymphocytes. Nature, *219*: 755–757, 1968.

203. Trubowitz, S., Masek, B., and Del Rosario, A. Lymphocyte Response to Phytohaemagglutinin in Hodgkin's Disease, Lymphatic Leukemia and Lymphosarcoma. Cancer, *19*: 2019–2023, 1966.

204. Turk, J. L. Delayed Hypersensitivity. Amsterdam, North-Holland Publishing Company, 1967.

205. Turk, J. L. (Ed.) Delayed Hypersensitivity. Specific Cell-mediated Immunity. Brit. Med. Bull., *23*: No. 1, pp. 1–97, 1967.

206. Turk, J. L., Cytology of the Induction of Hypersensitivity. Brit. Med. Bull., *23*: 3–8, 1967.

207. Uhr, J. W., and Baumann, J. B. Antibody Formation. I. The Suppression of Antibody Formation by Passively Administered Antibody. J. Exp. Med., *113*: 935–957, 1961.

208. Uhr, J. W., and Möller, G. Regulatory Effect of Antibody on the Immune Response. Adv. Immunol., *8*: 81–127, 1968.

209. Ure, D. M. J. Negative Association between Allergy and Cancer. Scottish Med. J., *14*: 51–54, 1969.

210. Valentine, F. T., and Lawrence, H. S. Lymphocyte Stimulation: Transfer of Cellular Hypersensitivity to Antigen *in vitro*. Science, *165*: 1014–1016, 1969.

211. Vernon-Roberts, B. The Effects of Steroid Hormones on Macrophage Activity. Int. Rev. Cytol., *25*: 131–159, 1969.

212. Volkman, A., and Collins, F. M. Recovery of Delayed-type Hypersensitivity in Mice Following Suppressive Doses of X-radiation. J. Immunol., *101*: 846–859, 1968.

213. Waksman, B. H. A Comparative Histopathological Study of Delayed Hypersensitive Reactions. *In* G. E. W. Wolstenholme and M. O'Connor (eds.), Ciba Foundation Symposium on Cellular Aspects of Immunity, pp. 280–322. London, J. and A. Churchill, 1960.

214. Wang, M. Delayed Hypersensitivity to Extracts from Primary Sarcomata in the Autochthonous Host. Int. J. Cancer, *3*: 483–490, 1968.

215. Ward, P. A., Remold, H. G., and David, J. R. Leukotactic Factor Produced by Sensitized Lymphocytes. Science, *163*: 1079–1081, 1969.

216. Warner, N. L., and Szenberg, A. Immunological Studies on Hormonally Bursectomized and Surgically Thymectomized Chickens: Dissociation of Immunological Responsiveness. *In* R. A. Good and A. E. Gabrielsen (eds.), The Thymus in Immunology, pp. 395–411. New York, Hoeber-Harper, 1964.

217. Weber, W. T. Qualitative and Quantitative Studies on Mixed Homologous Chicken Thymus Cell Cultures. Clin. Exp. Immunol., *6*: 919–940, 1970.

218. Weiser, R. S., Granger, G. A., Brown, W., Baker, P., Jutila, J., and Holmes, B. Production of Acute Allogeneic Disease in Mice. Transplantation, *3*: 10–21, 1965.

219. Wick, G., Kite, J. H., Jr., Cole, R. K., and Witebsky, E. Spontaneous Thyroiditis in the Obese Strain of Chickens. III. The Effect of Bursectomy on the Development of the Disease. J. Immunol., *104*: 45–53, 1970.

220. Williams, T. W., and Granger, G. A. Lymphocyte *in vitro* Cytotoxicity: Mechanism of Lymphotoxin-induced Target Cell Destruction. J. Immunol., *102*: 911–918, 1969.

221. Williams, T. W., and Granger, G. A. Lymphocyte *in vitro* Cytotoxicity: Correlation of Derepression with Release of Lymphotoxin from Human Lymphocytes. J. Immunol., *103*: 170–178, 1969.

222. Williams, T. W., and Granger, G. A. Comparisons of the Sensitivities of Various Cell Lines to Human Lymphotoxin. Fed. Proc., *29*: 306, 1970.

223. Winter, G. C. B., McCarthy, C. F., Read, A. E., and Yoffey, J. M. Development of Macrophages in Phytohaemagglutinin Cultures of Blood from Patients with Idiopathic Steatorrhoea and with Cirrhosis. Brit. J. Exp. Path., *48*: 66–80, 1967.

224. Wolstencroft, R. A., and Dumonde, D. C. *In vitro* Studies of Cell-mediated Immunity. I. Induction of Lymphocyte Transformation by a Soluble " Mitogenic "

Factor Derived from Interaction of Sensitized Guinea Pig Lymphoid Cells with Specific Antigen. Immunology, *18*: 599–610, 1970.

225. Wood, R. M., and Bick, M. W. The Effect of Heparin on the Ocular Tuberculin Reaction. Arch. Ophthalmol., *61*: 709–711, 1959.

226. Woodruff, M. F. A. Immunosuppression and Its Complications. Proc. Roy. Soc. Med., *62*: 411–416, 1969.

227. Zabriskie, J. B., and Falk, R. E. *In vitro* Reactivity of Lymphocytes to Particulate and Soluble Antigens. Nature, *226*: 943–945, 1970.

228. Zbar, B., Wepsic, H. T., Borsos, T., and Rapp, H. J. Tumor-graft Rejection in Syngeneic Guinea Pigs: Evidence for a Two-step Mechanism. J. Nat. Cancer Inst., *44*: 473–481, 1970.

229. Zbar, B., Wepsic, H. T., Rapp, H. J., Stewart, L. C., and Borsos, T. Two-Step Mechanism of Tumor Graft Rejection in Syngeneic Guinea Pigs. II. Initiation of Reaction by a Cell Fraction Containing Lymphocytes and Neutrophils. J. Nat. Cancer Inst., *44*: 701–717, 1970.

230. Zinsser, H. Studies on the Tuberculin Reaction and on Specific Hypersensitivities in Bacterial Infection. J. Exp. Med., *34*: 495–524, 1921.

231. Zinsser, H., and Mueller, J. H. On the Nature of Bacterial Allergies. J. Exp. Med., *41*: 159–177, 1925.

In Vitro Studies on Immunological Enhancement of Autochthonous and Syngeneic Tumors

Karl Erik HELLSTRÖM, and Ingegerd HELLSTRÖM

Departments of Pathology and Microbiology, University of Washington Medical School, Seattle, Washington U.S.A.

Most experimentally induced animal neoplasms have been found to possess tumor specific transplantation antigens (TSTA), which can be detected by the inability of transplanted tumor cells to grow in appropriately immunized hosts (*19, 25, 29, 30, 32*). Such antigens can be detected in spontaneous animal tumors as well (*28, 36*).

In vitro techniques are needed for attempts to analyze the immunological defense against antigenic tumor cells. We have taken a particular interest in those techniques by which cell-mediated immune responses can be monitored, because of the demonstration that the rejection of antigenic tumor cells is mediated primarily by immune lymphocytes (*26*). The colony inhibition assay (*7*) and a cytotoxic test closely related to it (*17, 35*), have been the tests of choice, since they permit quantitation and can be carried out with modest sized samples of target cells and lymphocytes.

Colony inhibition (CI) tests have by now been carried out with a large variety of tumors in animals, experimentally induced as well as spontaneous (*2, 5, 13, 14, 19, 22*). These tests have clearly shown that lymphocytes from immunized donors as well as from animals bearing progressively growing tumors can specifically destroy neoplastic cells of the types against which the lymphocyte donors have been immunized (or are carrying). It may appear surprising that lymphocytes from tumor-bearing animals have, in the doses so far tested, shown approximately the same reactivity as lymphocytes from animals whose tumors have been removed (or have regressed). A certain difference in lymphocyte reactivity between the two groups may yet exist and be detectable only after titration of the lymphocyte effect at various doses. Nevertheless, it is striking that tumors grow progressively *in vivo*, even when their cells can be killed by the tumor-bearing individuals' lymphocytes *in vitro*.

Several alternative hypotheses may be introduced to explain why antigenic

557

tumor cells sometimes escape from the immunological surveillance mediated by their hosts. For example, one may speculate that the number of immune lymphocytes is too low *in vivo* to fight a rapidly growing tumor, or that some mechanism is needed in addition to the lymphocytes for rejection of antigenic cells and is depressed, or that the tumor cells may be protected by a sialomucin coating, or that the tumor cells taking over *in vivo* have a low specific antigenicity following immunoselection (*19*).

We have taken a particular interest in the possibility that tumors grow progressively and kill because of the formation of enhancing (or blocking) serum factors, which can protect the neoplastic cells from the specific lymphocyte effect (*20*). Immunological enhancement (*24*) was first demonstrated in transplantation experiments performed with tumors grafted onto allogeneic hosts, which had either received antibodies directed against the foreign H-2 antigens of the graft or antigenic material stimulating the formation of such antibodies. Similar results were later obtained, when tumors were transplanted to syngeneic animals which had been inoculated with hyperimmune sera directed against the foreign tumor specific antigens (*1, 4, 27*). However, very little was known about enhancement of primary tumors when this work was started some 3–4 years ago.

Experiments were performed in which tumor cells were plated *in vitro* and exposed to sera to be tested for the presence of enhancing (blocking) activity, after which lymphocytes were added which were known to be immune to the specific antigens of the explanted cells. Controls were performed in which sera from untreated animals and from animals with unrelated types of neoplasms were added prior to the target cells being exposed to the immune lymphocytes.

The first system investigated was Moloney sarcoma in mice. The Moloney sarcoma virus induces sarcomas in mice of many strains, independently of the age of the inoculated animals. Tumors induced by a standard virus dose in BALB/c mice grow progressively and kill, if the mice are less than approximately 3 weeks old when inoculated with the virus. Sarcomas appearing in the older mice regress, on the other hand, and mice in which such regression has occurred have developed an immunity to transplants of Moloney sarcoma cells (*6*). A cell-mediated immunity can be detected with lymphocytes from both groups of mice, using the CI or the cytotoxicity tests.

We were able to demonstrate that sera from mice whose Moloney sarcomas were growing progressively could block tumor target cell destruction *in vitro* by lymphocytes immune to the specific antigens of Moloney sarcoma cells (*11, 12*). Animals whose tumors were going to regress contained such blocking factors as long as their sarcomas grew progressively, while no blocking effect was obtained with serum harvested after the onset of regression. On the contrary, such sera could de-block the blocking effect of serum from mice with progressively growing Moloney sarcomas so that the target cells were killed by immune lymphocytes in the presence of a 1:1 mixture between " progressor " and " regressor " sera.

A blocking effect similar to that detected in the Moloney sarcoma system has, by now, been demonstrated in a variety of experimental animal tumor systems, *viz.*, in rabbits with persistent Shope papillomas or Shope carcinomas (*9*), in mice with spontaneous mammary carcinomas (23), in mice and rats with methylcholan-threne induced sarcomas, primary or transplanted (16), in rats with polyoma virus induced sarcomas (31, 33), and in rats with Schmidt-Ruppin-Rous virus induced sarcomas (33). As shown in a separate contribution to this symposium, such an effect is very common in the human tumor system as well (10).

An important question is whether tumors grow because blocking factors are formed or whether these are detected because tumors are growing. The first alternative appears more likely for several reasons. A blocking effect of serum is detected prior to the appearance of palpable Moloney virus induced sarcomas (12) and often prior to the appearance of transplanted methylcholanthrene induced sarcomas (16). Mice whose Moloney sarcomas have regressed sometimes have recurrences, and blocking factors are by then seen immediately preceding the recurrence. Rats transplanted with polyoma tumor cells develop blocking serum activity. This activity decreases strongly after tumor removal (3), as it does after removal of growing methylcholanthrene induced sarcomas (16) but reappears before the recurrence of incompletely removed tumors (3). Although none of these observations conclusively proves that the blocking antibodies are responsible for tumor growth *in vivo*, they strongly indicate that such antibodies are the cause rather than the consequence of that growth and that they, anyhow, facilitate it.

There are a couple of aspects of this work which need some discussion. First, the ability of an individual to form blocking antibodies might serve a useful purpose under conditions not involving cancer. There is evidence that this is really the case in relation to pregnancy (21), as a possible guard against a graft-versus-host reaction in chimeric animals (18), and as a possible mediator of allograft tolerance (8), at least under certain conditions. This makes it likely that procedures capable of inducing and maintaining the production of blocking antibodies, as well as the passive administration of such antibodies, may be of great value in facilitating the take of transplanted allogeneic organs and tissues (34). One may also speculate that such procedures may be of value in decreasing autoimmunity, when that occurs.

Another aspect of this work is directly related to cancer prevention and therapy. Since methods now exist by which the formation of blocking antibodies can be monitored, such methods should be useful when trying—first in experimental animal systems-to develop immunoprophylaxis against certain types of tumors sharing common antigens, in order to avoid the development of enhancement. Furthermore, it appears likely that methods capable of depressing the organism's ability to form blocking antibodies, as well as methods by which such antibodies already formed can be removed, may be therapeutically beneficial. The possible depressing effect of drugs and radiation on blocking antibody formation needs to be investigated. Another lead, which seems to us to be even more straightforward, is to investigate to what extent non-blocking antibodies, like those discussed in relation to the Moloney sarcomas (12), are capable of depressing both the formation and the action of blocking antibodies *in vivo*. Since cell-mediated anti-tumor immunity is generally long lasting, and since the formation of blocking antibodies is interrupted shortly after the source of the antigen, the tumor, has been removed, it appears likely that antibodies, capable of binding to the same antigens without themselves blocking tumor cell destruction by immune lymphocytes, might be capable of decreasing the blocking effect of the same animal's serum and depressing further formation of blocking antibodies.; the de-blocking antibodies would also cancel the blocking activity of the blocking foctors already present. This hypothesis should be tested in systems, like the polyoma rat tumor system, where tumor virus is generally not released, so that it becomes possible to distinguish between the effect of a deblocking serum and simple neutralization of infectious tumor virus. Such distinctions cannot be made in the Moloney sarcoma system. Nevertheless, it is interesting that approximately 30% of mice can be cured of Moloney sarcomas after injection of (de-blocking) serum from mice whose Moloney sarcomas have regressed spontaneously (15), and one may speculate that the mice that were cured were so because an unblocking effect had been achieved (20).

REFERENCES

1. Attia, M. A. M., and Weiss, D. W. Cancer Res., 26: 1787–1800, 1966.
2. Baldwin, R. W. Int. J. Cancer, 7: 17–25, 1971.
3. Bansal, H., and Sjögren, H. O. Personal communication.
4. Bubenik, J., Adamcová, B., and Koldovský. P. Folia Biol. (Prague), 12: 11–16, 1966.
5. Datta, and Vandeputte, M. Cancer Res., 31: 882–889, 1971.
6. Fefer, A., McCoy, J. L., and Glynn, J. P. Cancer Res., 27: 1626–1631, 1967.
7. Hellström, I. Int. J. Cancer, 2: 65–69, 1967.
8. Hellström, I., Hellström, K. E., Allison, A. C., and Hellström, K. E. Nature, 230: 49–50, 1971. 1970.
9. Hellström, I., Evans, C. A., and Hellström, K. E. Int. J. Cancer, 4: 601–607, 1969.
10. Hellström, I., and Hellström, K. E., Evidence for Cell-mediated Immunity to Human Tumor Antigens. Proceedings of The 1st International Symposium of The Princess Takamatsu Cancer Research Fund, University of Tokyo Press, pp. 563, 1970.
11. Hellström, I., and Hellström, K. E. Int. J. Cancer, 4: 587–600, 1969.
12. Hellström, I., and Hellström, K. E. Int. J. Cancer, 5: 195–201, 1970.
13. Hellström, I., and Hellström, K. E. Science, 156: 981–983, 1967.
14. Hellström, I., Hellström, K. E., and Pierce, G. E., Int. J. Cancer, 3: 467–483, 1968.
15. Hellström, I., Hellström, K. E., Pierce, G. E., and Fefer, A. Transpl. Proc., 1: 90–94, 1969.
16. Hellström, I., Hellström, K. E., and Sjögren, H. O. Cell. Immunol., 1: 18–30, 1970.
17. Hellström, I., Hellström, K. E., Sjögren, H. O., and Warner, G. A. Int. J. Cancer, 7: 1–16, 1971.
18. Hellström, I., Hellström, K. E., Storb, R., and Thomas, E. D. Proc. Natl. Acad. Sci., 66: 65–71, 1970.
19. Hellström, K. E., and Hellström, I. Adv. Cancer Res., 12: 167–223, 1969.
20. Hellström, K. E., and Hellström, I. Ann. Rev. Microbiol., 24: 373–398, 1970.
21. Hellström, K. E., Hellström, I., and Brawn, J. Nature, 224: 914–915, 1969.
22. Hellström, I., and Sjögren, H. O. Int. J. Cancer, 3: 467–482, 1968.
23. Heppner, G. H. Int. J. Cancer, 4: 608–615, 1969.
24. Kaliss, N. Cancer Res., 18: 992–1003, 1958.
25. Klein, G. Ann. Rev. Microbiol., 20: 223–252, 1966.

26. Klein, G., Sjögren, H. O., Klein, E., and Hellström, K. E.   Cancer Res., *20*: 1561–1572, 1960.
27. Möller, G.   Nature, *204*: 846–847, 1964.
28. Morton, D. L.   Proc. Am. Assoc. Cancer Res., *3*: 346, 1962.
29. Old, L. J., and Boyse, E. A.   Ann. Rev. Med., *15*: 167–186, 1964.
30. Prehn, R. T., and Main, J. M.   J. Nat. Cancer Inst., *18*: 679–778, 1957.
31. Sjögren, H. O.   *In* Immunity and Tolerance in Oncogenesis, 4th Quadrennial Perugia Cancer Conf., 551–561, 1969.
32. Sjögren, H. O.   Progr. Exp. Tumor Res., *6*: 289–322, 1965.
33. Sjögren, H. O.   Cancer Res., *31*: 890–900, 1971.
34. Stuart, F. P., Saitoh, T., and Fitch, F. W.   Science, *160*: 1463, 1968.
35. Takasugi, M., and Klein, E.   Transplantation, *9*: 219–227, 1960.
36. Weiss, D. W., Faulkin, L. J., and DeOme, K. B.   Cancer Res., *24*: 632–741, 1964.

Evidence for Cell-mediated Immunity to Human Tumor Antigens

Ingegerd HELLSTRÖM, and Karl Erik HELLSTRÖM

Departments of Microbiology and Pathology, University of Washington Medical School, Seattle, Washington, U.S.A.

Increasing evidence has been obtained during the last decade that neoplasms originating in experimental animals possess tumor specific transplantation antigens (TSTA), which are absent from normal cells. Immune reactions against such antigens can, under appropriate conditions, lead to the death of the neoplastic cells. The tumor cell destruction is primarily mediated by lymphocytes. Humoral antibodies are sometimes cytotoxic to the neoplastic cells and sometimes protect them from destruction by immune lymphocytes through a mechanism of immunological enhancement. For further information and discussions of these points, the reader is referred to recent review articles (*13, 15–18*), as well as to a paper (*14*) presented at this symposium.

The animal experiments on tumor immunity have been obviously conducted so as to provide models for similar studies in man. *A priori*, it appears likely that at least some human tumors are antigenic and evoke cell-mediated immune responses. Direct experimental evidence that this is really the case has, however, started to appear only during the last few years. We would like to review some of this evidence here.

The well-known fact that some, albeit extremely few, human malignancies have been reported to regress spontaneously (*3*) suggests that mechanisms exist by which the human body may defend itself against cancer, and the finding that infiltration of tumors by lymphocytes and local lymph node reactions against them often correlate favorably with prognosis (*1*) has long suggested that these defense mechanisms may be, at least partially, of an immunological nature. Southam (*19*) was one of the first to provide more support to this line of argument by showing that tumor cells transplanted to autochthonous cancer patients are often rejected, unless the dose is very large, and that lymphocytes from such patients, mixed with neoplastic cells before transplantation, are able to further suppress their growth. Chu *et al.* (*2*), who studied postnasal carcinomas, made analogous observations: lymphocytes from the cancer patients had a somewhat greater ability to destroy cultivated autoch-thonous tumor cells than they had when tested against the same patients' skin fibro-blasts. Although the evidence from the studies of Southam (*19*) and of Chu *et al.* (*2*) gave some suggestive evidence in favor of cell-mediated anti-tumor immunity, alternative explanations of the findings could not be excluded.

The colony inhibition technique (*5*) has been much used in searches for lym-phocyte-mediated immunity against animal neoplasms. It provides distinct ad-vantages over the *in vivo* techniques utilized by Southam (*19*), as well as over the *in vitro* assays of Chu *et al.* (*2*) by providing better possibilities for quantitation. Col-ony inhibition (CI) studies performed on both experimentally, induced and spon-taneous animal tumors have clearly shown that lymphocytes from specifically im-munized, as well as from tumor-bearing, animals can specifically destroy neoplastic cells *in vitro*, the findings obtained with the CI assay showing the same degree of tumor-specificity as detected by transplantation tests to specifically immunized hosts *in vivo* (*13, 14*). The finding that immunity to autochthonous tumors could be easily detected (*5*) suggested that the CI technique was well suited to a search for human tumor immunity, mediated by the patients' lymphocytes.

The first tumor studied was neuroblastoma (*6, 8*). These tumors grow well *in vitro*, having a characteristic morphology, and they are of particular interest by being among the few groups of human neoplasms for which spontaneous regressions have been reported (*3*). Neuroblastoma specimens obtained from the operating room were explanted and kept *in vitro* during approximately 1–3 weeks. Normal skin fibroblasts from the donors of the tumor cells were obtained and cultivated as well. The experiments were conducted by exposing neuroblastoma cells (or skin fibroblasts in the controls), which had been plated onto 60 mm plastic petri dishes, to peripheral blood lymphocytes, obtained from either the autochthonous patients, from other patients with neuroblastoma, from patients with other malignancies, or from healthy subjects. The ability of the lymphocytes to suppress colony formation by the plated neuroblastoma cells was assessed after counting the colonies growing out from the tumor cells 3–5 days after exposure to lymphocytes. Percentage reduc-tion in colony numbers with lymphocytes from neuroblastoma patients, as com-pared to the controls, was calculated.

It was found that both autochthonous and allogeneic lymphocytes from neuro-blastoma patients, but not the control lymphocytes, inhibited the colony formation of plated neuroblastoma cells. Normal skin fibroblasts from the tumor donors were not affected. Furthermore, we observed that lymphocytes from certain relatives of neuroblastoma patients, most notably their mothers, had a colony inhibitory effect on neuroblastoma cells; this effect was seen also when a mother's lymphocytes were tested on neuroblastoma cells that were not derived from her own child (so that immunity to HLA antigens could be excluded as an explanation to these findings).

A somewhat paradoxical finding obtained was that lymphocytes from patients with actively growing neuroblastomas, in the doses tested, were approximately as inhibitory as were lymphocytes from patients who had become clinically symptom-free after therapy. This finding is, however, analogous to observations made with animal tumors and it appears to have the same explanation: It was found that serum from patients with growing neuroblastomas, but not from the cured ones, contained factors, presumably blocking antibodies, which could specifically protect cultivated neuroblastoma cells from destruction by lymphocytes immune to their antigens (6). Serum from relatives of neuroblastoma patients, whose lymphocytes were immune to neuroblastoma cells, did not contain any such blocking antibodies.

It was soon found that the observations made on neuroblastomas were not unique to that particular kind of neoplasm but that similar findings could be made on other human tumors as well (9). We have recently completed a fairly extensive survey of human malignancies with respect to cell-mediated anti-tumor immunity. The experimental protocol is similar to that used with neuroblastomas, except that we have, in addition, used a cytotoxicity test (9, 11), by which we demonstrate destruction of tumor target cells by immune lymphocytes; the advantage of that test is that smaller samples of lymphocytes and target cells can be used than in the colony inhibition assay. The major findings obtained were: Lymphocytes from patients with a large variety of tumors were capable of destroying cultivated autochthonous tumor cells, as compared to control lymphocytes, while normal cells from the tumor patients were not affected. The normal cells were most commonly skin fibroblasts; however, colon epithelial cells were used in experiments with colonic carcinomas and kidney epithelial cells in experiments with kidney tumors. Histologically similar tumors most commonly cross-reacted with respect to sensitivity to lymphocytes from tumor patients; there were, on the other hand, no cross-reactions between tumors of different types. Melanomas, colonic carcinomas, breast carcinomas, seminomas, ovarian carcinomas, and sarcomas represent some groups of neoplasms within which cross-reactions were observed.

Lymphocytes from tumor-bearing patients were approximately as inhibitory (cytotoxic) as were lymphocytes from patients who were clinically symptom free; this was also true when tumors other than neuroblastomas were studied. We, therefore, started to search for blocking antibodies against some of these tumors as well (7, 10, 12). It was found that patients with growing neoplasms almost invariably had a blocking serum activity. Such an activity was, on the other hand, seen very rarely with serum from patients who had no symptoms of growing tumors. An obvious question is, then: do the tumors grow because of the formation of blocking antibodies or do the blocking antibodies just represent a sign that tumors are growing? Although this question is not fully answered yet for human material, studies performed in animals (14) make it very likely that the presence of the blocking antibodies plays an important role in making possible (or at least facilitating) the growth of antigenic tumors.

We have repeatedly asked ourselves whether the findings so far obtained by searching for cell-mediated immunity to human neoplasms offer any future possibilities for tumor prophylaxis, diagnosis, and therapy. Some hope seems justified, particularly since groups of histologically similar tumors share antigens, so that some vaccination procedure—if we knew from animal experiments how to carry it out— might, one day, help prevent tumor formation; the obvious risks of achieving enhancement rather than a tumoricidal type of immunity naturally imply that more knowledge is needed about how one or the other type of immunity is achieved before any vaccination could be attempted, and then only in animal models to start with. As far as diagnosis goes, the demonstration of common antigens among similar types of tumors offers distinct possibilities, based on the work already begun on colonic carcinomas (20), following Gold and Freedman's discovery of a carcinoembryonic antigen among these (4). As therapy goes, finally, one may speculate that procedures aimed at increasing cell-mediated immunity and destroying blocking antibody formation, as well as physical removal of blocking antibodies already formed, may be therapeutically helpful; here, too, animal experiments are needed to provide the models. If one should dare a guess, one lead which seems worthwhile following is that of using (first in experimental animal systems) therapy with deblocking antibodies. However, a more immediate goal seems to be to study how the already existing types of therapy (surgery, radiation, drugs, and hormones) influence cell-mediated immunity and blocking antibody formation. Procedures are available by which this can be approached.

REFERENCES

1. Black, M. M., and Speer, F. D. Surg. Gynecol. Obstet., 106: 163–175, 1958.
2. Chu, E., Stjernswärd, J., Clifford, P., and Klein, G. J. Nat. Cancer Inst., 39: 595–618, 1967.
3. Everson, T. C., and Cole, W. H. Spontaneous Regression of Cancer. Saunders, Philadelphia, 1966.
4. Gold, P., and Freedman, S. O. J. Exp. Med., 122: 467–481, 1965.
5. Hellström, I. Int. J. Cancer, 2: 65–69, 1967.
6. Hellström, I., Hellström, K. E., Bill, A. H., Pierce, G. E., and Yang, J. P. S. Int. J. Cancer, 6: 172–188, 1970.
7. Hellström, I., Hellström, K. E., Evans, C. A., Heppner, G. Pierce, G. E., and Yang, J. P. S. Proc. Nat. Acad. Sci., 62: 362–369, 1969.
8. Hellström, I., Hellström, K. E., Pierce, G. E., and Bill, A. H. Proc. Natl. Acad. Sci., 60: 1231–1238, 1968.
9. Hellström, I., Hellström, K. E., Pierce, G. E., and Yang, J. P. S. Nature, 220: 1352–1354, 1968.
10. Hellström, I., Hellström, K. E., Pierce, G. E., and Yang, J. P. S. In Carcinomas of the Colon and Antecedent Epithelium, W. J. Burdette (ed.), pp. 176–188, C. C. Thomas, Publisher, Springfield, 1970.
11. Hellström, I., Hellström, K. E., Sjögren, H. O., and Warner, G. A. Int. J. Cancer, 7: 1–16, 1971.
12. Hellström, I., Hellström, K. E., Sjögren, H. O., and Warner, G. A., Int. J. Cancer, 7: 226–237, 1971.
13. Hellström, K. E., and Hellström, I. Adv. Cancer Res., 12: 167–223, 1969.
14. Hellström, K. E., and Hellström, I. Proceedings of the 1st International Symposium of The Princess Takamatsu Cancer Research Fund, pp. 557, University of Tokyo Press, Tokyo, 1971.
15. Klein, G. Ann. Rev. Microbiol., 20: 223–252, 1966.
16. Old, L. J., and Boyse, E. A. Ann. Rev. Med., 15: 167–186, 1964.
17. Sjögren, H. O. Progr. Exp. Tumor Res., 6: 289–322, 1965.
18. Smith, R. T. New Eng. J. Med., 278: 1207–1214; 1268–1275; 1326–1331, 1968.
19. Southam, C. M. Progr. Exp. Tumor Res., 9: 1–39, 1967.
20. Thomson, D. M. P., Krupey, J., Freedman, S. O., and Gold, P. Proc. Natl. Acad. Sci., 64: 161–167, 1969.

Discussion of Papers by Drs. Fujii, Nelson, K. Hellström, and I. Hellström

DR. NAKAHARA: I would like to ask Dr. Nelson and Dr. Hellström where they think the serum blocking factor comes from?

DR. K. HELLSTRÖM: Blocking factor is probably made by plasma cells but we don't have exact evidence. I would like to try to find out by transferring the blocking cell population and looking at the blockng effect.

Rather controversial observations have been presented. One group of investigators, Alexander and Mikulska and Barski, found that lymphoid cell populations from animals carrying tumors are not reactive, while in our case, the lymphocyte populations are reactive. This controversy may be solved; I think so because Dr. Heise, who was using the migration inhibition assay, is getting results closely similar to those of Mikulska and Alexander, although Barski found that lymphocyte populations from tumor-bearing individual peritoneal cell populations: lymphocytes, plasma cells, macrophages, *etc.*, were non-reactive, while those from individuals after tumor removal or spontaneous regression showed reactivity. That was quite opposite to our findings with the colony inhibition test. Then we found the blocking effect of serum that I referred to; the obvious type of experiment was to mix the cell population which was non-reactive with a reactive cell population to see if it could be rescued to reactivity or if the reactive population would become non-reactive, which would be the case in a cell population which either contained or produced blocking antibodies. We may now possibly have a cell population with which we can start to investigate this.

We also know that if we remove the spleen, we will get a decrease in the blocking effect of serum. So, some sort of cell population in the spleen plays a synthetic role; also, immunological enhancement by immunoglobulin often decreased after splenectomy.

What are the blocking antibodies? Unfortunately we do not know the correct full answer to that. They were present in the 7S fraction by Sephadex gel filtration but we don't know the exact class of immunoglobulin to which they belong. Presumably, they are immunoglobulins. They cannot be soluble antigens or non-specific factors because of their specificity. They also can't be antigen-antibody complexes.

DR. NELSON: My short anwser is plasma cells. But there is another comment from some of the earlier works on tumor allograft-enhancing antibody. The population of antibody-producing cells changes fairly consistently with time. If we take lymph nodes from an animal which rejected tumor, we could transfer to a non-immunized animal a capacity to reject tumor. After waiting a couple of weeks or months, if we take the lymph node, we could transfer immunological enhancement to non-immunized animals; that means that lymphnodes in the later stage were producing enhancing blocking antibody. It is similar to your experiments.

DR. NAKAHARA: It would be most instructive not only to myself but also to others who are present here, if either of you or both of you, could explain the mechanism by which cancer metastasis takes place so often in lymph nodes in an autochthonous system where the animals is supposed to have immunity but still develops metastasis.

DR. K. HELLSTRÖM: Because we have production of enhancing anti-body in lymph nodes, we have a high concentration of this blocking antibody in the lymph node. We have performed a similar type of *in vitro* experiment. We added a tremendous ratio of lymphocytes to target cells; when we added blocking serum, it blocked the effect of immune lymphocytes. Another possibility, not fully explored, is that we have specific anergy for tumor antigen by the original lymph nodes draining the tumor. In our system that we have, Shope carcinoma, we found original lymph nodes that were non-reactive. At this time, we don't know whether that was due to the production of enhancing antibody in the lymph node or whether all immune cells were exhausted from the lymph node.

DR. NAKAHARA: One more question. In the case of surgical operations where most of the original tumors are removed, so that animals or patients should have full immunity, sensitized lymphocytes and blocking antibody occur together. Why does recurrence take place so often?

DR. K. HELLSTRÖM: Where we have blocking antibody, the tumors should recur. If we have cell-mediated immunity and no blocking antibody, then one wonders why the tumor recurs. I think one should not be naive and believe that blocking antibody and cell-mediated immunity are the entire explanation. We have one situation that would not agree with this simplistic idea. That is Moloney sarcoma. Those tumors, as we showed, regressed, although the sera were not blocking and even showed an adverse effect on blocking antibody. Nevertheless, after a couple of months or so, some of the tumors have relapsed, at which time the serum has blocking antibody and cell-mediated immunity remains. In this particular case there are two possibilities: either new tomors appeared as a result of a new infection of normal cells that have later on become tumor cells, or some cells remained dormant; these may be seen from Dr. Klein's work, for example, as tumor antigens may vary with the state of cells in the cell cycles. Certain of these antigens on resting cells are present in much smaller quantities. That is something which needs to be studied.

DR. SOUTHAM: Dr. I. Hellström gave some data showing that cell-mediated immunity persisted for a long period of time. In either human or animal systems, do you have data on the duration or persistence of blocking antibody after a tumor regressed or was surgically removed?

DR. I. HELLSTRÖM: The blocking antibodies in animals varied a little bit but they disappeared fairly rapidly after the tumors were either surgically removed or after the tumor started regression. This is true in the Moloney sarcoma and also in the Shope papilloma systems. In a regression, in one or two days whole tumors disappeared; at that point, the blocking antibody titer drops. It is more difficult to study human cases. We have a melanoma patient we have followed now for a year. When tested the first time, she had tumor cells in a lymph node and cell-mediated immunity and blocking antibody. Then we tested once a month. Suddenly we could not find the blocking antibody in the serum. We felt rather disappointed at that time because the patient was due to come back to the clinician to take out a lymph node to give us tumor tissue. When the patient was operated, tumor cells in all the lymph nodes tested were gone. Since then, for eight months, she has been completely free from tumor. She has no blocking antibody, very strong cell-mediated immunity, 90–95% under our test conditions, and she had cytotoxic antibody using human complement.

DR. SOUTHAM: The rapid disappearance of the blocking antibody will confuse Dr. Nakahara and me even more, because blocking antibody should disappear rapidly after apparently complete surgical removal of the tumors. Then you should have only cellular immunity. That would be a major explanation.

DR. HO: Just now Dr. Nakahara asked about surgery. I think all these surgical operations removed many lymph nodes that had been the source for developing these antibodies.

DR. NAKAHARA: Regional lymph nodes are removed but you don't remove all lymph nodes.

DR. K. HELLSTRÖM: First of all, we found blocking antibody does disappear about a month or so following surgery as I. Hellström referred to. These are the patients with breast carcinoma and colonic carcinoma; surgeons are quite good at curing many of these patients. So at this moment, we can't say that it proves or disproves any of the arguments, but what has to be done is to tie these up and follow individual patients to see what happens with blocking antibody following treatment and offer any prognostically evaluable signs. That has not been done. Just to say many of these patients, I expected presumably to be cured from the disease. Then of course, one has also the possibility that when one does not find a blocking effect in the serum, still the blocking antibody is present, bound to the antigens of the tumor cells. Isaacs in Israel has done work on animal tumors; he was unable to elute blocking antibody from tumors in vivo. First, he had evidence that he could immunize and elute γ_2 globulin from mouse tumor *in vivo*. But at the meeting in Brussels, I claimed that this globulin would actively enhance such tumors on the standard type of test, and that, when mixed with the tumor cells *in vitro* and inoculated, the tumor grows better.

DR. NELSON: For the last few years, to return to the points raised yesterday, we have been consistently concerned with a viral etiology that demonstrates a common tumor-specific antigen in a particular type of tumor. Are there any tumors in man which don't have common tumor-specific antigen? Can we use this concept as suggestive of viral etiology at all, or not? Because of therapeutic points, it is great because you can use a variety of tumors that you have, but from the point of etiologic or basic knowledge, are we using too simple an interpretation or do you think viruses are widespread?

DR. I. HELLSTRÖM: All human tumors we have tested, and have found, are those as I described but I don't think that means necessarily that they are virus-induced. It could well be embryonic antigens or other antigens, we don't know. It could be that they are virus-induced but I don't think it has been proven at all.

DR. NELSON: As far as etiology is concerned, I would be very happy if we could turn up something in man which was like methyl-cholanthrene-induced tumor in animals, say presumably like lung carcinoma from cigarette smoking. Are there not any tumors that have no common antigens?

DR. I. HELLSTRÖM: I think maybe it is so; we can see the common, but they may have some individual antigens. We don't even know if the animal virus-induced tumors have individual antigen; but they actually have strong common antigens that have not been discovered. Also oppositely, the methyl-cholanthrene-induced tumors may have common antigens in addition to individual antigen. That may also be true in human tumors as well.

DR. HO: Following up Dr. Nelson's suggestion, why don't you test bladder carcinoma that has been thought to be induced by chemical carcinogens?

DR. K. HELLSTRÖM: Dr. Perlman in Stockholm tested bladder carcinoma in man with Takasugi and Klein's technique with a micro-test plate, similar or analogous to the test we have been using. With identical types of cells, namely blood lymphocytes from the bladder, cancer patients do kill bladder carcinoma cells. They do not kill normal bladder epithelial cells nor carcinoma cells of the prostate. So it is quite tumor-specific. Also, a blocking effect was found in the serum of the tumors whether they were chemically induced or not, but I think the chance that certain of these tumors is chemically-induced is likely.

Could I also mention that Lewis has evidence on some individually unique antigens in human melanoma? I do not think that is really controversial between whatever was found but the conclusion is more dependent on the technique. It is more likely that those tumors do have more than one group of antigens: individual unique antigens that may be perhaps reflect genetic variations, and common ones that may be carcinoembryonic or caused by virus infection. Maybe a certain tumor has organ-specific and tissue-specific antigens that happen to be present on tumor cells.

I think one should keep and open mind to a variety of antigens that could be either specific for on just associated with tumor cells as demonstrated by further improved techniques. Nevertheless, new findings of these antigens may have intrinsic value in relation to diagnosis, in relation to prevention, and in relation to therapy. At least I think the thesis is a most fruitful hypothesis until the opposite is found true.

DR. YOSHIDA: Is your blocking antibody quite a new type of antibody? Does it block only cell-mediated immunity or does it also block the cytotoxicity of circulating antibody? Does your blocking antibody require complement?

DR. K. HELLSTRÖM: The question you raised is whether blocking antibody has a blocking effect against cytotoxic serum antibody as well or only has a blocking effect against cell-mediated immunity. The answer is that we have to test it before we can say anything; this is a very important point to look into. Our blocking antibody does not require complement.

DR. FUJII: Could you tell me at what stage of cancer you got lymphocytes? How about in advanced cancer? What is the ratio of sensitized lymphocytes to target cells in your test?

DR. I. HELLSTRÖM: The stages of the patients were very different. Very advanced cancer patients, not on the days before dying but at stage of quite extensive tumor growth, still have cell-mediated immunity. As for the ratio between lymphocytes and target cells in our colony inhibition test, 5×10^6 lymphocytes were reacted with about 100 target cells. If we count the lymphocytes attached to the cell surface of target cells, it is not so many. Employing microtest tubes, we could lower the ratio of lymphocytes to target cells further, we are now testing that.

SUMMARY AND PROSPECTS

Chairmen:

Kusuya Nishioka, Chester M. Southam

Immunological Research in Human Neoplasia, Present Status and Prospects*

Chester M. SOUTHAM

Sloan-Kettering Institute for Cancer Research, New York, N.Y., U.S.A.

As the " anchor man " of this Symposium, I have been asked to attempt an integration of the material presented in these three days into the broad picture of tumor immunology. In using the word immunology I do not exclude the virologic studies that occupied our attention on the first day, for, truly, virology is inseparable from immunology. As we have seen, tumor virology is largely dependent on serologic techniques, but the relationship is more fundamental than that. Many tumor-specific antigens are viral components or a consequence of viral infection. The immunologic status and responses of the host largely determine whether or not an oncogenic virus is able to establish an infection or bring about neoplastic transformation of infected cells, and immunologic status also determines whether or not the transformed cells survive and propagate to produce a malignant neoplastic disease.

At the outset I wish to emphasize that cancer is a malignant neoplastic disease, not a laboratory phenomenon. The immediate pathogen of this disease is the cancer cell, not the etiologic virus or other oncogen. The pathogenesis of this disease is the consequence of the metabolism and propagation of the cancer cell, not its mere presence.

I hope that no one will misunderstand or take offense at this emphasis. You must not think that I am blind to the accomplishments or the promise of cellular and molecular biology, but I do want to point out that when fascinated by the beauty and precision of laboratory techniques we sometimes lose sight of our major objective (the objective of this Symposium and of our research efforts) which is cancer in man.

To be just slightly more specific, our objectives are to learn: how to prevent

---

* Summary paper for The First International Symposium of the Princess Takamatsu Cancer Research Fund, Tokyo, Japan, November 24–26, 1970.

cancer; how to detect it at such an early stage that available methods of treatment will be curative; and how to treat the established disease more effectively. Each of these objectives, in so far as they may be achieved through immunology, depends on the same fundamental knowledge. Let us consider those fundamental points and how they have been elucidated or left obscure by this Symposium.

Cancer-specific Antigens

The most basic concept in cancer immunology is that cancer cells are recognizable as foreign cells by the surveillance mechanisms of the autochthonous host, and that they elicit an immunologic reaction in that host. In other words, they are antigenic and immunogenic in the patient. Therefore, the detection of cancer-specific antigens was the first goal of cancer immunology reserach. To use the baseball metaphor with which Dr. Nakahara opened our scientific sessions, the demonstration of human cancer-specific antigens was " first base " in the ball game of tumor immunology.

Only five years ago a small group of investigators gathered in Tsukumi, USSR, to discuss the subjects of cancer immunology and virology under the leadership of the late Professor Lev Alexandravich Zilber. It was, I believe, the first international symposium devoted solely to these subjects, and the opening paper, which set the tone of the entire conference, was entitled " Do Specific Cancer Antigens Exist? " (*13*). That most fundamental question has now been aneswered repeatedly, confidently, and affirmatively. Characterization of these antigens is now a major need and one of our most immediate goals. Happily, we have evidence from this Symposium that this work is being pursued intensively and fruitfully.

Location of antigens

The location of cancer-specific antigens is of prime importance, because the cancer cell cannot be affected by antibodies or immunocytes unless the reacting antigen is at the surface of the living cancer cell. If a cancer-specific antigen developed only in dying cells, if it were secreted into extra-cellular fluids, or if it remained within the cell, it might have clinical importance for cancer detection and prognosis, but it is unlikely that host reactions with such antigens would have any influence upon tumor growth. Fortunately, the first conclusive demonstrations of tumor antigens rested on the development of specific resistance to the transplantation of syngeneic tumors in mice, so the existence of the antigens was proved and their location on the cell surface was immediately deduced (*16*). For human cancer however, the technique of transplantation has great limitations both in feasibility and in yield. Autotransplantation studies of human cancer in patients with incurable disease have given evidence that patients have some degree of resistance to autochthonous cancer and that cell-mediated mechanisms of specific immunity appear to be more important than serum antibody (*22*), but it seems unlikely that we can learn much more from these methods of human experimentation. Therefore, we must use less direct methods.

We may either seek *in vitro* evidence of tumor inhibitory reactions against autochthonous human cancer and then try to prove their specificity, or use immunochemical techniques of antigenic analysis to detect antigens specific for cancer and then try to determine their biological significance.

Both approaches are well illustrated in this Symposium.   The first by Ingegerd Hellström in studies which showed that the growth of human tumor cells in primary culture was inhibited by peripheral blood lymphocytes from the same patients. Earlier work by the Hellströms and their collaborators gave similar evidence of resistance to autochthonous cancer in patients with neuroblastoma (11).

The second approach is illustrated by work presented here by George Klein and the Henles on the antigens in cells of Burkitt's lymphoma (BL) and nasopharyngeal cancer (NPC) and the studies of antibodies to these antigens by the same investigators and by Hinuma, Hirayama, Lin, and Suzuki.   These reports leave no doubt that there are immunologic reactions against antigens of BL and NPC cells, some of which are located on the cell membrane.

Tumor specificity

The term " tumor-specific antigen " could be a semantic trap, and surely we do not want to compound our ignorance by confused terminology.   These antigens of BL and NPC are " specific " for these cancers as judged by their absence from normal cells and most other cancers, but they are not strictly tumor-specific because they occur in infectious mononucleosis (IM) cell lines, and because antibodies against them are found in the serum of patients with IM and Izumi fever (IF), which are non-neoplastic, or at least non-malignant, infectious diseases.   We face a similar semantic problem with the " tumor-specific antigens " which are normally present in fetal or embryonal life, but which are not found after birth except in tumor cells, as in primary hepatomas of rodents and humans (1) and in gastrointestinal tract adenocarcinomas of man (8).   However, these are all antigens which are clearly associated with certain cancers, and though we might be wise to avoid the term cancer-specific, it is certainly correct to call them " cancer-related."   An antigen which is cancer-related, but not truly cancer-specific, might nevertheless be of great importance in clinical medicine.   The presence of alpha-1 fetal globulin in the serum of an adult is almost certainly diagnostic of hepatoma, for this fetal antigen is not produced in adults, even by regenerating liver.   The " tumor-related " membrane antigens of BL and NPC are potential targets for immunotherapy in spite of the fact that they also occur in some non-malignant diseases, because they presumably do not occur on normal cells of the cancer patients.

Relation of antigens to virus

The relationship between the " tumor-specific " intracellular and membrane antigens of BL cells, and the presence of the herpes type virus (HTV) particle or its viral genome now seems firmly established, as discussed here by Werner Henle.   Some of these antigens are virion antigens, others (the membrane antigens) are part of the structure of the cell itself, although induced and probably maintained by the viral genome, and still others (the newly detected " early antigen " of the Henles and " new antigen " of Hinuma) are apparently not a part of the virion but an early consequence of the viral infection, possibly a part of the virus-producing machinery. These virus-determined antigens constitute strong evidence of a causal relationship of this herpes type virus to BL and NPC, but we must be aware that a similar distribution of a " coincidental " non-causal virus could give the same distribution of antigens.

In contrast to the common or cross-reacting tumor-specific antigens which are characteristic of all tumors caused by the same virus, the tumors induced in rodents by chemical carcinogens have individually unique antigens.   That is, immune reactions against the tumor-specific antigens of one chemically induced sarcoma do not cross-react with other tumors.   This uniqueness is so well documented that a demonstration of cross-reacting tumor-specific antigens has been cited as evidence of viral oncogenesis.   But we must beware of that trap.   Cross-reacting tumor antigens are characteristic of virus-induced tumors but they are not limited to such tumors.   The tumor-related antigens which presumably arise by depression of fetal antigens [the alpha 1 fetal antigens of hepatocellular carcinomas (1) and the carcinoembryonic antigens of colon cancer (5)] are common to many or all cancers of the same type, and there is no reason to suspect a common viral etiology.   Furthermore, recent studies suggest that there may occasionally be minor cross-reacting antigens even amongst the chemically induced sarcomas of mice (17).

The nature of tumor antigens

In this Symposium, we have also heard some fragmentary but interesting data relating to the chemical and structural nature of cell antigens and how they are altered by virus infection.

Nishioka and Tachibana reported studies of cell surfaces as revealed by the non-specific adherence of sheep erythrocytes which had been sensitized with IgG antibody, IgM antibody, or IgM antibody plus complement components 4 and 3 (IgG, IgM, and IA receptor sites respectively).   They found that various BL, NPC and IM cell lines differed characteristically in these immune adherence reactions, reflecting differences in cell surface characteristics, and that these characteristics are changed by virus infections.   Hayashi, using similar techniques, demonstrated changes in the cell surface characteristics of HeLa cells (which do not carry HTV) after injection with herpes simplex virus (HSV) and after treatment with acetone.

From Roizman's studies of the chemical changes in the surface membranes of HSV-infected cells we learned that the virus alters the glycoprotein composition of the cell surface, a change which might well affect immunological reactions and intercellular contacts.   Eva Klein observed that some lymphoid cell lines produced immunoglobulin which was incorporated into the cell surface, rather than secreted. George Klein showed us fluorescent antibody studies which clearly showed that the EBV-induced membrane antigen was distinct from normal cell surface (HLA) antigens, but that the two were located very close together on cell surfaces, suggesting that they may be distinct antigenic moieties on a common macromolecular complex.

Two other members of the Symposium made chance observations on the nature of cell antigens by serologic investigations.   Fujii found that antibodies produced in guinea pigs by the injection of xenogeneic cells cross-reacted with normal cell surface antigens (Forssman antigens) of the guinea pig—that is, autoantibodies were induced by a heterologous antigen.   Yoshida found anti-nuclear antibodies in many cancer patients, a phenomenon which might reflect an immune response to tumor-specific antigens which cross-react with normal cell components (which by themselves do not stimulate an immune reaction either because of their chemical structure or their intracellular location).   I wonder if long term observation of Fujii's guinea pigs would have revealed autoimmune disease, and whether Yoshida's anti-nuclear antibodies might contribute to the pathogenesis of cancer.

Aoki, in a discussion period, reported suppression of EBV-related antigens when Burkitt is tumor cells were cultivated in the presence of antibody—possibly an example in man of so-called antigenic modulation.

At present these various observations on the nature of cell surfaces and cell antigens seem mere curiosities, and for the most part they cannot be related to the biology of cancer, but they do give us reason to be confident that physicochemical characteristics of surfaces of living cells can be described and can be related to immunogenic and behavioral qualities.

Not mentioned in this Symposium, but pertinent to this subject, are attempts to isolate human tumor-specific antigens.   This is not surprising.   Attempts to obtain cell-free immunogenic preparations of TSTA's from experimental animal tumors have met with only limited success as yet (3, 15).   Attempts to extract normal human membrane antigens (HL-A) are very recent and as yet such cell-free preparations have not been shown to be immunogenic (18).   The desirability of purified human tumor-specific antigens for basic research and for clinical therapy and diagnosis is evident.   Recent progress in this field is encouraging (18) although the goal of clinical applicability is not in sight.

Perpetuation of tumor antigens

In my Abstract I mentioned the question of genetic versus epigenetic control of neo-antigens (" epigenetic " meaning control by some mechanism other than chromosomal DNA).   The outstanding examples of tumor antigens controlled by epigenetic mechanisms have been those induced by oncogenic RNA viruses.   If I understand correctly the work described by Dr. Greene, and other studies referred to by Dr. Moloney, this distinction is now meaningless, for even an RNA virus produces a complementary DNA template which functions like, or may actually be incorporated into, the genetic DNA of the cell.   I wonder if the molecular detectives might use similar methods to tell us by what modification of cellular chemistry the production of tumor-specific antigens is perpetuated in tumors induced by chemical carcinogens or plastics.   Is new genetic information introduced by chemical carcinogens?   Or are normal cell genomes modified?   I hope that someone, like Dr. Green, who can talk to molecules with fluency and understanding will find the time and the means to study this problem.

Immunologic Responses to Cancer

Coequal in importance with an understanding of tumor antigens is understanding of the immunologic responses which these antigens induce in the autochthonous host—that is, in the cancer patient.   Investigations of immune responses to human cancer have been slow and difficult.   Even the mere documentation that such responses do occur is recent, and rests on rather tenuous evidence.   The difficulty is not a lack of interest or effort, but the intrinsic nature of tumor biology.

Intrinsic obstacles to investigation

The possibilities for studying tumor-specific immunologic reactions in auto-chthonous systems are limited by technical problems and by the need for multiple tests and controls, so in studying animal tumors we usually resort to syngeneic tumor systems.   Sometimes we do use tumor systems in which there are immune reactions to foreign but normal tissue antigens, but the failure to recognize that such reactions are unrelated to cancer is the greatest pitfall in cancer immunology.

To study cancer-specific immune reactions in man is infinitely more difficult than to study them in experimental animals because two basic research necessities, syngeneic transplantation and normal controls, are unattainable.   We can study tumor growth in the patient himself (the autochthonous host) and may be able to observe a relationship between growth and immunologic factors, but there is no possibility of comparing the growth of the same tumor in another host.   Our cancer patients already have cancer before we can study them, and while that may seem too obvious to mention we should realize that in syngeneic animal systems almost all demonstrations of tumor-specific immunity are based on the stimulation of an immune response in a normal animal which, *subsequently,* is given a tumor transplant as a test of resistance.   We can sometimes grow a patient's tumor cells *in vitro* and see if they are affected by the presence of his own serum or immunocytes, but there is no source of genetically identical immunocytes for control studies (except for the rare patient who has an identical twin).

We still do not know how a tumor which carries neo-antigens on its surface and which elicits an immune response in the individual in which it arises can nevertheless grow progressively and kill its host.   Perhaps the amount of antigen in a few tumor cells is insufficient to elicit an immune response (the " sneaking through " hypothesis).   Perhaps the number of tumor-specific antigen sites on the tumor cell surface is too small to provide an adequate target.   Perhaps the type of immune response is ineffective—humoral rather than cellular, or blocking antibody rather than cytolytic antibody.

Immune responses to tumors provide only weak resistance to tumor growth. In studies of syngeneic tumors of mice and rats, tumor-specific immunization before tumor implantation increases by only 10-fold to 100-fold the minimum number of cells required to produce a growing tumor.   *In vitro* demonstration of cell-mediated inhibition of tumor cells requires immunocyte-to-tumor cell ratios of at least 10: 1 and, in some techniques 1,000: 1, which rarely, if ever, occur in nature.

Evidence for and nature of immune responses to cancer

Ingegerd Hellström reviewed for us the evidence of cell-mediated immune reactions against autochthonous human cancers which she and her co-workers obtained by use of the colony inhibition and cell inhibition techniques. Their extensive work on neuroblastoma seems to establish firmly the existence of tumor-inhibiting defenses against that tumor, and accumulating data indicates that the same is probably true of other human cancers. The Hellströms have been pioneers in developing these techniques and have shown tremendous energy and endurance in applying them to human cancer. Their achievements have been great, but they will not soon run out of work. I hope that they will soon find it possible to routinely study complement as a third major variable in their *in vitro* system so that it will more closely resemble the *in vivo* milieu, and will perhaps indicate the sum effect of immunocytes, blocking antibodies, and cytotoxic antibodies.

I know investigators in Japan, the United States, Canada, Italy, the Netherlands, and Sweden (and undoubtedly there are many others) who are also studying cell-mediated immune reactions to autochthonous human cancer and attempting to relate such reactions to the pathogenesis of the disease (*4, 5*, but mostly unpublished). Other pertinent studies of autochthonous human cancer by serologic techniques, autotransplantation, and skin tests have been recently reviewed (*19, 21*). Some success can be claimed by a variety of methods which measure tumor cell destruction or inhibition of cell propagation by immunocytes or serum, or simply reaction of antibody with cells or cell extracts. It must be admitted however, that to date success has been limited and the techniques are tedious, insensitive, and often unreliable. In total, these efforts provide some clear evidence of immune responses to autochthonous human cancer and a suggestion that such reactions reflect the pathogenesis of the disease. There is no direct evidence that they actually determine or influence the course of disease. Some data seem to justify the hope that immune mechanisms can eventually be manipulated as a means of therapy, but as yet there is no solid evidence of significant therapeutic responses to immunotherapy, although several clinical investigators are struggling valiantly toward this goal.

I have been greatly impressed and encouraged by increasing evidence of the multiplicity and interaction of the mechanisms of host defense. We have heard of this in Karl Erik Hellström's report of antibodies which block cell-mediated colony inhibition (suggesting a possible mechanism of immunologic tolerance) and in David Nelson's discussion of humoral factors in cell-mediated immunity. I consider this complexity encouraging because it may explain why the detection of immune responses eluded us so long, and because recognition of complexity often leads to unraveling, understanding, and control. It is already obvious that immune responses are not simply mediated by either antibodies or immunocytes. Specific antibodies may be directly cytotoxic if they initiate the complete chain reaction of complement fixation, or they may be indirectly cytotoxic (opsonins, cytophylic antibodies) by activating effector cells. Conversely, they may prevent immunocytes from reacting with target cells (blocking antibodies). Specifically sensitized immunocytes do not necessarily act directly on a target cell—indeed we now wonder if they ever do so. They release a variety of humoral mediators (lymphokines) which are the actual effectors or intermediaries in a chain of events.

Except for Nelson's review, the fact that host defenses include mechanisms other than antigenically specific reactions has not been mentioned in this conference—

presumably because it is not the current research interest of any of the speakers. We must not assume from this omission that non-specific mechanisms of host defenses are unimportant. The infiltrative capabilities of cancer cells and the fibroblastic encapsulation of tumors must have a major bearing on tumor pathogenesis, but have never attracted investigators because of the difficulty of observing, modifying and evaluating these processes. In another field of research, interest in non-specific defenses has been aroused by the anti-viral effect of natural and synthetic RNA-like polymers such as statalon and poly I.C, which appear to act through production of interferon or other non-specific host factors. Anti-tumor effects of various microbial and viral infections and microbial products, which are not antigenically related to the tumors, have been demonstrated convincingly in experimental tumor systems, even though they have not been sufficiently or consistently effective in treatment of human cancer. Incidentally, the RNA-like polymers poly I·C and poly A·U are impressively effective against herpes simplex virus infections in mice and rabbits and in human cell cultures (10), and certainly deserve to be tested against other herpes type viruses including the HTV of Burkitt's tumors and nasopharyngeal carcinoma.

Clearly, non-specific cellular, humoral and hormonal factors, as well as antigenically specific humoral and cellular reactions, all interplay and enter into the chain reactions which lead to consequences which generally assure the well-being of our bodies. It is indeed astounding that this immunologic homeostasis works so effectively so much of the time, and surely cancer is not exempted from its authority.

Immunologic consequences of cancer

The immunologic consequences of neoplastic disease were not within the scope of our discussions, so I will not attempt to discuss them, but I would remind you that many cancer patients are immunologically deficient—particularly in those cell-mediated reactions which appear to be the main mechanism of resistance to cancer (2, 14, 20). The deficiency occurs as a direct consequence of the neoplastic disease, but it is further increased by many of our anti-cancer treatments (chemotherapy, adrenal corticosteroids, and radiotherapy).

The immunosuppressive effect of cancer treatments have immediate pertinence to considerations of natural resistance to cancer and immunotherapy. Immunosuppression decreases resistance to tumor induction by viruses or by chemicals in laboratory animals, and it decreases resistance to implantation and growth of syngeneic or allogeneic tumor cells in animals and man. Is it reasonable to hope that we can enhance or retain immune resistance to tumors in the face of such depressed immune mechanisms? I think we can take some encouragement from studies (unpublished) by the late Dr. Reiner, in my laboratory, which showed that administration of cytoxan or fluoro-deoxyuridine (FDUR) in high sub-lethal doses did not abolish a previously established specific tumor resistance, even though it did diminish resistance to transplantation of syngeneic tumors in unimmunized mice. Cancer patients have obviously been exposed to their cancer and have, therefore, developed such resistance to their tumor as they can achieve, even though it was insufficient to prevent progressive tumor growth. Judging from our mouse experiments, that resistance, if any, would not be affected by clinically acceptable programs of chemotherapy and radiotherapy.

Prospects for Immunotherapy and Immunoprophylaxis

I have already pointed out that immunologic resistance to cancer is weak at best. Most studies of human cancer in which anti-tumor immune reactions were demonstrated were studies of patients with uncured cancer. That is, there was concurrent immunity and tumor growth, indicating that the immune reactions in these patients was quantitatively or qualitatively insufficient to completely suppress the tumor. What hope is there that such a weak resistance might have any clinically significant effect or any practical application in clinical medicine? Surely, our attempts would have a greater chance of success when the amount of residual cancer is very small. As judged by the experimental data, the amount of cancer that might be controlled by immunologic resistance is not in excess of 10^7 or 10^8 cells, which is about 10 to 100 mg of tumor tissue.

Can we even hope that such reactions can really accomplish a cure of cancer when chemotherapy which can eliminate many grams, even a kilogram, of tumor cells is almost never curative? Yes, I think it is a realistic hope because of the different nature of the two types of cell destruction. Chemotherapy kills a more or less constant proportion of cells—never 100%. Serologic reactions (and presumably cell-mediated reactions) do involve every accessible antigenic site if the antibody is present in excess. It is this fact which justifies the hope that if the total mass of tumor cells can be reduced by surgery or radiotherapy or chemotherapy to numbers below the magnitude of 10^8, the immune responses might be increased sufficiently to attack all of the remaining tumor cells. The optimistic immunologist must somehow explain, or explain away, the fact that in studies by the colony inhibition or similar techniques, destruction of 100 percent of the target cells is rarely achieved by immunocytes. One hopes that the explanation is not the absence of specific antigens on some of the cancer cells—as suggested by studies of antigenic modulation. It is possible, of course, that the number of specific antibody molecules (or antibody-like reactive sites on the immunocytes) is not in excess of the number of tumor antigen receptors. More likely, in such studies a considerable proportion of the target cells are normal stromal cells from the cultured tumor and that only these survive the immunologic attack.

Immunotherapy is too great an extension of the subject of this Symposium to attempt any further consideration of prospects or possible methods, but I will close with some personal thoughts about immunoprophylaxis because the possibility of vaccination with EBV-related antigens was raised and heatedly discussed during the first day of this conference.

In general there is no question that prophylaxis has a greater probability of success than does treatment. The greatest single problem is the availability of an effective antigenic preparation. A second very important problem is the need for suitable criteria to evaluate its efficacy. Ultimately of course we must evaluate in terms of lower cancer incidence or mortality, or later onset, but we would like an earlier indicator of immune response. The discovery of EBV and the mounting evidence that it may be a causal factor in Burkitt's tumor and nasopharyngeal cancer, as well as in infectious mononucleosis and Izumi fever, seems to open the way for an immediate clinical trial. Lending encouragement for such a trial are experiments with Marek's agent in which a virus vaccine protected chickens against subsequent exposure to live virus. That is, few tumors occurred in vaccinated birds during the observation period, while unvaccinated controls had a high incidence of tumors (6, 12). Similar experiments have also been reported with SV 40 virus in rats and hamsters (7, 9).

If such an experiment were tried in man with EBV-related antigens in an appropriate place and age group it should be possible to get a rapid indication of efficacy in preventing infectious mononucleosis or Izumi fever. Its efficacy for Burkitt's tumor could certainly be determined in ten years, and perhaps in five. Evaluation for nasopharyngeal carcinoma, however, might require two generations of investigators because of the later age of onset of that disease.

Should it be done? Should it be done now? I see two disconcerting observations which require careful consideration of pros and cons before making a decision.

The first is the serologic data presented by Doctors Hirayama, Kawamura, and Lin, which showed that nasopharyngeal cancer does occur in patients who have antibodies to EBV, and that populations with high anti-EBV titers had a greater statistical risk of NPC than populations with lesser or no antibody. As yet no one with antibodies to EBV has actually been observed to develop NPC. We do not know whether the NPC patients had the antibodies before they developed the cancer, but if so the antibodies obviously gave no protection against the cancer. Prospective studies may supply the missing data, but at present an investigator could not use antibody response to his vaccine as evidence that he had decreased the risk of tumor, and we have no other criterion for judging immunogenicity of an EBV (HTV) vaccine except the subsequent incidence of disease. The presence of anti-EBV antibody simply indicates exposure to the antigen, presumably by virus infection at some time in the past. The observation that the statistical risk of NPC was greater in groups with higher antibody levels may mean that the virus infection persists in the presence of antibody and increases both the cancer risk and the antibody level, or it may mean that formation of that antibody is stimulated by non-virion antigens of the tumor cells, but neither of these explanations would support the concept that the presence of that antibody is indicative of protection against NPC.

Second, and perhaps more disconcerting, was evidence reported by the Henles during discussions, that some of the steps of EBV-infection have been induced by x-irradiated cells, and that only a fragment of the total viral nucleic acid may be needed to perpetuate the lymphoblastoid character which is characteristic of established lymphoid cell lines (?neoplastically transformed). The later suggestion rests on the observation that the Raji cell line of Burkitt tumor, which contains no demonstrable virions or viral antigens, does show nucleic acid homology with EBV viral DNA. These concepts raise the possibility that a vaccine which is non-infectious by the usual criteria might contain sufficient of the viral genome to initiate neoplastic transformation rather than prevent it.

A third but lesser concern is our ignorance of the best vaccination procedures for producing immunologic resistance, as distinct from other immunologic responses. Numerous studies show that route, vehicle, and dosage schedule of a vaccine influence the kind and degree of immune response, and that for tumor inhibition circulating antibody is less effective than cell-mediated immunity and may in fact enhance tumor growth.

In short, when undertaking an experimental clinical trial of a vaccine for immuno-prophylaxis against a virus-induced tumor, we must face the possibility that we might induce cancer rather than prevent it, and that our vaccination procedures might enhance rather than inhibit a tumor if it should occur.

Any new procedure carries a potential risk. If we were unwilling to accept any risk we would never make any advances. You will recall that the early trials of poliomyelitis vaccines caused paralytic polio in several persons. They also resulted in the inoculation of infectious SV40 virus into tens of thousands of children and babies. SV40 virus is oncogenic in baby rats and hamsters and it causes transformation of human cells in culture. There is no indication to date of any ill effects from this exposure to SV40 virus, but it may be that we have not yet passed the incubation period of such an oncogen in humans. But, poliomyelitis vaccines prevented polio! The medical profession and the public have evaluated that clinical trial as well worth the risk. It is generally believed that the unfortunate personal tragedies of a few were an acceptable sacrifice, considering the benefits to mankind as a whole.

Should a clinical trial of vaccination with HTV-related antigens be undertaken? Yes. But only after fully evaluating the potential benefits and risks, and only under a protocol that will insure evaluatable data within a few years. This probably means that the trial should be made in populations at high risk of Burkitt tumor rather than NPC. In my own mind there is no doubt that the importance of the problem for all mankind fully justifies the theoretical risks of the vaccine trial.

Should it be done now? I think that it might be under taken very soon. The disconcerting problems which I have just discussed are susceptible to further epidemiologic and laboratory investigation, with rapid improvement in our knowledge of the safety of vaccine preparations and the type and efficacy of the immune response thereto. In my personal opinion, plans and preparations for a clinical trial could proceed concurrently with the necessary basic research, and thus the clinical trial could be initiated with a minimum of delay but with greater confidence of safety and adequacy.

Dr. Nakahara, in his opening words, warned that we should not expect to make a home run in the " game " we would be playing for these three days. I would also warn that a home run does not necessarily win the ball game. But I, for one, leave the field today feeling that at least some of the players have reached second base, and it is not the end of the ball game—it's still the first inning.

REFERENCES

1. Abelev, G. I. Production of Embryonal Serum Alpha-globulin by Hepatomas:

Review of Experimental and Clinical Data.   Cancer Res., *28*: 1344–1350, 1968.

2. Aisenberg, A. C. Hodgkin's Disease.   *In* M. Samter (ed.), Immunological Diseases. Little, Brown and Co., Boston, in press, 1971.

3. Baldwin, R. W. and Embleton, M. J.   Detection and Isolation of Tumor-specific Antigen Associated with a Spontaneously Arising Rat Mammary Carcinoma.   Int. J. Cancer, in press, 1971.

4. Bubenik, J., Perlmann, P., Helmstein, K., and Moberger, G.   Cellular and Humoral Immune Responses to Human Urinary Bladder Carcinomas.   Int. J. Cancer, *5*: 310–319, 1970.

5. Chu, E. H. Y., Stjernsward, J., Clifford, P., and Klein, G.   Reactivity of Human Lymphocytes Against Autochthonous and Allogeneic Normal and Tumor Cells *in vitro*.   J. Nat. Cancer Inst., *39*: 595–617, 1967.

6. Churchill, A. E., Payne, L. N., and Chubb, R. C.   Immunization Against Marek's Disease Using a Live Attenuated Virus.   Nature, *221*: 744–745, 1969.

7. Deichman, G. I., and Kluchareva, T. E.   Prevention of Tumor Induction in SV40 Infected Hamsters.   Nature, *1*: 1126–1128, 1964.

8. Gold, P., Kruper, J., and Ansari, H.   Position of the Carcinoembryonic Antigen of the Human Digestive System in the Ultrastructure of Tumor Cell Surface.   J. Nat. Cancer Inst., *45*: 219–225, 1970.

9. Goldner, H., Girardi, A. J., Larson, V. M., and Hilleman, M. R.   Interruption of SV40 Virus Tumorigenesis Using Irradiated Homologous Tumor Antigen.   Proc. Soc. Exper. Biol. and Med., *117*: 851–857, 1964.

10. Hamilton, L. D., Babcock, V. I., and Southam, C. M.   Inhibition of Herpes Simplex Virus by Synthetic Double-stranded RNA (Polyriboadenilic and Polyribouridylic Acids). Proc. Nat. Acad. Sci., *64*: 878–883, 1969.

11. Hellstrom, I., Hellstrom, K. E., Bill, A. H., Pierce, G. E., and Yang, J. P. S.   Studies on Cellular Immunity of Human Neuroblastoma Cells.   Int. J. Cancer, *6*: 172–188, 1970.

12. Kottaridis, S. D., and Luginbuhl, R. E.   Control of Marek's Disease by the Use of Inoculated Chick Embryo Fibroblasts.   Nature, *221*: 1258–1259, 1969.

13. Korngold, L.   Do Specific Cancer Antigens Exist?   *In* R. J. C. Harris (ed.), Specific Tumor Antigens, UICC Monograph Series 2, pp. 13–19. Medical Examination Publ. Co., Flushing, N.Y., 1967.

14. Miller, D. G.   The Immunologic Capability of Patients with Lymphoma.   Cancer Res., *21*: 1441–1441, 1968.

15. Oettgen, H. F., Old, L. J., McLean, E. P., and Carswell, E. A.   Delayed Hypersensitivity and Transplantation Immunity Elicited by Soluble Antigens of Chemically-induced Tumors in Inbred Guinea Pigs.   Nature, *220*: 295–297, 1968.

16. Old, L. J., and Boyse, E. A.   Immunology of Experimental Tumors. Ann. Rev. Med., *15*: 167–186, 1964.

17. Reiner, J., and Southam, C. M.   Further Evidence of Common Antigenic Properties in Chemically Induced Sarcomas of Mice. Cancer Res., *29*: 1814–1820, 1969.

18. Reisfeld, R. A., and Kahan, B. D.   Transplantation Antigens.   Adv. Immunol., *12*: 117–200, 1970.

19. Southam, C. M.   Evidence for Cancer-specific Antigens in Man.   Progr. Exper. Tumor Res., *9*: 1–39, 1967.

20. Southam, C. M.   Immunologic Status of Patients with Non-lymphomatous Cancer. Cancer Res., *21*: 1433–1440. 1968.

21. Southam, C. M.   Cancer Specific Antigens in Man.   *In* M. Samter (ed.), Immu-

nological Diseases. Little Brown and Co., Boston, in press, 1971.

22. Southam, C. M. Brunschwig, A., Levin, A. G., and Dizon, Q. Effect of Leukocytes on Transplantability of Human Cancer. Cancer, *19*: 174, 1753, 1966.

Closing Remarks

Waro Nakahara

In a recent review on the EB virus, Dr. Epstein called attention to the possibility of the virus being " an opportunistic passenger living as a commensal in lymphoid cell," a *wild goose*, to use his expression, which is, however, urgently necessary to *chase*. Dr. Espstein's *goose* has been a central subject in our symposium on human tumor virology and immunology.

The refinements of immunological methodology led us to the detection of formerly unrecognizable antigens and antibodies and to the analysis of membrane reactivity of infected tumor cells in tissue culture. At the same time, some papers presented have taken us to the studies on molecular and submolecular levels, involving the mechanism of cell gene expression, cell transformation by incorporation of viral genome, and possibly the concept of oncogene. It may not be too much to say that these studies on oncogenic viruses may introduce revolutionaly changes in our concept of carcinogenic mechanism. We may well be at the dawn of a new era of fundamental oncology.

One thing that has emerged most prominently may be the puzzling fact that the EB virus produces Burkitt's lymphoma, nasopharyngeal carcinoma, infectious mononucleosis and, lastly, Izumi fever. As far as can be ascertained by the finest immunological methods, the EB virus involved in all these diseases is a single species of virus, and it has not been possible to prove definitely the existence of specific variants of the EB virus to account for the various clinical and pathological manifestations. Moreover, the great majority of the population infected with the virus, as evidenced by a high antibody titer, remains without any clinically recognizable sign of disease.

How does a single species of virus produce lymphoma, carcinoma, monucleosis and even a febrile disease, while remaining entirely non pathogenic in the great majority of population infected with it? One may well wonder where this apparent confusion of observed facts may lead to.

Some papers presented at this symposium considered racial (genetic) and environmental factors, which may affect the clinical, immunological and oncological manifestations. Seroepidemiological studies spotlighted the role of racial background and climatic influences. It has not been possible to pick out any specific co-factor. It seems highly probable that there are may factors influencing degree and kind of the activity of the virus.

It is not at all strange that oncogenic virus may be widely distributed in a large population, producing tumors only in a very small proportion of the total. An important thing in cancer research is to discover the secondary factor or factors, which may either activate the otherwise latent virus, or produce such changes in cell genetic material as to summate with the weak oncogenic effect of the virus to bring it out in the form of manifest tumors. This last point is suggested from the theory of the summation of syncarcinogenic effects. Syncarcinogenesis means carcinogenesis brought about as the additive total effects of many different agents. To regard oncogenic viruses merely as another class of carcinogenic substances may be to offer a new approach toward the unification of our knowledge of carcinogenic mechanism.

I cannot close my remarks without expressing deepest gratitude to H. I. H. Princess Takamatsu and the officers and staff of the Princess Takamatsu Cancer Research Fund. It was indeed under the generous support of the Fund that this symposium was made possible. The results of the symposium were gratifying. I am confident that the success of this first symposium of the Fund will warrant holding symposia of similar scale in coming years to cover other subjects of importance in cancer research.

Finally, I extend my cordial thanks to each and all of you who have so actively participated in the symposium to make it such a success.